Normal and Abnormal Conduction in the Heart

Biophysics, Physiology, Pharmacology and Ultrastructure

Edited by

Antonio Paes de Carvalho, M.D., Ph.D.

Professor and Director, Instituto de Biofísica, Universidade Federal do Rio de Janeiro, Brazil

Brian F. Hoffman, M.D.

Professor and Chairman, Department of Pharmacology, Columbia University College of Physicians and Surgeons, New York, New York

Melvyn Lieberman, Ph.D.

Professor of Physiology, Duke University Medical Center, Durham, North Carolina

FUTURA PUBLISHING COMPANY
Mount Kisco, New York
1982

Published by:
Futura Publishing Company, Inc.
P.O. Box 330, 295 Main Street
Mount Kisco, New York 10549

LC #: 81-71154
ISBN #: 0-87993-172-8

Contributors

James F. Aiton, Ph.D., Department of Physiology, University of St. Andrews, St. Andrews, Scotland

Maurits A. Allessie, M.D., Biomedical Center, University of Limburg, Maastricht, The Netherlands

Bruce P. Bean, Ph.D., Department of Physiology, Yale University School of Medicine, New Haven, Connecticut

Rebecca L. Biegon, Ph.D., Department of Pharmacology, University of Connecticut Health Center, Farmington, Connecticut

Felix I.M. Bonke, M.D., Department of Physiology, Faculty of Medicine, Rijksuniversiteit Limburg, Maastricht, The Netherlands

Arthur M. Brown, M.D., Ph.D., Department of Physiology and Biophysics, University of Texas Medical Branch, Galveston, Texas

Edward Carmeliet, M.D., Ph.D., Physiology Laboratory, University of Leuven, Campus Gasthuisberg, Leuven, Belgium

Antonio Carlos Campos de Carvalho, M.D., M.Sc., Instituto de Biofísica da Universidade Federal do Rio de Janeiro, Rio de Janeiro, Brazil

Antonio Paes de Carvalho, M.D., Ph.D., Director, Instituto de Biofísica da Universidade Federal do Rio de Janeiro, Rio de Janeiro, Brazil

Marilene de Paula Carvalho, M.D., Ph.D., Instituto de Biofísica da Universidade Federal do Rio de Janeiro, Rio de Janeiro, Brazil

Charles J. Cohen, Ph.D., Department of Physiology, Yale University School of Medicine, New Haven, Connecticut

Ira S. Cohen, M.D., Ph.D., Department of Physiology and Biophysics, SUNY at Stony Brook, New York

Paul F. Cranefield, M.D., Ph.D., Laboratory of Cardiac Physiology, The Rockefeller University, New York, New York

Samuel Cukierman, M.D., M.Sc., Instituto de Biofísica da Universidade Federal do Rio de Janeiro, Cidade Universitária, Ilha do Fundão, Rio de Janeiro, Brazil

Kenneth H. Dangman, M.D., Department of Pharmacology, College of Physicians and Surgeons, Columbia University, New York, New York

W.C. De Mello, M.D., Department of Pharmacology, Medical Sciences Campus, San Juan, Puerto Rico

Frederick A. Dodge, Ph.D., IBM T. J. Watson Research Center, Yorktown Heights, New York

Paul C. Dolber, Ph.D., Department of Pathology, Duke University and Veterans Administration Medical Centers, Durham, North Carolina

Robin T. Falk, Ph.D., Department of Physiology and Biophysics, SUNY at Stony Brook, New York

John J. Fenoglio, Jr., M.D., Department of Pathology, College of Physicians and Surgeons, Columbia University, New York, New York

Harry A. Fozzard, M.D., Departments of the Pharmacological and Physiological Sciences and Medicine, The University of Chicago, Chicago, Illinois

David C. Gadsby, Ph.D., Laboratory of Cardiac Physiology, The Rockefeller University, New York, New York

Eduardo Antonio Conde Garcia, M.D., Ph.D., Instituto de Biofísica da Universidade Federal do Rio de Janeiro, Rio de Janeiro, Brazil

Peter Hess, M.D., Department of Physiology, University of Berne, Berne, Switzerland

Brian F. Hoffman, M.D., Department of Pharmacology, College of Physicians and Surgeons, Columbia University, New York, New York

C. Russell Horres, Ph.D., Department of Physiology, Duke University Medical Center, Durham, North Carolina

Michiel J. Janse, M.D., Ph.D., Departments of Cardiology and Clinical Physiology, University Hospital Wilhelmina Gasthuis, Amsterdam, and the Interuniversity Cardiological Institute, The Netherlands

Edward A. Johnson, M.D., Department of Physiology, Duke University Medical Center, Durham, North Carolina

Richard P. Kline, Ph.D., Departments of Pharmacology and Medicine, Mount Sinai School of Medicine, New York, New York

Wim Lammers, Ph.D., Department of Physiology, Rijksuniversiteit Limburg, Maastricht, The Netherlands

Kai S. Lee, Ph.D., Department of Physiology and Biophysics, University of Texas Medical Branch, Galveston, Texas

David N. Levin, M.D., Ph.D., Departments of the Pharmacological and Physiological Sciences and Medicine, The University of Chicago, Chicago, Illinois

Melvyn Lieberman, Ph.D., Department of Physiology, Duke University Medical Center, Durham, North Carolina

Albert J.C. Mackaay, M.D., Department of Physiology, University of Amsterdam, Amsterdam, The Netherlands

Masako Oya Masuda, Ph.D., Instituto de Biofísica da Universidade Federal do Rio de Janeiro, Centro de Ciencias da Saude, Ilha do Fundão, Rio de Janeiro, Brazil

Carlos Méndez, M.D., Department of Physiology, Centro de Investigación y de Estudios Avanzados del I.P.N., Mexico City, Mexico

Ernest Page, M.D., Departments of Medicine and of Pharmacological and Physiological Sciences, Pritzker School of Medicine, The University of Chicago, Chicago, Illinois

Achilles Pappano, Ph.D., Department of Pharmacology, University of Connecticut Health Center, Farmington, Connecticut

Trevor Powell, Ph.D., Department of Physiology and Biophysics, University of Texas Medical Branch, Galveston, Texas

Fidel Ramon, M.D., Ph.D., Department of Physiology, Duke University Medical Center, Durham, North Carolina

Walter R. Reber, M.D., Department of Physiology, University of Berne, Berne, Switzerland

Robert F. Reder, M.D., Department of Pediatrics, Mount Sinai Medical Center, and Departments of Pharmacology and Pediatrics, College of Physicians and Surgeons, Columbia University, New York, New York

Harald Reuter, M.D., Department of Pharmacology, University of Berne, Berne, Switzerland

Michael R. Rosen, M.D., Department of Pediatrics, Mount Sinai Medical Center, and Departments of Pharmacology and Pediatrics, College of Physicians and Surgeons, Columbia University, New York, New York

Teobaldo Antonio Saldeña, M.D., Ph.D., Instituto de Biofísica da Universidade Federal do Rio de Janeiro, Rio de Janeiro, Brazil
Norikazu Shigeto, M.D., Ph.D., Division of Cardiology, Hiroshima National Chest Hospital, Hiroshima, Japan
Victor A.J. Slenter, M.D., Biomedical Center, University of Limburg, Maastricht, The Netherlands
Joep Smeets, Ph.D., Department of Physiology, Rijksuniversiteit Limburg, Maastricht, The Netherlands
Joachim R. Sommer, M.D., Department of Pathology, Duke University and Veterans Administration Medical Centers, Durham, North Carolina
Madison S. Spach, M.D., Division of Pediatric Cardiology, Department of Pediatrics, Duke University Medical Center, Durham, North Carolina
Gerhard Steinbeck, M.D., Biomedical Center, University of Limburg, Maastricht, The Netherlands
Tetsuo Tashiro, M.Sc., Instituto de Biofísica da Universidade Federal do Rio de Janeiro, Rio de Janeiro, Brazil
Richard W. Tsien, D.Phil., Department of Physiology, Yale University School of Medicine, New Haven, Connecticut
Frans J.L. van Capelle, M.Sc., Department of Cardiology and Clinical Physiology, University Hospital Wilhelmina Gasthuis, Amsterdam, and the Interuniversity Cardiological Institute, The Netherlands
Marc Walton, M.D., Ph.D., Departments of the Pharmacological and Physiological Sciences and Medicine, The University of Chicago, Chicago, Illinois
Silvio Weidmann, M.D., Department of Physiology, University of Berne, Berne, Switzerland
Robert Weingart, Ph.D., Department of Physiology, University of Berne, Berne, Switzerland
David M. Wheeler, M.D., Ph.D., Department of Anesthesiology, University of Alabama Medical Center, Birmingham, Alabama
Andrew L. Wit, M.D., Department of Pharmacology, College of Physicians and Surgeons, Columbia University, New York, New York

Preface

Twenty years have gone by since the international meeting on "The Specialized Tissues of the Heart" convened in Rio de Janeiro, under the sponsorship of the Instituto de Biofísica. Cardiac microelectrophysiology was then only ten years old. We knew then much of what we know today about the varied contour of cardiac action potentials. We had learned of the ionic mechanism of the fast upstroke in Purkinje fibers, of the importance of potassium conductance changes during plateau and pacemaker potentials, and of the ionic mechanism of cholinergic inhibition in nodal and atrial tissues. On the other hand, we had no inkling of the existence of slow responses as a separate excitable entity, and, of course, we knew nothing about the role of calcium in its genesis. The mode of action of catecholamines was a mystery; and cell junctions were mostly considered as permanent, low resistance connections in health and disease, except for the "healing-over" of gross lesions of the cardiac tissue. With so much knowledge left out, we understood arrhythmias only in the crudest terms, and our explanations were based on the standard parameters of nerve excitability applied to the three-dimensional latticework of heart muscle.

Progress has been remarkable in these twenty years, both quantitatively and qualitatively. Classical electrophysiology of adult and cultured heart cells and the technique of voltage clamp have revealed a rich collection of unsuspected phenomena. Ultrastructure research has progressed to the point where it can add significant data to clarify the finer biophysical and physiological arguments. Other biophysical methods are now emerging as potential sources of useful information. The Organizing Committee was therefore eager to call a new meeting, involving many of the colleagues from the Americas and Europe who have contributed most to the field. Our only regret is that we could not bring all of them together. The Instituto de Biofísica of the Universidade Federal do Rio de Janeiro, together with the Academia Brasileira de Ciências, agreed to sponsor this revival of their early 1960 enterprise. Thanks to them, this book collects the beautiful work of many laboratories and the best piece of mind of our guests during the lively discussions. We feel the volume is a most appropriate and critical representation of the present state of basic electrophysiological knowledge of both normal and abnormal excitation of the heart.

A.P.C.
M.L.
B.F.H.

Acknowledgments

The Organizing Committee wishes to express its gratitude for the generous financial support provided by: Conselho Nacional de Desenvolvimento Científico e Tecnológico (SEPLAN/CNP$_q$, Brasil), Coordenação do Aperfeiçoamento de Pessoal de Nível Superior (MEC/CAPES, Brasil), Financiadora de Estudos e Projetos SA (SEPLAN/FINEP, Brasil), Companhia Brasileira de Petróleo Ipiranga, Shell Brasil Petróleo SA, IBM do Brasil Ltda., União de Construtoras SA, Salicultores Mossoro´-Macau SA, Banco Boavista SA, Banco Itaú SA, Unibanco SA, Laboratório Knoll SA, Laboratório Schering SA, and Laboratório Silva Arajo-Roussel SA.

We are also grateful for the excellent assistance of Ms. Lilian Oswaldo Cruz, Ms. Gilda Paes de Carvalho and the Members of the Instituto de Biofisica in planning the local arrangements for the meeting. It is a pleasure to acknowledge the skillful copyediting of Ms. Patricia Spivey and the fine index provided by David Piwnica-Worms and Leslie D. Anderson.

Antonio Paes de Carvalho
Brian F. Hoffman
Melvyn Lieberman

Contents

Chapter 1

Cardiac Muscle: Ultrastructure of Its Cells and Bundles

Joachim R. Sommer and Paul C. Dolber

Cardiac muscle is no exception to the general principle that functional properties of a system are dictated by its geometry at all levels of resolution. Anatomical enquiries are therefore fundamental to define that geometry.

Our aim over the past two decades has been to describe the structure of cardiac muscle and to interpret the anatomy in physiologic terms. Alternatively, we have taken the impetus from physiologic observations to search the anatomy for functional explanations. This dual approach is mutually beneficial. For example, the old controversy whether or not cardiac muscle is a syncytium seemed resolved when it was discovered that all cardiac muscle cells were separated from each other by individual cell membranes. But this observation was contradicted by physiologists who stated categorically that cardiac muscle behaves electrically as a syncytium. Subsequently, and without having to abandon their previous dictum, the anatomists discovered membrane patches, the nexuses, that intimately join adjacent cardiac muscle cells, readily accounting for electrical coupling between cells. A similar interaction between physiologic and anatomic observations has provided new insights into the properties of the conduction system: Electronmicroscopic studies have shown that the cells of the conduction system have no transverse tubules. Hence, they can be expected to have electrical properties different from those of ventricular cells, which do have transverse tubules, all other parameters of importance being equal. Likewise, the definition of the geometry of cell appositions in bundles of conducting cells in small versus large mammals has provided an anatomical explanation for otherwise puzzling electrophysiologic records and has raised important questions regarding the contribution to measured electrical activity of narrow intercellular clefts. Thus, anatomical studies have succeeded in defining the conditions of geometry that permit the success of certain voltage-clamp experiments on cardiac muscle. Furthermore, the significance of the difference between loose (small mammals) and tight (large mammals) packing of conduction cells has been especially illuminating in studies on dog hearts. Several years ago, we showed that the conduction-cell bundles in the dog heart assume an intermediate position: in the dog heart, the cells are loosely packed, but many of the fibers are tightly packed. Accordingly, in appropriate electrophysiologic studies on

---

This work was supported by NIH 12486 and the VA Research Service.

conduction-cell bundles in the dog we encounter both properties: those attributable to loose packing and those attributable to tight packing, varying from one bundle to the next.

In the following we shall present a brief review of the ultrastructure of cardiac muscle as it has been disclosed through the efforts of many laboratories. We can afford to be brief, because there are several thorough reviews of the matter to which we can refer the reader (McNutt and Fawcett, 1974; Sommer and Waugh, 1976; Tranum-Jensen, 1976; 1978; Masson-Pevet, 1979, Dolber, 1980; Challice and Viragh, 1973; Sommer and Johnson, 1979; Page and Fozzard, 1973; Sommer et al., 1972).

COMMON VENTRICULAR CELLS OF MAMMALS

Plasma Membrane

The common ventricular cells make up the bulk of the muscle mass of the ventricles. Throughout the mammalian kingdom, an individual cell will have an average diameter between 10 to 20 μm, but its length will vary considerably, ranging from about 30 to 160 μm. The geometry of the cells is quasi-cylindrical: the surfaces are curved, and the cells are much longer than they are thick, but the surfaces are sculptured into several step-like terraces that jut out at right angles to the longitudinal axis of the cells and provide the rabbets for joining one cell with the next (Figs. 1 and 2). At each terrace is an intercalated disc that provides the end-to-end joint between cells. The intercalated disc is composed of three junctional complexes: the intermediate junction, the desmosome, and the nexus *(macula communicans)*. All three junctions are clearly defined anatomically. These junctional complexes, interrupted by segments of common (not further specialized) plasma membrane, form conical protrusions that dovetail with similar projections from the adjacent cell and, thus, make for an effective joint between cells (Figs. 3 and 4). Cardiac cells, on the whole, do not branch. Rather, the branching geometry observed with the light microscope is the result of whole cells separating from one another but remaining attached to each other in one area. Of all the junctional complexes forming the intercalated disc, the nexus (Figs. 3 through 6) is most consistently oriented in longitudinal direction; that is, it is parallel to the long axis of the cells (Figs. 3 and 4). Often the "riser" connecting two transverse portions of the intercalated discs of two adjacent cells is a nexus (Fig. 2). In such a case, two adjacent cells will seem to be continuous with each other when observed with the light microscope, which is incapable of resolving the nexus. There are also a few junctional complexes between cells along their long sides, as opposed to the typical location of intercalated discs at cell ends. All three junctional complexes may participate in such lateral contact regions but not necessarily be combined the way they are in the intercalated disc. Elsewhere, the plasma membrane shows grooves that coincide with the location of Z lines. The Z lines are anchored to the plasma membrane by 10-nm fibrils, which, as parts of a cytoskeleton, hold in the plasma membrane (Figs. 7 and 8). Although transverse tubules invaginate from such grooves, these grooves are also seen in muscle cells that do not have transverse tubules. On the extracellular side, the plasma membrane of cardiac muscle cells is covered by a laminar coat, which usually can clearly be demonstrated to extend into transverse tubules (Fig. 7).

Transverse Tubules

The transverse tubules (Figs. 7 and 10 through 13) are plasma-membrane invaginations that cross the cardiac cells mainly in transverse direction. But many tubular connections are oriented in a longitudinal direction as well (Fig. 12). The transverse tubules show great variations in diameter. More commonly, they are about 200 nm wide, with considerable differences found between species and from one region of one cell to the next. The transverse tubules often form pouches separated by stretches of tubules that may be as narrow as 30 nm. The static pictures taken with an electron microscope do not exclude the possibility that the geometry of the transverse tubules as revealed in these pictures may be the result of dynamic events taking place along the transverse tubules in vivo. It remains to be seen whether their intricate geometry interferes with accumulation and depletion of ions within the extracellular spaces that they enclose. In contrast to skeletal muscle (Fig. 10), the transverse tubules of cardiac muscle carry a large number of caveolae (Fig. 13), which are also quite numerous elsewhere along the plasma membrane, both in cardiac and skeletal muscle. The plasma membrane of the transverse tubules, and that covering the cell's periphery, is attached periodically to specialized portions (the junctional SR) of the sarcoplasmic reticulum (SR), forming couplings. These quasi-attachments (or couplings) are accomplished by periodic processes, or feet, between the junctional SR and the plasma membrane and seem to be quite strong, because even in severely disrupted cells the structure of the couplings usually remains intact. Exceptions to this are the cardiac cells of the bird, which do not have transverse tubules, and the cardiac cells of several species of mammals at birth. But, all common ventricular cells of adult mammals have transverse tubules.

Sarcoplasmic Reticulum

The sarcoplasmic reticulum (SR) is a tubular network of membranes whose function is to sequester calcium. Anatomically, the SR has two major compartments: the free SR and the junctional SR (Figs. 7, 8, 10, and 11). The free SR consists of the smooth tubules surrounding the contractile material. The free SR may form fenestrated retes in the center of the sarcomere at M lines (M rete) and at Z lines (Z rete). The retes in cardiac muscle are not as well developed as they are in skeletal muscle. The free SR is continuous with the junctional SR (called terminal cisterna in skeletal muscle; for comparison see Figs. 7 and 10), which contains granular material usually in the form of an interrupted electron-dense line, and makes contact with the inside of the plasma membrane via junctional processes. Such couplings are seen at transverse tubules (interior couplings) and at the external plasma membrane (peripheral couplings). Analogous structures occur in skeletal muscle in both locations. At particular Z lines in cardiac muscle at which transverse tubules are missing, the SR often has rounded outpouchings (corbular SR, Figs. 7 through 9), which also contain granular material and carry junctional processes at their surfaces. The junction between the junctional SR and the plasma membrane, both at transverse tubules and at the cell periphery, is thought to represent the anatomical site where electrical activity originating at the cell surface is translated into calcium release from the nearby junctional SR, at least in skeletal muscle. By analogy, such a relationship might exist in cardiac muscle as well. But this quite attractive structure-function relationship is complicated by certain anatomical observations in bird heart muscle, where between 70 and 80% of all SR specializations, indistinguishable from junctional SR, are not in contact with the plasma membrane.

Other Cellular Organelles in Cardiac Cells

Cardiac cells contain organelles usually seen in other eucaryotes, such as some rough endoplasmic reticulum, some lysosomes, a few coated vesicles, often several

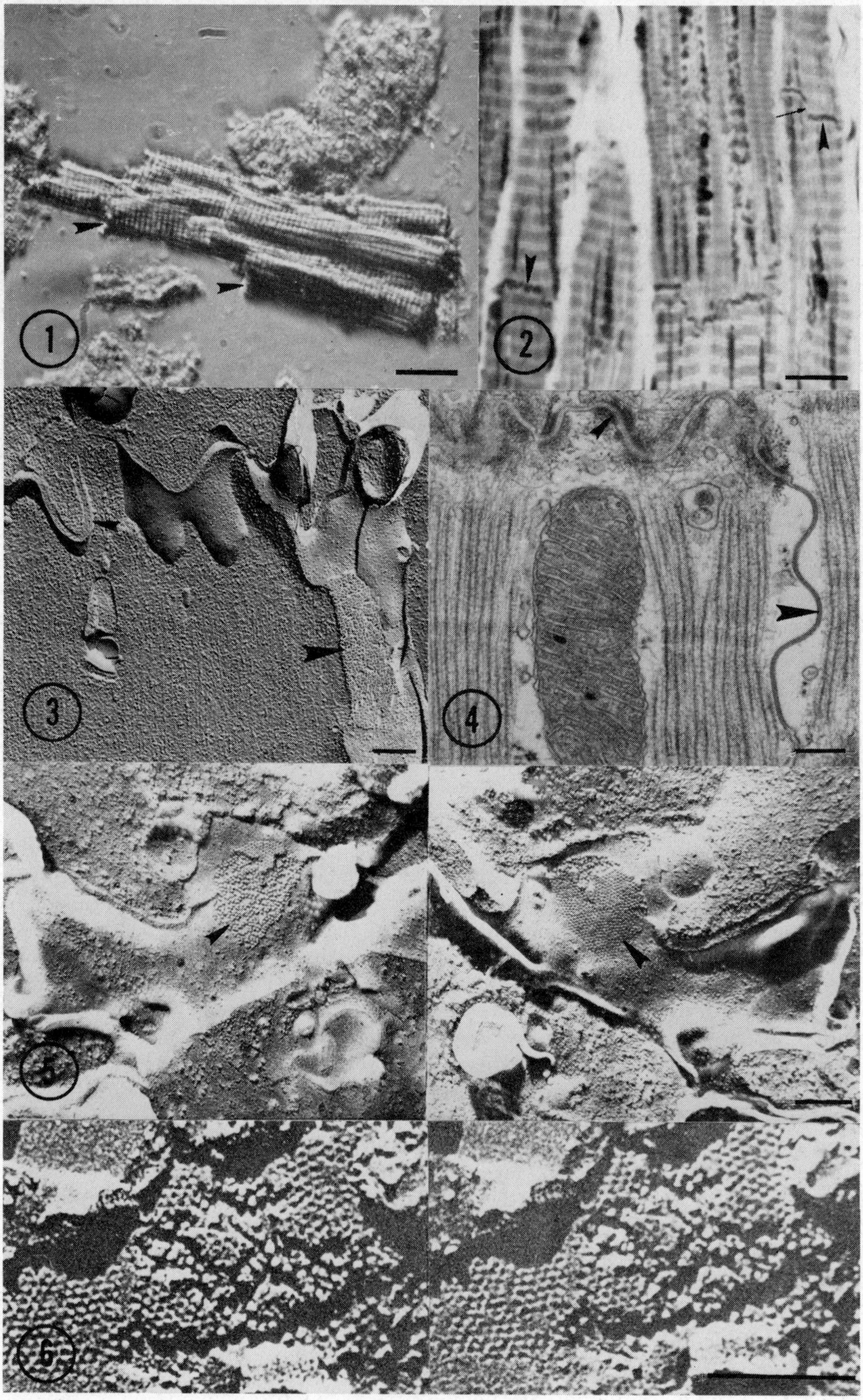
1
2
3
4
5
6

Figure 1. Isolated rat heart muscle cell. The cell surface is sculptured into terraces (arrowhead) at right angles to the long axis of the cell. Nomarski interference contrast. The scale bar represents 10 μm. The original magnification is ×1000.

Figure 2. Strand of conduction cells from the rabbit left ventricle. In this light microscopic view, the intercalated discs (arrowheads, thin arrow) traverse the cells at right angles to their longitudinal axis and reveal the rabbet-like joints between cells. The scale bar represents 8 μm. The original magnification is ×800.

Figure 3. Freeze-fracture preparation through an intercalated disc. This view shows the conical dovetails between two adjacent cells, and the particulate P face of the nexus (large arrowhead), which is arranged in longitudinal direction and often represents the riser of the step between two adjacent terraces (see Fig. 2, thin arrow). The small arrowhead points to a desmosome, which is one of the junctional complexes forming the intercalated disc. The scale bar represents 150 nm. The original magnification is ×42,500. (From Sommer and Johnson, 1979.)

Figure 4. A thin section of a region of a cardiac muscle cell similar to that seen in Fig. 3. The scale bar represents 150 nm. The original magnification is ×53,500. (From Sommer and Johnson, 1979.)

Figure 5. Complementary double replica of a freeze-fracture through a nexus of a cardiac cell from the dog. The small arrowhead on the left points to the particles of the P face of one of the plasma membranes forming the nexus. The large arrowhead on the right points to the complementary fracture face (E face) pulled off from the P face of the opposite during fracturing. The pits in the E face are in register with the particles on the opposite side. The scale bar represents 120 nm. The original magnification is ×59,000. (From Sommer et al., 1972.)

Figure 6. The structure of the nexus as seen in a stereo pair of a freeze-fracture preparation. The scale bar represents 0.15 μ. The original magnification is ×150,000. (From Steere and Sommer, 1972.)

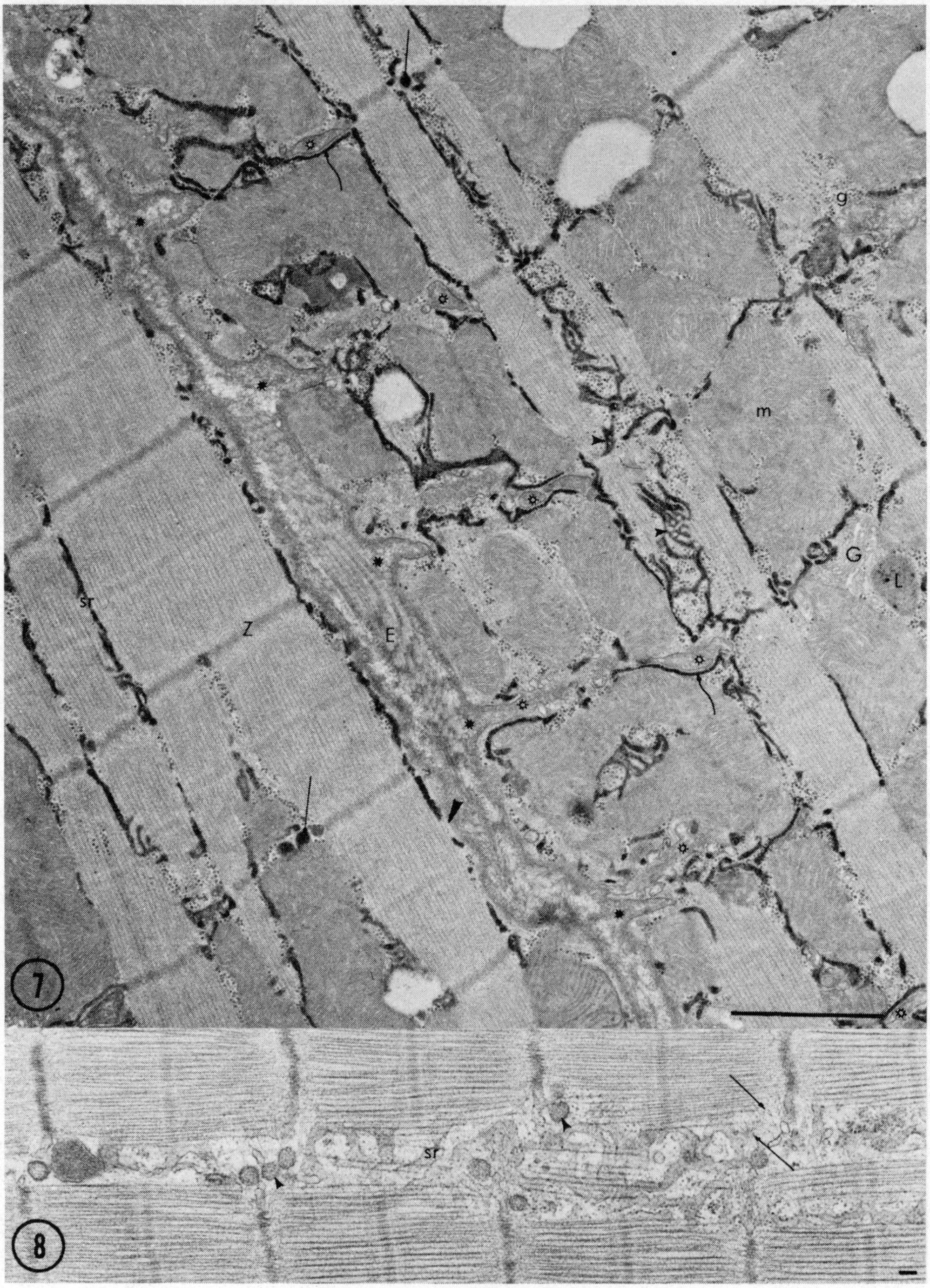
g
m
G
L
sr
Z
E
7
sr
8

Golgi regions, and many mitochondria. The mitochondria make up about 35% of the cell volume. The contractile material appears very similar to that observed in skeletal muscle. The sarcomere length is defined by the distance between two successive Z lines. This distance varies with the state of contraction as the actin filaments, which are attached to the Z line material, are pulled into the lattice of myosin filaments. The H band, which represents the distance between the free ends of the actin filaments emanating from successive Z lines within one sarcomere, also varies in width with the state of contraction, but it is often obscured in cardiac muscle cells. In contrast, the H band of some skeletal muscle cells (for example, frog) is very prominent and clearly defined. The M line is very prominent in cardiac muscle cells and, as in skeletal muscle, is flanked by a lighter zone, which is referred to as the L or the pseudo-H zone. The proportion of multinucleated cardiac cells remains an open question.

GEOMETRY OF CELL AND CELL BUNDLE APPOSITIONS

Individual cardiac muscle cells are electrically connected with each other through nexuses. Because most nexuses in cardiac muscle are part of the intercalated disc, which is visible with the light microscope, serial sections of about ½- to 1-μm thick through a muscle bundle provide a feasible way to obtain a rough measure of the number of cell-to-cell connections between cells and cell bundles over a given distance down the length of a strand of cells. Although our studies are preliminary, a certain pattern of the distribution of such connections emerges (Fig. 14, views A and B). Heart

---

Figure 7. Electron photomicrograph showing parts of two adjacent cardiac cells from the hamster. The extracellular space (E) separating the two cells from each other is filled with collagen. Z grooves are prominent (asterisks) and extend into the interior of the cell as transverse tubules (open asterisks). The sarcoplasmic reticulum (SR) is selectively stained in dark contrast revealing to good advantage the intricate network that it forms. The SR is continuous with the junctional SR (curved arrows), which attaches to the transverse tubules via junctional processes (barely visible). The junctional SR of cardiac muscle is much smaller in diameter than that in skeletal muscle is (see Fig. 9). The junctional SR forms interior couplings with transverse tubules, and peripheral couplings with the external membrane. Within a sarcomere (from one Z line to the next), the free SR forms a rete, each at the Z lines and M line (small arrowheads), although the rete at the Z line is frequently quite rudimentary. Note the large number of mitochondria (m). L = lysosome; G = Golgi; g = glycogen; straight arrows = corbular SR; arrowhead = plasma membrane. The scale bar represents 8 μm. The original magnification is ×26,000. (From Sommer and Waugh, 1976.)

Figure 8. A section showing the appearance and the distribution of corbular SR (arrowheads), which is always located at Z lines. The straight arrows point to anchor fibers, which are part of the cytoskeleton that attaches the SR to Z lines, and Z lines to plasma membrane. sr = sarcoplasmic reticulum. The scale bar represents 65 nm. The original magnification is ×31,000. (From Sommer and Johnson, 1979.)

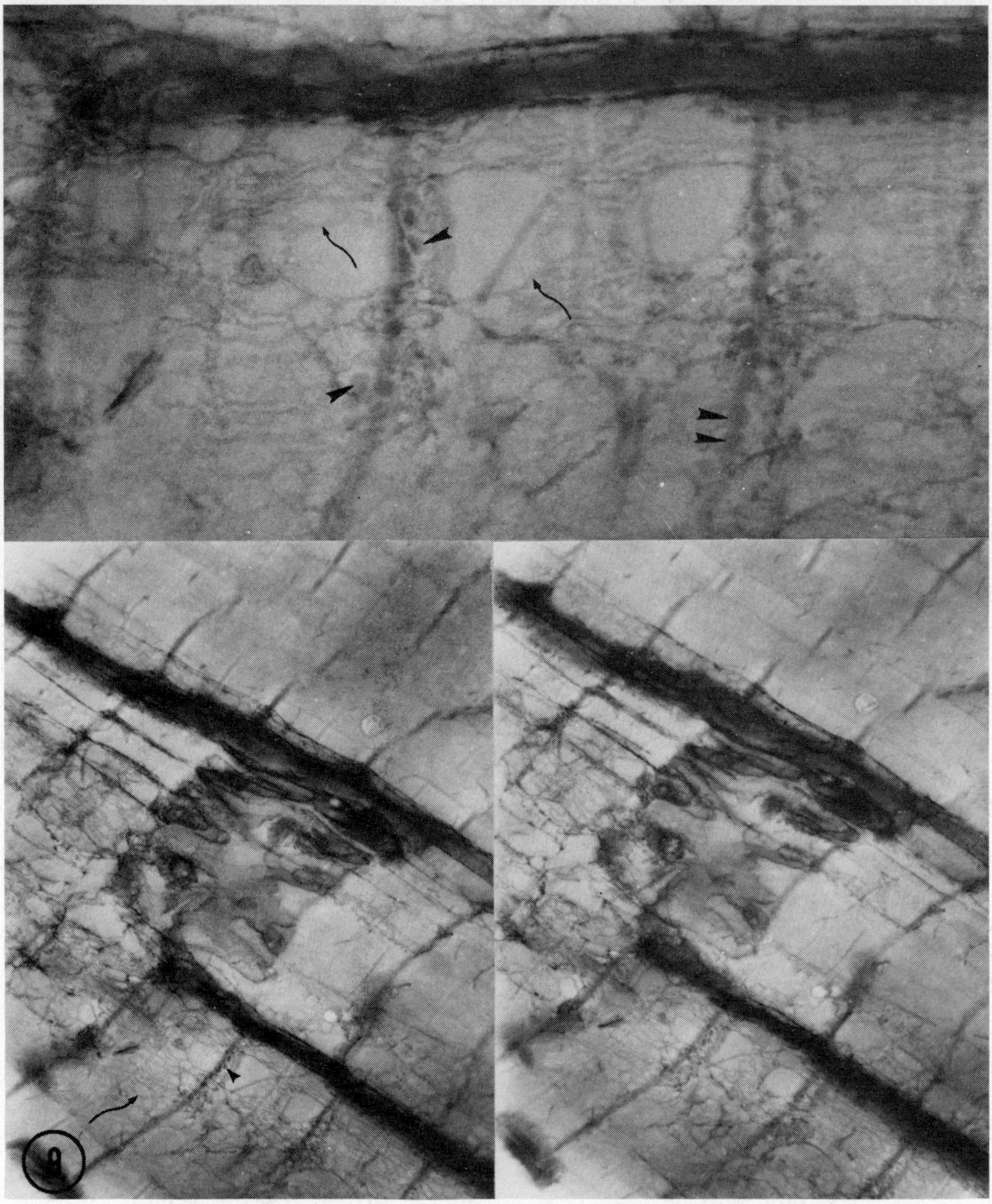

Figure 9. Top: High voltage electronphotomicrograph of hamster cardiac muscle in which the SR is stained selectively. Note the corbular SR at the Z lines lined up like a string of beads (arrowheads). SR = curved arrows. Bottom: A stereo pair of the above region. (Courtesy of Dr. R.A. Waugh).

muscle is apparently composed of what we tentatively call "unit bundles," each comprising between 2 and 30 cells. We use the term unit bundle because all its constituent cells are connected with each other within a space of 30 to 50 μm down the length of the strand. These unit bundles eventually join with one another at longer intervals, about every 100 to 150 μm, to form fascicles. These, in turn, make contact with other fascicles at still greater intervals to form larger bundles, and so on. Each of the cell-to-cell and bundle-to-bundle connections occurs, of course, via a nexus. Sometimes, only a single connection between two cells, each belonging to one of two adjacent bundles of fascicles, may be formed before more widespread joining of such bundles or fascicles may take place further down the strand (Fig. 14, view B). Such an arrangement may have unexpected consequences for the spread of excitation, especially when the cell-to-cell connections are viewed as finite resistors. This geometry is consistent with Spach's findings reported in these proceedings (see chapter 9). It will be interesting to see whether there is a difference in the geometry between bundles of conduction, common ventricular, and atrial cells but at this preliminary stage of our studies there does not seem to be one. Additional geometric features of bundles of cardiac cells are discussed below.

CONDUCTION CELLS

Tawara observed that the His bundle is but the beginning of an uninterrupted branching system of connected cells, the terminal branches of which are the cells originally described by Purkinje. Tawara suggested that this network serves as a conduction system for the spread of excitation to both ventricles. His own and many subsequent anatomical studies, notably those of Truex, established that the constituent cells of this network vary in morphology both within the system itself and between species. The classical Purkinje cells of the heart are very large, have little and peripherally located contractile material, and are found mainly in the large mammals. On the other side of the morphologic spectrum are the conduction cells that cannot be distinguished from common ventricular cells by light microscopy. These occur mainly in the smaller mammals. Between the large classical Purkinje cells and those that are indistinguishable by light microscopy from the common ventricular cells are the cells of intermediate morphology, the transitional cells of Truex. Macroscopically, the conduction system (from the His bundle to its end ramifications) can sometimes be located by treatment with iodine solutions that stain glycogen, which in a few animals (for example, in the dog) is plentiful. In most animals, however, much of the conduction system is visible macroscopically because the conduction cells usually travel within so-called *chordae tendineae spuriae* (false tendinous cords) that traverse the ventricular cavity. Every now and then, these strands also contain admixtures of common ventricular cells, especially in the large mammals.

We have found by electron microscopy that all conduction cells lack transverse tubules. This observation led to our working hypothesis, that, at least in adult mammals, the distinguishing feature between conduction and common ventricular cells would be the absence of transverse tubules in the former. The morphogenesis of these two types of cardiac cells remains unexplained. But one suggestions is that the absence of transverse tubules is related to cell size. The notion here is that the development of transverse tubules automatically follows the increase in cell diameter beyond a critical value (about 8 μm). Another suggestion is that cells are coded for transverse tubules in addition to, and independent from, cell size. Indeed, many cardiac cells *without* transverse tubules are much larger than 15 μm in diameter, and, on the other hand, many cells *with* transverse tubules are much below 8 μm in diameter. Even with the

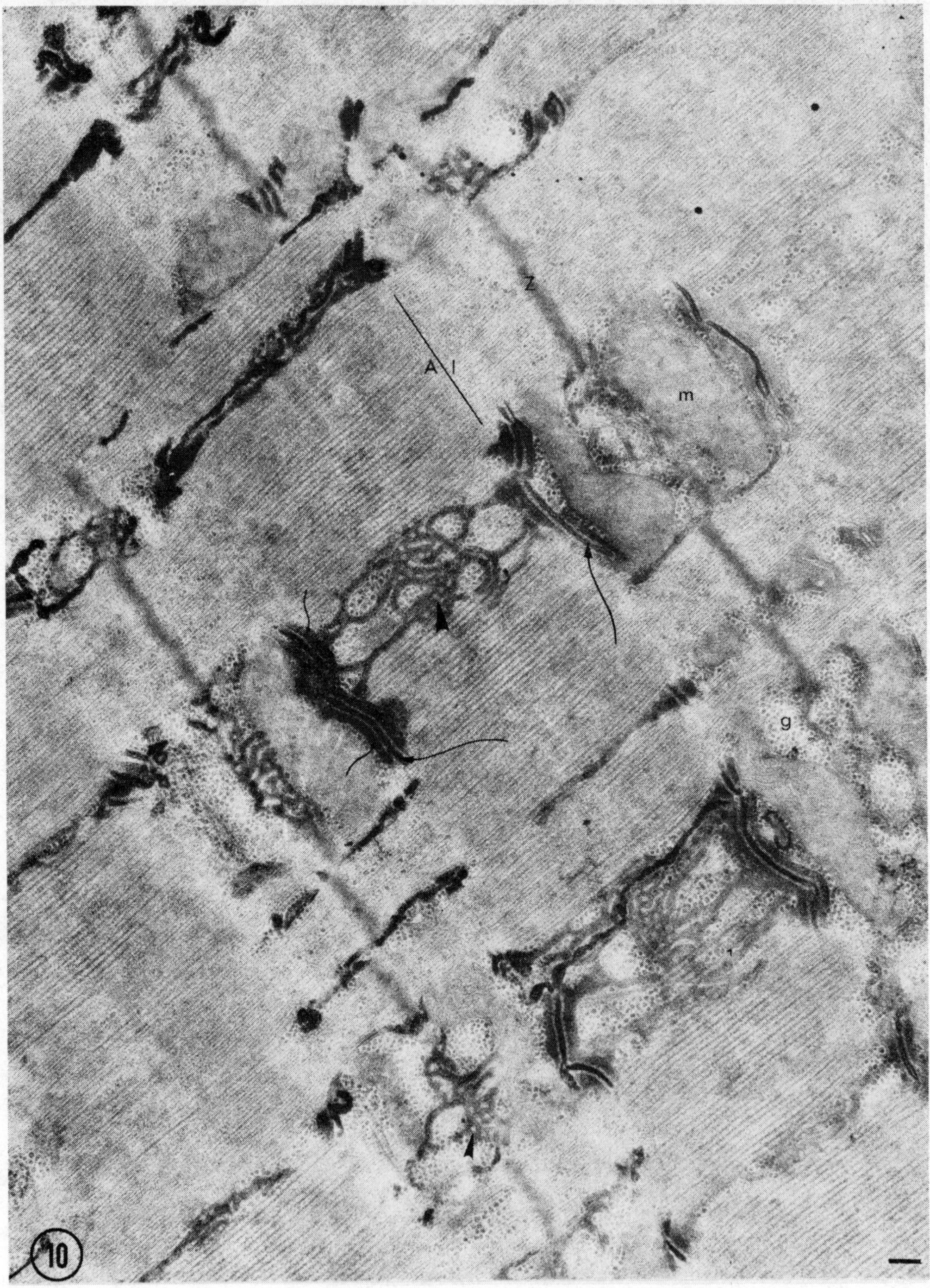
Z
A
I
m
g
10

supposition that all other parameters of importance be equal (for example, specific membrane properties), these differences in cell geometry clearly spell differences in overall electrical properties, for instance, those concerning conduction velocity. Unfortunately, it is not yet possible to make a direct structure-function correlation between the electrical properties of a cell with and another cell without transverse tubules. The reason is that isolated cardiac cells are very difficult to study electrophysiologically (see chapter 10 by Brown et al.). Such studies on isolated cells are imperative, however, because it is not possible to elucidate the electrical properties of a single cell as long as that cell remains a part of a network of electrically coupled cells. The electrical records obtained from such a cell would reflect some average, at that point, of the electrical properties of the whole network within a few space constants from the cell being investigated.

The importance of the influence of geometry on certain electrical properties of the conduction system is further illustrated by the following observations. In studying strands of conduction cells in several mammals, we have been impressed by the variety of ways the component cells are assembled (Figs. 14 through 19). Briefly, in the small mammals (mouse, cat, rabbit, etc.), the conduction cells (that is, those without transverse tubules) are packed with contractile material and are loosely assembled into bundles (Fig. 16). In the larger mammals (ungulates, elephant, whale, etc.), the component cells of the conduction bundles are tightly packed and are of the classical Purkinje cell type; that is, they have very large diameters (up to 100 μm) and very little contractile material (Figs. 15 and 17 through 19). The conduction cells in the small mammals are separated from each other by distances mostly exceeding 1 μm. In contrast, conduction cells in the large mammals are separated by narrow intercellular clefts (about 30 nm wide). Although the conduction cells in smaller mammals are covered throughout by a laminar coat, only that part of each conduction cell facing the very surface of the entire bundle is covered by this coat in the larger mammals. The intercellular clefts between the cells have no laminar coat, except for pockets here and there where the clefts widen over short distances (Fig. 19). But, estimates of the width of these clefts are made on *fixed* tissue. In vivo, the width of the clefts may be even smaller or may fluctuate. The very absence of a laminar coat may facilitate the very tight apposition of the adjacent membranes. A recent observation for the sarcoplasmic reticulum is that the inner lamellae of its envelope may actually merge, leading to complete obliteration of the SR lumen (Sommer et al., 1980). The maintenance of close apposition of the cells is aided by desmosomes, which are especially numerous in strands of classical Purkinje cells (Fig. 18). There are, of course, many nexuses between all conduction cells. Physiologically, the very tight packing of the cells causes a momentary decrease in the effective membrane capacitance during depolarization, because a large proportion of the plasma membranes of the individual cells of such a bundle is depolarized through a series resistance residing in the narrow clefts, thus

---

Figure 10. Section through mouse diaphragm. In this skeletal muscle, the SR shows a distribution similar to that seen in cardiac muscle, except that there are two transverse tubules (curved arrows) for each sarcomere. Each transverse tubule is flanked by junctional SR (small curved arrows), all three structures making up a triad. The triads in this type of skeletal muscle are located at the A/I junction. Arrowheads = retes of the free SR; g = glycogen; m = mitochondrion; Z = Z lines. Scale bar represents 60 nm; original magnification is ×68,000. (From Waugh et al., 1973.)

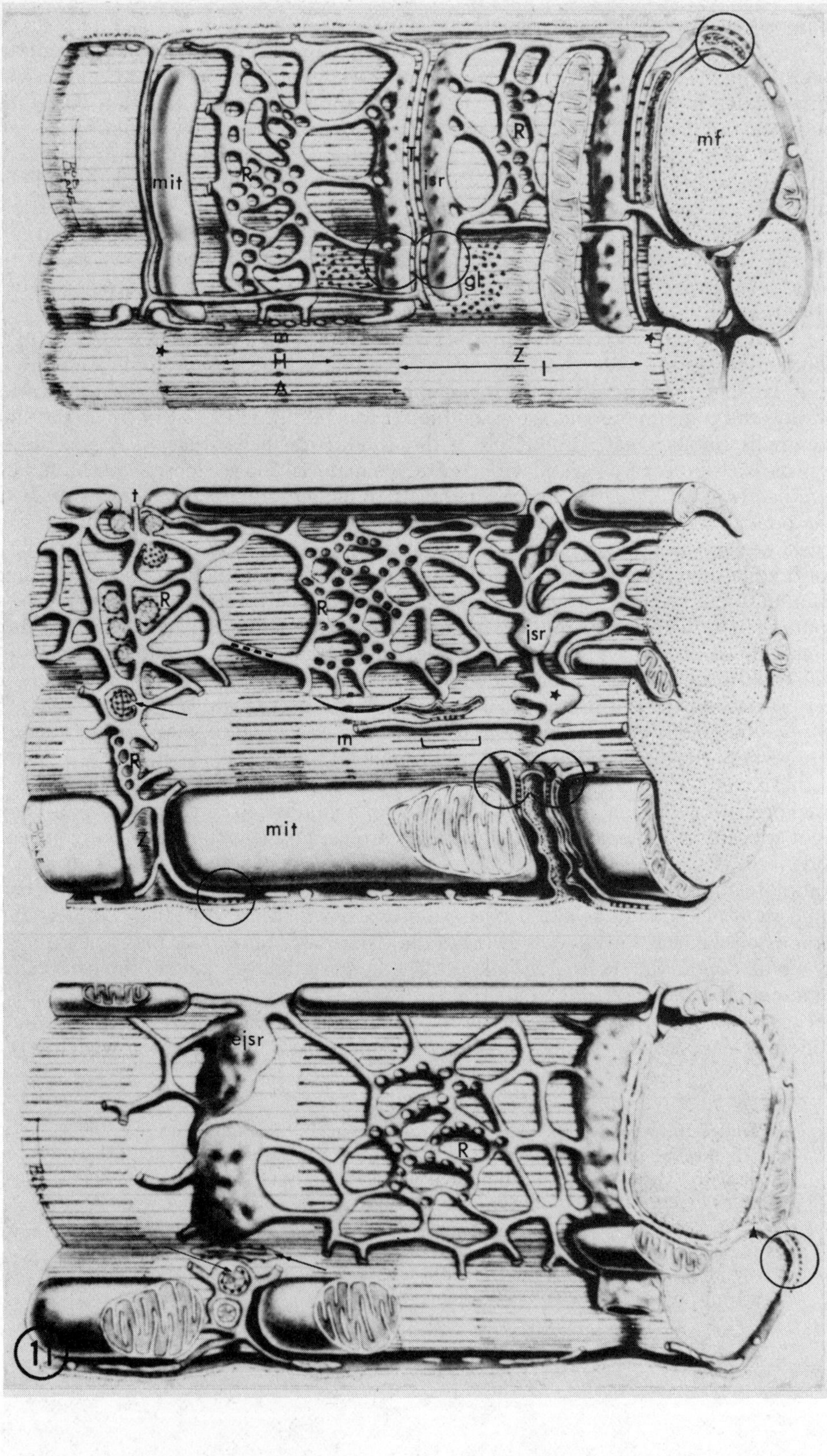
mit
R
T
jsr
R
mf
gl
m
H
A
Z
I
t
R
R
jsr
m
R
Z
mit
ejsr
R
11

Figure 11. Relationships between sarcoplasmic reticulum (SR) and myofibrils in skeletal muscle (top panel), mammalian cardiac muscle (middle panel), and avian cardiac muscle (bottom panel). Free SR is all the SR except the junctional SR (jsr; terminal cisterna). The junctional SR forms peripheral couplings (circles) and interior couplings (double circles) with plasma membrane of cell surface and of transverse tubules, respectively. Two couplings make a triad (double circles); one coupling makes a dyad (single circles and jsr with underlying transverse tubule in middle panel). Junctional SR has processes that make quasi-contact with transverse tubules. Free SR is differentiated into two retes (R) at M and Z lines, respectively. Z rete includes Z tubule (t, middle panel), which is a tubule of SR in mammalian cardiac muscle that is found on most Z lines as if attached to it. Retes have many fenestrations that are also seen in junctional SR of skeletal muscle. M rete is connected to junctional SR by longitudinal tubules (broken line); in skeletal muscle the general region of transition between longitudinal tubules and junctional SR is called intermediate cisterna. This region in cardiac muscle may be represented by structures seen in freeze-fracture preparations. In avian cardiac muscle (bottom panel), the general disposition of SR is similar, except that SR specializations indistinguishable from junctional SR in other striated muscles occur deep in the interior of muscle fibers at Z lines without contact with plasma membrane (ejsr, double-headed arrow). Sometimes an extended junctional SR extends into the interior (continuous form, arrowhead), but more commonly the extended junctional SR is connected to the junctional SR of peripheral couplings via tubules of free SR (discontinuous form, ejsr). On cross section (double-headed arrow), the extended junctional SR appears as a flattened tubule, which is bisected by a central dense line and which has junctional processes on either side. Corbular SR (arrows, middle and bottom panels) is a specialization of SR in the region of the Z rete and is found especially where transverse tubules are absent, such as in mammalian atrial muscle, in fibers of the conduction system, and in some avian hearts in which the extended junctional SR is not well developed (for example, in chickens). Corbular SR has only one connection with free SR in contrast to extended junctional, which has two or more. Corbular SR often occurs in clusters, contains electron-dense granular material, and has processes on its surface. In skeletal muscle (top panel), transverse tubules (T) are small in diameter as compared with those in cardiac muscle and are situated at either A-I junctions (stars) or at Z lines (Z). In mammalian cardiac muscle, they are at Z lines, and in avian cardiac muscle (bottom panel) they are absent. Transverse tubules form interior couplings with junctional SR. Transverse tubules in cardiac muscle are very polymorphous in size and shape with bulbous outpouchings in many places (star, middle panel; see also Fig. 12). Fuzzy coat over plasma membrane, the laminar coat, extends into transverse tubules of cardiac but apparently not of skeletal muscle. mit = mitochondria; gl = glycogen; m = M line; A = A band; I = I band; H = H band; Z = Z line. (From Bossen et al., 1978.)

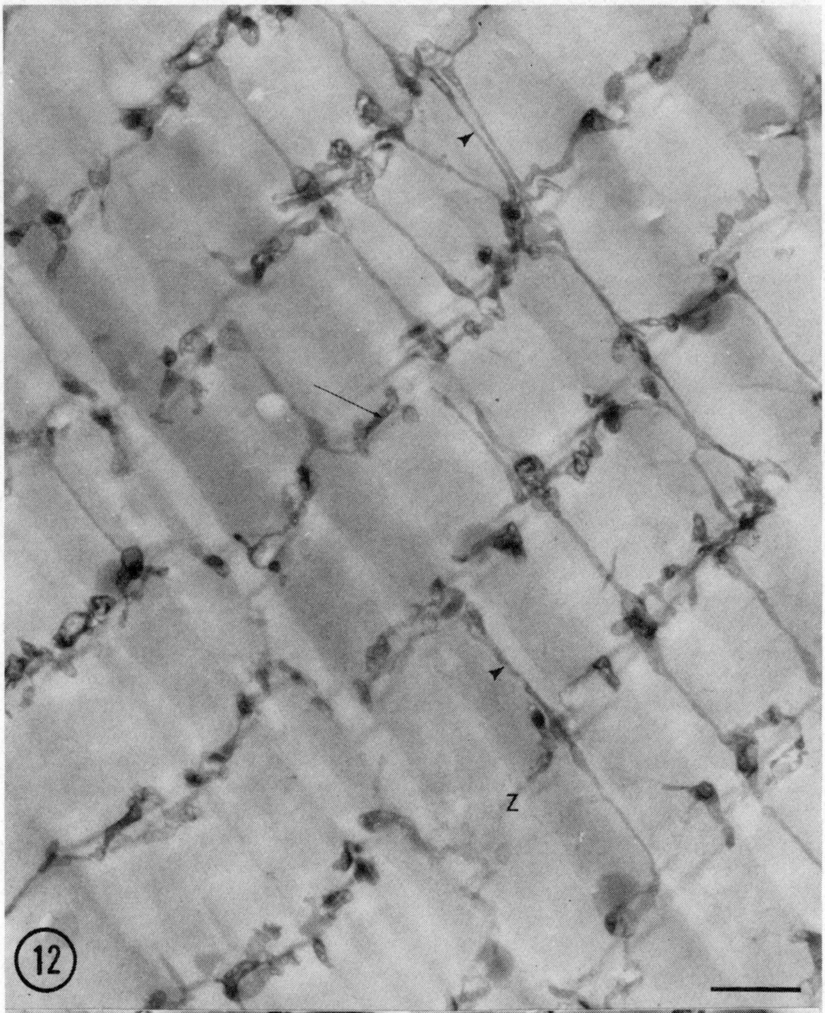
Z
12

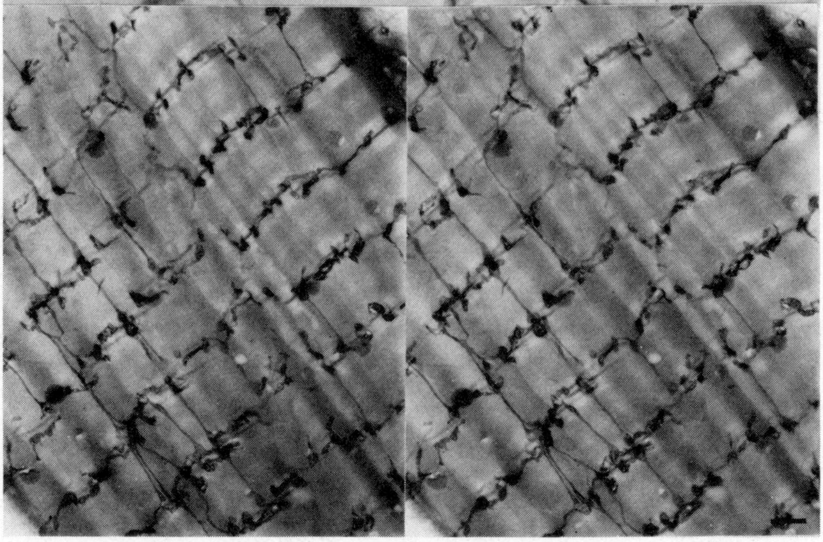

further increasing the conduction velocity in such a bundle. The geometry of the conduction system of the dog takes a position intermediate between the small and the large mammals, in that the constituent cells of the conduction strands in the dog are both loosely and tightly packed. Tight packing of the conduction cells, as apposed to the common ventricular cells, seems to be more prominent in immature dogs (versus mature dogs).

The conduction system in all likelihood is meant to program the sequence of the heart's contraction in a direction opposite to that in which excitation would proceed without a conduction system, the reason being to prevent premature closure of the cardiac outflow tract. In such a scenario, our observations of the conduction system reveal a spectrum of morphologic adaptations that may have evolved to negotiate with appropriate speed the different distances encountered in hearts of different sizes. The anatomy of the bird heart illustrates well the general applicability of the notion that there may be an obligatory geometric differential favoring fast conduction in conduction cells over that of common ventricular cells, if we disregard other contributing factors in the two populations, such as different membrane properties. The bird heart, like the mammalian heart, is composed of two populations of cardiac cells, the common ventricular and the conduction cells. The common ventricular cells have an average diameter of about 8 μm and, in contrast to their mammalian relatives, have no transverse tubules. Surprisingly, the conduction cells of bird cardiac muscle are not like those observed in mammals of comparable size and heart rate, for example, in the mouse. Instead, they are indistinguishable, both by light and electron microscopy, from the classical Purkinje cells: they are very large in diameter, have little and peripherally located contractile material, and are very tightly packed as, for example, in the ungulate, elephant, and whale hearts. It is tempting to suggest that in the bird heart the postulated geometric differential between conduction cells and common ventricular cells is sustained by the differences in cell size and cell packing between the two populations, neither of which has transverse tubules, whereas in the mouse that differential resides merely in the presence or absence of transverse tubules.

COMMON ATRIAL CELLS

The common atrial cells are all the muscle cells in the atria, excluding those found in the sinoatrial (SA) and atrioventricular (AV) nodes (Fig. 20). They are quite similar in morphology to the muscle cells in the ventricles, except that they often have atrial-specific granules, the function of which remains enigmatic. As in the ventricles, two different cell populations can be distinguished among the common atrial cells, one with, the other without transverse tubules. In the ventricles, the cells without transverse tubules are found in the entire conduction system, from the bundle of His to its

---

Figure 12. (top) Thick sections of the part of a cardiac muscle cell in which the transverse tubules have been contrasted with colloidal lanthanum hydroxide and photographed with a high-voltage electron microscope. The transverse tubules (arrow) have a varied geometry, ranging between thin tubules and large irregular pouches. On occasion, thin tubules that connect transverse tubules lie in the longitudinal direction (arrowheads). The scale bar represents 1 μm. The original magnification is ×13,000. (From Sommer and Waugh, 1976.)
(bottom) A stereo pair of the above illustrations. The scale bar represents 1 μm. The original magnification is ×6000. (From Sommer and Waugh, 1976.)

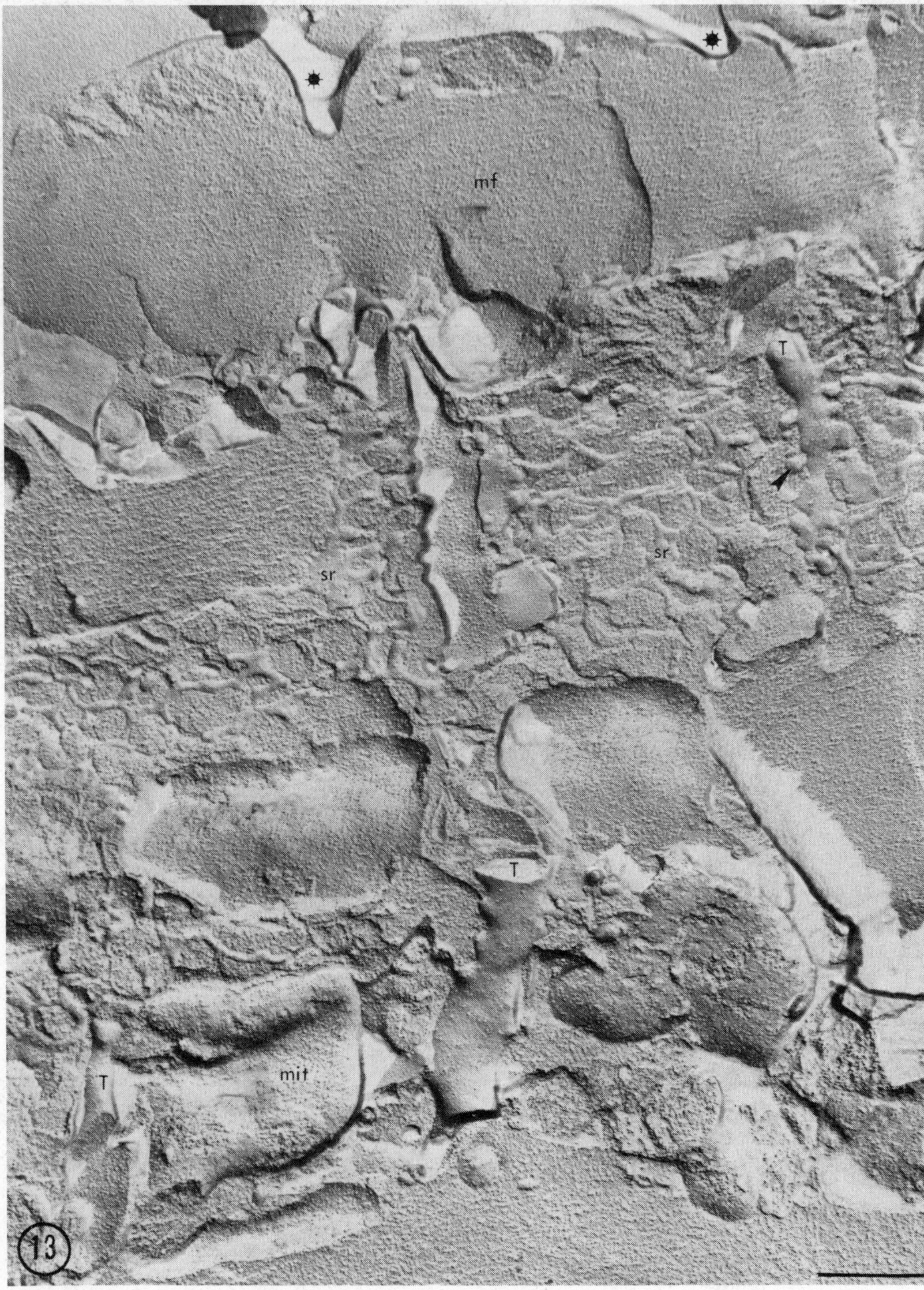
mf
T
sr
sr
T
T
mit
13

peripheral ramifications, but the common ventricular cells all have transverse tubules. In the ventricles, at least in some animals, these two cell populations can be distinguished electrophysiologically, but in the atria this is not possible because a great variety of action potentials characteristically are observed in different regions. Also, it is not possible in the atria to identify anatomically the topographic conditions analogous to those observed in the ventricles. Discrete tracts of continuous cells of unique morphology that are isolated, indeed insulated, from the rest of the atrial wall, analogous in every respect to the topography of the bundles and branches of the conduction system in the ventricles, do not exist in the atrium. At this point, no direct, rigorous ultrastructural correlation between "specialized fibers" as defined electrophysiologically has been accomplished, if only because electrical measurements so far have been possible only on cells that are part of an electrically coupled network, precluding the identification of the electrical properties of a single cell. The occurrence of pale or clear cells in electron micrographs of atrial cells does not allow a unique interpretation regarding their nature. In most instances, these cells show plain evidence of preparation artifacts; in other cases, large perinuclear regions, notoriously poor in contractile material, are nothing more than normal variations in the size of these spaces. In some instances, a case could be made that the observed morphology might remotely resemble Purkinje cells or cells usually seen only in the nodes. To obtain a measure of possible local variations in cell composition, we examined the volume fractions of various cell components in over 1,000 cells from different regions of the right atrium, including the SA node, and also from ventricular muscle (Fig. 21). We found that the volume fractions of intracellular components are virtually identical in all regions of the atrium studied, with the exception of the SA node, and that, significantly, these volume fractions did not differ from those observed in the ventricle. This further indicates the absence of accumulations of clear or pale cells anywhere outside the nodes. The few clear cells in the atrium that may be difficult to dismiss as either artifacts or as normal variations in cell composition seem to be randomly distributed throughout the atrium. These cells may be vestiges of either nodal or conduction tissue, the functional expression of which may be distorted or rendered ineffectual by the overall geometry of their integration among all atrial cells. Nevertheless, as in the ventricles, there is unequivocal anatomical evidence for the presence of two different cell populations that are distinguished by the absence or presence of transverse tubules. But, in contrast to the situation in the ventricles, in the atrium these two populations are diffusely integrated anatomically; albeit with the cells without transverse tubules being situated more toward the endocardium, a location where the ventricular conduction cells are also usually found.

Whether the cell population without transverse tubules represents derivatives of a conduction tissue anlage remains hypothetical, of course. Nevertheless, circumstantial evidence is not in conflict with the possibility that the atrial cells without transverse tubules may, in fact, be vestigial descendants of a putative conduction system anlage having lost the same rigorous anatomical isolation, indeed insulation, from the remainder of the common atrial cells, which is so characteristic of the separation between the ventricular conduction cells and the common ventricular cells. The case for the

---

Figure 13. Freeze-fracture preparation of cardiac muscle. The transverse tubules (T) are in register with the Z grooves (asterisks). The myofibrils (mf) are surrounded by the SR network (sr). The transverse tubules have many caveolae that jut out, berry-like (arrowhead). mit = mitochondria. The scale bar represents 0.5 μm. The original magnification is ×38,000.

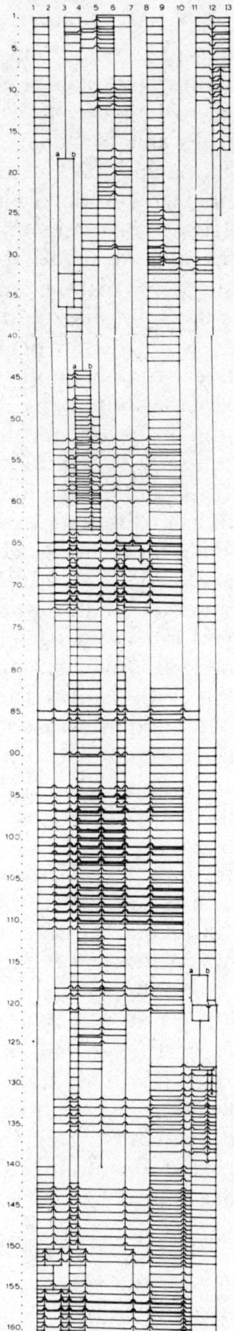

14A

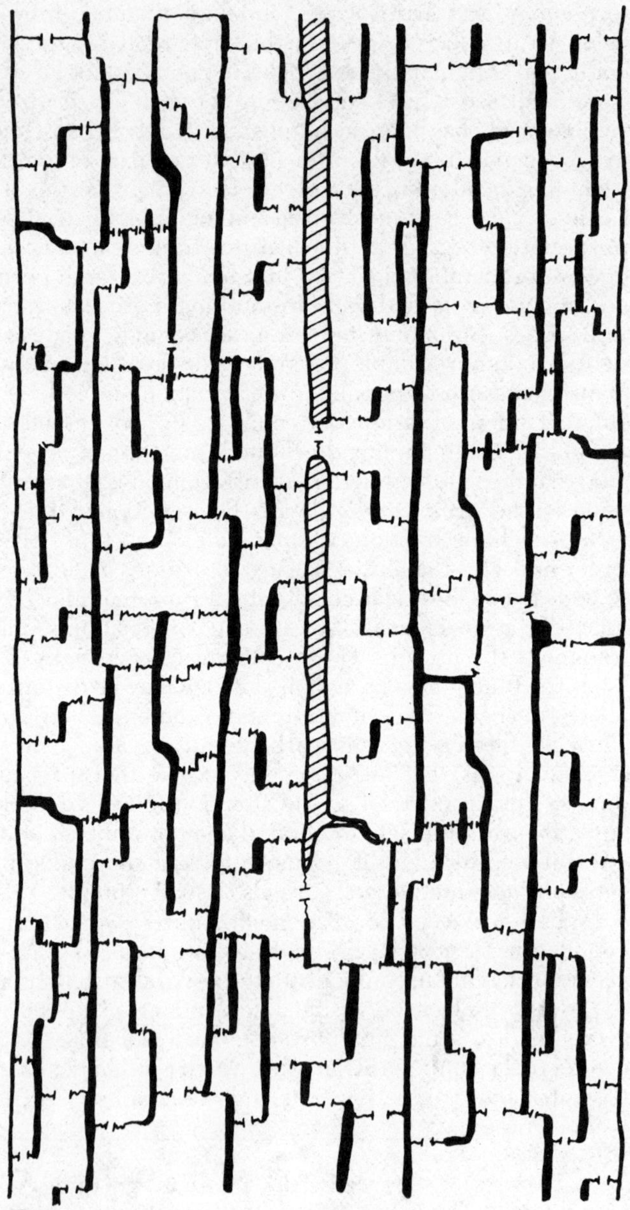

14B

existence in the atria of at least two cell populations, each of different provenance, can be strengthened by the following observations. There is agreement that although the "classical" Purkinje cells are conduction cells *par excellence*, anatomical variations of these cells are found in the ventricular conduction system of, especially, the small mammals. Therefore, the absence, or extreme paucity, in the atrium of unequivocally identifiable "classical" Purkinje cells is no objection, *per se*, to suggesting that derivatives of the conduction tissue may occur in the atria. For one, there is one population of cells in the atria that shares its absence of transverse tubules with ventricular conduction cells. More recently, evidence for substantial differences between atrial, conduction and ventricular cells has been reported. The evidence comes from studies using fluorescent antibodies and protein electrophoresis (Sartore et al., 1978, Thornell and Eriksson, 1981). Moreover, we recently found that the volume fraction of SR in mouse atrial cells is three times that found in common ventricular cells of that animal. Furthermore, there are twice as many cells without transverse tubules in the right as in the left atrium, which may reflect the topography of the conduction tissue anlage (Anderson, 1974). Finally, it is, perhaps, legitimate to anticipate conduction tissue derivatives in the atria of mammals simply by analogy to the situation found in birds *(natura non facit saltum)*. The atria of birds are pervaded by sometimes single, more often multiple connected cells that are indistinguishable from "classical" Purkinje cells. They are identical in morphology, both light and electron microscopically, to those seen in the conduction system in bird ventricles, and to those encountered in the ventricles of large mammals. They are very large cells with little peripherally located contractile material, and they are often very tightly packed into bundles. Thus, the bird heart has an anatomically, if not electrophysiologically, defined conduction system in the atria. It should be pointed out, however, that, although searched for, direct connections between the SA and the AV node by continuous bundles of such cells have never been observed. It remains to be seen whether in the mammalian atria more subtle geometric conditions prevail, such as tight packing of common atrial cells (analogous to our earlier findings in sheep and goat Purkinje cells), that would establish an anatomical basis for differences in the conduction of excitation from one region of the atrium to the next. According to our preliminary studies, that does not seem to be

---

Figure 14A. A quasi-wire diagram of intercellular contacts within a bundle of conduction cells of the rabbit over a distance of 160 μm down the strand at about 1-μm intervals. Note the common intercellular contacts among all cells within relatively short distances (about 50 μm). This column of 13 cells, which was an entire false tendinous cord, represents a "unit bundle." (From Johnson and Sommer, 1967.)

Figure 14B. A schematic drawing of two adjacent "unit bundles" of cardiac muscle cells as they are connected with one another by either a single cell connection at about 100 μm down the strand, or by more extensive fusion between the bundles farther down in the drawing. Extracellular spaces between cells are denoted by the black lines of different thickness. Extracellular spaces between "unit bundles" are denoted by the shaded areas. The nexuses between individual cells are indicated by perforations in the wavy lines representing intercalated discs. Current flow going laterally from one "unit bundle" into the next must proceed in a labyrinthine path, whereas current flow in a longitudinal direction can proceed in a straight line.

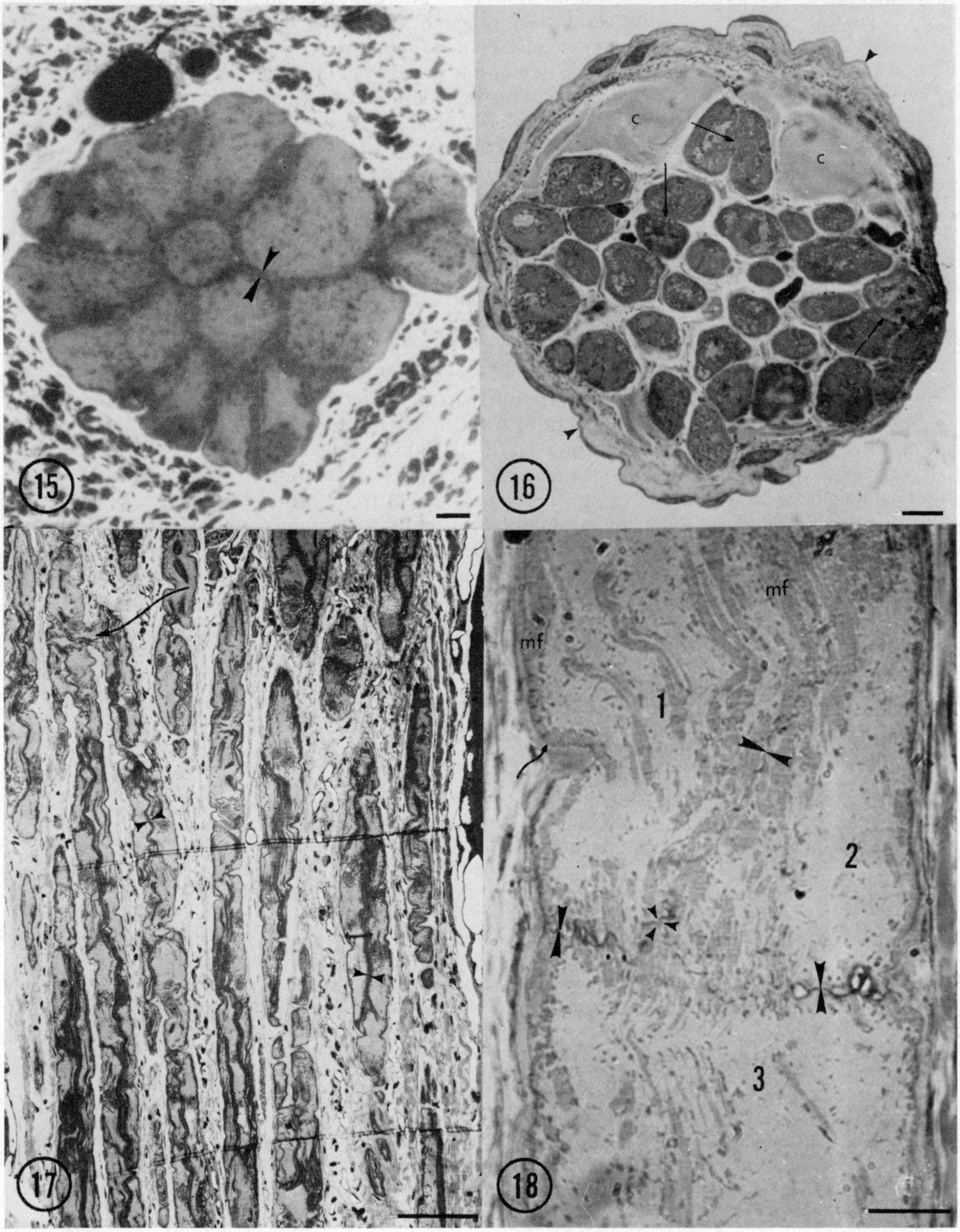
15
16
c
c
17
mf
mf
1
2
3
18

Figure 15. Light microscopic view of a classical bundle of tightly packed goat Purkinje cells. The cells are large, have a clear cytoplasm, and little peripherally located contractile material, which is stained dark (between arrowheads). The plasma membranes of both adjacent cells run between the two thin layers of myofibrillar material (see Fig. 17). The bundle of cells is surrounded by collagen; between the collagen fibers are a few blood vessels. The scale bar represents 10 μm. The original magnification is ×450. (From Sommer and Johnson, 1968.)

Figure 16. Transverse section through a *chorda tendinea* of the rabbit's left ventricle. The strand is surrounded by endocardium (arrowheads) and contains some collagen (c). A few cells are shown to be connected by junctional complexes as seen in the intercalated disc (arrows). This is one of hundreds of serial sections cut to study the geometry of cell-to-cell connections. Note that the cytoplasm is crowded with contractile material except for the centrally located nucleus in several cells. The scale bar represents 10 μm. The original magnification is ×700.

Figure 17. Longitudinal thick section through a classical strand of Purkinje cells from a sheep. Each of the cell columns is composed of several cells. The border between the tightly packed cells is usually between two layers of peripherally located contractile material (opposed arrowheads, see also Figs. 16 and 17). The curved arrow shows a connection between two adjacent columns of cells. Because of the multiple connections between the cells within one column, such a bundle would be like a unit bundle. The scale bar represents 80 μm. The original magnification is ×140.

Figure 18. Higher magnification of a column like the one shown in Fig. 15. The cell borders between the constituent cells are indicated by two opposed arrowheads. The small arrowheads indicate the junction of the three cells (1, 2, 3) that make up this particular column. The curved arrow points to the plasma membrane. mf = myofibrils that are a thin layer in the periphery of cells. The scale bar represents 10 μm. The original magnification is ×1,400.

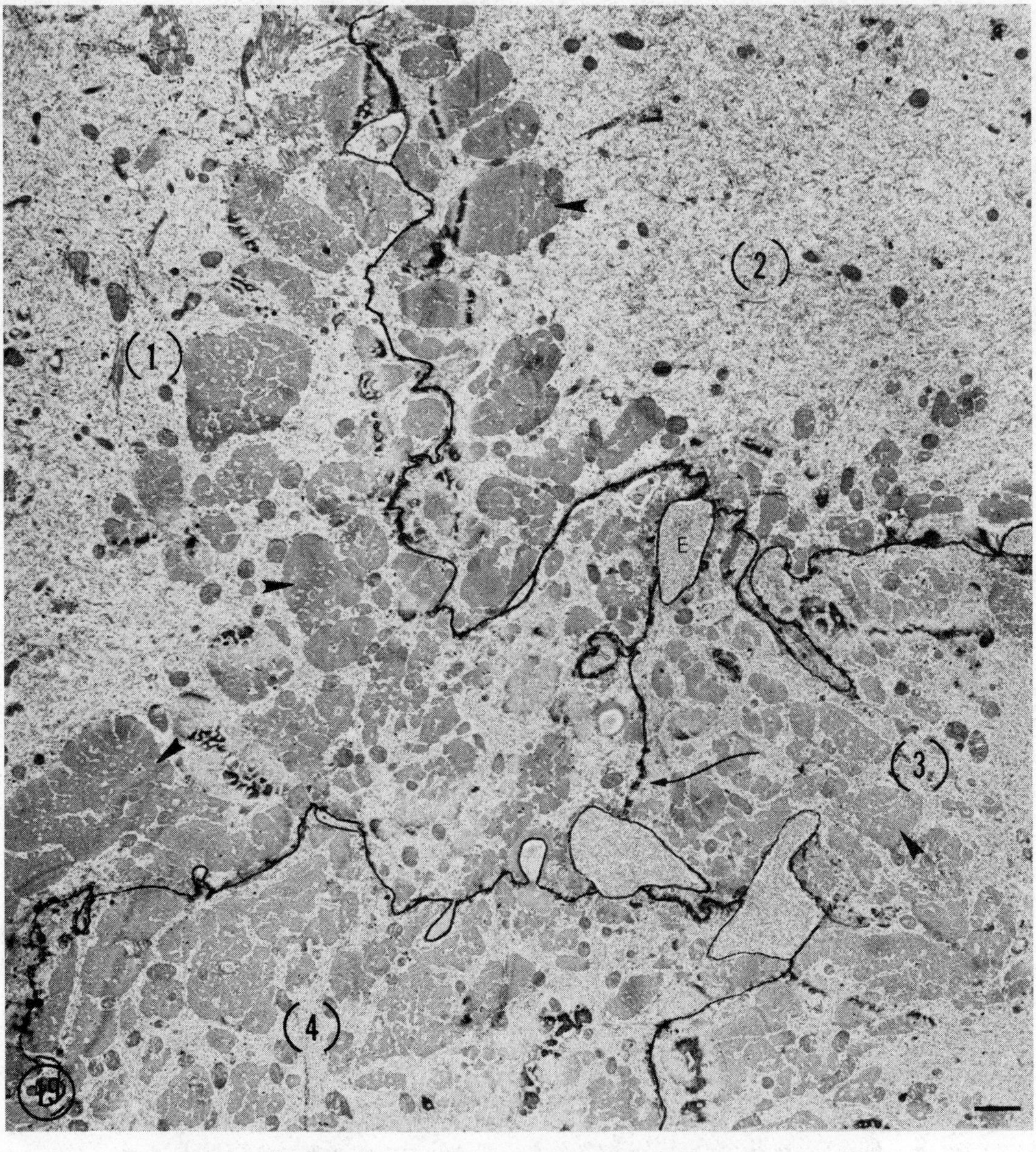

Figure 19. Electronmicrograph of a junction between four classical Purkinje cells of the sheep (1, 2, 3, 4). The cell borders between the four cells have been blackened with India ink. The distance between these adjacent plasma membranes is about 20 to 30 μm, although larger pockets of extracellular space (E) here and there remain. The curved arrows show a row of desmosomes. The arrowheads point to contractile material, which, as usual, is located in the periphery of the cells. The remainder of the cytoplasm is filled with haphazardly arranged fibrillar material. The scale bar represents 1 μm. The original magnification is ×7,500.

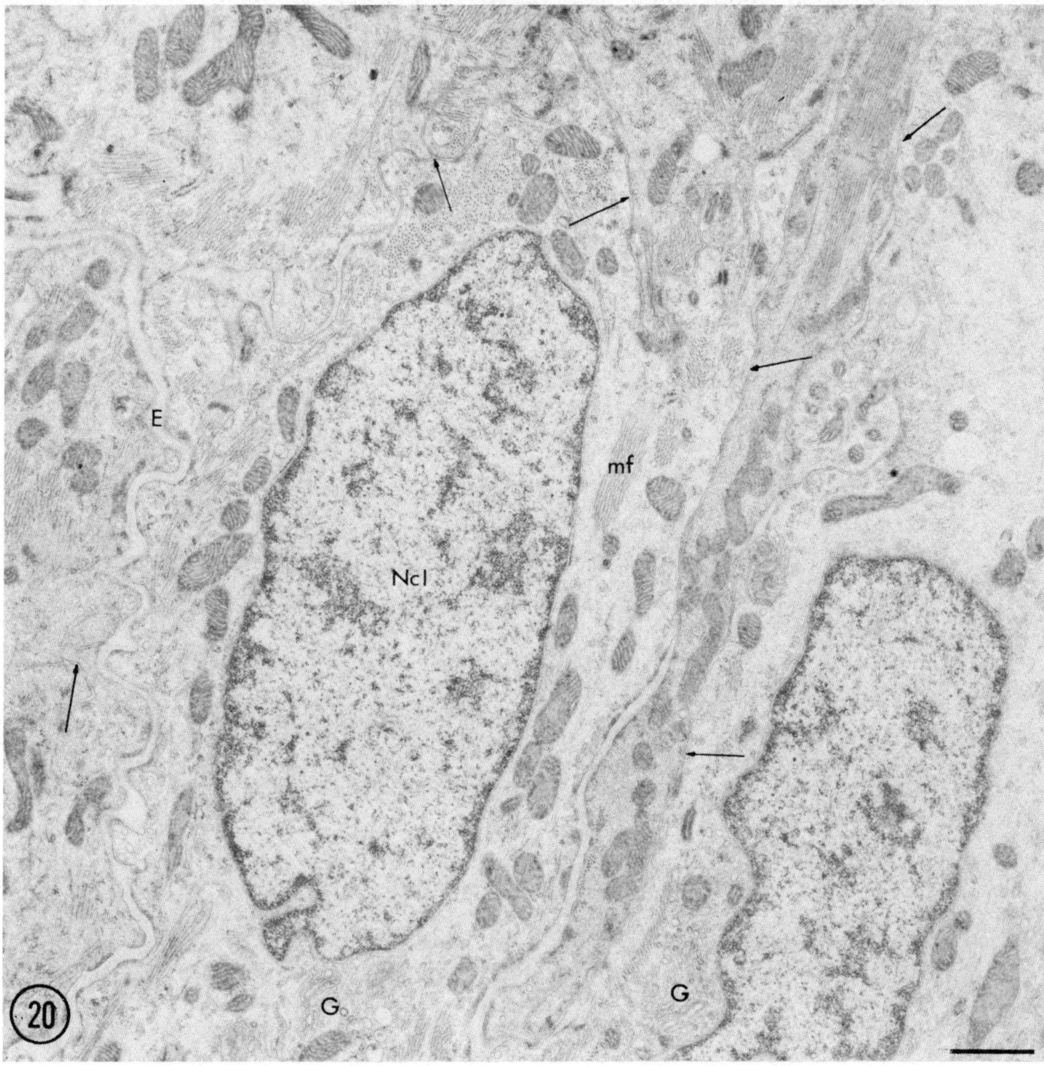

Figure 20. SA nodal cell. Several cells are apposed by either very narrow (thin arrows) or larger intercellular spaces. Note the small amount of contractile material (mf). G = Golgi complex. The scale bar represents 1 μm. The original magnification is ×13,300.

the case. Whether the anatomical difference in the two populations spells different membrane properties between the two cannot be answered at this time. The possibility that geometry of cell apposition may influence, if not determine, some or all of the observed physiologic properties must be excluded. Teleologically, there may be good reason that in the atria the working cells are diffusely integrated with conduction cells whereas in the ventricles the two cell populations are geometrically separated, with the separation being maintained over long stretches. For in the atrium, the main

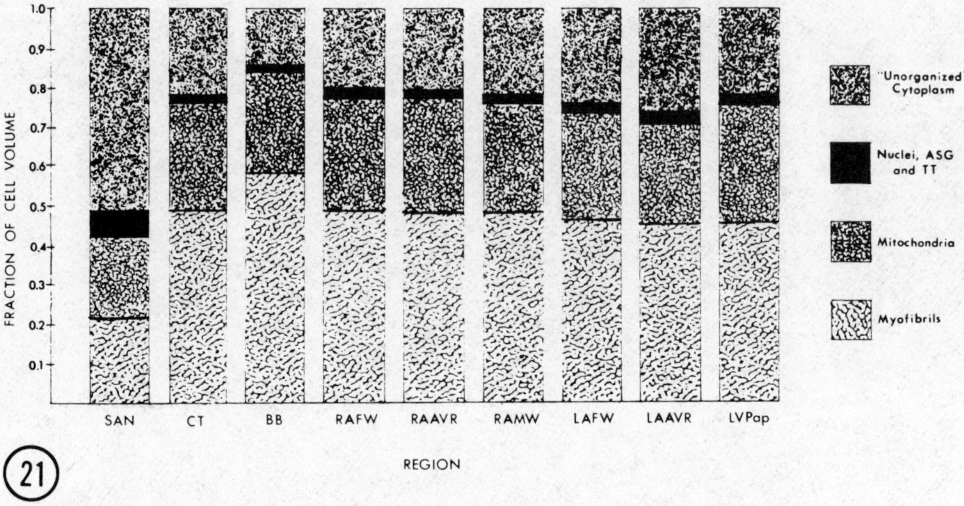

Figure 21. Volume fractions of some structures in cardiomyocytes (Dolber, 1980). ASG = atrial specific granules, TT = transverse tubules, "unorganized" cytoplasm = all that is not myofibrils, mitochondria, nuclei, ASG, nor TT (including some organized structures; for example, Golgi complexes, rough ER, etc.). Nine regions were sampled: Sinoatrial node (SAN), crista terminalis (CT), Bachmann's bundle (BB), right atrial free wall (RAFW), right atrial AV ring (RAAVR), right atrial medial wall (RAMW), left atrial free wall (LAFW), left atrial AV ring (LAAVR), and left ventricular papillary muscle (LVPap). For the data in each region, perfusion-fixed hearts of two 6.5-lb. rabbits were used; from each heart, five blocks were sectioned from each region, and ten micrographs (magnification ×13,880) were taken (total of 100 micrographs per region).

objective is to get the electrical impulse to the AV node safely, which is assured by geometrically integrating conduction and working cells in such a way that the whole atrium would act as the conductor, indiscriminately. In the ventricles, safety is compromised in favor of the overriding requirement of programming the spread of excitation in such a way that the wave of contraction proceeds from the tip of the heart toward the base; hence, electrical isolation of the conduction fibers from the working fibers, at least over long stretches, becomes mandatory.

The size distribution of rabbit atrial cells overall seems to indicate two clusters of cell diameters, one around 7 μm and the other around 15 μm. This is especially true for the larger muscle bundles; that is *crista terminalis*, Bachmann's bundle, pectinate muscle, and *limbus fossae ovalis*. The medial wall of the right atrium, exclusive of the *limbus fossae ovalis*, the sinoatrial ring bundle, and the roof of the right atrium are occupied predominately by cells of the smaller diameter.

NODAL CELLS

In the sinoatrial (SA) and atrioventricular nodes (AV), one finds characteristic nodal cells as well as common atrial cells and cells of intermediate appearance. The characteristic nodal cells in both nodes are quite similar (Torii, 1962; Tranum-Jensen,

1976; 1978). Despite extensive morphologic study of the AV node, including serial sectioning by thin sections for electron microscopy, no rigorous and universally accepted structure-function correlation has proved possible, most likely because the geometry of the AV node and its adjacent regions is so complex, in part due to the so-called overlay fibers (Anderson et al., 1974; Tranum-Jensen, 1976; Marino, 1979). In contrast, the geometry of the SA node is less complex and thus more conducive to structural analysis (Fig. 20). The cells of the SA node (and a large proportion of the AV nodal cells) differ greatly in morphology from other cardiac muscle cells (Torii, 1962; Tranum-Jensen, 1976; Masson-Pevet, 1979). Most notable is the paucity of organized myofilaments and, correspondingly, the abundance of relatively empty cytoplasm containing disorganized strands of actomyosin filaments. Moreover, nodal cells have very few atrial specific granules and transverse tubules. The often reported scarcity of nexuses requires cautious functional interpretation. The frequency of this important junctional complex between cells is easily underestimated because of the extremely small area that it covers in these cells. Moreover, from the physiologic point of view, it is important to recall that in very small cells, as the nodal cells are, the input resistance is very high. Therefore, effective electrical coupling between these very small cells can be accomplished even with a relatively high coupling resistance if that is what small nexuses are to imply. At present, the relationship between the size of a nexus and its electrical resistance is not known. Being small and irregular in shape, the SA nodal cells have a high surface-to-volume ratio, which is about twice that of other atrial cells (Dolber, 1980). The presence of a very large number of caveolae at the plasma membrane doubles their surface-to-volume ratio further (Masson-Pevet, 1979). The nodal cells share some common features with "classical" Purkinje cells: they have little organized contractile material, no transverse tubules, and are tightly packed. They are different from Purkinje cells in that they are much smaller in diameter. The close apposition between cells occurs in clusters, adjacent clusters being separated from one another by collagenous connective tissues.

Aside from specific membrane properties, about which rigorous data are lacking, two structural factors contribute to the electrophysiologic behavior of nodal tissue—the geometry of cellular connections, and the geometry of individual cells with their associated extracellular space. The relatively low conduction velocity within the nodal tissue might be accounted for in large part by the scarcity of nexuses (but see above) within and between cell clusters. The effects of cellular geometry and that of the extracellular space are much harder to gauge. Because nodal cells have both a high surface-to-volume ratio and also a high surface-to-volume ratio of the associated extracellular clefts, the action potential could be controlled, in part, by ion accumulation and depletion acting to change both the driving force for ion flow and the rate of electrogenic pumping (Johnson, 1979). In addition, in cells with a high surface-to-volume ratio, intracellular metabolic events could modify significantly the shape of the action potential if any of the products or reactants affect ionic channels directly, or alter the energy supply for the pumps. The question of the morphologic substratum of pacemaking properties remains unresolved; it has not been possible to identify morphologic features that make a cell a pacemaker cell. It may be significant, however, that those tissues most often associated with pacemaking properties (SA and AV nodes, Purkinje cells) are those that invariably show tight cellular packing and, thus, very narrow intercellular spaces.

In the preceding paragraphs, we have given a brief review of, and added some more recent data to, the present status of the ultrastructure of heart muscle, especially as it pertains to the conduction tissue. There is no doubt that ultrastructural investigations, tempered by close collaboration with physiologists and, I might add, *vice versa*, have greatly enhanced our knowledge of how cardiac muscle works. But these studies have also shown the limits of each method of inquiry. In the immediate future, it is safe to say, there is a need for the morphologist to study in greater detail the geometry of cell appositions, especially in the right atrium, and to apply the ultrarapid freezing technique to the study of cardiac muscle in an attempt to evaluate the ultrastructure as close to its in vivo condition as this technique will allow and especially with respect to the geometry of intercellular spaces, and with respect to the elucidation of transitory events at the plasma membrane and adjacent compartments, such as the SR. The acquisition of such data will provide the constraints within which physiologic interpretations, as well as mathematic modelling, must operate.

Acknowledgments

We wish to acknowledge the technical contribution of Mr. I. Taylor, Mrs. B. Scherer and E. Whitted. We are also grateful for the photographic work performed by Mrs. J. Calder and the staff of the VA Medical Illustration Department, Durham, N.C., as well as for the secretarial help rendered by Ms. L. Pace.

REFERENCES

Anderson RH, Janse MJ, Van Capelle FJL, Billette J, Becker AE, Durrer D (1974) A combined morphological and electrophysiological study of the atrioventricular node of the rabbit heart. Circ Res **35**:909–922

Bossen FH, Sommer JR, Waugh RA (1978) Comparative stereology of the mouse and finch left ventricle. Tissue Cell **10**:773–784

Challice CE, Viragh S (eds) (1973) Ultrastructure of the Mammalian Heart. New York, Academic Press

Dolber PC (1980) A morphological approach to some problems of rabbit cardiac atrial physiology. Ph.D. Thesis, Duke University

Johnson EA (1979) The genesis of the cardiac action potential: Chemical and electrical considerations. Proc Austral Physiol Pharmacol Soc **10**:59–72

Johnson EA, Sommer JR (1967) A strand of cardiac muscle: Its ultrastructure and the electrophysiological implications of its geometry. J Cell Biol **33**:C103–C129

Marino TA (1979) The atrioventricular node and bundle in the ferret heart: A light and quantitative electron microscopic study. Am J Anat **154**:365–392

Masson-Pevet MA (1979) The fine structure of cardiac pacemaker cells in the sinus node and in tissue culture. Ph.D. Thesis, University of Amsterdam

McNutt NS, Fawcett DW (1974) Myocardial ultrastructure. *In* The Mammalian Myocardium, edited by GA Langer, AJ Brady. New York, Wiley, pp. 1–49

Page E, Fozzard HA (1973) Capacitive, resistive and syncytial properties of heart muscle: Ultrastructural and physiological conditions. *In* The Structure and Function of Muscle, vol II, Structure, Part 2, edited by GH Bourne. New York, Academic Press, pp. 91–158

Sartore S, Pierobon-Bormioli S, Schiaffino S (1978) Immunohistochemical evidence for myosin polymorphism in the chicken heart. Nature **274**:82–83

Sommer JR, Johnson EA (1968) Cardiac muscle: A comparative study of Purkinje fibers and ventricular fibers. J Cell Biol **36**:497–526

Sommer JR, Johnson EA (1979) Ultrastructure of cardiac muscle. *In* Handbook of Physiology, sec 2: The Cardiovascular System, vol I, The Heart, edited by RM Berne. Bethesda, MD, American Physiological Society, pp. 113–186

Sommer JR, Wallace NR, Junker J (1980) The intermediate cisterna of the sarcoplasmic reticulum of skeletal muscle. J Ultrastruct Res **71**:126–142

Sommer JR, Steere RL, Johnson EA, Jewett PH (1972) Ultrastructure of cardiac muscle. A comparative review with emphasis on the muscle fibers of the ventricles. *In* Hibernation and Hypothermia, Perspectives and Challenges, edited by FE South, JP Hannen, JR Willis, ET Pengelley, NR Alpert. Amsterdam, Elsevier, pp. 255–291

Sommer JR, Waugh RA (1976) The ultrastructure of the mammalian cardiac muscle cell with special emphasis on the tubular membrane systems. Am J Pathol **82**:192–221

Steere RL, Sommer JR (1972) Stereo ultrastructure of nexus faces exposed by freeze-fracturing. J Microscopie **15**:205–218

Thornell LE, Eriksson A (1981) Filament systems in the conducting cells of the heart. Physiol Rev (in press)

Torii H (1962) Electron microscopic observations of the S-A and A-V nodes and Purkinje fibers of the rabbit. Jpn Circ J **26**:39–77, 1962

Tranum-Jensen J (1976) The fine structure of the atrial and atrioventricular (AV) junctional specialized tissues of the rabbit heart. *In* The Conduction System of the Heart: Structure, Function and Clinical Implications, edited by HJJ Wellens, KI Lie, MJ Janse. Philadelphia, Lea and Febiger, pp. 55–81

Tranum-Jensen J (1978) The fine structure of the sinus node: A survey. *In* The Sinus Node: Structure, Function, and Clinical Relevance, edited by FIM Bonke. Boston, Martinus Nijoff Medical Division, pp. 149–165

Waugh RA, Spray TL, Sommer JR (1973) Fenestrations of sarcoplasmic reticulum. J Cell Biol **59**:C254–C260

Discussion

OLIVEIRA CASTRO: How can you explain the presence of lanthanum in the central channel of the connexon? Lanthanum distribution is restricted to the extracellular fluid, and the channel should be entirely isolated from this fluid.

SOMMER: I have no explanation for the presumed presence of lanthanum within the connexons. I should like to point out, however, that we do not find an electron-dense dot in the center of the connexon when we leave out osmium tetroxide as part of the preparative procedure (Steere, and Sommer, 1972). Thus, the presence of lanthanum in the connexons is in doubt. I believe no one has been able to convincingly demonstrate the presence of a channel in the connexons with tracers. The best evidence for a special domain within the connexon that may be suitable for the transfer of ions from one cell to the other comes from the work of Unwin and Zampighi (Nature 283:545–549, 1980) on diffraction studies of isolated gap junctions.

PAGE: Caspar et al. and Unwin and Zampighi, which you cite, did not use osmium in the fixation procedure. And their observations were made by X-ray diffraction, low-dosage electron microscopy, image analysis, and other methods quite independent from those that are used to prepare freeze-fracture specimens. Yet, they find clear evidence for the existence of a channel in the center of the connexon. They also find conformational alterations of this channel that are not completely unlike those that occur when junctional function is interfered with. I think that there are several lines of distinct evidence for the existence of a central channel in the middle of the connexon. True, this channel has still not been delineated in a desirable way, but on the other hand the evidence that it is an artifact is perhaps less strong than the evidence obtained by multiple techniques in favor of the existence of something that looks like a channel in the center of the connexon.

JOHNSON: Why are there transverse tubules in cardiac muscle?

SOMMER: I actually do not know. Interestingly, however, the surface-to-volume ratio of bird cardiac cells is the same as that of mouse cardiac cells. Correspondingly, the cell diameter of bird cardiac cells, which do not have transverse tubules, is about half that of mouse cardiac cells, which do have transverse tubules. But remember that many mammalian cardiac cells, although having no transverse tubules, have large diameters. Nystroem, who described the transverse tubules in heart muscle in the late nineteenth century, called them "saftkanälchen," channels for juices. We have speculated that they may have evolved to permit survival under conditions in which cardiac hypertrophy develops. In hypertrophy, heart muscle cells increase in diameter at least twofold, creating potential diffusion problems.

WEIDMANN: Is there a need to postulate transverse tubules to explain a fast activation of the contractile system by calcium inflow?

SOMMER: No, I don't think so. Many years ago, Nelson and Benson (J Cell Biol *16*:297–313, 1963) and, more recently, we (Sommer and Johnson, J Cell Biol *36*:497–526, 1968) made calculations that assumed calcium release from somewhere near the cell surface, and we measured the delay between stimulation and the first occurrence of contraction as seen on a television. From this, there seems to be ample time for calcium diffusion—even given heart rates of 1000 per minute, which both cell types, the bird cells without and the mouse cells with transverse tubules, are capable of. But, not knowing the diffusion parameters of calcium in muscle cytoplasm , we made these calculations, for a water medium. Our understanding of the activation process is further complicated by the nature of the junctional SR found in the bird. The heart muscle cell of the bird does have junctional SR, but most does not make contact with the plasmalemma.

Chapter 2

Structural Approaches to Permeability of Cardiac Gap Junctions

Ernest Page

The permeability of gap junctions in intact cardiac preparations does not lend itself to precise measurement by electrophysiological or isotopic measurements (Weidmann 1965; 1966). On the one hand, the geometrical arrangement of the junctions in a multicellular syncytium, as well as the membrane properties of both junctional and non-junctional plasmalemma, render difficult the sharp electrophysiological separation of junctional membrane conductance from that of non-junctional plasmalemma; on the other hand, the rate of sarcoplasmic diffusion in the axial direction does not permit a sharp kinetic separation from that of tracer solute permeation across the gap junctions between cells. These technical difficulties notwithstanding, the permeability of cardiac gap junctions is important for several physiologically interesting questions. Does gap junctional permeability in cardiac cells vary during physiological fluctuations in sarcoplasmic ionized Ca activity (a_i^{Ca})? To what extent does the apparent difference between the intracellular-specific axial resistance (R_i) of Purkinje fibers and ventricular muscle (Weidmann, 1952; 1970) result from differences in gap junctional permeability? What role, if any, does variation in gap junctional permeability play in the disturbances of impulse conduction associated with cardiac glycoside toxicity and with other pathophysiological conditions? Does gap junctional permeability change during the embryonic development of the heart? The resolution to these and other questions requires new and better methods for determining gap junctional permeability.

One approach is to develop ultrastructural criteria for judging the permeability of gap junctions. Recently, the basis for this approach has been reviewed (Page and Shibata, 1981), and experiments that apply it to cardiac gap junctions are beginning to appear (Baldwin, 1979; Dahl and Isenberg, 1980; Shibata and Page, 1980; Page and Upshaw-Earley, 1980a; Quertermous et al., 1980a; 1980b). In this chapter, I will present some examples of ultrastructural methods that have already been applied to this problem and consider additional methods potentially useful for understanding gap junctional permeability in heart muscle.

Supported by Grants HL 10503 and HL 20592, awarded by the National Heart, Lung and Blood Institute and the U.S. Public Health Service.

ULTRASTRUCTURAL METHODS AIMED AT QUANTIFYING GAP JUNCTIONAL PERMEABILITY IN HEART MUSCLE

Current Techniques

Rigorous and well-standardized ultrastructural criteria for quantifying the permeability of gap junctions between cardiac cells are not yet established. Current attempts to correlate cardiac gap junctional structure with junctional permeability rely predominantly on quantitative analysis of membrane replicas obtained from freeze-fractured cardiac nexuses (Baldwin, 1979; Dahl and Isenberg, 1980, Shibata and Page, 1980; Page and Upshaw-Earley, 1980a; 1980b; Quertermous et al., 1980a; 1980b) and, to a much lesser extent, on measurements made on thin-sectioned material.

The structural criteria for determining the gap junctional permeability in heart muscle were initially those that Peracchia used for freeze-fractured crayfish synapses and epithelial cells from vertebrate stomach, hepatocytes, and lens (see review by Peracchia, 1980). According to Peracchia, the calcium-induced transformation of a permeable junction into an impermeable junction is associated with (1) a transition from a random distribution of gap junctional particles and pits in the lipid bilayer in the permeable state to a highly ordered, quasicrystalline array in the impermeable state; and (2) an aggregation of junctional particles and pits that cause a leftward shift in the frequency distribution of center-to-center distances to a new distribution with a smaller mean distance. In addition, Peracchia described a decrease in the width of the junctional gap, which he determined from thin-sectioned tissues of electrically decoupled junctions.

But these criteria cannot be applied indiscriminately to cardiac gap junctions. The methodologic problems that may affect the results of measurements on replicas of freeze-fractured gap junctions must be considered. A partial list of these considerations includes the changes in junctional structure resulting from the methods used to cross-link, glycerinate, quick-freeze, or otherwise preserve the junctional structure for freeze fracture; the difficulties in interpreting the location of the fracture planes through the junctions (Sjöstrand, 1979); the degree of plastic deformation; the undulation or tilt of the junctional fracture faces; and the precision, the validity of sampling, and the reproducibility of the measurements made on the electron micrographs of the junctional replicas.

The extent to which the junctional structure is perturbed by the methods of preserving it needs to be assessed cautiously. To date, no gap junction in any tissue has been visualized in its native state. For this reason, all interpretations of what the native structure is like are extrapolations beset by substantial uncertainty. To evaluate errors in such interpretations: it is desirable to compare several methods of preserving the tissue (e.g., glutaraldehyde fixation, rapid freezing with liquid helium or liquid propane, freeze substitution); to analyze the structures thus preserved by several different structural approaches (e.g., transmission electron microscopy of thin-sectioned, positively stained junctions, optical and electron diffraction of negatively stained junctions, X-ray diffraction of junctions in the hydrated state, freeze fracture of in situ junctions and of isolated fractions of junctional membrane); and to attempt quantitative analysis of the data thus obtained. If the properties of the structure appear similar with several preparative and analytical techniques, one may be dealing with something close to the native structure, or at least with an artifact stable enough to serve as a point of departure for further studies. For critical discussions of structural methodologies and interpretations, see the recent monograph edited by Rash and Hudson (1979) and the recent reviews by Sjöstrand (1979), Pinto da Silva and Kachar (1980), and Peracchia (1980).

In heart muscle, problems that are to some extent peculiar to this tissue compound the methodologic difficulties. Exposing the cardiac gap junctions to an increased a_i^{Ca} changes their structure (Dahl and Isenberg, 1980; Shibata and Page, 1980, 1981; Page and Upshaw-Earley, 1980a; 1980b) and decreases their permeability (De Mello, 1975; Délèze, 1970; Nishiye, 1977; Weingart, 1977; Dahl and Isenberg, 1980). Therefore, it is essential that any structure-preserving method avoid raising the a_i^{Ca}, or that it at least stabilize the gap junctional structure before any elevation of a_i^{Ca} can change that structure. This is not merely a hypothetical issue. For example, concentrations of glutaraldehyde commonly used to fix heart muscle depolarize the tissue (Fozzard and Dominguez, 1969). They may therefore release calcium from the sarcoplasmic reticulum. Conceivably they may also affect mitochondrial and plasmalemmal calcium transport mechanisms in such a way as to raise the a_i^{Ca}.

My laboratory has compared several methods currently used to determine the structure of gap junctions. We have preserved rat ventricular myocardial cells and sheep Purkinje fibers by glutaraldehyde fixation, by rapid freezing with a liquid helium-cooled copper probe (Shibata et al., 1980), and by rapid freezing in dichlorodifluoromethane (Freon) slush (Shibata and Page, 1981). We have also preserved the hearts of rats and rabbits by glutaraldehyde fixation or quick freezing so that junctional structures in situ could be studied under different conditions: in hearts contracting at 37° C on the Langendorff cannula, during in vitro perfusion at 0° C, at a pH of 9.0, and after calcium depletion (Page and Upshaw-Earley, 1980a; 1980b). Under all of these conditions, both the pitted fracture face of the junction (the extracellular or E face) and the particulate face (the cellular or P face) were present as arrays, not as widely spaced scattered units like those found in lens (Peracchia, 1980). Conceivably, all the procedures that we used for preparing the heart muscle for freeze-fracture produced a redistribution of junctional particles, which in their native distribution either are not present in discrete arrays or are much more widely spaced. We believe that this interpretation is excessive and improbable because our measurements can detect large and reproducible differences in particle diameter and in interparticle spacing between impermeable and control (probably permeable) junctions (Shibata and Page, 1981). Even though it is very likely that the membrane replicas of the presumably permeable control junctions deviate to some extent from the native structure of the junction, such deviations do not apparently obscure significant structural differences between permeable and impermeable junctions in cardiac muscle and Purkinje fibers.

So far, there are three methods for quantifying the information in electron micrographs of gap junctional fracture faces. All have been applied to membrane replicas of freeze-fractured heart muscle and Purkinje fibers. The first method is optical diffraction of the negative film of the electron micrograph (Page and Upshaw-Earley 1980a). It yields a first-order diffraction pattern that provides information about mean center-to-center distance and its standard deviation, the latter being a rough index of the degree of short-range order. The results of this procedure are most easily interpreted when the gap junctional structure is highly regular.

The second method is to measure the distributions of center-to-center spacings between P-face particles and between E-face pits directly on enlarged projections of the negative films of the replica with an instrument like the Nikon Model 6C-2 Profile Projector (Shibata et al., 1980; Shibata and Page, 1981). This procedure can also be used to determine the distribution of P-face particle diameters (Dahl and Isenberg, 1980; Shibata and Page, 1981) the apparent height of P-face particles (Dahl and Isenberg, 1980), the apparent lattice angles, assuming a quasihexagonal lattice (Dahl and Isenberg, 1980), and the relative width of the junctional gap (Dahl and Isenberg, 1980).

The third method is a statistical analysis of the spatial distribution of P-face particles and E-face pits in the plane of the junctional fracture faces. The procedure is to digitize the *X-Y* coordinates of the centers of each particle (or pit) and to subject these data to a modification of the analysis of nearest-neighbor distances introduced by Clark and Evans (1954). Gilula et al. (1980a; 1980b) and Schneider et al. (1980) of the Department of Statistics at the University of Chicago have modified the statistical treatment of Clark and Evans to take into account four considerations that affect its application to membrane replicas of gap junctions from rat myocardial cells and sheep cardiac Purkinje fibers: (1) the nonindependence of nearest-neighbor distances (Diggle et al., 1976), (2) the effects of the boundary of the field covered in the electron micrograph or of the structural limits of the junction, (3) the effects resulting from the appreciable (that is, non-negligible) size of membrane particles relative to the particle density (number of particles per unit area of gap junctional fracture face), and (4) the artifactual increase in membrane particle diameters resulting from the deposition of platinum and carbon on them. We have so far applied the Clark-Evans criteria with modifications 1 through 4 to P-face particle distributions of gap junctions from controls and from rat left ventricles perfused with low-calcium EGTA. Although the gap junctional arrays under both conditions appeared, qualitatively, to be rather regular and closely spaced, statistical analysis revealed that the distribution was indistinguishable from a random array. (In this analysis, we used measured values for particle diameters and computed the statistical distributions for thicknesses of shadowing metal of 0.5 to 3.0 nm.) This analysis suggests that because the particle diameters are finite (not negligible compared with the area of lipid bilayer in which they were embedded), particle distributions that superficially appear regular may in fact be intrinsically random. If a random particle distribution is equated with the permeable state of the junction (Peracchia, 1980; Kistler and Bullivant, 1980), then, at least by statistical criteria, the apparently regular but intrinsically random distributions seen in the closely packed gap junctions of heart muscle and Purkinje fibers may be permeable rather than impermeable. This analysis reconciles to some extent Peracchia's insistence that particle distributions in permeable junctions must be random with our observation that membrane replicas obtained from presumably permeable cardiac gap junctions appear qualitatively to be nonrandom arrays.

Structural Features of Gap Junctional Sealing in High a_i^{Ca}

The electrophysiologic features of gap junctional sealing after injury in solutions containing a high calcium concentration are defined well by the studies of Délèze (1965; 1970), De Mello (1972), and Nishiye (1977). These studies indicate that, at 37° C and in the presence of millimolar calcium concentrations comparable to those in blood plasma or interstitial fluid, the transformation of permeable to impermeable gap junctions approaches completion within 1 minute after their exposure to high a_i^{Ca}. Gap junctional sealing under these conditions should thus be a useful experimental model for studying the concomitant ultrastructural events of a decrease in junctional permeability.

Figure 1 (replotted from Shibata and Page, 1981) graphs the time course of the changes in mean diameter of the P-face particles (upper graph) and of the mean center-to-center spacing between P-face particles (lower curve) for gap junctions from sheep Purkinje fibers that were cut and incubated for 1 to 30 minutes at 37° C in Tyrode's solution (calcium concentration, 1.8 mM; pH, 7.3). Control values at "zero-time" were obtained by cutting the fibers in a similar solution containing 2% glutaraldehyde (pH, 7.3), so that the junctions were cross-linked before a structural change could be induced by calcium. Figure 1 shows that the diameter of the P-face particles underwent a highly significant increase of about 10% ($2P < 0.001$) in the first minute

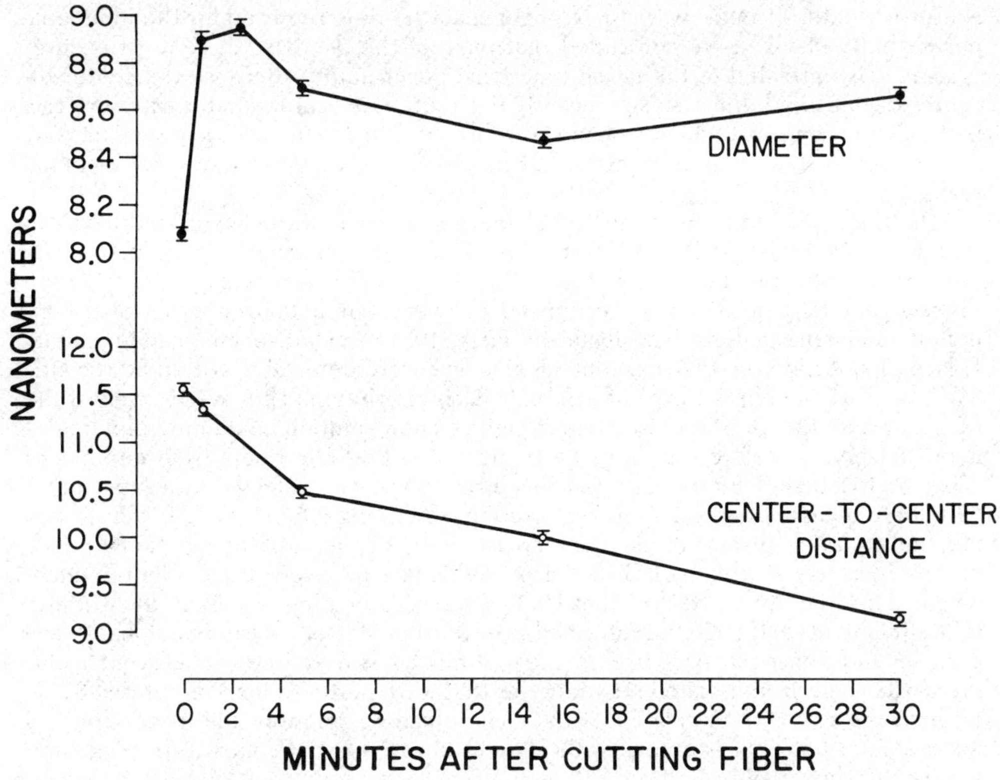

Figure 1. Changes in mean gap junctional P-face particle diameter (upper graph) and mean gap junctional center-to-center distance between P-face particles (lower graph) of sheep Purkinje fiber gap junctions from fibers that were cut in Tyrode's solution containing 1.8 mM calcium at t = 0 minutes. Data replotted from Tables I and II of Shibata and Page (1981). Dispersions are ± SEM.

after the junction was exposed to high calcium by cutting the fiber. The diameter remained significantly larger than the control value for 30 minutes, declining slightly from the initial maximal value after 2 minutes. This change was irreversible. When Purkinje fibers that had been cut and incubated for 5 minutes in Tyrode's solution containing 1.8 mM calcium were subsequently incubated for 10 minutes in calcium-free Tyrode's containing 0.5 mM EGTA, the mean diameter remained high (8.80 ± 1.22 nm). These experiments support the conclusion that the diameter of the gap junctional P-face particles in Purkinje fibers increases irreversibly in a high calcium solution with a time course similar to that for the sealing of gap junctions (Délèze, 1970; Nishiye, 1977).

The time course of the calcium-induced change in center-to-center distance between P-face particles (Fig. 1, lower graph) differed from that for the change in particle diameter. The mean center-to-center distance decreased continuously for 30 minutes, each point on the graph being significantly smaller than the control ($2P < 0.001$) and smaller than each point immediately preceding or following it ($2P < 0.001$). Because the junctions are known to seal within 1 minute, the duration of the decline in center-to-center distance was much longer than the time required for the junctional permeability change. We concluded that most of the decrease in center-to-center spacing was unrelated to the fall in junctional permeability. Because the center-to-center distance did diminish significantly during the first minute after exposure to a high calcium concentration, it remains possible that the decline in spacing reflects two separate processes, with only the earlier process correlating in time with junctional sealing.

During our studies on structural changes associated with calcium-induced gap junctional sealing in cut Purkinje fibers, we observed an unexpected and previously undescribed phenomenon: characteristic gap junctional E-face pits lying outside the discrete junctional arrays and widely dispersed over the lipid bilayer of the apparently nonjunctional plasmalemma (Shibata and Page, 1981). Such dispersed gap junctional E-face pits outside the discrete junctional arrays were detectable within 30 seconds after the Purkinje fibers were cut in a high calcium solution. They were absent if the fibers were cut in an otherwise similar high calcium solution containing glutaraldehyde. Dispersed E-face pits brought about in cut Purkinje fibers by 5 minutes of exposure to a high (1.8 mM) calcium concentration were not affected by a subsequent 10-minute incubation in calcium-free solution containing 0.5 mM EGTA; that is, the junctional particle dispersal, like the increase in the diameter of the junctional P-face particle, was irreversible by EGTA. Dispersed E-face pits were also evident in intact (uncut) Purkinje fibers after calcium-loading the cells in a high-calcium, low-sodium solution (Shibata and Page, unpublished). In addition, dispersed gap junctional P-face particles and E-face pits have been found (but much less frequently) in left ventricular myocardial cells from isolated rat ventricles that were perfused for 3 minutes at 37° C through the coronary circulation with calcium-loading solutions (39 mM sodium, 8 mM calcium; pH, 7.3; isosmolal with plasma) to the point of contracture (Page and Upshaw-Earley, 1980b).

We cannot yet be certain about the origin of the dispersed gap junctional pits and particles. Our working hypothesis is that they are derived by the dispersal of junctional channel assemblies (connexons) originally located on the periphery of the discrete junctional arrays. If so, the connexons evidently disperse in the polymerized state, because peptide subunits of disassembled connexons are probably too small to be detected by freeze fracture. Other interpretations are possible. For example, high calcium concentrations conceivably may stimulate the assembly of connexons from peptide precursors of the connexons that may be present in nonjunctional plasma membrane. In that case, the dispersed connexons might be on their way to the discrete junctional arrays rather than being breakdown products derived from such arrays. Further experiments are required to exclude this and other mechanisms. Interestingly, in this connection, dispersed gap junctional particles have recently been described during the in vivo disappearance of gap junctions in an insect (Lane and Swales, 1980).

Our data on ultrastructural changes in gap junctions from cut sheep Purkinje fibers exposed to high ($\sim 10^{-3}$ M) calcium concentrations supports the results of Dahl and Isenberg (1980), obtained on intact sheep Purkinje fibers in which the cytoplasmic calcium activity was raised but to much lower levels (4 to 36 $\times$ 10^{-6} M). Dahl and Isenberg did not examine the time courses of the structural variables. But, the stability of the calcium-induced changes in the diameters of the P-face particles (Fig. 1) makes it possible to compare our data with theirs with respect to this structural variable. When Dahl and Isenberg raised a_i^{Ca} experimentally to 8 $\pm$ 2 μM, they observed that the mean diameter of the P-face particles increased to 9.1 nm. Moreover, the distribution of the diameters of the P-face particles changed from symmetrical and unimodal to bimodal, with peaks at 8.2 and 9.6 nm. Figure 2, taken from Shibata and Page (1981), shows the

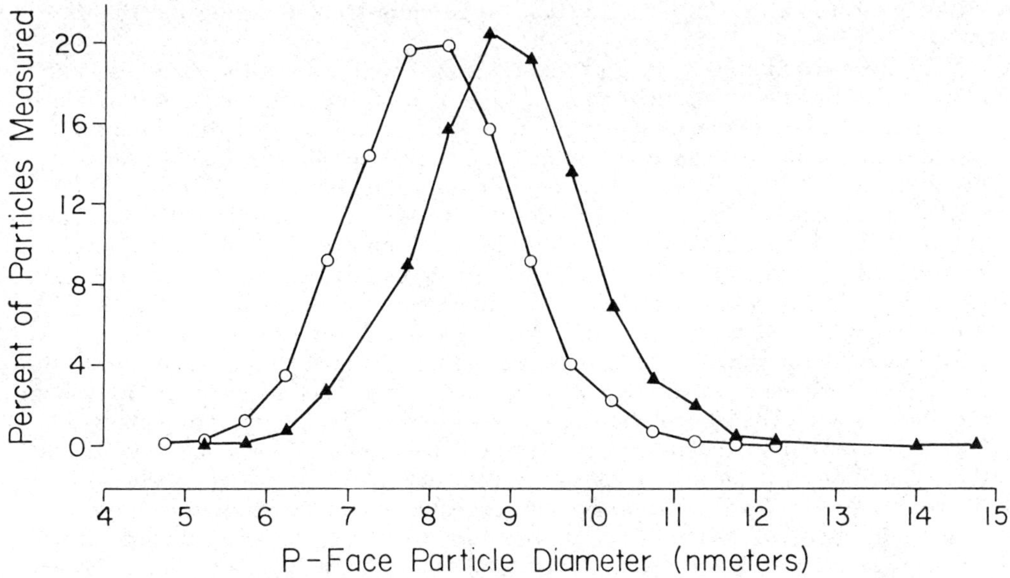

Figure 2. Frequency distribution of the diameters of gap junctional P-face particles from Purkinje fibers cut in Tyrode's solution (1.8 mM calcium) containing glutaraldehyde (open circles denoting zero-time values) compared with distribution in otherwise identical glutaraldehyde-free solution and fixed after 1 minute with glutaraldehyde (triangles). Reproduced from Shibata and Page (1981).

distribution of the diameters of the P-face particles from Purkinje fibers cut in Tyrode's solution (calcium concentration, 1.8 mM) at zero time and after 1 minute of exposure to the high calcium concentration. At this very high calcium concentration, the entire distribution is shifted to the right, yielding a new unimodal distribution with a higher mean of 8.90 ± 0.03 nm, compared with a control value of 8.07 ± 0.02 nm. In any case, the existence of two populations of P-face particle diameters at $\sim 10^{-5}$ M calcium and their shift to a unimodal distribution grouped symmetrically around a single higher mean (Fig. 2) are suggestive. This shift is consistent with the existence of two populations of channels at a_i^{Ca} of $\sim 10^{-5}$ M: one population of impermeable channels that has undergone a conformational change, a second population of permeable channels that has not undergone such a change. According to this logic, at 10^{-3} M a_i^{Ca} all channels would be impermeable and would have undergone a conformational change, perhaps because the calcium-selective sites relevant to sealing and to the conformational change were saturated at this concentration.

The decreases in gap junctional permeability caused by elevations of a_i^{Ca} to 5×10^{-5} M or less are characteristically reversible by reducing the cytoplasmic calcium concentration to normal values (Loewenstein, 1978; De Mello, 1975). Although no data are available on this point, it seems probable that the ultrastructural changes that cardiac gap junctions undergo over this range are similarly reversible. But, after the junctions are exposed to a 1.8 mM calcium solution, both the increase in the diameter of the gap junctional P-face particles and the dispersal of E-face pits are irreversible (Shibata and Page, 1980). This finding suggests that the high (extracellular) calcium concentrations that irreversibly seal the junctions bring about additional structural changes that are not evoked by exposure to lower calcium concentrations.

Structural Features of Gap Junctions in Calcium-Depleted Purkinje Fibers

Figure 3 (replotted from Shibata and Page, 1981) shows the changes in the diameter of the P-face particle and the center-to-center distance between P-face particles in gap junctions of sheep Purkinje fibers cut and incubated for up to 30 minutes at 37° C in an oxygenated, simulated, cytoplasmic electrolyte solution containing less than 10^{-7} M calcium. The composition of this solution, taken from Délèze (1970), was, 6.2 mM sodium, 75 mM sucrose, 150 mM potassium, 0.5 mM EGTA, 4 mM chloride, 73 mM sulfate, 6 mM bicarbonate, 0.2 mM phosphate, and 5.6 mM glucose. Before being cut in this solution, the fibers were depleted of calcium by preincubation for 30 minutes in calcium-free Tyrode's solution containing 0.5 mM EGTA. The preincubation in a solution with such a low external calcium concentration undoubtedly altered the permeability of nonjunctional plasmalemma, but was necessary to avoid a transient exposure of the gap junctions to a high calcium concentration when the fiber was cut. The control at zero time was obtained by incorporating glutaraldehyde into the simulated cytoplasmic electrolyte solution used for incubation. Under these conditions, the mean control value for the diameter of the P-face particle of cut fibers at zero time (7.89 ± 0.02 nm) was lower than that for zero-time controls cut after 30 minutes of preincubation in Tyrode's solution containing 1.8 mM calcium (8.07 ± 0.02 nm, $n = 2608$). The difference was significant ($2P < 0.001$) and presumably reflected the cellular calcium depletion resulting from preincubation in EGTA-containing Tyrode's solution. Thereafter, the diameter decreased continuously (Fig. 3), showing no sign of approaching a constant value after 30 minutes.

The zero-time control value of 10.55 ± 0.04 nm for center-to-center distance of fibers cut after preincubation in EGTA-Tyrode's was significantly smaller ($2P > 0.001$) than was the corresponding figure of 11.56 ± 0.06 nm for fibers cut after preincubation in normal Tyrode (calcium 1.8 nmoles). Figure 3 shows that center-to-center distance was constant for the first 5 minutes after cutting; thereafter it declined significantly. The constant or diminishing center-to-center distance in very low ($< 10^{-7}$ M) calcium solutions is not readily reconcilable with the hypothesis that at low a_i^{Ca} gap junctional particles in cardiac cells become more widely spaced. Perhaps preincubation in EGTA-Tyrode somehow decreased gap junctional permeability before cutting, but that would not explain why the spacing did not increase after cutting in EGTA.

Structure and Permeability of Isolated Cardiac Gap Junctions

Gap junctional membranes have recently been isolated and purified to a variable extent from homogenates of heart muscle, starting with ventricular muscle of the guinea pig (Nishiye et al., 1980), mouse (Kensler and Goodenough, 1980), rabbit (Quertermous et al., 1980a; 1980b), and sheep (Manjunath, Goings and Page, 1981). Similar preparations of gap junctions isolated from lens have already been used to examine the effects of calcium ions on the structure of freeze-fractured junctions (Peracchia, 1978; 1980; Kistler and Bullivant, 1980). Isolated gap junctions also may be expected to play an increasingly important role in the study of the structural basis for changes in permeability of cardiac gap junctions.

The extraction of quantitative information from cardiac gap junctions visualized by the electron microscopic techniques heretofore used (freeze fracture and conventional transmission electron microscopy of thin sections opacified by "staining" with heavy metals) is inherently limited by several factors. The image is distorted, and structural resolution is lost by radiation damage resulting from the rather high electron-beam densities used, as well as by the need to opacify the junctions by depositing

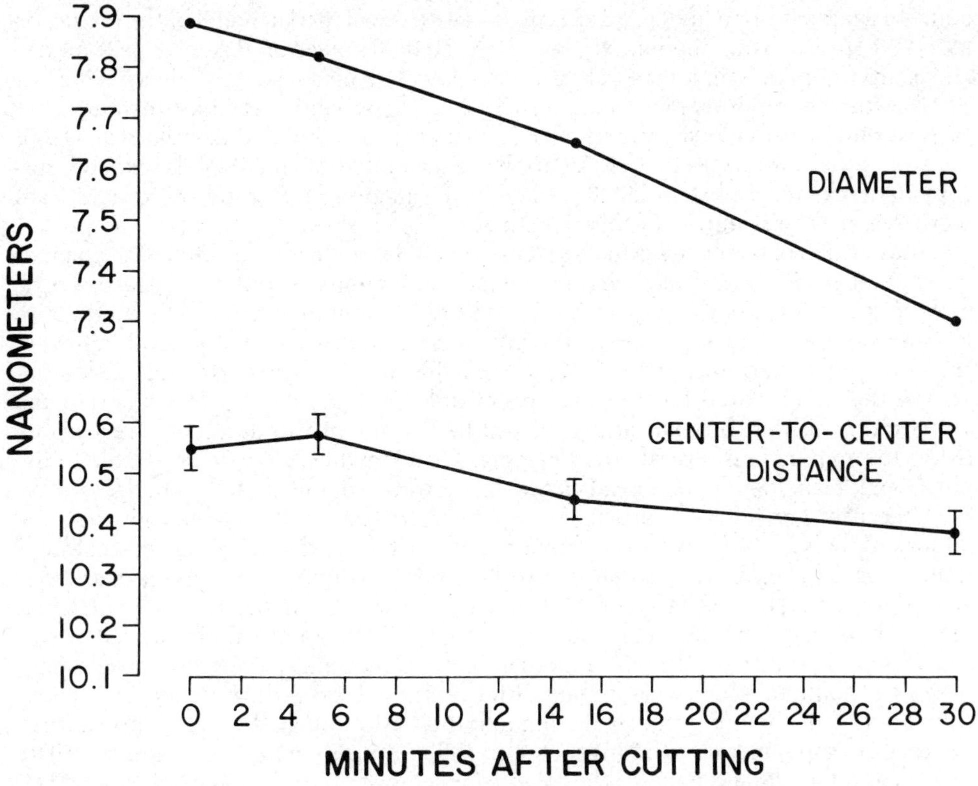

Figure 3. Changes in mean gap junctional P-face particle diameter (upper graph) and center-to-center distance (lower graph) of gap junctions of sheep Purkinje fibers cut in a low ($< 10^{-7}$ M) calcium solution. Dispersions are ± SEM. See text for discussion. Data replotted from Tables I and II of Shibata and Page (1981).

layers of heavy metal on them. In addition, plastic deformation of freeze-fractured material may produce artifactual disorder in the P-face of the gap junction (Caspar et al., 1977). Moreover, the dehydration to which all gap junctions are subjected during the preparation of thin-sectioned or negatively stained specimens for electron microscopy may alter junctional structure to an indeterminate extent.

The pioneering studies of hepatocyte gap junctions isolated with the use of enzymes (Caspar et al., 1977; Makowski et al., 1977), as well as recent extensions of this work, which used enzyme-free methods to isolate the junctions (Zampighi and Unwin, 1979; Unwin and Zampighi, 1980; Henderson et al., 1979), have clearly pointed the way to a more complete and sensitive analysis of cardiac gap junctional structure. Caspar et al. (1977) combined optical diffraction and subsequent image analysis of electron micrographs of negatively stained junctions with analysis of X-ray diffraction data on glutaraldehyde-fixed and unfixed junctions. This combined study succeeded in distinguishing variable from invariant parts of the junction, and it generated a low-resolution, three-dimensional representation of the junction. More recently, Zampighi and Unwin (1979) found two configurations of the channel unit or connexon. The two configurations were interconvertible by dialyzing the detergent-extracted junctions against distilled water, a conversion that could be reversed by re-adding detergent. In a later study, Unwin and Zampighi (1980) developed a model of the connexon based on studies using moderately low (10 to 20 e/Å^2) electron doses, densitometry, and computer processing. By combining even lower electron dosages, electron diffraction, and further refinements in image processing, it may well be feasible to extend the ~ 20 Å resolution provided by the study of Caspar et al. (1977) and Makowski et al. (1977) to resolutions of from 9 Å to 3–4 Å. Applying scanning transmission electron microscopy (Ohtsuki and Crewe, 1980) to isolated gap junctions may also lead to significant increases in the resolution of this structure.

Resolution of the changes in junctional channel structure associated with changes in channel permeability may require major refinements of present ultrastructural techniques. With respect to the published applications of available techniques to isolated gap junctions, it seems worthwhile to point out two additional problems that are not simply questions of resolution: *(1)* It has not been experimentally demonstrated that the isolated junctions are permeable; and *(2)*, it is unclear whether the structural transition brought about by distilled water in the detergent-treated hepatocyte gap junctions described by Zampighi and Unwin (1979) is comparable to the physiologic transition in junctional channel structure brought about by changes in a_i^{Ca}.

Because gap junctions isolated from heart muscle will undoubtedly become important tools in the correlation of junctional structure with junctional permeability, it seems useful to enumerate some of the difficulties in working with these preparations and in evaluating results based on experiments with them. In mammalian ventricular myocardium, gap junctions make up about 1% of the plasma membrane area (Stewart and Page, 1978; Page, 1978) and less than 0.3% of total plasma membrane + sarcoplasmic reticulum, which cosediment with the gap junctions during differential centrifugation. It is therefore not surprising that the best published isolation procedures for cardiac gap junctions (Nishiye et al., 1980; Kensler and Goodenough, 1980; Manjunath, Goings and Page, 1981) have so far achieved only partial purification. The major structural contaminants identified by Kensler and Goodenough were fragments of the fascia adherens region of the intercalated disk. Moreover, rather drastic procedures were required to achieve the highest degree of partial purification, including exposure of the membrane to extremes of ionic strength, ranging from near zero to greater than 0.6 M, as well as extensive extraction with three detergents (Kensler and Goodenough, 1980). Although cardiac gap junctions can perhaps be isolated more readily with exogenous proteases (Nishiye et al., 1980), evidence from other tissues suggests that this procedure degrades the junctional proteins (Henderson et al., 1979; Herzberg and Gilula, 1979). Kensler and Goodenough's procedures yielded a membrane product that appeared heptalaminar in thin sections. This heptalaminar junctional complex therefore contained the junctional contributions from the plasmalemmas of both cells making up the junction, as well as the junctional gap between them. It remains to be determined whether this isolated junctional complex is permeable in the same way that junctions between intact myocardial cells are permeable, and whether the complex can undergo calcium-mediated changes in permeability and structure. The successful insertion of isolated gap junctional complexes into lipid bilayers has not yet been described, and permeability measurements on gap junctional vesicles have not been reported. At present there is no critical technique for comparing the permeability of isolated cardiac gap junctions with their in situ permeability.

SUMMARY

This paper reviews the application of quantitative ultrastructural techniques as a tool for studying the permeability of gap junctions between cardiac cells. Experiments by Shibata and Page on the cut Purkinje fiber preparation of Délèze (1970) were used to examine the concomitant ultrastructural events of gap junctional sealing by high (1.8 mM) calcium concentration. Measurements on membrane replicas of freeze-fractured fibers showed that, within 1 minute after exposure to high calcium, the mean diameter of the gap junctional P-face particles increased significantly, and junctional E-face pits were widely dispersed over the fracture face of nonjunctional plasmalemma. The diameter distribution at high calcium concentrations remained unimodal and approximately symmetrical. Neither the increased diameter nor the dispersal of E-face pits was reversed by subsequent exposure to EGTA. Mean center-to-center spacing between P-face particles decreased in high calcium concentrations, but the time course of this process differed significantly from that of the diameter change. Thus, the time course of the calcium-induced diameter change and the dispersion of E-face particles coincided approximately with that of junctional sealing, but the change in interparticle spacing did not. Dispersed junctional E-face pits and P-face particles were also demonstrable after calcium loading of intact Purkinje fibers. The use and limitations of structural studies on isolated cardiac gap junctional membranes are discussed, with emphasis on increased resolution and on the lack of criteria for determining the permeability of such preparations.

REFERENCES

Baldwin KM (1979) Cardiac gap junction configuration after an uncoupling treatment as a function of time. J Cell Biol **82**:66–75

Caspar DLD, Goodenough DA, Makowski L, Phillips WC (1977) Gap junction structures: I. Correlated electron microscopy and X-ray diffraction. J Cell Biol **74**:605–628

Clark PJ, Evans FC (1954) Distance to a nearest neighbor as a measure of spatial relationships in populations. Ecology **35**:23–30

Dahl G, Isenberg G (1980) Decoupling of heart muscle cells: Correlation with increased cytoplasmic calcium activity and with changes in nexus ultrastructure. J Membrane Biol **53**:63–75

Délèze J (1970) The recovery of resting potential and input resistance in sheep heart injured by knife or laser. J Physiol (Lond) **208**:547–562

De Mello WC (1972) The healing over process in cardiac and other muscle fibers. *In* Electrical Phenomena in the Heart, edited by WC De Mello, New York, Academic Press, pp 323–351

De Mello WC (1975) Effect of intracellular injection of calcium and strontium on cell communication in heart. J Physiol (Lond) **250**:321–345

Diggle PS, Besoz J, Gleaves JF (1976) Statistical analysis of spatial point patterns by means of distance methods. Biometrics **32**:659–667

Fozzard HA, Dominguez G (1969) Effect of formaldehyde and glutaraldehyde on electrical properties of cardiac Purkinje fibers. J Gen Physiol **53**:530–540

Gilula Z, Karrison T, Meier P (1980a) The effect of diameter on zones of inhibition in the analysis of spatial patterns. Technical Rept. No 116, Dept. of Statistics, Univ. of Chicago

Gilula Z, Karrison T, Meier P (1980b) On the edge (boundary) effect on the nearest neighbor distribution. Technical Rept., Dept. of Statistics, Univ. of Chicago

Henderson D, Eibl H, Weber K (1979) Structure and biochemistry of mouse hepatic gap junctions. J Mol Biol **132**:193–218

Hertzberg L, Gilula NB (1979) Isolation and characterization of gap junctions from liver. J Biol Chem **254**:2138–2147

Kensler RW, Goodenough DA (1980) Isolation of mouse myocardial gap junctions. J Cell Biol **86**:755–764

Kistler J, Bullivant S (1980) The connexon order in isolated lens gap junctions. J Ultrastruct Res **72**:27–38

Lane NJ, Swales S (1980) Dispersal of junctional particles, not internalization, during the in vivo disappearance of gap junctions. Cell **19**:579–586

Loewenstein WR (1978) Cell-to-cell communication: Permeability, formation, genetics, and functions of the cell-to-cell membrane channel. *In* Membrane Physiology, edited by TE Andreoli, FJ Hoffman, DD Fanestil, New York, Plenum Medical Book Co, pp 335–356

Makowski L, Caspar DLD, Phillips WC, Goodenough DA (1977) Gap junction structure: II. An analysis of the X-ray diffraction data. J Cell Biol **74**:629–645

Manjunath CK, Goings GE, Page E (1981) Isolation and protein composition of gap junctions from rabbit hearts (abst). J Cell Biol **91**:100a

Nishiye H (1977) The mechanism of Ca^{2+} action on the healing-over process in mammalian cardiac muscles: A kinetic analysis. Jpn J Physiol **27**:451–466

Nishiye H, Mashima H, Ishida A (1980) Ca binding of isolated cardiac nexus membranes related to intercellular uncoupling. Jpn J Physiol **30**:131–136

Ohtsuki M, Crewe AV (1980) Optimal imaging techniques in the scanning transmission electron microscope: Application to biological macromolecules. Proc Natl Acad Sci USA **77**: 4051–4054

Page E (1978) Quantitative ultrastructural analysis in cardiac membrane physiology. Am J Physiol 4:C147–C158

Page E, Shibata Y (1981) Permeable junctions between cardiac cells. Annu Rev Physiol **43**: 431–441

Page E, Upshaw-Earley J (1980a) Gap junctional particle distributions in rat ventricle (abst). Federation Proc. **39**:298

Page E, Upshaw-Earley (1980b) Order and dispersal of rat heart gap junctional arrays (abst). J Cell Biol **87**:1920

Peracchia C (1978) Calcium effects on gap junction structure and cell coupling. Nature **271**: 669–671

Peracchia C (1980) Structural correlates of gap junction permeation. Int Rev Cytol **66**:81–146

Pinto da Silva P, Kachar B (1980) Quick freezing vs. chemical fixation: Capture and identification of membrane fusion intermediates. Cell Biol Int Rep **4**:625–640

Quertermous T, Shibata Y, Page E (1980a) Effect of calcium on cardiac gap junctions (abst). Abst Am Heart Assn

Quertermous T, Shibata Y, Page E (1980b) Effects of high Ca^{2+} concentration on gap junctions isolated from rabbit hearts (abst). J Cell Biol **87**:192a

Rash JE, Hudson CS (eds) (1979) Freeze Fracture: Methods, Artifacts, and Interpretations. New York, Raven Press

Schneider M, Karrison T, Meier P (1980) Correction for packing and edge effects in nearest neighbor distances. Technical Report No 124, Department of Statistics, University of Chicago

Shibata Y, Page E (1980) Ca^{2+}-induced dispersal of gap junctional arrays in sheep cardiac Purkinje fibers (abst). J Cell Biol **87**:192a, 1980

Shibata Y, Page E (1981) Gap junctional structure in intact and cut sheep cardiac Purkinje fibers: a freeze-fracture study of Ca^{2+}-induced resealing. J Ultrastruct Res **75**:195–204

Shibata Y, Nakata K, Page E (1980) Ultrastructural changes during development of gap junctions in rabbit left ventricular myocardial cells. J Ultrastruct Res **71**:258–271

Sjöstrand FS (1979) The interpretation of pictures of freeze-fractured biological material. J Ultrastruc Res **69**:378–420

Steward H, Page E (1978) Improved stereological techniques for studying myocardial cell growth: Application to external sarcolemma, T-system, and intercalated disks of rabbit and rat hearts. J Ultrastruct Res **65**:119–134

Unwin PNT, Zampighi G (1980) Structure of the junction between communicating cells. Nature **283**:545–549

Weidmann S (1952) The electrical constants of Purkinje fibres. J Physiol (Lond) **118**:348–360

Weidmann S (1965) The functional significance of the intercalated disks, *In* Electrophysiology of the Heart, edited by B Taccardi, G Marchetti, Oxford, Pergamon Press, pp 149–152

Weidmann S (1966) The diffusion of radiopotassium across intercalated disks of mammalian cardiac muscle. J Physiol (Lond) **187**:323–342

Weidmann S (1970) Electrical constants of trabecular muscle from mammalian hearts. J Physiol (Lond) **210**:1041–1054

Weingart R (1977) The actions of ouabain on intercellular coupling and conduction velocity in mammalian ventricular muscle. J Physiol (Lond) **264**:341–366
Zampighi G, Unwin PNT (1979) Two forms of isolated gap junctions. J Molec Biol **135**:451–464

Discussion

JOHNSON: Two aspects must be considered in intercellular uncoupling. The first is electrical and the second is morphologic. There seems to be a clear electrical effect before there is a clear morphologic effect. Is the failure of correlation due to the time taken to complete the freeze-fracture procedure? Are there other artifacts in these measurements of size and position of the junctional particles?

PAGE: The quality of the data shown here is commensurate with the present state of the art in freeze fracture. I should like to point out that we have taken extreme care in preparing our specimens, even going to the point of quick freezing the tissue by touching it to a copper probe cooled with liquid helium. This is not to deny, however, that in the freeze-fracture method itself there can be steps that may give rise to artifact. But, we have adopted the pragmatic view that we should try to look for correlations between freeze-fracture structure and physiologic function whenever these point in an interesting direction, as was the case with the data shown in the present paper.

SOMMER: How can one be sure that fixation with glutaraldehyde is not altering terribly the tissue structure? In my experience, glutaraldehyde is very harmful to several structures, especially membranes.

PAGE: I am well aware of that. Several controls show that the smallest concentration of glutaraldehyde you use, and the briefest exposure to this agent, give the best preservation of membrane structure. We have gone to the point of using 1.0% glutaraldehyde for only 1 minute, which is quite different from what people mostly do, which is to use 3 to 5% glutaraldehyde for a very long time. Still we are not working in an area where you can be really dogmatic about anything. I would say only that this is the present state of the art.

VASSALE: Do you think that the rhythmic change of free intracellular calcium with activity can alter the structure of the junctional subunit during the cardiac cycle? Could it do so in a cumulative beat-to-beat basis over several succeeding cycles?

PAGE: I have no data that indicate a possible effect during a given cycle. But a progressive loading of the cytoplasm with calcium due to any functional derangement should be expected to alter coupling and gap junctional structure eventually.

WEIDMANN: Some ten years ago, I attempted to detect such cycle-dependent changes (J Physiol **210**:1041–1054, 1970). Subthreshold square pulses were passed through electrodes situated at both ends of calf ventricular trabeculae in silicon oil to minimize extracellular conductance. Microelectrodes were used to record the longitudinal voltage gradient in the midinterpolar region where no membrane current is expected to flow. This voltage gradient did not noticeably change during a cycle of activity. Although the method is relatively insensitive, it nevertheless should have revealed any major change of internal longitudinal resistance (>30%). This negative result may mean that the rise of intracellular calcium in the course of an action potential is insufficient to have a major effect on disc resistance. Alternatively, the result may indicate that the increase of internal calcium is restricted to compartments well separated from the discs.

LIEBERMAN: Functional uncoupling due to high intracellular calcium should be reversible if one lowers intracellular calcium. You mentioned that you were able to carry your preparations from high to low calcium, and yet the structural effects that you associate with uncoupling were irreversible. How do you explain this?

PAGE: The structural effects shown here were indeed irreversible. We have no particular explanation for it. Perhaps you are speaking of a small perturbation of calcium inside the cell whereas I am speaking of a very large perturbation. This may be a difference.

Chapter 3

Low Resistance Contacts and the Propagation of the Cardiac Action Potential

Silvio Weidmann

Propagation velocity along a cardiac preparation depends not only on properties of the excitable membrane but often enough on the coupling between cells. This may sound like a trivial statement, and yet the role of the coupling resistance has often been overlooked in the past. I propose to start by giving the functional evidence suggesting that cardiac cells are coupled by low-resistance junctions. Then I will focus on a few special problems that are either not generally known or have not been solved to a satisfactory degree.

Internal Longitudinal Resistance

In one of his remarkable papers, Engelmann (1875) described morphologic and functional similarities between heart muscle and what today is called smooth muscle of the intestinal type. Thus, in frog ventricle, as in rabbit ureter, stimulation of any site would be followed by contraction invading eventually all other sites, wherever situated and however thin the connecting bridge of tissue. Engelmann concluded, "Die einzelnen Zellen vermögen sich während des Lebens den Erregungsvorgang durch Contakt mitzuteilen."

In fact, the concept of the heart as a morphologic syncytium was widely taken for granted until Sjöstrand and Andersson (1954), using high-resolution electron microscopy, described cardiac muscle as composed of well-defined individual cells, their regions of contact being specially organized cell boundaries (intercalated disks).

In the late 1940s cable analysis was used as a method to obtain values for some essential electrical properties of nerve fibers: the resistance and capacity of the surface membrane, and the internal and external longitudinal resistance (Hodgkin and Rushton, 1946; Davis and Lorente de Nó, 1947). While working with A.L. Hodgkin and A.F. Huxley, it became possible for me to apply this method to a preparation of cardiac origin, the false tendon of newly born goats (Weidmann, 1952). Within a given false tendon are often single Purkinje fibers (strands of Purkinje cells), either alone or visibly isolated from one another over a distance of several millimeters.

Purkinje had described false tendons (1839; 1845) as crossing the ventricular cavities of ungulate hearts, and he admittedly had ignored the function of these "cartilage-like" fibers. But their functional significance must have been clear as early as 1854 to von Hessling because he had drawn their terminations with a pattern of cross-striations and had shown them to fuse with ventricular fibers.

Figure 1 shows changes of membrane resting potential due to the flow of hyperpolarizing current. The electrotonic effect spreads for a distance that is many times the length of a single cell, conveying the impression of a tight electrical coupling. From the space constant (λ), the input resistance ($\Delta V/\Delta I$), and the diameter of the fiber, I calculated the electrical parameters, using Hodgkin's equation (Weidmann, 1952). The resistivity of the internal longitudinal pathway (R_i) turns out to be as low as 100 to 200 Ωcm (Weidmann, 1952; 1970). When this value is compared with that of Tyrode's solution (52 Ωcm), it becomes clear that after having allowed for the resistivity of myoplasm alone there is very little resistance left for the membranous structures seen between adjoining cells, and thus the conclusion of low-resistance coupling.

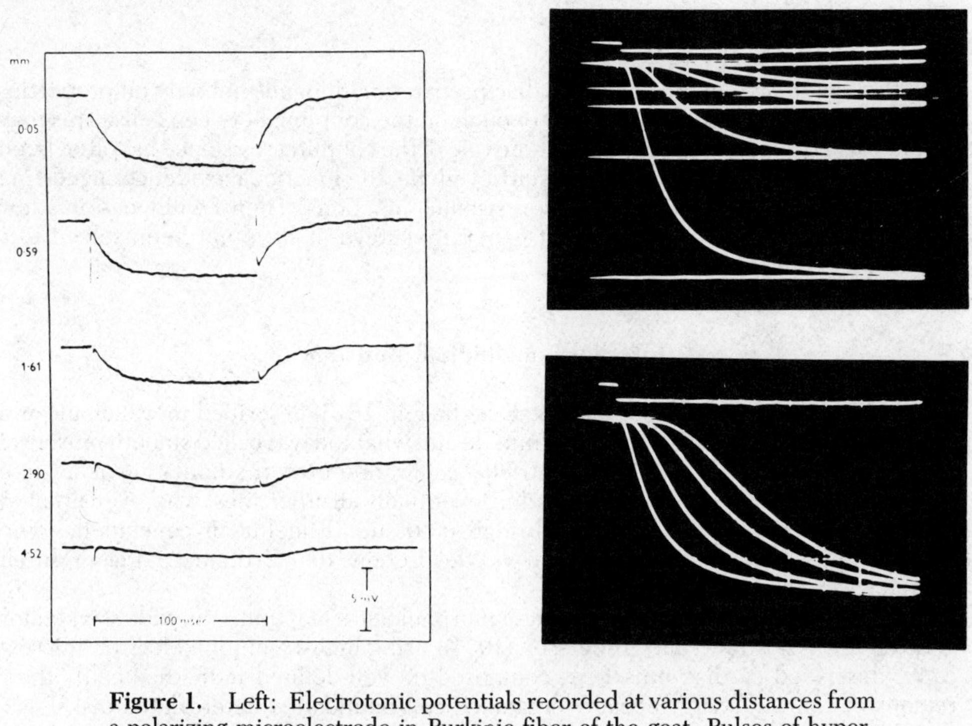

Figure 1. Left: Electrotonic potentials recorded at various distances from a polarizing microelectrode in Purkinje fiber of the goat. Pulses of hyperpolarizing current lasting for 100 msec are switched on and off. The spikes are artefacts due to stray capacities. (From Weidmann, 1952) Right: The responses of a "cable" made of capacitors and resistors. Potential changes following the "make" of a constant current are recorded at the following distances from the site of current injection: 1.59 λ, 2.38 λ, 3.18 λ, and 3.97 λ. The behavior of the cable is shown (upper records) using constant amplification and (lower records) variable gain to scale all potential variations to reach the same steady-state amplitude. The time constant of the "membrane" is 47 msec. The time taken to reach half-maximal amplitude is seen to propagate at a constant speed, as predictable from theory (Hodgkin and Rushton, 1946).

Cell-to-cell Diffusion of Tracers

An isotope of potassium (^{42}K) and various other tracer molecules (radioactive or fluorescent) will redistribute by diffusion if introduced into part of a bundle. This is possible only if cell communications are considerably more permeable than surface membranes. Figure 2 illustrates an experimental procedure that Weingart (1974) used with ventricular trabeculae and [^{14}C]-tetraethylammonium [^{14}C]-TEA. In this case, he mounted the preparation in a double chamber, exposing the left side to the tracer for a short period of time (10 minutes). There evidently was redistribution, in this case of a nonsteady-state nature. From the shape of this curve at a given time, he could calculate a longitudinal diffusion coefficient and, making some reasonable assumptions for diffusion in myoplasm, as well as for the percentage of nexus-type membrane on a straight cross section, an estimate of a permeability coefficient of intercalated disks or nexal area.

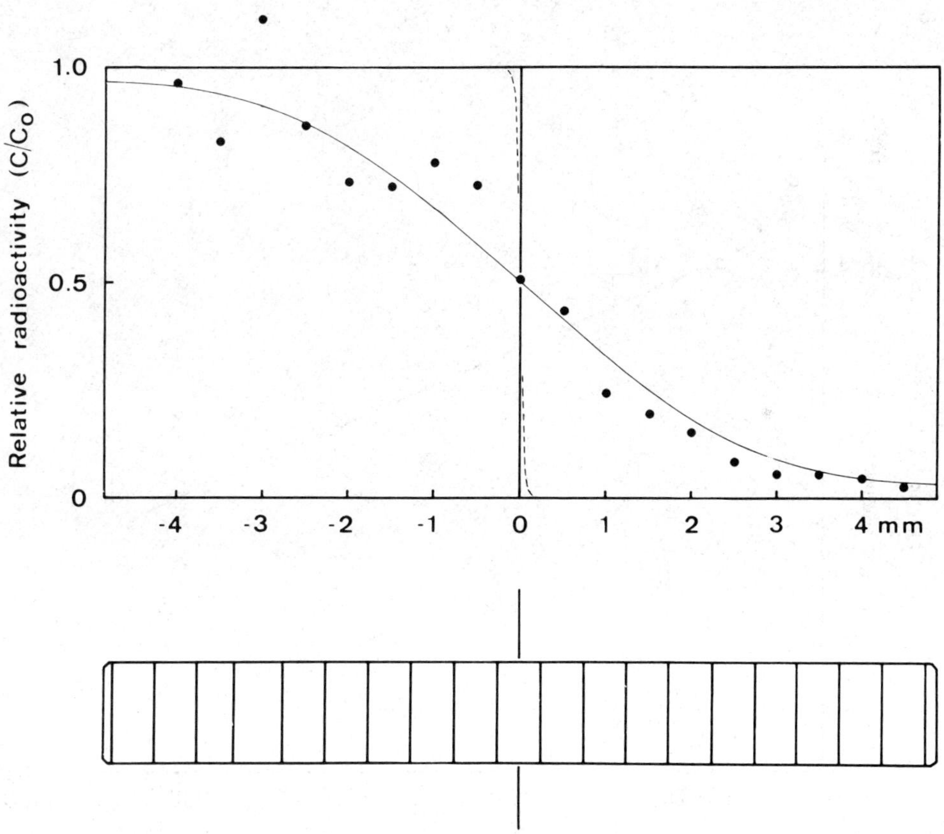

Figure 2. Distribution of [^{14}C]-TEA within a bundle of a calf ventricular trabecula exposed to the tracer in the left-hand compartment between t = 0 and t = 10 min. There is nonsteady-state distribution as counted in slices (see below) 240 minutes after the start of the experiment. The values are fitted by a theoretical curve assuming a longitudinal diffusion coefficient of 1.75×10^{-6} cm^2/sec. The interrupted curve in the upper panel shows the distribution of radioactivity as expected at the end of the loading period. (From Weingart, 1974)

Figure 3 shows a plot of nexal permeability versus molecular weight of various tracers for which quantitative data are available. From ^{42}K to digoxin (molecular weight, 781 daltons), the permeability drops by two orders of magnitude, and there is reason to assume that molecules larger than 1000 daltons cannot pass the nexal channels (Imanaga, 1974).

Having thus documented once again the reasons for assuming a low resistance between adjoining cells, I propose to focus attention on a few special problems.

Internal Resistance and Conduction Velocity

A slow conduction is generally attributed to changes of the properties of the surface membrane; namely, to its reduced ability to pass inward ionic current when depolarized. This is indeed the situation we are faced with most frequently.

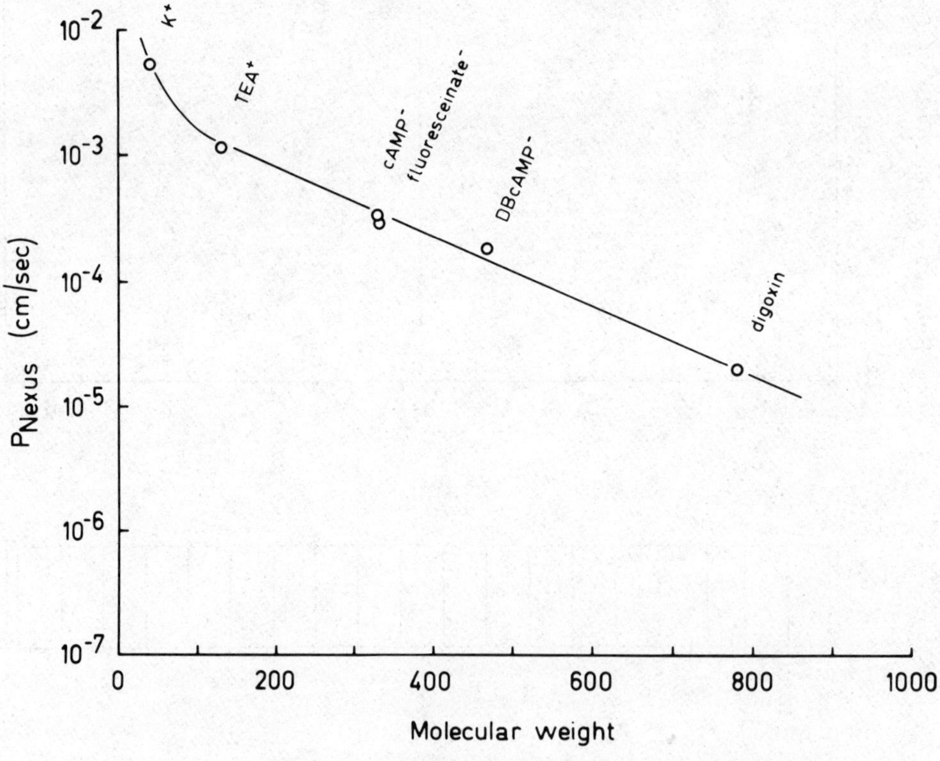

Figure 3. Permeability of the nexal membrane of mammalian ventricular preparations to substances of various molecular weight: ^{42}K (from Weidmann, 1966), TEA (from Weingart, 1974), cAMP and DBcAMP (from Tsien and Weingart, 1976), fluoresceinate (from Pollack, 1976) and digoxin (from Hess and Müller, 1982). Diffusion coefficients have been expressed as nexal permeabilities on the ground of reasonable assumptions for geometry and for diffusion within myoplasm. (From Weingart, 1981)

Several interventions will result in a more or less reversible decrease of cell coupling, for instance, exposure to hypertonic solutions (Barr et al., 1965), digitalis poisoning (Weingart, 1977), or hypoxia (Wojtczak, 1979). It would be tempting to correlate the measured changes of conduction velocity to changes of internal resistance. But, all these interventions change the response of the surface membrane, maybe by a common underlying mechanism (internal ionic activity). It would thus be difficult to sort out the effect of internal resistance and of membrane responsiveness as being responsible for a decrease of conduction velocity.

Two reports in the literature possibly suggest that conduction velocity can increase above "normal" and that this probably is the result of tighter electrical coupling. Rosen et al. (1972) observed the conduction velocity of dog false tendons to increase at an unchanged shape of the action potential upstroke when dog blood was used as a superfusing medium instead of Tyrode's solution. They did not attempt to look for a concomitant drop of internal resistance, which indeed would have been difficult under their experimental conditions. Hermsmeyer (1980) reported angiotensin II to increase conduction velocity above normal (in Tyrode's solution), and indeed he found a concomitant fall of internal resistance with trabeculae of mammalian hearts. The relationship he reported is close to that expected on theoretical grounds; namely that θ is inversely proportional to $\sqrt{r_i + r_o}$, where θ is the conduction velocity, r_i is the internal longitudinal resistance per unit length, and r_o is the external longitudinal resistance per unit length. In his publication, Hermsmeyer did not mention the absence of an influence of angiotensin II on the shape of the upstroke of the intracellular action potential. He assures me, however, that the relevant records exist and that no difference of upstroke shape can be detected at a reliability level of $< 5\%$.

The Nonisotropic Case

Several types of cardiac preparations are made up of longitudinally oriented cells (crista terminalis, papillary muscles, trabeculae, and the moderator band of ungulates). With such preparations, the experimentor may use two modes of bulk stimulation and compare longitudinal to transverse conduction (Clerc, 1976). If short stimulating pulses are used, the action potential invariably starts near the cathode and propagates towards the former anode. With nonisotropic preparations, there is now a possibility to study the influence of internal resistance on propagation velocity because the surface membrane to be excited keeps the same properties. Using ventricular trabeculae of the sheep, Clerc (1976) found the transverse r_i to be 9.4 times the longitudinal r_i. Conduction velocity transverse was three times lower than conduction velocity longitudinal, in good agreement with predictions. The shape of the upstroke looked the same (Fig. 4).

It is often useful to figure out the spatial distribution of transmembrane potential in the case of conduction at uniform speed. For instance, with an upstroke duration of 1 millisecond and a longitudinal conduction velocity of 1.0 mm/msec, the front of the action potential extends over 1 mm or some 8 to 9 cell lengths of 120 μm each. For transverse conduction at a velocity of 0.3 mm/msec, the upstroke extends over 0.3 mm or some 15 cell diameters of 20 μm each.

Current Flow during Propagation

Figure 5 shows the upstroke of a Purkinje fiber action potential plotted against distance. Assuming a propagation velocity of 2.0 mm/msec and an upstroke duration of

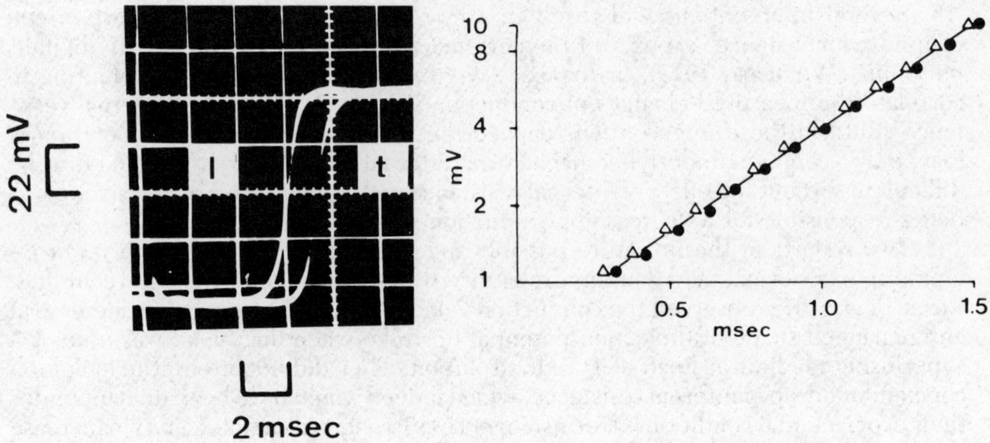

Figure 4. The upstroke of an action potential made to propagate longitudinally (l) or transversely (t) within the same trabecular muscle from the right ventricle of a calf heart. The graph illustrates the method used for graphical analysis of the "foot" of the action potential. In this case, the time constant of the foot was 530 μsec for both longitudinal (open symbols) and transverse (filled symbols) propagation. (From Clerc, 1976)

0.5 msec, I calculated that as many as 12 cells (80 μ in length) were simultaneously involved in passing membrane current as well as longitudinal currents, inside the cable and outside.

Again, some essential properties of propagating action potentials are generally known (for example, from the work of Hodgkin and Huxley, 1952) but on occasions not realized. The maximal upstroke velocity (dV/dt_{max}) in the voltage trace does not coincide with the maximal inward current. The inversion point in the voltage trace has the only merit that longitudinal charge movement to a given site and charge movement from that same site cancel out, making the rate of potential displacement entirely dependent on instantaneous membrane inward current and membrane capacity. In the instance of Figure 5, maximal inward transmembrane current would flow after dV/dt had gone through its maximum, at a membrane potential near 0 mV.

Is There a Capacity Shunting the Disk Resistance?

An answer to this question has repeatedly been sought. Within the disk there are two cell membranes coupled in series, and the double layer capacity of 1 cm^2 of unfolded disk may be predicted to be of the order of 0.5 μF. This, combined with a resistor estimated to be 2 Ωcm^2 (Weidmann, 1966), suggests a possible time constant of the order of 1 μsec. If reliable experimental evidence could be obtained confirming a value of that order, we need not worry; for, in the course of impulse propagation, practically no longitudinal current would be required to change the charge on so small a capacity.

Two methods for measuring longitudinal impedance have been used. The first makes use of constant current steps applied to the ends of a trabecula (in silicon oil). The voltage transient recorded between two microelectrodes near the middle of the preparation where no membrane current is expected to flow should give an indication

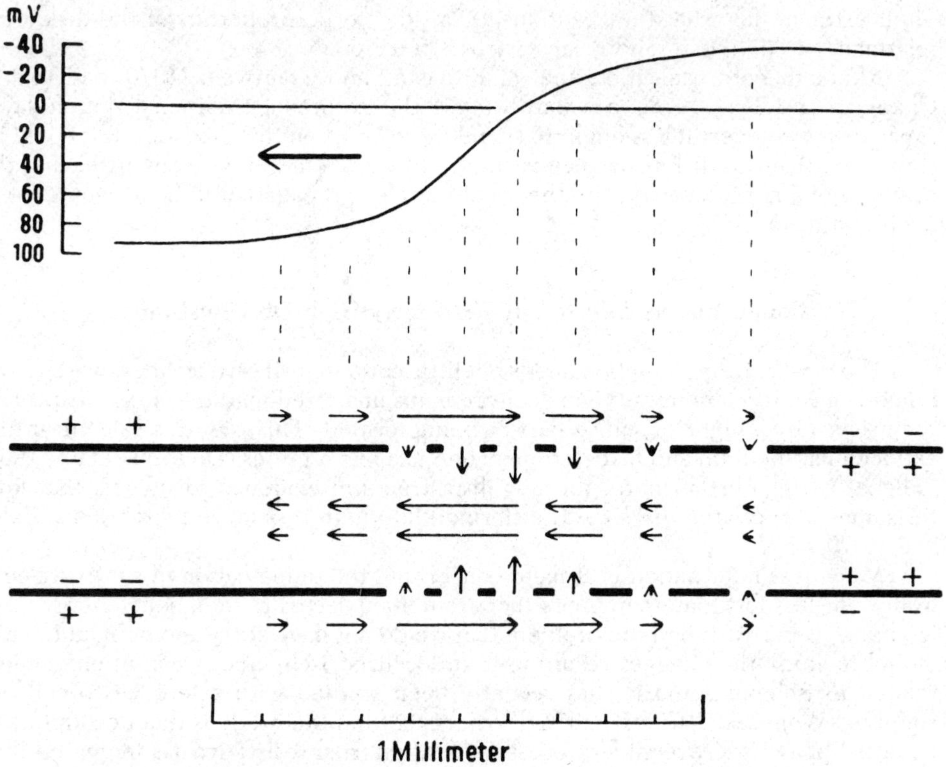

Figure 5. Upstroke of an action potential propagating at uniform velocity from right to left along a Purkinje fiber. The following assumptions have been made: fiber diameter = 76 μm; internal and external resistivity in the longitudinal direction = 100 Ωcm each; membrane capacity = 6 μF/cm^2; conduction velocity = 2.0 m/sec. The lower panel shows longitudinal and transmembrane flow of charge, with 1 mm of arrow length corresponding to a current density of 7.0 mA/cm^2. (From Weidmann, 1956)

of the disk time constant when corrections are made for the resistors not shunted by capacitors (extracellular space, myoplasm). In records obtained by the use of old-fashioned cathode followers (Weidmann, 1970), there was no clearly visible jump of the voltage trace (resistive components alone) followed by an exponential part signaling the filling of capacitors. Yet, the input probes connected to high-resistance microelectrodes responded with a time constant of as much as 10 to 20 μsec. Thus, it would not have been possible to recognize parallel coupled resistors and capacitors having time constants of 1 μsec or even 10 μsec.

Another method currently used for circuit analysis is the impedance-locus diagram. The frequency of a sine wave is varied. Total impedance and phase angle are measured at any one frequency. From an analysis of the high-frequency end of impedance-locus diagrams, Freygang and Trautwein (1970) calculated that there are elements oriented longitudinally and in series with the surface membrane, their time constant being 60 to 70 μsec, their resistive component being 0.18 Ωcm^2, and their nominal capacity being thus 360 μF/cm^2. Chapman and Fry (1978), also using longitudinal impedance measurements, calculated elements with time constants of 320 μsec to be spatially arranged in the longitudinal direction of frog ventricular trabeculae.

Their estimate for what they cautiously consider to be properties of the disk are a resistance of 0.93 Ωcm^2 and a capacity of 370 $\mu F/cm^2$.

Although both capacities, that of Freygang and Trautwein (1970) and that of Chapman and Fry (1978), can hardly have the nature of traditional double-layer capacities, we nevertheless ought to spend more effort on this problem. If it could be confirmed that the disk resistance is shunted by any kind of an element having the property of a large capacity, the theory of impulse propagation in heart would be in need of a major revision.

Conduction as Affected by Extremely High Disk Resistance

The most extreme situation needs but little comment. If cardiac fibers are cut, the functional contact among surviving cells remains unaltered, and the survivors protect themselves by a high-resistance barrier being formed. This requires calcium in the extracellular medium and takes a time of one to a few minutes (De Mello et al., 1969; Délèze, 1970). Furthermore, there is ultrastructural evidence to suggest that low-resistance intercalated disks are transformed into high-resistance membranes (Baldwin, 1970).

Much less information is at hand concerning the demarcation of surviving cells from their less fortunate neighbors that are denied access to metabolic energy. Our ignorance is partly due to the problem that we do not have at the moment an in vitro model to study the changes resulting from localized ischemia. A condition vaguely related to ischemia, anoxia, has recently been studied with reference to cell decoupling (Wojtczak, 1979). One result emerging from this study is that decoupling in its initial phase is a reversible process, even if internal resistivity has increased by a factor of 3, provided that oxygen is readmitted after a reasonably short delay (when structures essential for metabolism are still intact?). Impulse conduction in anoxia considerably outlasts the critical time for recoupling. It is only when internal resistivity has risen by a factor of the order of 20 that it becomes impossible to set up a conducted action potential. With reference to a border zone between an ischemic and a well-perfused region, this is precisely the situation we dislike: cells that will never have a chance to recover, yet refuse to uncouple.

REFERENCES

Baldwin KM (1970) The fine structure and electrophysiology of heart muscle cell injury. J Cell Biol **46**:455–476

Barr L, Dewey MM, Berger W (1965) Propagation of action potentials and the structure of the nexus in cardiac muscle. J Gen Physiol **48**:797–823

Chapman RA, Fry CH (1978) An analysis of the cable properties of frog ventricular myocardium. J Physiol **283**:263–282

Clerc L (1976) Directional differences of impulse spread in trabecular muscle from mammalian heart. J Physiol **255**:335–346

Davis L Jr, Lorente de Nó R (1947) Contribution to the mathematical theory of the electrotonus. *In* A Study of Nerve Physiology, edited by R Lorente de Nó, Stud Rockefeller Inst Med Res **131**:442–496

Délèze J (1970) The recovery of resting potential and input resistance in sheep heart injured by knife or laser. J Physiol **208**:547–562

De Mello WC, Motta GE, Chapeau M (1969) A study on the healing-over of myocardial cells of toads. Circ Res **24**:475–487
Engelmann TW (1875) Ueber die Leitung der Erregung im Herzmuskel. Pflügers Arch **11**: 465–480
Freygang WH, Trautwein W (1970) The structural implications of the linear electrical properties of cardiac Purkinje strands. J Gen Physiol **55**:524–547
Hermsmeyer K (1980) Angiotensin II increases electrical coupling in mammalian ventricular myocardium. Circ Res **47**:524–529
Hess P, Müller P (1982) Extracellular versus intracellular digoxin action on bovine myocardium, using a digoxin antibody and intracellular glycoside application. J Physiol **322**:199–210
von Hessling T (1854) Histologische Mittheilungen. Z Wissensch Zool (Leipzig) **5**:189–200
Hodgkin AL, Huxley AF (1952) A quantitative description of membrane current and its application to conduction and excitation in nerve. J Physiol **117**:500–544
Hodgkin AL, Rushton WAH (1946) The electrical constants of a crustacean nerve fibre. Proc R Soc Lond B **133**:444–479
Imanaga I (1974) Cell to cell diffusion of Procion Yellow in sheep and calf Purkinje fibers. J Membr Biol **16**:381–388
Pollack GH (1976) Intercellular coupling in the atrioventricular node and other tissues of the rabbit heart. J Physiol **255**:275–298
Purkyně JE (1839) Nowe spostrzezenia i badania w przedmiocie fizyologii i drobnowidzowéj anatomii. Rocznik wydzialu lekarskiego w universitecie Jagiellonskim Kraków **2**:44–67
Purkinje JE (1845) Mikroskopisch-neurologische Beobachtungen. Arch anat Physiol wissensch Med (Leipzig) 281–295
Rosen MR, Gelband H, Hoffman BF (1972) Effects of blood perfusion on electrophysiological properties of isolated canine Purkinje fibers. Circ Res **30**:575–587
Sjöstrand FS, Andersson E (1954) Electron microscopy of the intercalated discs of cardiac muscle tissue. Experientia (Basel) **10**:369–370
Tsien RW, Weingart R (1976) Inotropic effect of cyclic AMP in calf ventricular muscle studied by a cut end method. J Physiol **300**:489–504
Weidmann S (1952) The electrical constants of Purkinje fibres. J Physiol **118**:348–360
Weidmann S (1956) Elektrophysiologie der Herzmuskelfaser. Bern, Huber
Weidmann S (1966) The diffusion of radiopotassium across intercalated disks of mammalian cardiac muscle. J Physiol **187**:323–342
Weidmann S (1970) Electrical constants of trabecular muscle from mammalian heart. J Physiol **210**:1041–1054
Weingart R (1974) The permeability to tetraethylammonium ions of the surface membrane and the intercalated disks of sheep and calf myocardium. J Physiol **240**:741–762
Weingart R (1977) The actions of ouabain on intercellular coupling and conduction velocity in mammalian ventricular muscle. J Physiol **264**:341–365
Weingart R (1981) Cell-to-cell coupling in cardiac tissue. Proc 28th Int Congr Physiol Sci **8**:59–68. Budapest, Akadémiai Kiadó
Wojtczak J (1979) Contractures and increase in internal longitudinal resistance of cow ventricular muscle induced by hypoxia. Circ Res **44**:88–95

Discussion

PAES DE CARVALHO: What value would you ascribe to the specific resistance of the junctional membrane? Shouldn't disc resistance be represented by a lumped parameter in series with cytoplasmic resistance?

WEIDMANN: I agree with you that a model closer to reality would have to represent in series a succession of myoplasmic and junctional resistances. Although there have been attempts to do this, I find no need to discern between these two in my model. What I have said once is that a disc plus one cell equivalent of cytoplasm would have a specific resistance of about 3 Ωcm^2. I have not, however, given a value for disc alone (J Physiol **187**:323–342, 1966).

MÉNDEZ: In studying propagation perpendicular to the long axis of the fibers, how much should we take into account the possible zig-zag geometry of the pathway?

WEIDMANN: The pathway for transverse excitation is almost certainly a zig-zag one, and the internal resistance is about nine times larger transversely than longitudinally, according to L. Clerc, (1976). In his calculations, Clerc thought that he did not really need lateral gap junctions between cells and could explain all his data by a zig-zag pathway.

JOHNSON: Dr. Spach will show later on in this meeting that it was necessary to postulate some kind of discontinuous propagation in heart muscle to explain the results he obtained when comparing propagation along the longitudinal axis of the fibers versus propagation perpendicular to this axis. Modeling of electrical coupling in the transverse direction required some reactive impedance capable of introducing a time constant of the order of 60 μsec.

Chapter 4

Ionic Factors Controlling Cell Communication in Heart

W.C. De Mello

Ionic coupling is an important mechanism for cell-to-cell communication in embryonic tissues, epithelia, nervous tissue, and also in heart muscle (see review, De Mello, 1980a). Through low-resistance junctions, ions can diffuse without hindrance from cell to cell, and molecules can be shared by the functional units, making possible metabolic cooperation (Pitts and Finbow, 1977). The intercellular channels in cardiac fibers are permeable to potassium ions (Weidmann, 1966), fluorescein (molecular weight, 320) (Pollack, 1973; De Mello, 1979a), Procion yellow (MW 625) (Imanaga, 1974); Lucifer yellow (De Mello, 1979b), and tetraethylammonium (MW 130) (Weingart, 1974). Indirect evidence also suggests that sodium ions diffuse from cell to cell in cardiac Purkinje fibers (De Mello, 1976).

Knowledge of the factors involved in the generation of gap junctions is still scanty. It is known, however, that these junctions are not permanent structures, at least during development (Bennett and Trinkaus, 1970). Conceivably, the synthesis or destruction of gap junctions in heart muscle represents an important regulatory factor for cell communication, but the plasticity of intercellular junctions in adult tissues, and particularly in the heart, is not known.

Nevertheless, the permeability of the hydrophylic channels between cells can be modulated by variations of the intracellular calcium concentration $[Ca^{2+}]_i$. When calcium ions are injected iontophoretically inside a cardiac cell, the electrical coupling is gradually diminished, and cell decoupling is achieved in about 400 sec. (De Mello, 1975) (see Fig. 1). As the coupling coefficient (V_2/V_1) declines, the input resistance increases. This seems to indicate that the diameter of the permeable channels or their number is reduced when the free $[Ca^{2+}]_i$ is increased.

The use of the photoprotein aequorin as a calcium ion indicator shows that when calcium is injected into the cell and reaches the area of the intercellular junction, the electrical coupling is reduced or abolished in Chironomus salivary gland cells (Rose and Loewenstein, 1975). The effect of high $[Ca^{2+}]_i$ on electrical coupling of heart cells is totally reversible. The reestablishment of cell-to-cell communication is probably related to the uptake of the ion by the sarcoplasmic reticulum and mitochondria or to its extrusion through the surface cell membrane. Caffeine, a drug that releases calcium from terminal vesicles and inhibits its uptake by these structures (Herz and Weber, 1965) causes a marked decline in the rate of cell recoupling in fibers previously injected

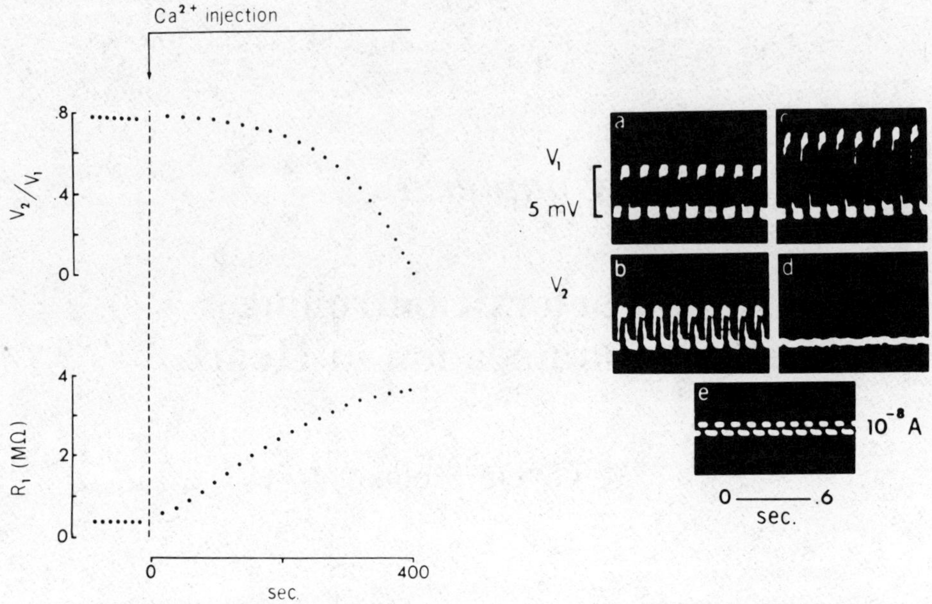

Figure 1. Effect of intracellular calcium injection on the electrical coupling of Purkinje cells.
At right—typical effect of intracellular calcium injection on electrical coupling. a) and b) show controls V_1 and V_2; c) and d) recorded after 410 seconds of calcium injection, showing cell decoupling. e) outward current pulses (60 msec in duration, 5 Hz, 10^{-8} A).
At left—influence of intracellular calcium injection on the coupling coefficient (V_2/V_1) and on input resistance (R_1) of Purkinje cells (average from six experiments). Temperature—37° C.

with calcium (see De Mello, 1975). On the other hand, recent studies (De Mello, 1978) indicate that caffeine (6 mM), by itself, increases the intracellular longitudinal resistance (r_a) in canine Purkinje fibers. The increment in r_a can be interpreted as due to a rise in free $[Ca^{2+}]_i$.

Because the free $[Ca^{2+}]_i$ increases during the excitation process in cardiac fibers, an obvious question arises: Is the junctional conductance reduced during the plateau of the action potential? Weidmann (1970) did not detect any change in intracellular longitudinal resistance during the action potential. Although further studies are required to elucidate this subject, it is conceivable that the low diffusion coefficient of calcium ions in the cytoplasm (Kushmerick and Podolsky, 1969) prevents a change in $[Ca^{2+}]_i$ at the gap junctions.

How much calcium is necessary to abolish cell-to-cell communication? Measuring the amount of calcium injected into a cardiac cell and using a transfer number of 0.32 (Gorman and Herman, 1979) indicates a value of 1.5×10^{-13} moles. Assuming a cell volume of 0.3×10^{-9} liters, the calcium concentration at the moment of cell decoupling is about 10^{-4} M. This is only an approximation value of $[Ca^{2+}]_i$ because part of the calcium injected is taken up by the sarcoplasmic reticulum and mitochondria and part is extruded through the nonjunctional membrane. This value of $[Ca^{2+}]_i$ is similar to that required to suppress the electrical coupling in Chironomus salivary gland (5 to 8×10^{-5} M; Loewenstein et al., 1967).

The mechanism by which calcium abolishes electrical coupling is not known. Two possibilities can be considered. *(1)* Calcium binds to negative sites probably located at the cytoplasmic end of the channel and blocks the diffusion of small ions like potassium (see Fig. 2). This hypothesis is supported by the finding that lanthanum and other strongly charged cations injected intracellularly suppressed cell communication (see below). Because phospholipids are present in gap junctions (Goodenough and Stoeckenius, 1972), their negative polar groups might represent the binding sites for calcium. *(2)* The other possibility is that calcium activates enzyme processes, such as the adenosine triphosphatases, and triggers conformational changes in the protein

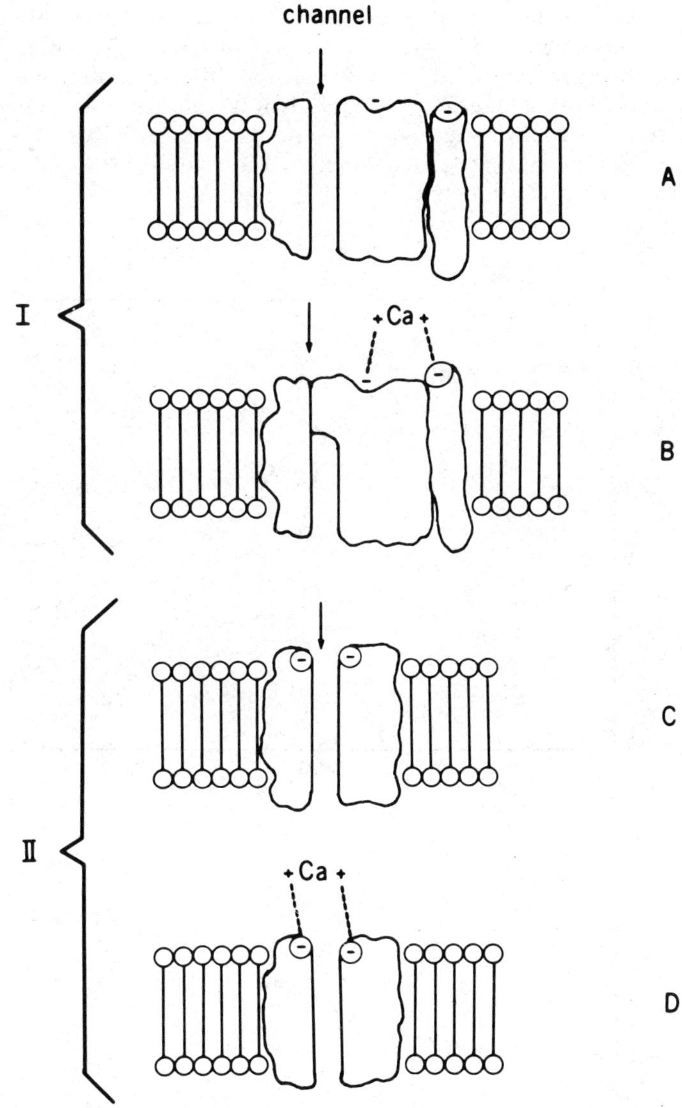

Figure 2. Possible mechanisms of heart cell decoupling elicited by calcium. I) A—channel before the rise in $[Ca^2]_i$; B—binding of calcium to charged ligand and consequent conformation change of protein molecule, closing the gate. II) C—control; D—binding of calcium to negative sites closing the gate to molecules and to small monovalent cations.

molecules present in gap junctions. As a consequence, the channel is closed (see Fig. 2). Nevertheless, the uncoupling process can be activated by several cationic species (De Mello, 1980a) indicating that the first hypothesis described above, is more likely.

Because calcium influx in heart cells increases when intracellular sodium concentration increases (Glitsch and Reuter, 1970), I thought it important to test the calcium hypothesis by injecting sodium inside a heart cell and following its effect on electrical coupling and input resistance. I used microelectrodes filled with 1 M sodium chloride to electrophoretically inject the ion into the cytosol. Figure 3 shows the effect of an intracellular sodium injection on the coupling coefficient (V_2/V_1) and on input resistance (R_1) of Purkinje cells. The rise in intracellular sodium concentration ($[Na^+]_i$) causes electrical uncoupling and increases the input resistance (De Mello, 1974; 1976). By determining the space constant, I could calculate the separate changes in membrane resistance per unit of length (r_m) and of the intracellular longitudinal resistance per unit of length (r_a). Table 1 shows that r_a was increased by 250%, whereas r_m was reduced by 23%; this means that a rise in junctional resistance is the main cause for cell decoupling when sodium is injected.

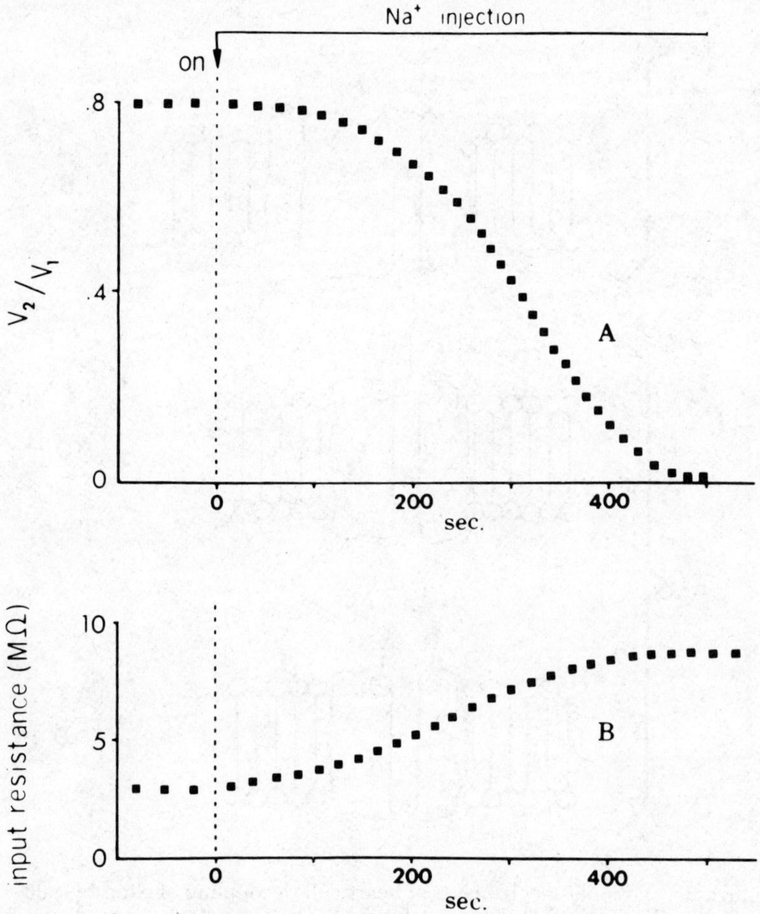

Figure 3. Influence of intracellular sodium injection on the electrical coupling and input resistance of Purkinje cells (average from five experiments).

Table 1
Effect of Intracellular Sodium Injection on Input Resistance (R_o), Space Constant (λ), Membrane Resistance per Unit Length (r_m), and Axial Resistance per Unit Length (r_a)

	R_o ($\times 10^6$)Ω		λ (mm)		r_m (KΩcm)		r_a (MΩ/cm)	
	Normal	After Na^+ injection	Normal	After Na^+ injection	Normal	After Na^+ injection	Normal	After Na^+ injection
Fiber 1	2.5	5	1.3	0.5	650	500	38	200
Fiber 2	3	4.3	1.4	0.58	840	498	40	140
Fiber 3	2	6	1.6	0.51	640	600	25	230

*Values of R_o and λ were determined experimentally. Values of r_m and r_a were calculated as described in De Mello, 1976.
†Determinations of λ and R_o were made after 250 to 300 seconds of sodium injection.

The question then arises: Is sodium alone able to decrease the junctional conductance? The answer seems to be no. When sodium is released into the cell in the presence of a low extracellular calcium concentration ($[Ca^{2+}]_o$), the electrical coupling is barely reduced. If $[Ca^{2+}]_o$ is suddenly increased, the cell previously injected with sodium is quickly decoupled (see Fig. 4). Therefore, the decoupling action of a sodium

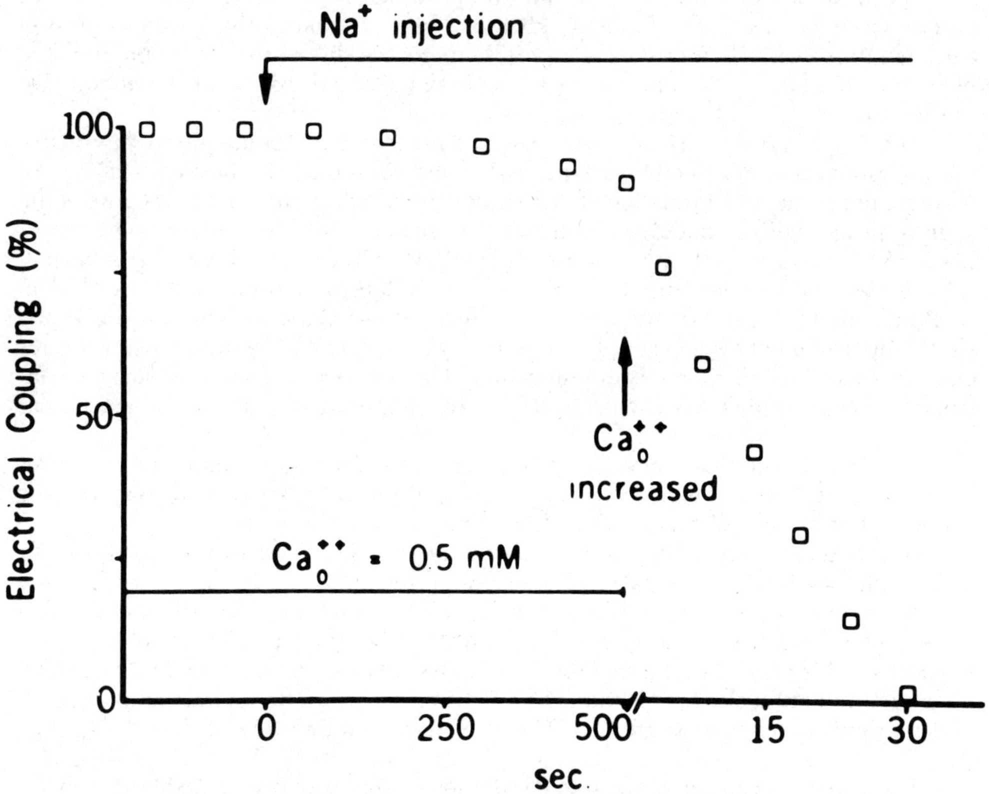

Figure 4. Effect of extracellular calcium concentration on the decoupling action of intracellular sodium injection (average from five experiments). The normal coupling coefficient (V_2/V_1) was taken as 100%. Arrow, at right, indicates increase in $[Ca^{2+}]_o$. (From De Mello, 1976, with permission of Cambridge University Press).

injection must be due to a rise in $[Ca^{2+}]_i$. The maintenance of a low $[Na^+]_i$ is then essential for the preservation of intercellular communication. This conclusion is supported by ouabain's ability to increase r_a and to cause cell decoupling in heart fibers (De Mello, 1976; Weingart, 1977) (see Fig. 5 and Table 2). The effect of the glycoside on cell-to-cell communication seems related to the increment in free $[Ca^{2+}]_i$. In fact, Weingart (1977) showed that the decoupling action of ouabain is accelerated by increasing $[Ca^{2+}]_o$. On the other hand, the electrical coupling abolished by the drug can be reestablished by injecting EDTA into the cell (see Fig. 6 and De Mello, 1979b).

Previous observations of Page et al. (1964) and Ellis (1977) indicate that the removal of potassium ions from the extracellular fluid leads to inhibition of the sodium-potassium pump and to an increase of the intracellular sodium concentration. It seems, then, that a potassium-free solution may have an effect similar to that of ouabain on the electrical coupling. This is, indeed, the case. The removal of potassium ions from the extracellular fluid causes depolarization and oscillation of the membrane potential (see Carmeliet, 1961). The electrical coupling gradually declines, and in about 90 minutes total cell decoupling is found (see Fig. 7, average data from five experiments). Simultaneously with the change in cell communication, the input resistance increases notably (see Fig. 7).

Because the inhibition of sodium extrusion leads to cell decoupling, the question arises, can the activation of the sodium pump improve cell communication? Under certain circumstances, yes. Norepinephrine, which stimulates the sodium pump in cardiac fibers (Vassalle and Barnabei, 1971) increases the resting potential and the electrical coupling in Purkinje fibers partially depolarized by recent dissection (De Mello, 1977a).

The conclusion drawn from these experiments is that the sodium pump modulates the junctional conductance by varying $[Na^+]_i$ and consequently the free $[Ca^{2+}]_i$. An increase in the rate of stimulation of cardiac fibers leads to an increase in the rate of the sodium pump, with a concurrent increment in respiration. More adenosine triphosphate (ATP) is consumed, but also the rate of ATP synthesis is enhanced. In normal, well-oxygenated cardiac muscle, ATP synthesis is determined mainly by the rate of ATP utilization. It can be envisaged that a marked tachycardia in the presence of a slight impairment of oxygen supply might result in a fall in ATP synthesis with serious consequences for cell-to-cell communication. The free $[Ca^{2+}]_i$ is indeed largely controlled by active uptake mechanisms at the mitochondrial and sarcoplasmic reticular level.

In nerve, 2-4-dinitrophenol, an uncoupler of oxydative phosphorylation, causes the release of calcium from mitochondria and other intracellular stores, thus increasing the free $[Ca^{2+}]_i$ (Blaustein and Hodgkin, 1969).

In cardiac Purkinje fibers, 2-4-dinitrophenol (0.5 mM) increases the intracellular longitudinal resistance (see Table 3), causes cell uncoupling (De Mello, 1979a) (see Fig. 8), and suppresses the cell-to-cell diffusion of fluorescein. This effect of dinitrophenol seems related to the rise in free $[Ca^{2+}]_i$. There are two pieces of evidence supporting this view: *(1)* the metabolic inhibitor causes contractures in myocardial fibers; *(2)* the intracellular injection of EDTA immediately after cell uncoupling elicited by dinitrophenol reestablishes 70% of control coupling (De Mello, 1979a) (see Fig. 9).

These results can be summarized as follows: the oxydative phosphorylation is inhibited, and the cell ATP content is reduced by dinitrophenol (see McDonald and MacLeod, 1972) with a consequent increase in free $[Ca^{2+}]_i$ and cell decoupling. The synthesis of high-energy phosphate bonds is then essential for the maintenance of a low free-$[Ca^{2+}]_i$ and consequently for the preservation of high junctional conductance in heart fibers.

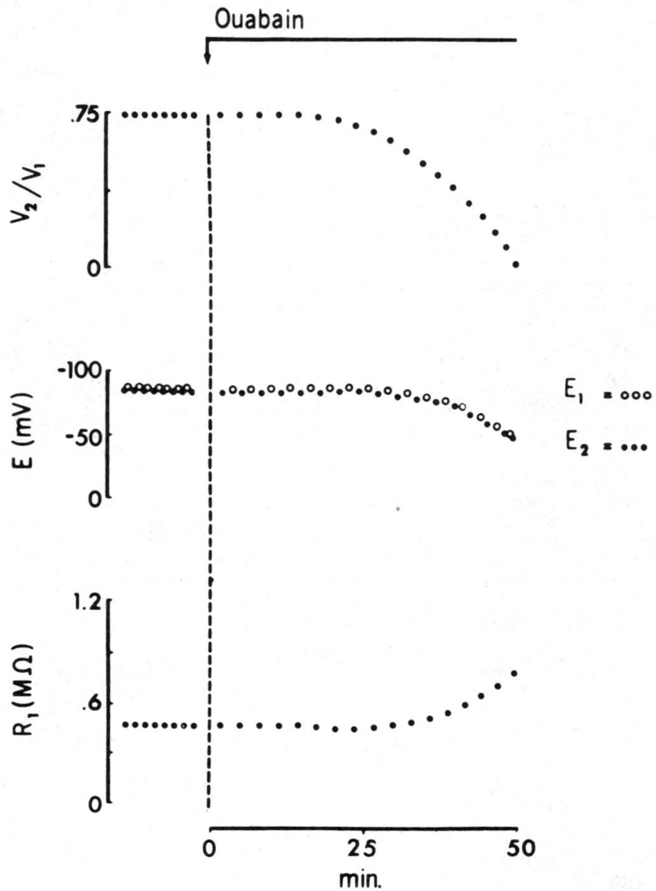

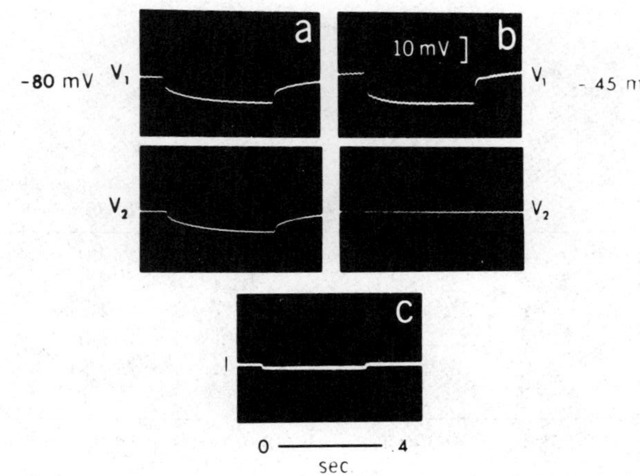

Figure 5. Effect of ouabain on the electrical coupling of Purkinje cells. At right—typical effect of ouabain (2×10^{-6} M) on the electrical coupling. a) V_1 and V_2 recorded before ouabain; b) V_1 and V_2 55 minutes after the addition of ouabain. I—current pulse (10^{-8}A).
At left—influence of ouabain (2×10^{-6} M) on the coupling coefficient (V_2/V_1), membrane potential (E_1, E_2), and input resistance (R_1) (average from six experiments).

Table 2

Effect of Ouabain (2×10^{-6} M) on Space Constant (λ), Input Resistance (R_1), Membrane Resistance per Unit Length (r_m), and Intracellular Longitudinal Resistance per Unit Length (r_a) of Purkinje Fibers

Expt. No.	λ*(mm)		V_o/I_o (R_1*) (KΩ)		r_m (KΩcm)		r_a (MΩ/cm)	
	Control	Ouabain	Control	Ouabain	Control	Ouabain	Control	Ouabain
6	1.35	0.25	450	680	117	34	6.9	54.4
7	1.43	0.30	530	780	148	46.8	7.5	52
8	1.25	0.25	390	600	93	30	6.5	48
9	1.62	0.22	400	550	128	24.2	5	50
10	1.55	0.29	210	310	63	17.9	2.8	21.3
Mean + SEM	1.44 ± 0.05	0.26 ± 0.08	396 ± 54	584 ± 74	109 ± 21	30.5 ± 4.8	5.7 ± 0.8	45 ± 6

*Measurements of space constant and input resistance were made after an exposure of 40 minutes to ouabain. Distance between polarizing and voltage recording microelectrodes at V_1 (about 50 μm).

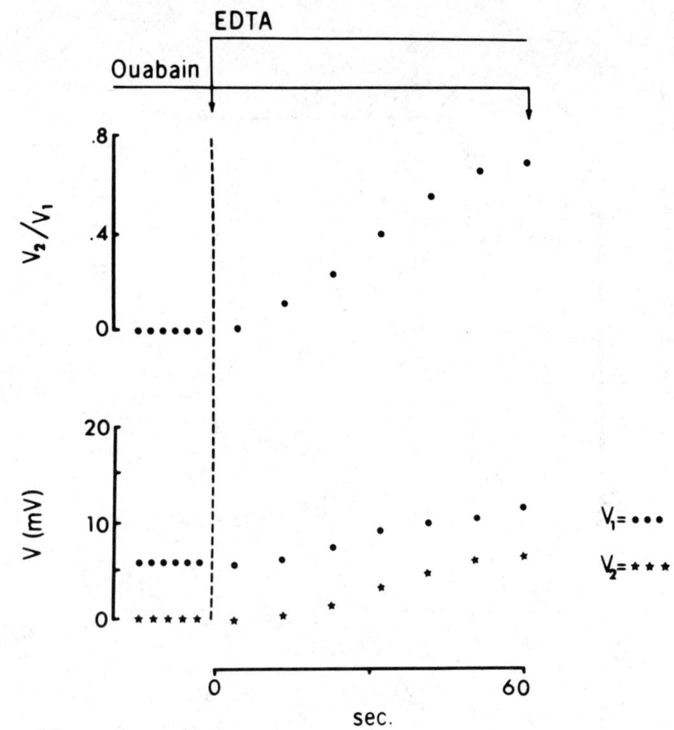

Figure 6. Recoupling action of EDTA on Purkinje fiber previously exposed to ouabain (2×10^{-6} M). I—2×10^{-9} A, 600 msec in duration, 0.5 Hz.

Influence of other ions on the electrical coupling of cardiac cells.

Other cations also influence the cell-to-cell communication in heart fibers. Strontium has effects similar to those of calcium and causes cell decoupling when injected intracellularly (De Mello, 1975). Recent studies indicate that lanthanum is as effective or even more efficient than calcium is in abolishing the electrical coupling (see Fig. 10) (De Mello, 1979c). The injection of the ion inside the cell elicits a hyperpolarization, a reduction in V_2/V_1, and an increase in input resistance. Similar results are produced by manganese injection, but the effect of this ion seems smaller than that of lanthanum (De Mello, 1979c). Lanthanum's marked effect on electrical coupling is probably due to its nonhydrated ionic radius (within 0.02 Å of calcium's ionic radius) and also to its strong positive charge.

The possibility that hydrogen ions are involved on the control of junctional conductance has been discussed by Turin and Warner (1977). They found that when cells of Xenopus embryos are exposed to 100% carbon dioxide, the input resistance is augmented and the electrical coupling is abolished. In cardiac muscle, the iontophoretic injection of hydrogen ions inside the cell increases r_a by 650% (De Mello, 1980b) and causes cell decoupling to occur in about 10 min. The input resistance of the injected cell is increased concurrently with the fall in V_2/V_1 (see Fig. 11). On the other hand, a notable increment in coupling coefficient is seen when hydroxyl ions are injected into the cytosol of a Purkinje cell (De Mello, unpublished observations). These findings are indicative that intracellular pH influences the junctional resistance. The possible interactions between changes in intracellular hydrogen ion concentration ($[H^+]_i$) and $[Ca^{2+}]_i$ will be discussed by Dr. Weingart.

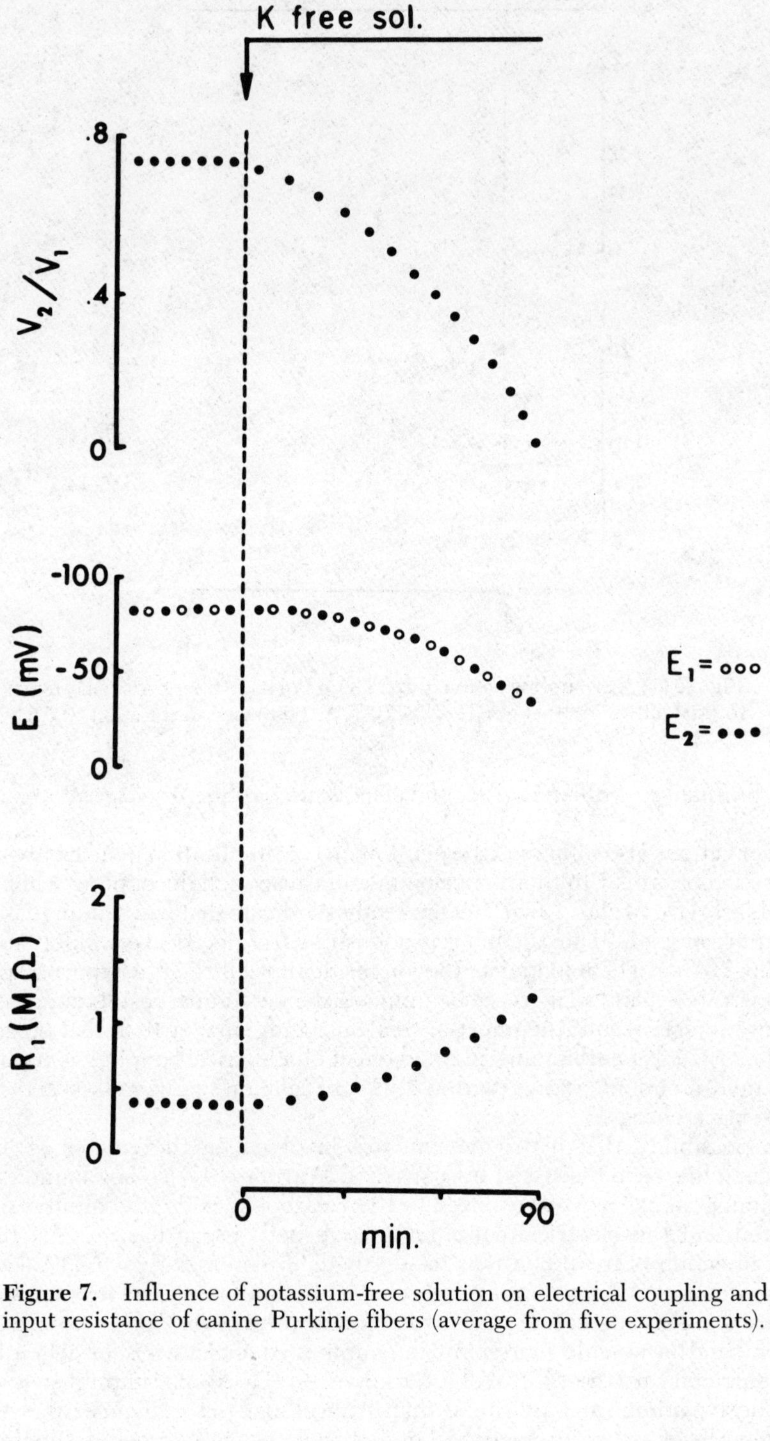

Figure 7. Influence of potassium-free solution on electrical coupling and input resistance of canine Purkinje fibers (average from five experiments).

Table 3

Effect of 2-4-dinitrophenol (DNP) on Membrane Resistance per Unit Length (r_m), Intracellular Longitudinal Resistance per Unit Length (r_a), Space Constant (λ), and Input Resistance (R_1) of Purkinje Fibers Immersed in Normal Tyrode's Solution

	λ(μm)		$R_o(\times 10^6)\Omega$		r_m (KΩcm)		r_a (MΩ/cm)	
	Normal	DNP	Normal	DNP	Normal	DNP	Normal	DNP
Fiber 1	1500	950	2	3	600	570	26	63
Fiber 2	1575	830	2	3.3	600	547	26.6	79.5
Fiber 3	1685	900	2	2.3	640	414	25	51.1
Fiber 4	1700	1010	2.8	3.4	952	680	32.9	68
Fiber 5	1600	980	1.9	2.4	608	470	23.7	48.9

[a]Values of R_o and λ were determined experimentally. Values of r_m and r_a were calculated as described in De Mello, 1979a. Measurements of λ and R_o were performed between 7 and 10 minutes after DNP was introduced into the bath. From De Mello, 1979a, with permission of Springer-Verlag.

Physiologic implications of changes in junctional conductance.

When the heart muscle is damaged, the spread of injury current is fortunately quickly suppressed by the establishment of ionic barriers between injured and non-injured cells (the healing-over process). Two feasible sites for the location of these barriers are the surface cell membrane or the intercellular junctions.

In skeletal muscle fibers, the outflow of protoplasm through the injured area is prevented by the formation of a film (surface precipitation reaction; Heilbrunn, 1956). Because this reaction does not represent an efficient mechanism of electrical sealing (De Mello, 1973), it seems reasonable to think that in heart muscle the probable location of the ionic barrier is the intercellular junction. Recent studies of fluorescein diffusion in healed Purkinje fibers show that the high-resistance barrier is localized not at the cut end, but 150 to 200 μm away (De Mello, 1980a). This site presumably corresponds to gap junctions facing the damage. As calcium is essential for the healing-over process (Délèze, 1965; De Mello et al., 1969), a rise in calcium concentration, due to the lesion, may reduce markedly the junctional conductance. This hypothesis is supported by the finding that the rise in free $[Ca^{2+}]_i$ causes electrical decoupling (De Mello, 1975). Thanks to the healing-over process, large masses of cardiac cells are protected from the depolarizing effects of injury current originating in the damaged areas.

A fall in junctional conductance produced by ischemia or drugs, such as ouabain, may play an important role on the generation and cardiac arrhythmias. An increase in junctional resistance produces a reduction in conduction velocity as has been found when $[Na^+]_i$ is increased or ouabain is used (see De Mello, 1976; Weingart, 1977).

In the atrioventricular node, the cells are electrically coupled, but the spread of the electrotonic potentials is reduced by a small space constant (430 μm; De Mello, 1977b). In this tissue, the intracellular longitudinal resistance (r_a) is much higher than it is in atrial muscle (De Mello, 1977b). This finding is probably related to the rare occurrence of a gap junction in the atrioventricular node (James and Scherf, 1968). The high value of r_a not only contributes to the delay of impulse conduction in this tissue but also makes propagation of the impulse extremely vulnerable to variations in resistance of the nonjunctional membrane. A small decrease in this resistance can elicit A-V block. This seems to be the mechanism by which acetylcholine suppresses the atrioventricular conduction (De Mello, 1977b).

The synaptic inhibition of the sinoatrial node seems also due to a marked rise in conductance of the nonjunctional membrane without a necessary increment of the

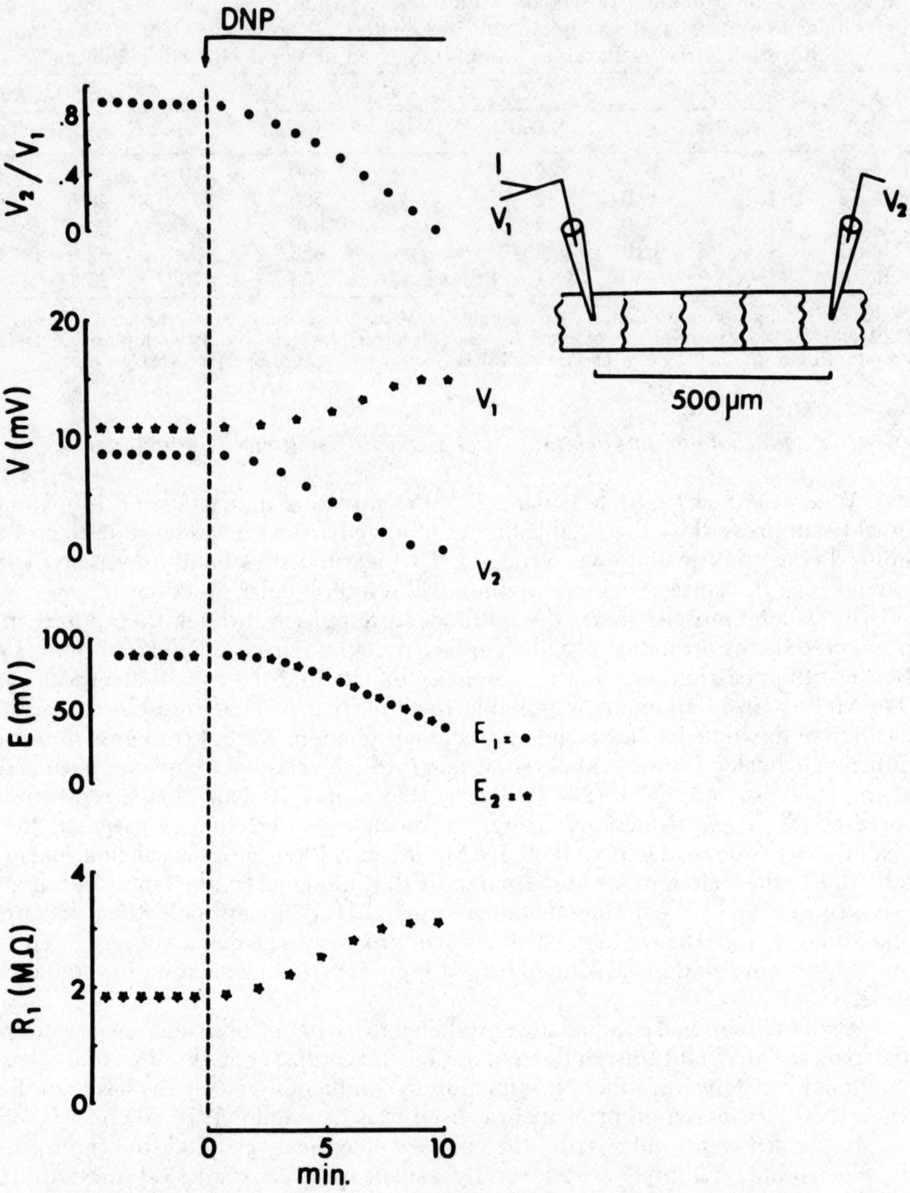

Figure 8. Effect of DNP on intercellular communication in dog Purkinje fibre. Time-course of R_1 (input resistance of cell 1), V_1 and V_2 (changes in membrane potential in cells 1 and 2, respectively), E_1 and E_2 (membrane potentials of cells 1 and 2 at zero current, taking outside minus inside potential) and coupling coefficient (V_2/V_1). Arrow indicates start of treatment with DNP (0.5 mM). At right—drawing (not an exact scale) shows experimental procedure used during this experiment, and distance between cells 1 and 2. Cells impaled were not located at the end of strand. Temperature—37°C. From De Mello, 1979a, with permission of Springer-Verlag.

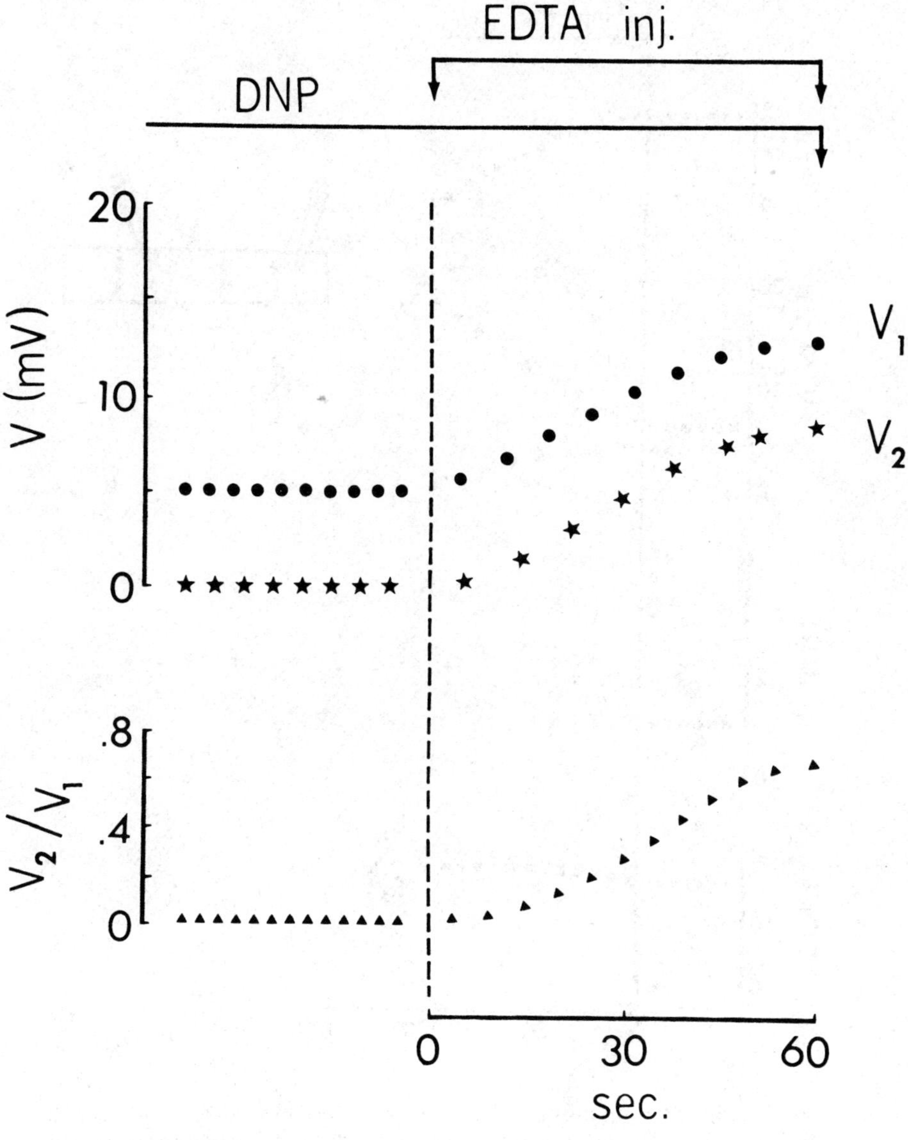

Figure 9. Influence of intracellular injection of EDTA on electrical coupling of Purkinje cells exposed to DNP for 10 to 12 minutes (average from five experiments). Arrow shows start of EDTA injection. I—2 × 10^{-9} A, 600 msec, 0.5 Hz. Temperature—37° C. From De Mello, 1979a, with permission of Springer-Verlag.

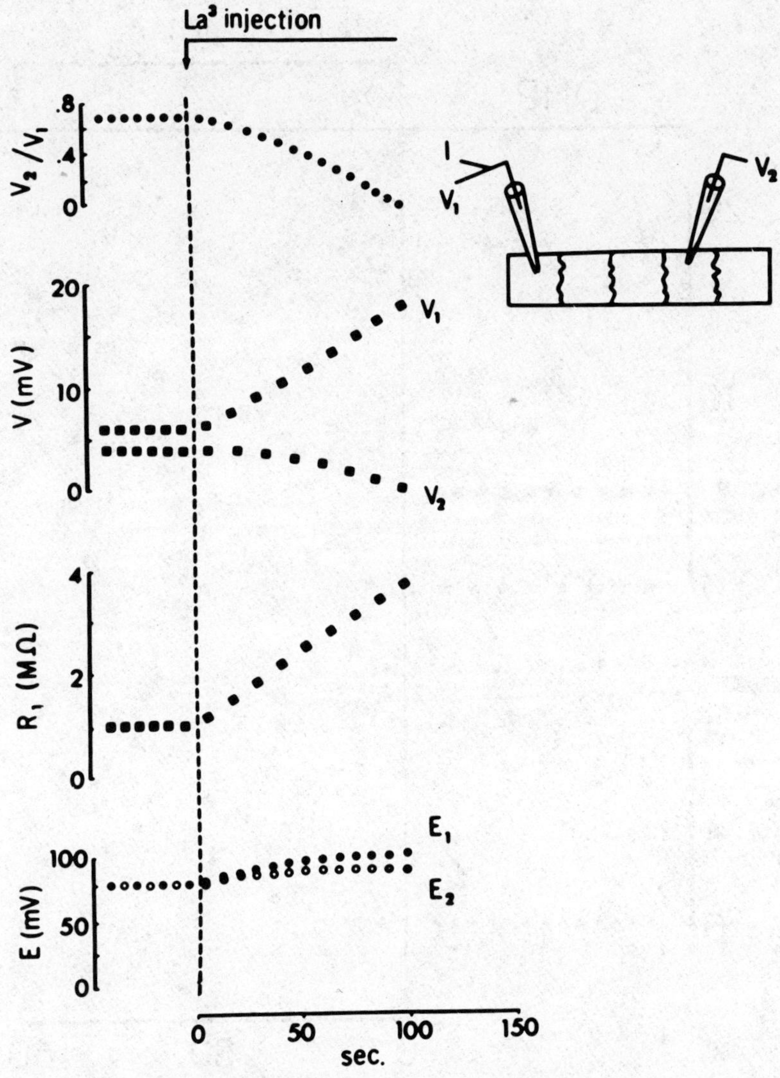

Figure 10. Decoupling of Purkinje cells produced by intracellular injection of lanthanum. Time-course of V_1, V_2, E_1, and E_2 and coupling coefficient (V_2/V_1). Arrows show start of lanthanum injection. The points before lanthanum injection represent control values of each of the electrical parameters. I—10^{-8} A; 50 msec in duration, 3 Hz. At right, diagram showing experiment procedure. From De Mello, 1979c—with permission of Academic Press, London.

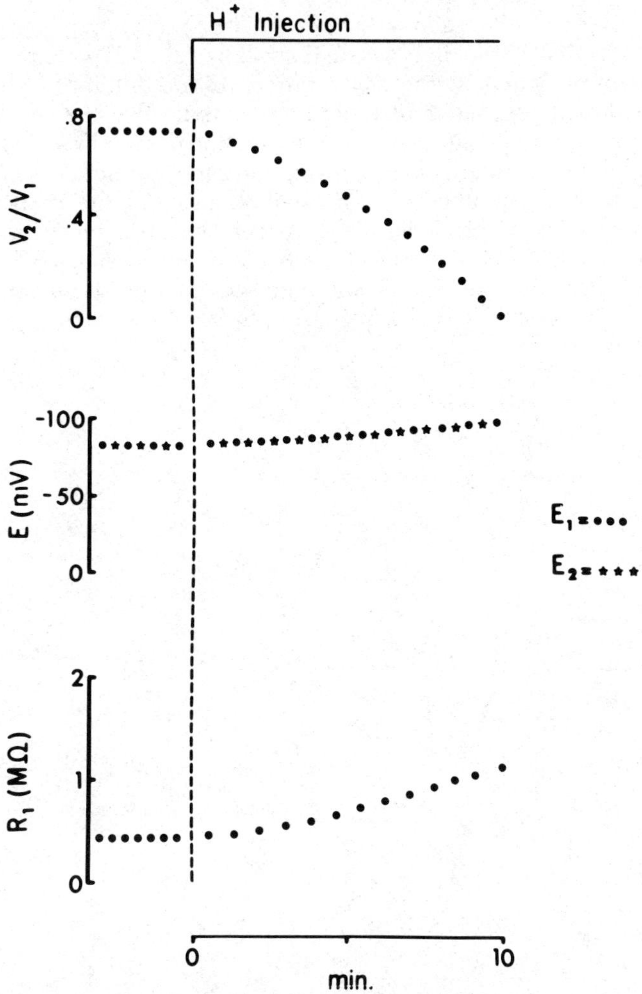

Figure 11. Effect of intracellular injection of hydrogen ions on the electrical coupling of canine Purkinje cells (average from five experiments). Time-course of input resistance (R_1), E_1, E_2 and coupling coefficient (V_2/V_1). Arrow shows start of hydrogen ion injection. The points before hydrogen ion injection represent control values of each of the electrical parameters. I—10^{-8} A; 60 msec in duration, 5 Hz. R_1 was measured with voltage-recording microelectrode impaled about 50 μm away from polarizing electrode. Measurements of R_1 made with a balanced bridge circuit showed changes in the same direction. From De Mello, 1980b, with permission of Academic Press, London.

junctional resistance. The nodal cells are electrically coupled (Dudel and Trautwein, 1958), but the mean area of the gap junction (5×10^{-2} μm²) is smaller than that found in atrial muscle (54×10^{-2} μm²) (Masson-Pevet, 1979). I must add that the injection of fluorescein in true pacemaker cells is not followed by widespread diffusion of the dye like that seen in atrial or in Purkinje fibers (De Mello, 1980a). These observations might indicate that the diameter or number of the hydrophylic channels in the pacemaker is smaller than those present in atrial muscle.

In true pacemaker cells, the resting potential is smaller than it is in pacemaker cells located near crista terminalis (Paes de Carvalho et al., 1959). How can these cells be electrically coupled and at the same time present different values of resting potential? A reasonable explanation would be to assume that the active extrusion of ions (sodium, for instance) through the nonjunctional membrane is dissimilar in different areas of the node and keeps the membrane potential at different levels despite the presence of gap junctions. The maintenance of ionic gradients inside the node seems essential for the physiology of the pacemaker, but only further studies will dilucidate the meaning of this electrical heterogeneity in the sinoatrial node. Finally, Figure 12 shows the influence of ionic and metabolic factors on junctional resistance and the major consequences of cell decoupling to heart function.

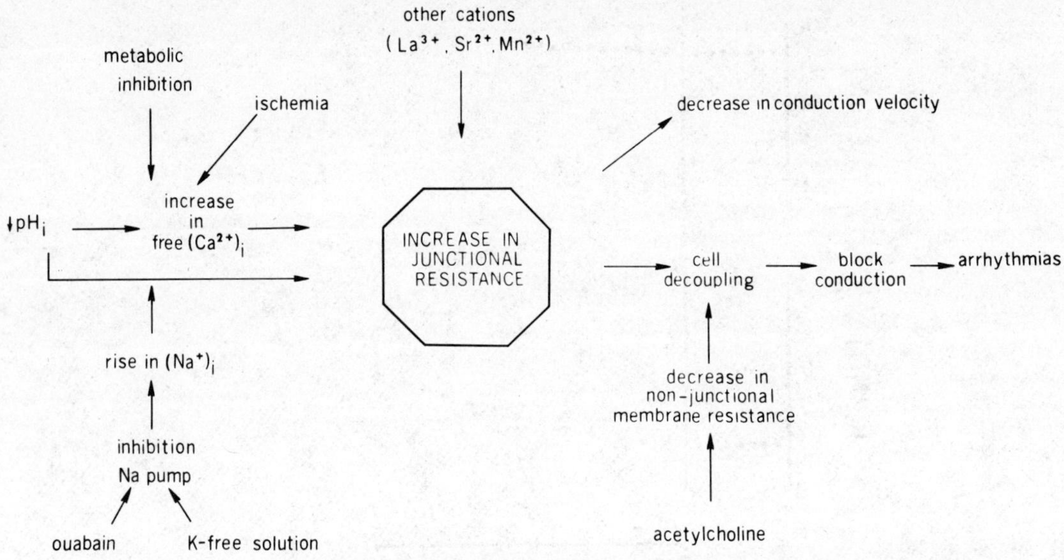

Figure 12. Factors that influence the junctional resistance in cardiac muscle and the major consequences of cell decoupling.

REFERENCES

Bennett MVL, Trinkaus JP (1970) Electrical coupling between embryonic cells by way of extracellular space and specialized junctions. J Cell Biol **44**:592–610

Blaustein MP, Hodgkin AL (1969) The effect of cyanide on the flux of calcium from squid axons. J Physiol **200**:497–527

Carmeliet EE (1961) Chloride and potassium permeability in cardiac purkinje fibres. Brussels: Presses Académiques Europeenes.

Délèze J (1965) Calcium ions and the healing-over of heart fibres. *In* Electrophysiology of the Heart, edited by B. Taccardi, G Marchetti, London, Pergamon Press, pp. 147–148

De Mello WC (1973) Membrane sealing in frog skeletal muscle fibers. Proc Natl Acad Sci USA **70**:982–984

De Mello WC (1974) Electrical uncoupling in heart fibres produced by intracellular injection of Na or Ca. Physiologist **17**:3

De Mello WC (1975) Effect of intracellular injection of calcium and strontium in cell communication in heart. J Physiol **250**:231–245
De Mello WC (1976) Influence of the sodium pump on intercellular communication in heart fibres: Effect of intracellular injection of sodium ion on electrical coupling. J Physiol **263**: 171– 197
De Mello WC (1977a) Factors involved on the control of junctional conductance in heart. Proc Int Union Physiol Sci **12**:319 (Abst.)
De Mello WC (1977b) Passive electrical properties of the atrioventricular node. Pfluegers Arch **371**:135–139
De Mello WC (1978) Cell-to-cell diffusion of fluorescein in heart fibers. Fed Proc **37**:3
De Mello WC (1979a) Effect of 2-4-dinitrophenol on intercellular communication in mammalian cardiac fibers. Pfluegers Arch **380**:267–276
De Mello WC (1979b) On the decoupling action of ouabain. Physiologist **22**:4
De Mello WC (1979c) Effect of intracellular injection of La^{3+} and Mn^{2+} on electrical coupling of heart cells. Cell Biol Int Rep **3**:113–119
De Mello WC (1980a) Intercellular communication and junctional permeability. *In* Membrane Structure and Function, vol. 3, edited by EE Bittar, New York, John Wiley and Sons, pp. 127–170
De Mello WC (1980b) Influence of intracellular injection of H^+ on the electrical coupling in cardiac Purkinje fibres. Cell Biol Int Rep **4**:51–55
De Mello WC, Motta G, Chapeau M (1969) A study on the healing-over of myocardial cells of toads. Circ Res **24**:475–487
Dudel J, Trautwein W (1958) Der mechanismus der automatischen rhythmischen Impulsbildung der Herzmuskelfaser. Pfluegers Arch **269**:553–565
Ellis D (1977) The effects of external cations and ouabain on the intercellular sodium activity of sheep heart Purkinje fibres. J Physiol **273**:211–240
Glitsch HG, Reuter H (1970) The effect of internal sodium concentration on calcium fluxes in isolated guinea-pig auricles. J Physiol **209**:25–43
Goodenough DA, Stoeckenius W (1972) The isolation of hepatocyte gap junctions. J Cell Biol **54**:646–656
Gorman ALF, Herman A (1979) Internal effects of divalent cations on potassium permeability in molluscan neurons. J Physiol **296**:393–410
Heilbrunn LV (1956) The Dynamics of Living Protoplasm. New York, Academic Press
Herz R, Weber A (1965) Caffeine inhibition of Ca uptake by muscle reticulum. Fed Proc **24**:208 (Abst.)
Imanaga I (1974) Cell-to-cell diffusion of Procion Yellow in sheep and calf Purkinje fibers. J Membr Biol **16**:381–388
James TN, Scherf L (1968) Ultrastructure of the human atrioventricular node. Circulation **37**:1049–1070
Kushmerick MJ, Podolsky RJ (1969) Ionic mobility in muscle cells. Science, NY 166:1297
Loewenstein WR, Nakas M, Socolar SJ (1967) Junctional membrane uncoupling: Permeability transformation at cell membrane junction. J Gen Physiol **50**:1865–1891
Masson-Pevet M (1979) The fine structure of cardiac pacemaker cells in the sinus node and in tissue culture. Thesis. Amsterdam, Rodopi Press
McDonald TF, MacLeod DP (1972) The effect of 2-4-dinitrophenol on electrical and mechanical activity, metabolism and ion movements in guinea-pig ventricular muscle. Br J Pharmacol **44**:711–722
Paes de Carvalho A, De Mello WC, Hoffman B (1959) Electrophysiological evidence for specialized fiber types in rabbit atrium. Am J Physiol **196**:483–488
Page E, Goerke RJ, Storm SR (1964) Cat heart muscle in vitro: IV. Inhibition of transport in quiescent muscles. J Gen Physiol **47**:531–543
Pitts JD, Finbow ME (1977) Junctional permeability and its consequences. *In* Intercellular Communication, edited by WD De Mello, New York, Plenum Press, pp 61–86
Pollack GH (1973) Intercellular coupling in the atrioventricular node and other tissues of the rabbit heart. J Physiol **255**:275–298
Rose B, Loewenstein WR (1975) Permeability of cell junction depends on local cytoplasmic calcium activity. Nature (London) 254:250

Turin L, Warner A (1977) Carbon dioxide reversibly abolishes ionic communication between cells of early amphibian embryo. Nature (London) 270:56

Vassalle M, Barnabei O (1971) Nor-epinephrine and potassium fluxes in cardiac Purkinje fibres. Pfluegers Arch **322**:287–303

Weidmann S (1966) The diffusion of radiopotassium across intercalated discs of mammalian cardiac muscle. J Physiol **187**:323–342

Weidmann S (1970) Electrical constants of trabecular muscle from mammalian heart. J Physiol **210**:1041–1054

Weingart R (1974) The permeability to tetraethylammonium ions of the surface membrane and intercalated disks of sheep and calf myocardium. J Physiol **240**:741–762

Weingart R (1977) The actions of ouabain on intercellular coupling and conduction velocity in mammalian ventricular muscle. J Physiol **264**:341–365

Discussion

FOZZARD: Dr. De Mello's second model suggests that a negatively charged gap junction channel allows positive particles to pass through. Calcium ions, by shielding these negative charges, would change the selectivity of the channel. Dr. Weidmann showed in his presentation the relationship between molecular size and apparent permeability for the gap junction. Interestingly, the same line fits positively and negatively charged particles. This suggests to me that electrostatic sieving is not important in the gap junction channel. I suspect therefore that the concept of calcium ions shielding these negative charges and altering the selectivity of the channel is probably not correct. Whatever calcium is doing is more likely to occur at a distance from the channel itself and probably involves some conformational change.

REUTER: How much hydrogen and hydroxyl ions did you have to inject to overcome the buffer capacity of the cell?

DE MELLO: One has to inject very large quantities in a very quick way to obtain effects. I have tried to calculate the concentration of hydrogen ions inside the cell during the experiments but there are great difficulties in this calculation. Hydrogen ions are highly mobile and diffuse longitudinally across the gap junctions, as well as across the plasma cell membrane.

HOFFMAN: Could you tell us some more about the possible effects of changes in membrane potential on coupling? If one changes the membrane potential by altering external potassium or by passing a small hyperpolarizing current, it appears that one can greatly modify the effect of calcium on coupling. I tend to think that these alterations in membrane voltage do not necessarily entail a conformational change at the level of the gap junctional channels.

DE MELLO: In 1971, Rose and Loewenstein found that salivary gland cells that were uncoupled by several procedures could be recoupled by hyperpolarization. We got similar results in canine Purkinje fibers. Two reasonable explanations might be considered: *(1)* changes in the electrical field would reestablish the junctional conductance or *(2)* the intracellular free-calcium concentration would be reduced by hyperpolarization. Brinley and Mullins (Ann NY Sci **242**:406–433, 1974) showed that an increment in membrane polarization in squid axon causes a drop of free $(Ca^{2+})_i$. We think that our results can be interpreted according to the second alternative.

GADSBY: Returning again to the question of cell recoupling upon hyperpolarization, could an alternative explanation for your results be that the applied hyperpolarizing current results in a depletion of potassium ions just outside the cell and, consequently, a decrease in membrane potassium conductance? This effect would cause an apparent improvement in cell coupling because the amplitude of the electrotonic potentials would increase and it would provide an explanation for the time courses of onset and offset of the changes that you see.

DE MELLO: That is not impossible here, but further studies are required to elucidate the mechanism of cell recoupling by hyperpolarization.

BROWN: In isolated cells like red blood cells or neurons, the injection of calcium causes an increase in the potassium ionic conductance of the membrane. On the other hand, if other bivalent ions like barium or strontium are injected, this is not observed. The ion sequence for this effect is, I think, similar to that with which divalent ions block the calcium channel. Is it possible that when you look at the effects of calcium injections you are looking at two effects; namely, uncoupling with increased axial resistance and an increase of potassium conductance with decreased resistance through the plasma membrane? In this context, when you experiment with the injection of other divalent cations like manganese or lanthanum, you may be looking at different net results of the action of the ions on those two aspects of the calcium effect.

DE MELLO: During our studies on the intracellular injection of calcium we found a slight decrease in membrane time constant. Assuming that the membrane capacity is not changing, it is reasonable to conclude that the resistance of the nonjunctional membrane was slightly reduced. However, the very large increase in input resistance of the injected cell favours the interpretation that the junctional resistance was markedly increased. Now take, for instance, the data recently obtained by us on lanthanum injections inside cardiac cells. The injection results in hyperpolarization and shortening of the action potential, which is exactly what you would expect from an increase in potassium conductance like that shown by Isenberg with calcium injections.

RAMÓN: We have studied the junctional mechanism in crayfish axons. After the axons are perfused internally, the junctions are no longer sensitive to either calcium or hydroxyl ions. This result substantiated our claim that calcium is not directly responsible for the blockade of junctional communication in these axons. We believe that calcium acts indirectly when blocking junctional permeability.

DE MELLO: I have read your paper, and I have a few doubts in my mind. Is calcium really reaching the junction? Can you prove, using aequorin for instance, that calcium is getting to the junction? On the other hand, you mention that there must be something inside the cell capable of blocking the junction when activated by calcium. In our old experiments on the healing-over process in cardiac muscle, I noticed that a decrease in temperature causes a decrease in the healing-over process, even if the calcium concentration is the same. This might indicate that calcium is not the whole story and that there may be some other factor involved in the action of calcium on the junction. The Q_{10} for healing-over is 4.7, which points to an important metabolic component in the process.

JOHNSON: In your hyperpolarization experiments on AV nodal cells, a sort of notch is seen in the upstroke of the action potential. Do you get this result often?

DE MELLO: Yes. Also, the same observation was reported by Brian Hoffman (1961) for similar experiments.

JOHNSON: Did you use unidimensional cable theory to analyze the results of the AV node polarization experiments?

DE MELLO: Yes. The polarization of node cells was made using a suction electrode in an attempt to reduce the problem to one spatial dimension.

JOHNSON: In such a bulky structure such as the AV node, the unidimensional theory may not be the appropriate theory to use. If the tridimensional geometry is taken into consideration, your estimate of 0.5 mm for the space constant may even fall short of the true value. This is a puzzling result because as you know I favor the idea that slow conduction within the AV node is in a large portion due to an increased longitudinal internal resistance. The values that you find for the space constant give the idea that the coupling resistance between cells in the AV node may not be different or at least not different enough from that in the atrium. How then do you explain the tremendous slowing of conduction within the AV node?

DE MELLO: In Hoffman and Cranefield's book (1960), results on AV nodal cell hyperpolarization show a decrease in the maximum rate of rise of the action potential instead of the increase one would expect from removal of inactivation of the fast sodium channel. This finding favors the concept that the upstroke mechanism in AV nodal cells is indeed different from the fast sodium response normally found in other parts of the heart. Other findings involving ionic environment changes and pharmacologic responses also favor this concept. It would thus seem logical to explain slow conduction in the AV node as resulting importantly from a different and much slower depolarizing mechanism in the AV nodal cell. On the other hand, an increase in internal longitudinal resistance may be expected from the smaller cell size within the AV node. This would result in some shortening of space constant even if cell coupling is of low resistance. I agree with you that longitudinal resistance should also be an important factor in the AV node, especially because conduction of activity depends on a weak-current-generating mechanism.

MÉNDEZ: Our experiments on AV nodal polarization also confirm the results of Hoffman and Cranefield and the data shown by Dr. De Mello more recently. Hyperpolarizing nodal cells cause a slowing of the action potential upstroke instead of the increase in rate of rise expected from a fast sodium response. My question to Dr. De Mello concerns the space-constant measurements. Could the passage of large currents or the use of microelectrodes capable of passing such currents cause some degree of lesion in the AV nodal cell and therefore tend to decrease coupling and shorten the space constant?

DE MELLO: The point made in your question may be important. Many investigators are becoming aware that the frequent puncturing of a cell usually leads to membrane leakage and lesion and resulting perhaps in uncoupling. But, I do not think that this was a significant factor in our experiments.

Chapter 5

Influence of Intracellular pH on Cell-to-Cell Coupling in Sheep Purkinje Fibers

Robert Weingart, Peter Hess, and Walter R. Reber

Cell-to-cell coupling by means of junctional membrane channels of high conductance is a feature common to many tissues. In heart, morphologic and functional evidence shows that nexal structures between adjacent cells exist for the working myocardium, as well as for the specialized tissues, such as the Purkinje fibers, and the atrioventricular and sinoatrial nodal tissue (for references, see Pollack, 1976; De Mello, 1977; Irisawa, 1978; Pévet-Masson, 1979).

For some time, we have known that the "transfer" properties of the junctional membrane show a degree of plasticity. Loewenstein, working on insect salivary glands, suggested that the junctional conductance might be controlled by the intracellular calcium concentration ($[Ca^{2+}]_i$) in a graded fashion (Rose and Loewenstein, 1975; Loewenstein, 1978). And, several workers have since demonstrated a similar mechanism in cardiac tissue (for references, see De Mello, 1980a). The picture of the junctional channel that emerges from the functional studies is complemented by ultrastructural observations. Morphologic studies reveal that the junctional channel, or connexon, is composed of six protein subunits, whose molecular weight is of the order of 25,000 to 30,000 daltons (Caspar et al., 1977; Makowski et al., 1977; Hertzberg and Gilula, 1979; Kensler and Goodenough, 1980). Unwin and Zampighi (1980), using Fourier methods to analyze electronmicrographs, find two different configurations of the connexons, presumably corresponding to the open and closed state of a junctional channel. The transition from the open to the closed configuration of the hexagon seems to be produced by a radial inward movement of the inclined subunits.

Although the model by Unwin and Zampighi provides data for a mechanistic explanation of the changes in channel porosity, the molecular basis of the underlying mechanism remains obscure. For example, how do calcium ions interact with the structural units of the channel to induce the functional changes? Chemically, it has the capability of a wide range of selective interactions with polypeptides (Williams, 1971; Urry, 1978). It is tempting, therefore, to assume that the divalent cation is able to modify the conformation of the proteins composing the junctional channel and, thus, that it might control the conductance of the connexon.

Because hydrogen ions compete with Ca^{2+} for binding sites at functional groups of membrane polypeptides (Hille et al., 1978), perhaps they also influence intercel-

This work was supported by the Swiss National Science Foundation (No. 3.071-0.76 and 3.565-0.79).

lular coupling. Recently, two groups of investigators reported evidence supporting this hypothesis. They found that intracellular acidosis impairs the current flow between cells of early Xenopus embryos (Turin and Warner, 1980; Rink et al., 1980) and of mouse pancreas (Iwatsuki and Petersen, 1979). Rose and Rick (1978), who performed the experiments on insect salivary glands, did not find a correlation between uncoupling and changes in pH_i.

This chapter reports the experiments that we carried out to determine the effects of altering intracellular pH (pH_i) on the cell-to-cell communication in sheep cardiac Purkinje fibers. Because the junctional channels are only accessible from the intracellular surface of the cells, we chose experimental interventions that exclusively altered pH_i.

METHODS

Purkinje fibers were dissected from the ventricles of calf and sheep hearts. For an experiment, a preparation was placed in a small Perspex chamber (volume, 1 ml) that was temperature-controlled at 35° C. Preheated solution entered the chamber via a multiway tap that allowed fast solution changes. The Tris-buffered Tyrode's solution was composed of 150 mM $NaCl$, 4 mM KCl, 1.8 mM $CaCl_2$, 0.5 mM $MgCl_2$, 10 mM Tris (pH, 7.4), 10 mM glucose and was gassed with 100% O_2. In bicarbonate-buffered Tyrode's solution, Tris was replaced by HCO_3^-. The pH was kept at 7.4 by adding 24.5 mM HCO_3^- when the Tyrode's solution was equilibrated with 6% CO_2 ($P\text{CO}_2$, 40 mm Hg), and by adding 61.2 mM bicarbonate when it was gassed with 15% CO_2 ($P\text{CO}_2$, 100 mm Hg). Tonicity was maintained by reducing the Cl^- concentration. No osmotic compensation was made when 15 mM NH_4Cl was added to the Tris-buffered Tyrode's solution. The calcium activity was kept constant by adjusting all solutions to that of the Tris-buffered Tyrode's solution, which had been measured with a Ca^{2+}-sensitive macroelectrode. Carbon dioxide loss between the fluid reservoir and the experimental chamber was minimized by the plastic (Teflon™) tubing and a high flow rate (5 ml/min).

Cable parameters were extracted from one-dimensional cable analysis (Weidmann, 1952). Hyperpolarizing current pulses (duration, 200 to 300 msec; frequency, 0.5 to 1 Hz) were passed through a current electrode filled with 1.5 M potassium citrate and located at the very end of the preparation. The resulting deflections of the membrane voltage (V_m) were measured with two voltage electrodes filled with 3 M KCl potassium chloride and positioned at constant distances from the current electrode.

Intracellular pH measurements were made with recessed-tip glass microelectrodes. These electrodes were composed of an insulating aluminosilicate glass (tip size, 0.5 μm or less) and a sealed-in tip made from pH-sensitive glass (code 0150) and their construction was similar to that described by Thomas (1978). Each electrode was individually tested by exposing it to a series of calibrating solutions. These solutions, varying in pH (Tris or Hepes) from 6.5 to 7.5, contained a constant ionic background, chosen to simulate the cytoplasmic composition. This "internal solution" was composed of 120 mM KCl, 7 mM $NaCl$, 1 mM $MgCl_2$. The pH electrodes that had slopes ranging from 50 to 56 mV/pH unit were accepted for the experiments.

Intracellular Ca^{2+} was measured with liquid ion-exchanger microelectrodes sensitive to Ca^{2+}, which were manufactured as follows: Micropipettes pulled from glass (Pyrex™) capillary tubing were beveled on an air-driven rotating disc coated with aluminium oxide. Optical examination was performed to select pipettes with a tip size of 1 μm or slightly less. A series of selected pipettes, kept in a metal block, was first preheated to 200° C in an oven, before a droplet of *N,N*-dimethyltrimethylsilylamine was added for silanization. The Ca^{2+} sensor, provided by Dr. Ammann, was then introduced into the tip of the electrode from the back. The sensor consisted of 10% (wt/wt) neutral ligand ETH 1001 and 1% sodium tetraphenylborate in (o-nitrophenyl) octylether (Oehme et al., 1976). The shank of the electrode was then filled with "internal solution" (for composition, see below) whose *pCa* was set to 6.4 by 4 mM EGTA. Calibration of the electrodes was performed using the "internal solution" buffered to a pH of 7.2 with either 10 mM Tris or Hepes. The Ca^{2+} was varied between 10 mM and 40 n*M*. The lower concentrations were buffered with either 4 mM total NTA, HEDTA, or EGTA. The resulting calibration curves gave a 5- to 10-mV response between *pCa* 7 and 6. The electrodes showed no significant response to protons over a pH range from 6.5 to 7.5.

The ion-sensitive microelectrodes (10 to 100 GΩ) were connected to a high-impedance electrometer (WPI, model F 223A), and the conventional microelectrodes (10 to 15 MΩ) were connected to standard-unity gain electrometers (WPI, model 750 and M701). The signals were continuously recorded on a chart recorder (Brush 2400). To reduce the noise, the signals from the ion-sensitive electrodes were often filtered with a low-pass filter (corner frequency, 10 Hz).

RESULTS

Several methods have been described in the literature to manipulate the intracellular pH. In this study, we have chosen two experimental interventions, exposure to CO_2 and to NH_4Cl. Both methods lead to rapid shifts in pH_i.

Figure 1 shows the effect on the membrane potential (V_m; upper trace) and pH_i (lower trace) when a Purkinje fiber is exposed for short periods to Tyrode's solution of varying PCO_2. The lower trace represents the difference signal (V_{diff}) obtained by electronically subtracting V_m (the membrane resting potential, measured with a 3 M *KCl* microelectrode) from V_{HE} (the signal measured by the pH microelectrode). V_{diff} is a measure of the free-H^+ concentration. Changing from Tris-buffered Tyrode's solution ($PCO_2 \approx 0$ mm *Hg*) to bicarbonate-buffered Tyrode's solution equilibrated with 5% CO_2 (PCO_2, 40 mm *Hg*) produced a rapid intracellular acidification. Starting from a control value of 7.22, pH_i was altered by 0.27 pH units. After superfusion with Tris Tyrode's solution was resumed, pH_i fully recovered within 4 minutes. Exposure to bicarbonate-buffered Tyrode's solution equilibrated with 15% CO_2 (PCO_2, 100 mm *Hg*) led to a larger pH_i shift, 0.5 pH units in this case. Again, this change was reversible by washing out the solution containing the CO_2. The upper trace in Figure 1 illustrates that the intracellular acidification was accompanied by a slight hyperpolarization of the resting membrane potential V_m.

Similar shifts in pH_i induced by CO_2 have been described by Ellis and Thomas (1976) for cardiac tissue. These intracellular alterations are explained by the following sequence of steps. Carbon dioxide diffuses rapidly across the sarcolemma and equilibrates with the intracellular space. It undergoes hydration, which is catalyzed by carboanhydrase. The subsequent dissociation, producing H^+ and HCO_3^-, leads to the acidification.

Figure 2 illustrates the response of V_m (upper trace) and pH_i (lower trace) when 15 mM NH_4Cl was added to the Tris-buffered Tyrode's solution for a period of

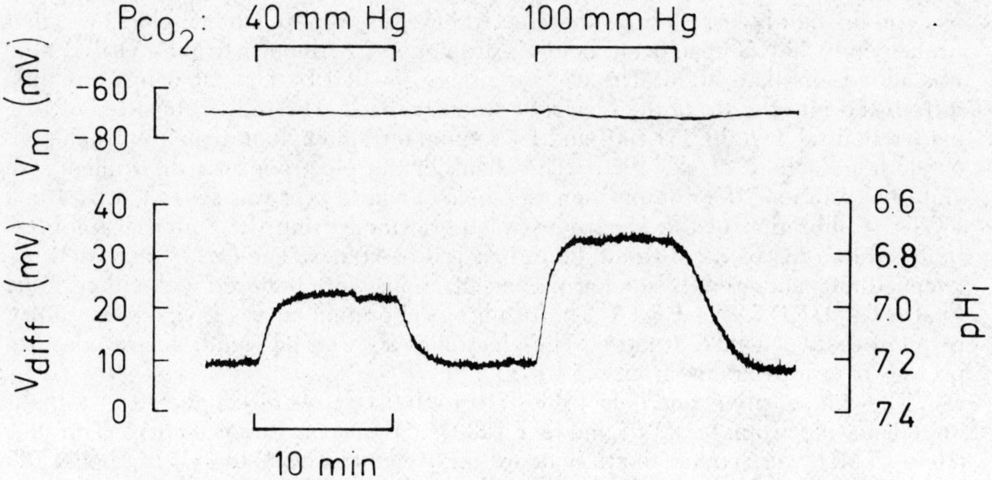

Figure 1. The effect of CO_2 on intracellular pH (pH_i). Tris-buffered Tyrode's solution (nominally CO_2-free) was replaced for 10-minute periods by bicarbonate-buffered Tyrode's solution equilibrated either with 5% CO_2 (PCO_2 = 40 mm Hg) or 15% CO_2 (PCO_2 = 100 mm Hg). The extracellular pH (pH_o) was kept at 7.4 throughout. The Purkinje fiber was impaled with a reference microelectrode filled with 3 M KCl and a pH microelectrode. The distance between the electrodes was about 0.5 mm. The upper trace shows the membrane resting potential, V_m, recorded with the reference electrode. The lower trace shows the signal of the difference between the electromotive force seen by the pH electrode and the reference electrode, V_{diff}. At the end of the run, the pH electrode was calibrated using "internal solutions" with different pH values (see Methods section).

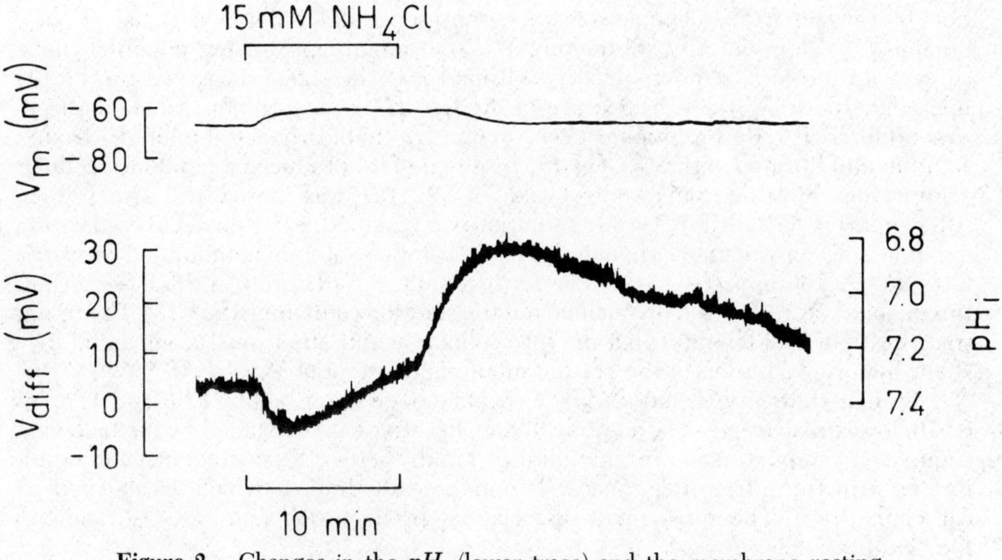

Figure 2. Changes in the pH_i (lower trace) and the membrane resting potential, V_m (upper trace), produced by a 10-min exposure to 15 mM NH_4Cl. For further details, see legend to Figure 1.

10 minutes. Perfusion with the NH_4Cl produced an initial alkalinization (phase 1); that is, the pH_i increased from 7.33 to 7.49 within 2.5 minutes. Thereafter, pH_i gradually declined (phase 2) and eventually reached a value above control. Washing out the NH_4Cl after 10 minutes led to a rapid acidification (phase 3) in that pH_i decreased to 6.84 within 7 minutes. The recovery from this low pH_i value (phase 4) occurred over the next 30 to 40 minutes. The upper trace in Figure 2 shows that exposure to NH_4Cl induced a reversible membrane depolarization of 5 mV. This might be explained by the potassium-like effect of NH_4^+ (Van Bogaert et al., 1978).

In cardiac tissue, similar biphasic changes in pH_i induced by NH_4Cl have also been observed by Deitmer and Ellis (1980). It has been proposed that phase 1 is due to the fast diffusion of ammonia across the sarcolemma and the subsequent hydration and dissociation into NH_4^+ and OH^- (Jacobs, 1940). Boron and DeWeer (1976) suggested that phase 2 is caused by slow influx of NH_4^+ into the cells, thus reducing the concentration of OH^-. Phase 3 is governed by the rapid diffusion of NH_3 out of the cells, leaving behind an excess of protons. Phase 4 is presumably brought about via activation of a proton pump (Aickin and Thomas, 1977; Deitmer and Ellis, 1980).

Using these two methods, we have carried out experiments to investigate the possible effects of pH_i on the cell-to-cell coupling (Weingart and Reber, 1979). Figure 3 shows the analysis of an experiment in which the effect of a reduction of CO_2 on the linear cable properties of a long Purkinje fiber was examined. The internal longitudinal resistance (r_i) of 1 cm of fiber length and the membrane resistance (r_m) of 1 cm of fiber length were calculated from the space constant (λ) and from the input resistance (R_{in}). The calculated values of r_i and r_m were plotted as percentage changes, relative to the averaged control values. At 0 minute, the bicarbonate-buffered Tyrode's solution that was equilibrated with 5% CO_2 was replaced by the Tris-buffered Tyrode's solution. This caused a decrease in r_i of about 45% (upper panel). Concomitant with this change, r_m increased by some 40% (middle panel). The lower panel shows that the withdrawal of the CO_2 also produced a depolarization of the membrane resting potential (V_m) by about 5 mV. At 11 minutes, when the bicarbonate-buffered Tyrode's solution was reinstated, all three parameters (r_i, r_m, and V_m) slowly returned towards their control values.

The effect of an increase of CO_2 on the cable properties was studied by, first, superfusing the preparation with Tris-buffered Tyrode's solution, which was then replaced by bicarbonate-buffered Tyrode's solution equilibrated with 15% CO_2. This treatment, which induces an intracellular pH load in the acidic direction (see Fig. 1, right hand side), produced an increase in r_i from between 20 to 40%.

The effect of a short exposure to 15 mM NH_4Cl on the linear cable properties of another Purkinje fiber is shown in Figure 4. The upper panel shows a biphasic change of r_i induced by this treatment. Addition of NH_4Cl at 0 minute produced a decrease in r_i over the first 2 minutes. The maximum decrease was 8%. This early decrease gave way to a gradual increase in r_i towards control value. Withdrawal of the NH_4Cl at 15 minutes led to a transient increase in r_i. A maximal increase of 17% was reached 5 minutes after washout. Recovery to the control value was achieved after 40 minutes. The middle panel shows that the change in r_m had a different time course. During the exposure to NH_4Cl, r_m decreased by about 18% and did not show any sign of a recovery. The recovery only took place when NH_4Cl was washed out. During the washout, r_m transiently overshot by some 12% before it approached the control level. The response of V_m is illustrated in the lower panel. As in Figure 2, V_m depolarized by 2 to 3 mV during the exposure to NH_4Cl. Removal of the NH_4Cl produced a transient hyperpolarization.

In all experiments performed with NH_4Cl, the initial decrease in r_i was found to vary between 8 and 25% whereas the late increase in r_i reached values ranging from 17 to 43%.

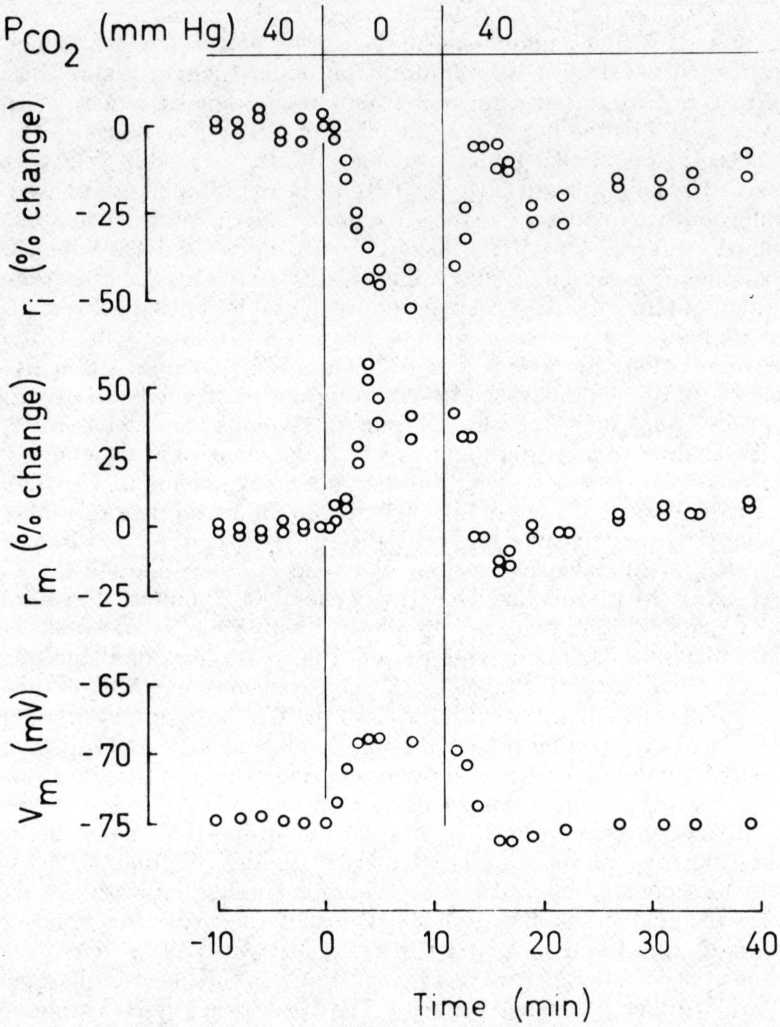

Figure 3. The effect of CO_2 on the internal longitudinal resistance of 1 cm fiber length, r_i (upper panel), the membrane resistance of 1 cm fiber length, r_m (middle panel), and the membrane resting potential, V_m (lower panel). Bicarbonate-buffered Tyrode's solution equilibrated with 5% CO_2 (PCO_2 = 40 mm Hg) was replaced with Tris-buffered Tyrode's solution (nominally CO_2-free) for a short period of time (11 min). The changes in r_i and r_m are plotted as a percentage of the averaged control values. Each point represents an individual determination. Length of fiber: 6 mm.

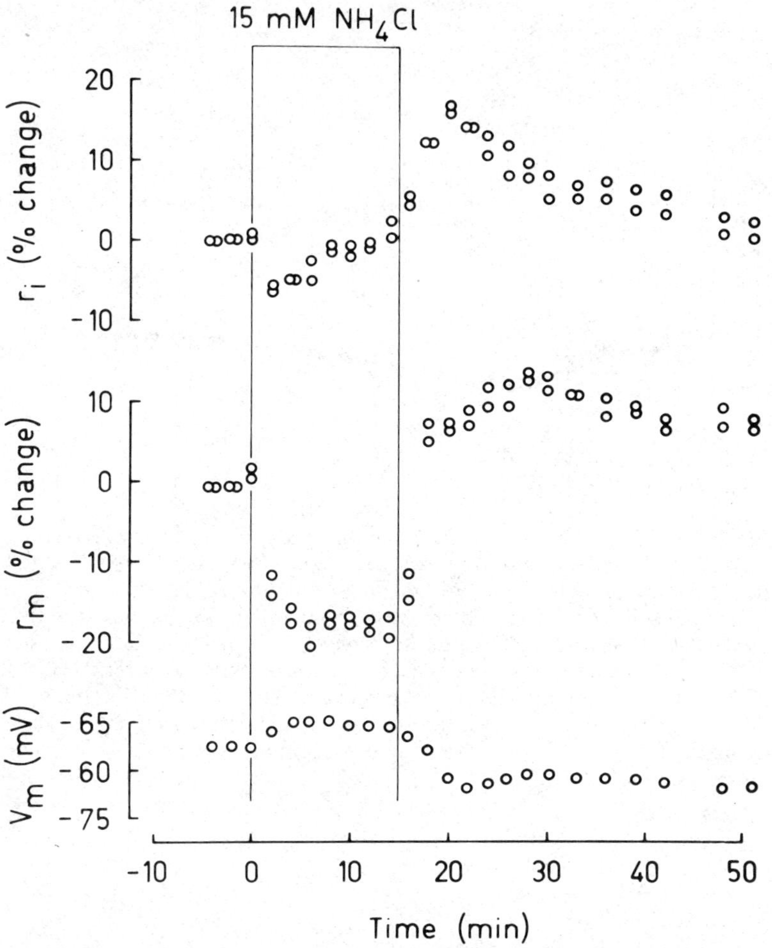

Figure 4. Changes in the cable parameters r_i (upper panel) and r_m (middle panel), and V_m (lower panel), induced by exposing a Purkinje fiber to 15 mM NH_4Cl for a period of 15 minutes. As in Figure 3, each point represents a single determination. Length of fiber: 7.1 mm.

To rule out the possibility of an involvement of Ca^{2+} in the observed changes in r_i, we have attempted to measure the free intracellular Ca^{2+} under the pH interventions (Hess and Weingart, 1980), using the Ca^{2+}-sensitive microelectrodes. Figure 5 shows the original records of an experiment in which the influence of carbon dioxide on pCa_i was studied. For a short period of time, the Tris-buffered Tyrode's solution was replaced by the bicarbonate-buffered Tyrode's solution equilibrated with 15% CO_2. The lower trace shows the difference signal, V_{diff}, obtained by subtracting V_m (the membrane resting potential measured with a 3 M KCl microelectrode) from V_{CaE} (the signal measured with the Ca^{2+}-sensitive electrode). V_{diff} is a measure of the free Ca^{2+} concentration. The V_{diff} trace shows that the free intracellular Ca^{2+} concentration was reversibly decreased during the treatment with CO_2. It decreased from 0.87 to 0.53 μM.

Figure 6 illustrates a similar experiment. This time the influence of NH_4Cl on pCa_i was investigated. Exposure to 15 mM NH_4Cl caused the free Ca^{2+} to increase

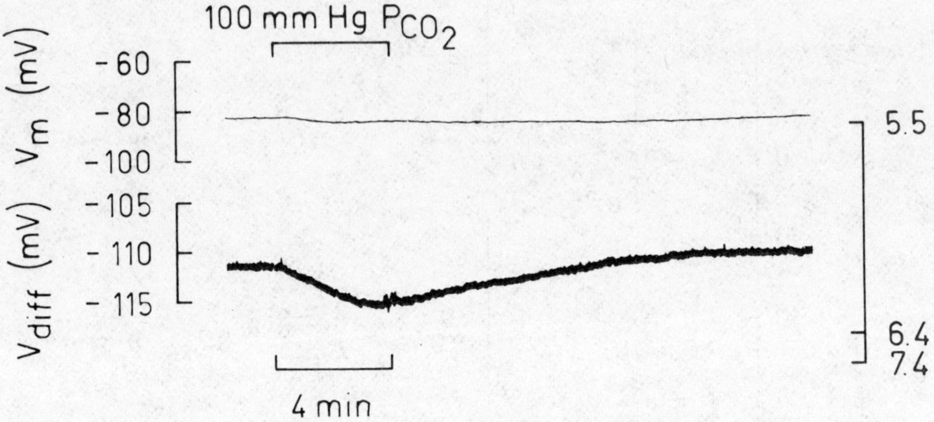

Figure 5. The effect of the intracellular pH (pH_i) on the intracellular free-Ca^{2+}. The preparation was exposed to a bicarbonate-buffered Tyrode's solution equilibrated with 15% CO_2 (Pco_2, 100 mm Hg) for 4 minutes. The upper trace shows the membrane resting potential, V_m, recorded with a conventional microelectrode, and the lower trace shows the difference signal, V_{diff}, obtained by subtracting V_m from the signal seen by the Ca^{2+} electrode. Calibration of the Ca^{2+} electrode using "internal solutions" of different pCa, was performed after the experimental run. This enabled us to relate the V_{diff} scale to a pCa scale. The experiment was performed at room temperature (22° C).

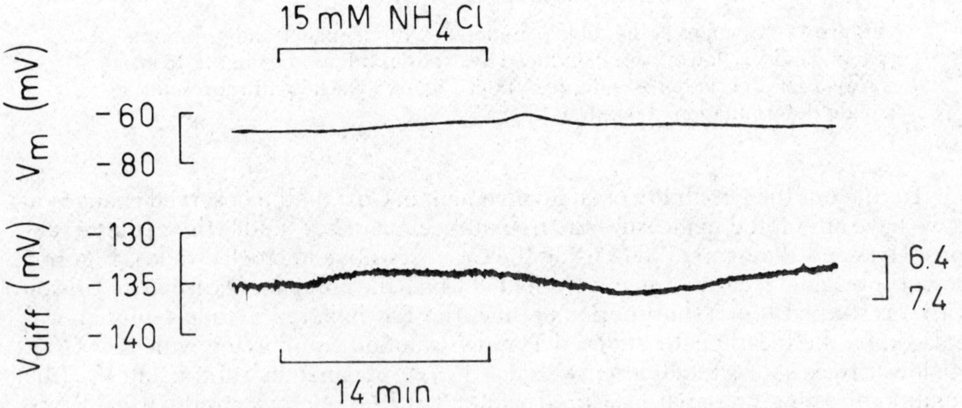

Figure 6. Changes in V_m (upper trace) and in pCa_i (lower trace) during a 14-minute exposure to 15 mM NH_4Cl. The experiment was carried out at room temperature (22° C). For further details, see legend to Figure 5.

from 0.09 to 0.18 μM. When the NH_4Cl was washed out, there was the suggestion of a transient undershoot of the Ca^{2+} signal.

The Ca^{2+} measurements revealed that the intracellular free-Ca^{2+} increased when the proton concentration was decreased, and that it decreased when the proton concentration was increased. In other words, the observed response of Ca^{2+} to the intracellular pH loads cannot be explained by a simple competitive interaction.

DISCUSSION

The purpose of this study is to test the hypothesis that protons are involved in controlling the conductance of the nexal membrane in cardiac tissue. The linear cable analysis that we have performed with sheep Purkinje fibers reveals that the internal longitudinal resistance, r_i, can be modified by established experimental interventions that induce intracellular pH shifts. Our results show, on the one hand, that the intracellular *alkalosis* induced by withdrawal of CO_2 (Fig. 1) or perfusing with NH_4Cl (Fig. 2) is accompanied by a *decrease* in r_i (Figs. 3 and 4). On the other hand, intracellular *acidosis* imposed by raising the CO_2 (Fig. 1) or by NH_4Cl washout (Fig. 2) is associated with an *increase* in r_i (Fig. 4). The correlation between pH_i and r_i is further substantiated by their similar time course during the experimentally induced pH loads. Although the two parameters seem to reach stable values during the short CO_2 interventions (Figs. 1 and 3, respectively), they both display phasic changes in the course of exposure to NH_4Cl (Figs. 2 and 4, respectively). Recently, De Mello (1980b) found a similar increase in r_i when he injected protons into Purkinje fibers.

Because the internal longitudinal resistance, r_i, reflects the contribution of two resistive elements in series, the cytoplasmic resistance, r_c, and the nexal resistance, r_n, the changes in r_i may be due to either an altered r_c or an altered r_n. But, the pH-dependent changes in r_c appear to go in the wrong direction to account for the observed alterations in r_i. Meves and Völkner (1958), working with frog skeletal muscle, demonstrated that intracellular acidification gives rise to a decrease of r_c. This suggests that the alterations in r_i that we have observed in the Purkinje fibers likely reflect genuine modifications of the nexal resistance, r_n.

Protons may act directly on the nexal membrane to cause the observed changes in r_i, or indirectly through changes in intracellular free-Ca^{2+}. But, a competitive interaction between H^+ and Ca^{2+} like that which may occur with the intracellular proteins (Fabiato and Fabiato, 1978), the sarcoplasmic reticulum (Nakamaru and Schwartz, 1972; Fabiato and Fabiato, 1978), or the mitochondria (Carafoli and Lehninger, 1972) seems unlikely because of what we found with the Ca^{2+} microelectrodes. In these experiments, *alkalosis*, which *decreased* the r_i, was associated with an *increase* in the $[Ca^{2+}]_i$ (Fig. 6); and *acidosis*, which *increased* r_i, was associated with a *decrease* in $[Ca^{2+}]_i$ (Figs. 5 and 6). The Ca^{2+} hypothesis predicts changes in the opposite direction. Our observations are thus consistent with a *direct* action of protons on the cell-to-cell coupling. The measured changes in r_i during the pH manipulations may be, if anything, underestimated because of the concomitant but opposite changes caused by the change in $[Ca^{2+}]_i$.

CONCLUSION

Calcium ions and protons are probably able to modify, independently, the electrical properties of the nexal membrane in cardiac tissue. This view gains support by recent morphologic observations. Peracchia and Peracchia (1980) investigated the effects of protons on the gap junctions isolated from fiber cells of the calf lens. At a pH of 6.5 or lower, they observed a transition from a disorderly to a crystalline packing of particles. These modifications turned out to be different from those induced by high Ca^{2+} concentrations (Peracchia and Dulhunty, 1976).

REFERENCES

Aickin CC, Thomas RC (1977) An investigation of the ionic mechanism of intracellular pH regulation in mouse soleus muscle fibres. J Physiol **273**:295–316

Boron WF, De Weer P (1976) Intracellular pH transients in squid giant axons caused by CO_2, NH_3, and metabolic inhibitors. J Gen Physiol **67**:91–112

Carafoli E, Lehninger AL (1972) A survey of the interaction of calcium ions with mitochondria from different tissues and species. Biochem J **122**:681–690

Caspar DLD, Goodenough DA, Makowski L, Phillips WC (1977) Gap junction structures: I. Correlated electronmicroscopy and X-ray diffraction. J Cell Biol **74**:605–628

Deitmer JW, Ellis D (1980) Interactions between the regulation of the intracellular pH and sodium activity of sheep cardiac Purkinje fibres. J Physiol **304**:471–488

De Mello WC (1977) Passive electrical properties of the atrioventricular node. Pflüg Arch **371**:135–139

De Mello WC (1980a) Intercellular communication and junctional permeability. *In* Membrane structure and function, Vol 3, edited by EE Bittar, New York, John Wiley & Sons, pp 127–170

De Mello WC (1980b) Influence of intracellular injection of H^+ on the electrical coupling in cardiac Purkinje fibres. Cell Biol Int Rep **4**:51–58

Ellis D, Thomas RC (1976) Direct measurement of the intracellular pH of mammalian cardiac muscle. J Physiol **262**:755–771

Fabiato A, Fabiato F (1978) Effects of pH on the myofilaments and the sarcoplasmic reticulum of skinned cells from cardiac and skeletal muscles. J Physiol **276**:233–255

Hertzberg EL, Gilula NB (1979) Isolation and characterization of gap junctions from rat liver. J Biol Chem **254**:2138–2147

Hess P, Weingart R (1981) Intracellular free calcium modified by pH_i in sheep cardiac Purkinje fibres (abstr). J Physiol **318**:14–15

Hille B, Woodhull AM, Shapiro BI (1978) Negative surface charge near sodium channels of nerve: divalent ions, monovalent ions, and pH. Philos Trans R Soc Lond [Biol] **270**:301–318

Irisawa A (1978) Fine structure of the small sinoatrial node specimen used for the voltage clamp experiment. *In* The Sinus Node, edited by FIM Bonke Ed, The Hague, Martinus Nijhoff, pp 311–319

Iwatsuki N, Peterson OH (1979) Pancreatic acinar cells: The effect of carbon dioxide, ammonium chloride and acetylcholine on intercellular communication. J Physiol **291**:317–326

Jacobs MH (1940) Some aspects of cell permeability to weak electrolytes. Cold Spring Harb Symp Quant Biol **8**:30–31

Kensler RW, Goodenough DA (1980) Isolation of mouse myocardial gap junctions. J Cell Biol **86**:755–764

Loewenstein WR (1978) Cell-to-cell communication. *In* Physiology of Membrane Disorders, edited by TE Andreoli, JF Hoffman, DD Fanestil, New York, Plenum Press, pp 335–356

Makowski L, Caspar DLD, Phillips WC, Goodenough DA (1977) Gap junction structures. II. Analysis of the X-ray diffraction data. J Cell Biol **74**:629–645
Meves H, Völkner KG (1958) Die Wirkung von CO_2 auf das Ruhemembranpotential und die elektrischen Konstanten der quergestreiften Muskelfaser. Pfluegers Arch **265**:457–476
Nakamaru Y, Schwartz A (1972) The influence of hydrogen ion concentration on calcium binding and release by skeletal muscle sarcoplasmic reticulum. J Gen Physiol **59**:22–32
Oehme M, Kessler M, Simon W (1976) Neutral carrier Ca^{2+}-microelectrode. Chimia (Aarau) **30**:204–206
Peracchia C, Dulhunty AF (1976) Low resistance junctions in crayfish. J Cell Biol **70**:419–439
Peracchia C, Peracchia LL (1980) Gap junction dynamics: Reversible effects of hydrogen ions. J Cell Biol **87**:719–727
Pévet-Masson MA (1979) The fine structure of cardiac pacemaker cells in the sinus node and in tissue culture. PhD Thesis, University of Amsterdam
Pollack GH (1976) Intercellular coupling in the atrioventricular node and other tissues of the rabbit heart. J Physiol **255**:275–298
Rink TJ, Tsien RY, Warner AE (1980) Free calcium in Xenopus embryos measured with ion-selective microelectrodes. Nature **283**:658–660
Rose B, Loewenstein WR (1975) Permeability of cell junction depends on local cytoplasmic calcium activity. Nature **254**:250–252
Rose B, Rick R (1978) Intracellular pH, intracellular free Ca, and junctional cell-cell coupling. J Membrane Biol **44**:377–415
Thomas RC (1978) Ion-Sensitive Intracellular Microelectrodes. London, Academic Press
Turin L, Warner AE (1980) Intracellular pH in early Xenopus embryos: Its effect on current flow between blastomeres. J Physiol **300**:489–505
Unwin PNT, Zampighi G (1980) Structure of the junction between communicating cells. Nature **283**:545–549
Urry DW (1978) Basic aspects of calcium chemistry and membrane interaction: on the messanger role of calcium. Ann NY Acad Sci **307**:3–27
Van Bogaert PP, Vereecke JS, Carmeliet EE (1978) The effect of raised pH on pacemaker activity and ionic currents in cardiac Purkinje fibers. Pflüg Arch **375**:45–52
Weidmann S (1952) The electrical constants of Purkinje fibres. J Physiol **118**:348–360
Weingart R, Reber WR (1979) Influence of internal pH on r_i of Purkinje fibres from mammalian heart (abst). Experientia **35**:929
Williams RJP (1971) Biochemistry of group IA and IIA cations. Adv Chem Ser **100**:155–173

Discussion

JOHNSON: The Ca^{2+} microelectrode is also sensitive to Na^+. How much of a change in internal Na^+ would be necessary to obtain a change of Ca^{2+} electrode potential of the order shown in your data?

WEINGART: The Ca^{2+} microelectrodes show indeed some sensitivity towards Na^+. To explain our data in terms of an altered intracellular Na^+ concentration we would need a change of the order of 5 to 10 mM. But, this type of interference would be small at the levels of internal Na^+ changes occurring in our experiments. We also should worry about H^+, but the calibration curves for our electrodes show that we do not need to be concerned about this point either. Therefore, I feel confident in saying that the signals recorded with the Ca^{2+} electrodes reflect changes in intracellular Ca^{2+}.

JOHNSON: Is it conceivable that you might have changes in internal Na^+ due to interference with the Na^+-K^+ transport?

WEINGART: Yes, provided the Na^+-K^+ transport is affected by pH. As a matter of fact, control experiments revealed that there are no such changes in internal Na^+ during the short time pH interventions studied.

REUTER: I suppose you had the KCl electrode in one cell and the Ca^{2+} electrode in another cell. Now, if you have decoupling between these two cells, is it still justified to rely on the measurements of Ca^{2+} concentration in one of them as representing what goes on in both? Could deviations of resting potential between the two uncoupled cells affect your results?

WEINGART: During our experimental interventions, the electrical coupling was only moderately changed, there was nothing like totally uncoupled cells. For this reason, I would expect uniformity of the membrane resting potential over the whole preparation.

I. COHEN: It seems that you have ruled out the possibility that the effect of pH on R_i can occur through a Ca^{2+}-mediated mechanism. What about the possibility that a Ca^{2+} effect on R_i can be mediated through a pH-change mechanism?

WEINGART: I do not think this happens. When intracellular Ca^{2+} is substantially increased, there is only a very modest decrease in intracellular pH. Even though both pH and pCa are well buffered, experimentally it seems much easier to induce large changes in intracellular Ca^{2+} than it is to change the intracellular pH.

C. COHEN: Your experiments suggest an alternative explanation for the effects of 2,4-DNP on cell coupling to that given earlier by Dr. De Mello. Because 2,4-DNP acts as a carrier for proton transport, the addition of this substance might lower intracellular pH, and thereby reduce cell coupling. This hypothesis predicts that the effect of 2,4-DNP would be decreased if the external pH were made more alkaline.

DE MELLO: We have done this experiment by adding NH_4Cl to the outside solution a few minutes after adding 2,4-DNP. There has been no recovery from the 2,4-DNP effect in spite of the expected alkalinization of the cytoplasm. Another point about H^+ release by intracellular Ca^{2+} should be considered. La^{3+}, a well-known inhibitor of Ca^{2+}-H^+ transport in mitochondria, also produces cell decoupling. This shows that you do not need a high H^+ concentration in the cell for decoupling to occur.

OLIVEIRA CASTRO: Birgit Rose shows in salivary glands results for the influence of pH in cell coupling that are different from those shown here. Would you care to comment?

WEINGART: Rick and Rose (J Membr Biol **44**:377–415, 1978) could indeed not find any evidence for a proton-mediated control of the cell-to-cell coupling. But, bear in mind that their conclusions were based mainly on their aequorin data. Because the Ca^{2+} response of this photoprotein is pH-dependent (Blinks et al., Pharmacol Rev **28**:1–93, 1976), it might be difficult to differentiate between effects due to H^+ changes and those due to Ca^{2+} changes.

Chapter 6

Prolonged Action Potentials from Squid Axons

Fidel Ramón

Although cardiac muscle has been extensively studied over the past three to four decades, our understanding of how cells behave as a functional syncytium and propagate action potentials is still incomplete (McAllister et al., 1975). A better understanding of the processes associated with excitation and propagation has been limited by the small size of cardiac cells and the complicated geometry of their assembly (Sommer and Johnson, 1968; Mobley and Page, 1972). Therefore, studies were begun with an axon preparation having prolonged (cardiac-like) action potentials but without the complicating factors such as cell geometry, electrogenic pumps, automatism, and electrotonic coupling.

Action potentials from squid axons perfused internally with solutions containing tetraethylammonium (TEA), a drug that affects the membrane potassium channels in a complex way (Armstrong and Binstock, 1965), are very similar in shape to those from cardiac muscle (Tasaki and Hagiwara, 1957). In this chapter, I will describe some membrane properties responsible for these prolonged action potentials from axons. I will show that the characteristic "plateau" is due to a slowly inactivating sodium conductance (Chandler and Meves, 1970a; 1970b; 1970c; 1970d) rather than to a decrease in potassium conductance, and that repolarization occurs when the potassium current finally overcomes the slowly inactivating sodium current.

METHODS

Experiments were performed on axons dissected from squids (*Loligo pealei*) available at the Marine Biological Laboratory at Woods Hole, Massachusetts. Axons were excised and cleaned of most adhering connective tissue and small fibers, and the axoplasm was squeezed out with a rubber roller by the technique of Baker et al. (1962a). Axons were reinflated with internal solution (see below) and placed in an experimental chamber.

A small "space-clamped" region of squid axons was studied by skewering it with a type of axial electrode known as "piggyback" (Wu and Narahashi, 1973). The external electrodes were small blocks of silver platinized at the surface facing the axon. Action potentials recorded under these conditions are known as membrane action potentials (MAP's), to distinguish them from unrestricted propagated action potentials (PAP's). The voltage-clamp electronic circuit was conventional except for a "gated logic switch" that allowed changes from the current-clamp to the voltage-clamp mode, and vice versa, in about 1 μsec (Bezanilla et al., 1970). Series resistances of about 3 to 4 Ωcm^2 were compensated for.

PAP's were studied by, first, perfusing the axon trunk and its two main branches and placing them in another experimental chamber (Ramón and Moore, 1979). A pair of small external hook electrodes were then placed on the axon to stimulate action potentials. Voltage recordings were made by intracellular microelectrodes filled with 2.5 M KCl for final resistances of about 10 MΩ.

The external perfusion solution was artificial sea water (ASW), composed of 450 mM Na, 10 mM K, 50 mMCa, and 576 mM Cl and buffered with 5 mM HEPES to a pH of 7.3. The internal perfusion medium was standard internal solution (SIS), composed of 320 mM K, 50 mM Na, 50 mM F, 320 mM glutamate, 333 mM sucrose and buffered with 15 mM phosphate to a pH of 7.4. Internal solution free of potassium ions was obtained by replacing K glutamate with 275 mM CsF (isosmolarity kept with sucrose). Temperature of the experimental chamber was kept between 8° and 12° C by a thermoelectric device controlled by an electronic feedback circuit. Added to the SIS were 20 mM tetraethylammonium chloride (TEA) and 0.2 mM N-bromoacetamide (NBA). NBA was perfused for about 1 minute.

Individual ionic conductances during the plateau phase of action potentials from axons perfused with TEA were studied with an electronic circuit that turned the membrane potential control on and off. A complete description of this technique and its application to squid axons perfused with normal solutions has been given by Bezanilla et al., (1970). Briefly, the technique consists of alternatively clamping the membrane potential to the sodium and potassium equilibrium potentials at different times during the action potential, and measuring individual potassium and sodium ionic currents developed after capacitative transients. Ionic conductances can then be calculated with the following equations:

The total membrane current (I_m) is the sum of the individual sodium (I_{Na}), potassium (I_K), and leak (I_l) components (Hodgkin and Huxley, 1952),

$$I_m = I_{Na} + I_K + I_l \tag{1}$$

because each ionic current component is equal to the product of the channel conductance (G) and the driving force ($V - V_e$),

$$I_m = G_{Na}(V - V_{Na}) + G_K(V - V_K) + G_l(V - V_l) \tag{2}$$

Also, because $G_l << G_{Na}$ and G_K, we can eliminate G_l from Eq. 2, and get

$$I_m = G_{Na}(V - V_{Na}) + G_K(V - V_K) \tag{3}$$

Thus, when the membrane potential is held near the potassium or sodium equilibrium potentials,

$$G_K = \frac{I_m(V_{Na})}{V_K - V_{Na}} \tag{4}$$

and

$$G_{Na} = \frac{I_m(V_K)}{V_{Na} - V_K} \tag{5}$$

where $I_m(V_{Na})$ and $I_m(V_K)$ are the membrane currents at the corresponding reversal potentials.

The advantage of this technique over regular voltage-clamp studies for obtaining membrane ionic conductances is that individual ionic conductances are obtained during the action potential examined.

RESULTS

Voltage Clamp

Ionic currents from squid axons, both intact and perfused with normal solutions or with solutions containing sodium fluoride and TEA, have been studied with voltage-clamp techniques (Hodgkin and Huxley, 1952; Chandler and Meves, 1970a; Armstrong, 1975). Thus, only the voltage-clamp data directly relevant to interpreting the prolonged action potentials used in this study will be presented.

Internal Solutions Free of Potassium Ions

Axons perfused with potassium-free solutions are ideal for measuring the remaining sodium currents. A family of voltage-clamp pulses applied to K^+-free perfused axons elicits sodium currents that show an initial transient component and a steady-state component (Fig. 1H).

The initial transient (fast) sodium currents have characteristics of the activation, the inactivation, and the reversal potential described by Hodgkin and Huxley (1952). The steady-state (slow) current component, on the contrary, is different in that it is inactivated with a very slow time constant (Fig. 1, A–G; see also Chandler and Meves, 1970c). Both current components are equally sensitive to TTX (Chandler and Meves, 1970a; Oxford, personal communication). A plot of the current-voltage relationships of these two sodium current components, fast (filled circles) and slow (open circles), is shown in Figure 2. The slow sodium current is inward in the range ±40 mV and reverses in sign at about the same potential as the fast transient sodium current does.

Inactivation characteristics of sodium currents can be obtained by conventional two-pulse experiments (Hodgkin and Huxley, 1952). A plot of the fast-sodium inactivation parameter (h-inf; Fig. 3), obtained during perfusion of the axons with potassium-free solutions, shows that a fraction of sodium current is not inactivated at membrane potentials up to +25 mV. This, again, is the slowly inactivating (steady-state) sodium current component (Chandler and Meves, 1970b; 1970c).

Internal Solutions Containing TEA

Voltage-clamp currents resulting from TEA added to SIS are shown in Figure 4 (inset). Current-voltage relationships show that normal peak sodium currents are unaffected by TEA, whereas potassium currents are blocked in a characteristic way (see also Armstrong and Binstock, 1965). Current-voltage relationships 80 msec after the beginning of the clamp pulse show inward currents in the region −30 to +10 mV (Fig. 4; open circles).

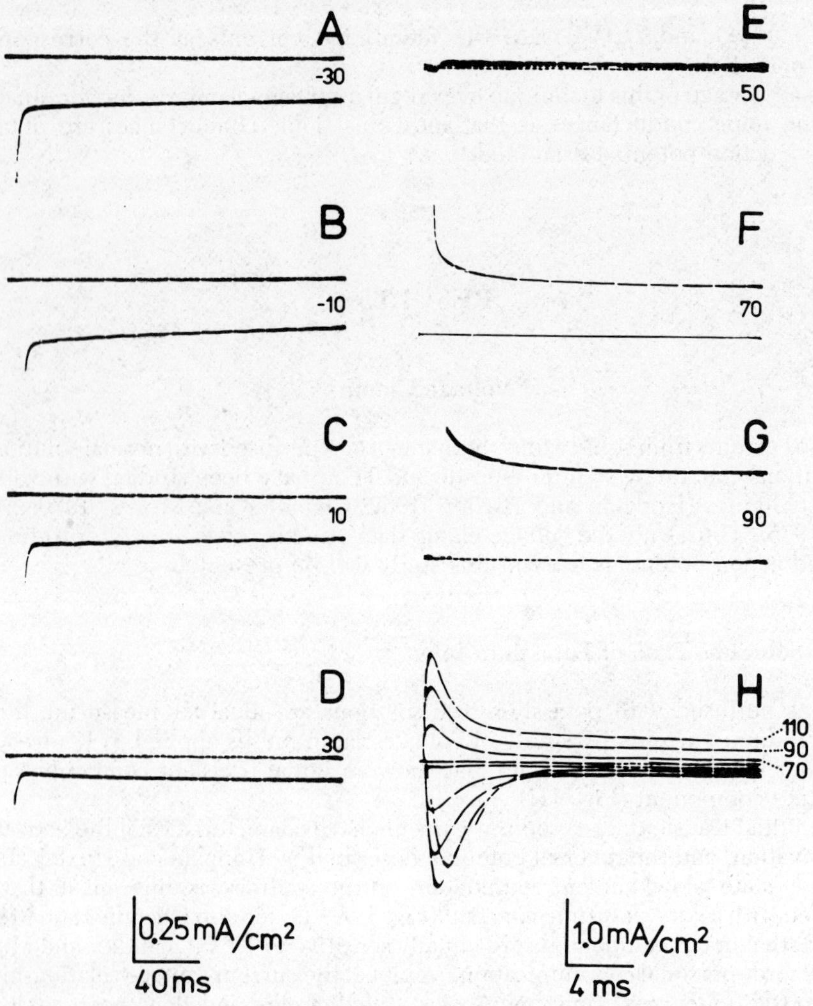

Figure 1. Sodium currents obtained from voltage-clamped squid axons internally perfused with solutions free of potassium ions. The membrane potential during the clamp pulse is given at the right of each trace. Holding potential was −70 mV. Graph H (calibration bars at the bottom right) shows peak currents and the beginning of steady-state currents. These slow currents are seen better in graphs A through G (calibration bars at the bottom left). Note that around 0 mV there is a significant steady-state inward sodium current.

Membrane Action Potentials

Prolonged Action Potentials

Two methods of producing prolonged action potentials in squid axons were used: *(1)* blocking the potassium channels with TEA, and *(2)* blocking the fast-sodium inactivation with NBA. Both drugs were perfused internally.

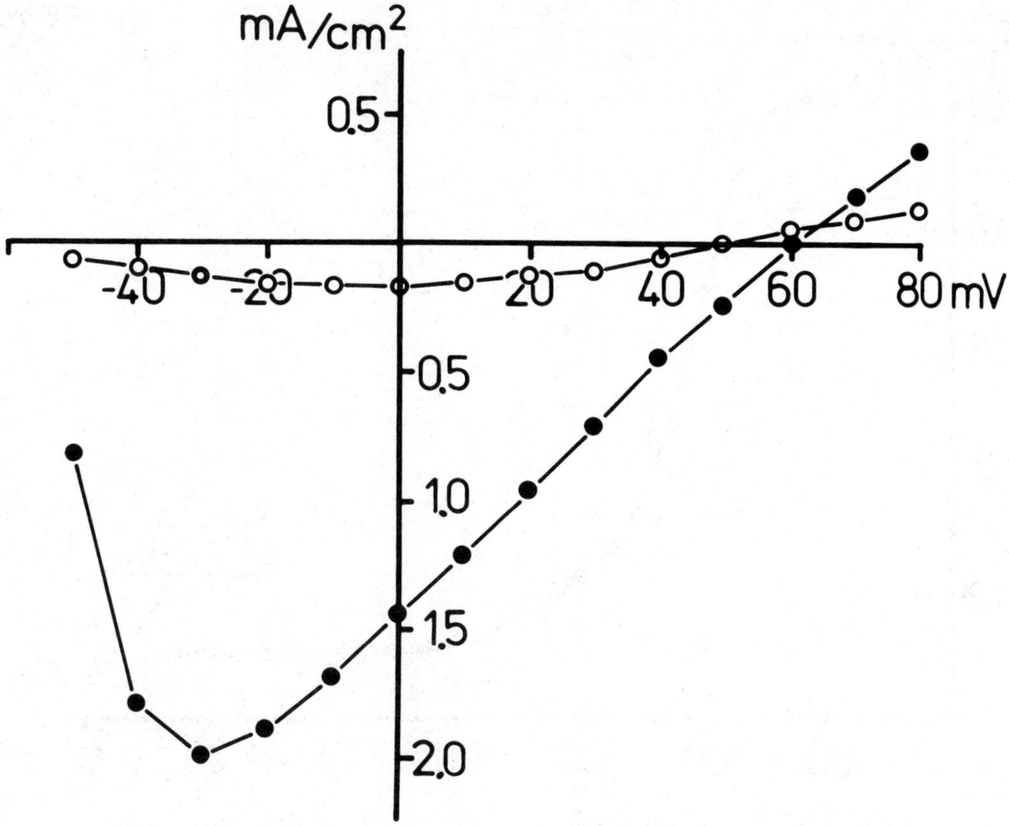

Figure 2. Current-voltage relationships of the sodium currents shown in Fig. 1. Peak currents (filled circles) and steady-state currents (open circles) are inward in the region ±40 mV.

(1) Blocking potassium channels. Action potentials recorded from squid axons internally perfused with TEA (Fig. 5) consisted of a fast upstroke, typically about 300 V/sec at 16° C, followed by a phase of sustained depolarization, the "plateau." The spike led to the plateau in a smooth transition without the "dip" seen in some cardiac muscles (Vassalle, 1966). These action potentials retained their configuration as long as perfusion was maintained. The effects of TEA were completely reversible.

(2) Blocking sodium inactivation. NBA is a drug that destroys inactivation of the sodium conductance in squid axons (Oxford et al., 1978). Partial elimination of sodium inactivation would be expected to prolong the action potentials (Weidmann, 1951; Takenaka and Yamagishi, 1969).

Figure 6B shows an MAP obtained during perfusion of a squid axon with NBA at a concentration of 0.250 mM for about 1 minute. The prolonged action potential had a spike and a phase of sustained depolarization separated by a "dip." The spike was sharp, and the initial repolarization was fast. This led to a plateau at an almost constant potential around −15 mV. Prolonged exposure of the axon to NBA led to small action potentials of seconds in duration and eventually to spontaneous activity. These effects were irreversible.

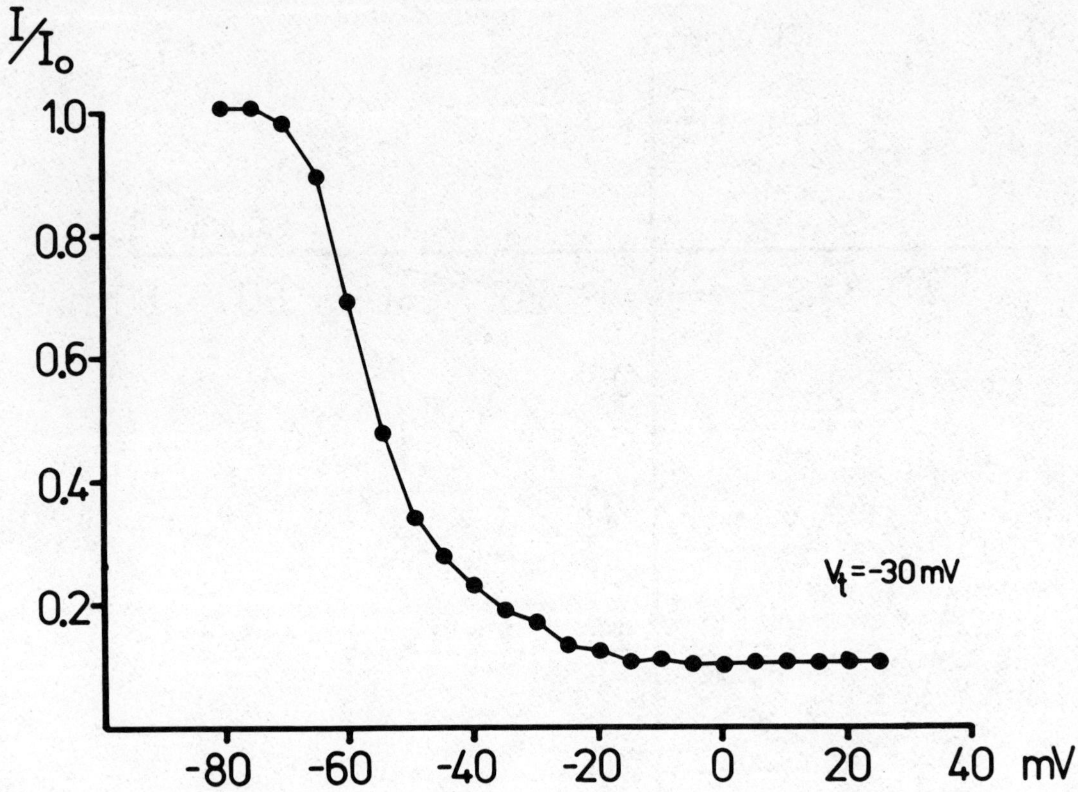

Figure 3. Inactivation curve of sodium currents from axons perfused with solutions free of potassium ions. Note that inactivation does not reach 0 at any membrane potential, and around 0 mV has values of about 0.1. Test pulse was to −30 mV.

Duration of the Action Potential and Refractory Period

The duration of TEA action potentials was very sensitive to stimulus frequency. Figure 5 shows action potentials elicted by two stimuli separated by a short interval. When a first action potential was allowed to follow its normal course, a second stimulus applied immediately after produced a brief response. But, when the first action potential was terminated abruptly by a brief voltage-clamp pulse (see below), a second stimulus elicited an action potential of almost normal duration.

The dependence of MAP's on the frequency of stimulus also provided a convenient way to set their duration. Experiments reported here were performed for convenience, with action potentials whose duration was relatively short. But, similar results could have been obtained regardless of the duration of the action potential.

Membrane Resistance during the Plateau Phase

Membrane voltage changes produced by the injection of square pulses of current during the plateau phase of MAP's were proportional to the membrane slope resis-

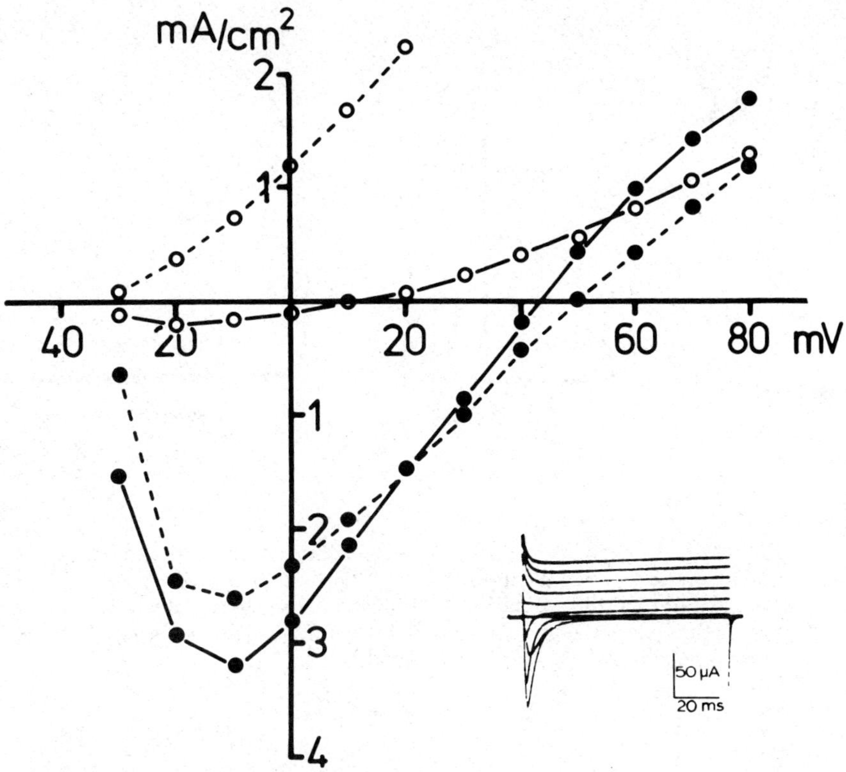

Figure 4. Current voltage relationships of axons perfused internally with TEA (20 mM) showing control curves (dotted lines) and the effect of TEA on these relationships. Peak transient currents (filled circles) are slightly affected, whereas steady-state currents (open circles) are blocked by the drug. Note that there is a remaining component of inward current around −20 mV. Inset shows current records.

tance in space-clamped axons. Figure 6 shows these voltage changes during MAP's from axons perfused with TEA (Fig. 6A) and with NBA (Fig. 6B). In both cases, the amplitudes of the voltage changes were small at the beginning of the plateau, then increased towards the end of the action potential, reaching values close, but not equal, to those at rest. The two superimposed traces in Figure 6B show different MAP's durations due to differences in frequency of stimulation. These results indicate that the membrane resistance during the plateau was lower than it was at rest, a finding opposite to that generally described for cardiac muscle (Fozzard and Sleator, 1967; Goldman and Morad, 1977a; 1977b).

Experiments were conducted in an attempt to observe changes in membrane resistance during the plateau of PAP's (Fig. 6C). Square pulses of current were injected by a microelectrode, and propagated action potentials were recorded with a microelectrode nearby. The lack of change in the amplitude of voltage responses could be interpreted as indicating that membrane resistance (strictly, input impedance) did not change throughout the phase of sustained depolarization (see Discussion).

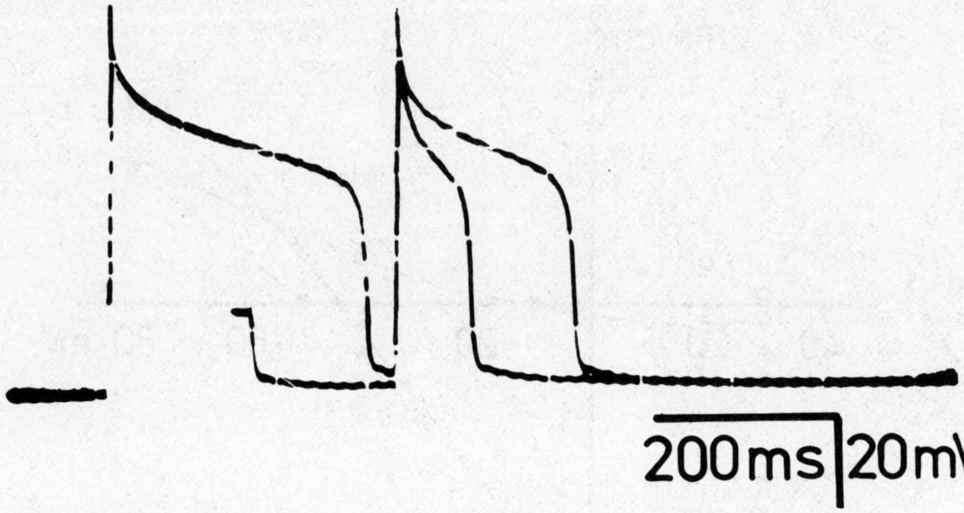

Figure 5. Effect of the duration of a TEA action potential on another action potential elicited by a second stimulus. When the first action potential is of normal duration, the second one is brief and with a short plateau. But, if the first action potential is interrupted by a brief voltage-clamp pulse, the duration of the second one is prolonged.

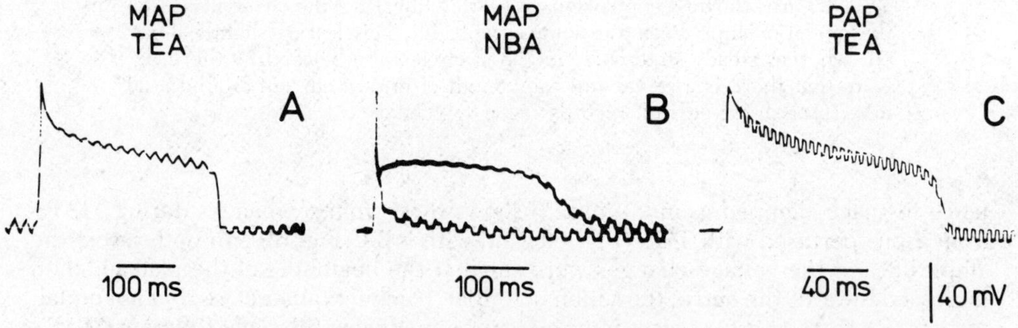

Figure 6. Effect of small square current pulses delivered during prolonged duration action potentials from squid axons. In graph A the axon was perfused with TEA; in graph B, with a short (about 1 min) application of NBA; and in graph C, with TEA. MAP stands for membrane action potential; and PAP, for propagated action potential. Note that, in graphs A and B, the amplitude of voltage changes in response to current pulses is lower at the beginning of the plateau than it is at the end. In graph C, there is no change in the amplitude of voltage changes in response to current pulses. See text for further details.

Ionic Conductances during the Plateau

Figure 7, A and B, shows the results obtained when the potential control was turned on and off as axons were being perfused with standard solutions (see also Bezanilla et al., 1970). In Figure 7A, the membrane potential was clamped to −70 mV at different times during the action potential, and current records in response to several voltage pulses were superimposed. Because the transmembrane voltage was constant, the time course of an increase in sodium conductance during the action potential could be seen by interpolating the beginning of those current records. In Figure 7B the voltage-clamp pulse displaced the membrane potential to +50 mV (a value that approximated the sodium equilibrium potential); thus, traces show only potassium currents. The time course of the increase in potassium conductance was also obtained by interpolating the beginning of the current traces.

Figure 7, C and D, shows the results of perfusing squid axons internally with TEA. When the membrane potential was clamped to −70 mV during the action potential, the current traces demonstrate the sodium conductance decreased. When the membrane potential was clamped to +50 mV, the potassium conductance remained nearly constant throughout the plateau of the action potential (Fig. 7D).

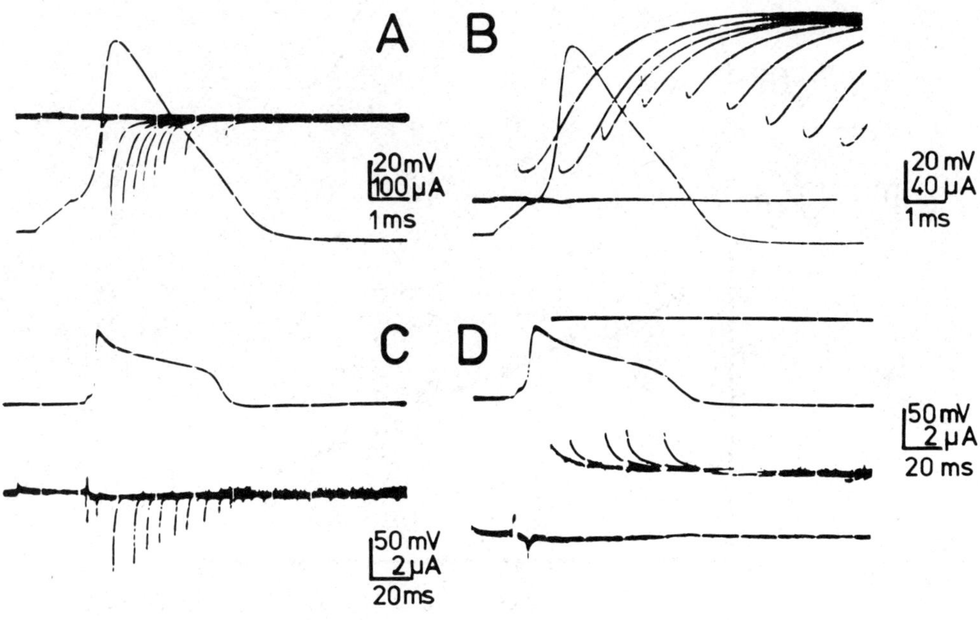

Figure 7. Results of turning the potential control on and off in squid axons perfused with normal solutions (graphs A and B) and solutions containing TEA (graphs C and D). Conductance curves for individual ionic components of the action potential can be obtained from these records as described in the text and are plotted in Fig. 8. Resting potentials were −64 mV in graphs A and B and −60 mV in C and D.

Figure 8 shows the values of sodium and potassium conductances obtained during action potentials recorded from axons perfused internally with TEA. The upper part of the figure provides, for reference, a trace of a TEA action potential. The large increase in sodium conductance responsible for the initial depolarization would be off scale in the figure, and it is not shown. After the initial transient increase, sodium conductance decreased during the plateau of the action potential whereas potassium conductance remained at a nearly constant level. These results provide the basis for explaining the changes in membrane resistance during the plateau phase of action potentials illustrated in Figure 6A.

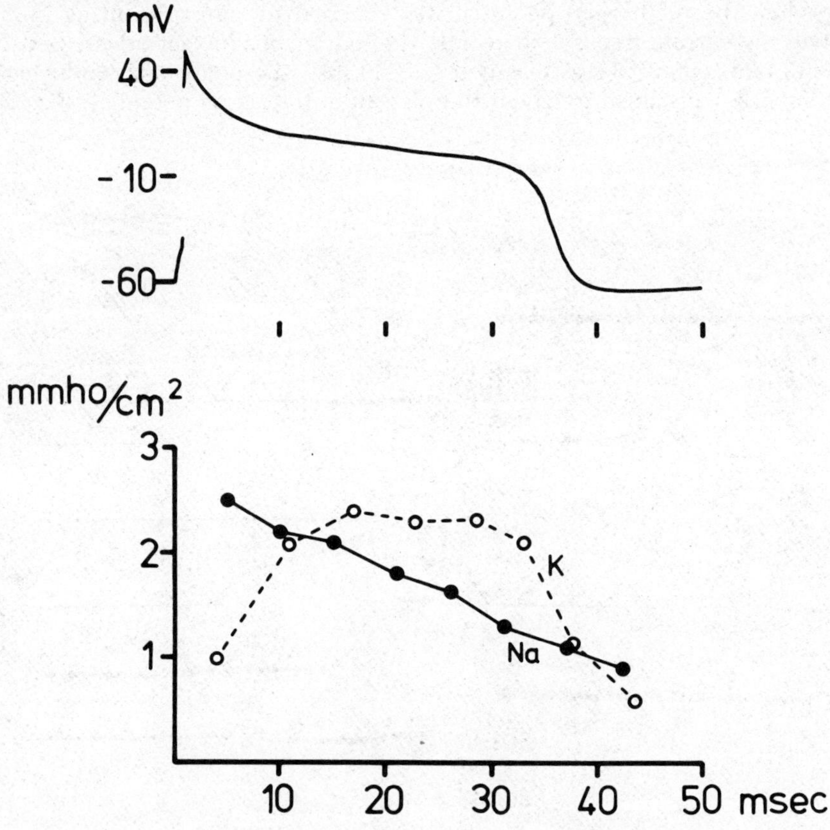

Figure 8. Sodium and potassium conductances during a TEA action potential obtained by turning the potential control on and off. The upper part of the figure shows the trace of an action potential for reference. The lower part of the figure shows the ionic conductances calculated as described in the text. Note that sodium conductance decreases during the plateau phase of the action potential, whereas potassium conductance remains constant.

All-or-Nothing Repolarization of the Action Potential

Action potentials interrupted by a brief voltage-clamp pulse during the plateau phase repolarized at the end of the pulse if the membrane potential was displaced below a certain voltage threshold. Figure 9, A–D, shows TEA MAP's interrupted at different times by voltage-clamp pulses to various levels. Voltage pulses above a threshold minimally perturbed the action potential, which continued its normal course after release by the clamp. Voltage pulses below that threshold resulted in sudden repolarization of the action potential.

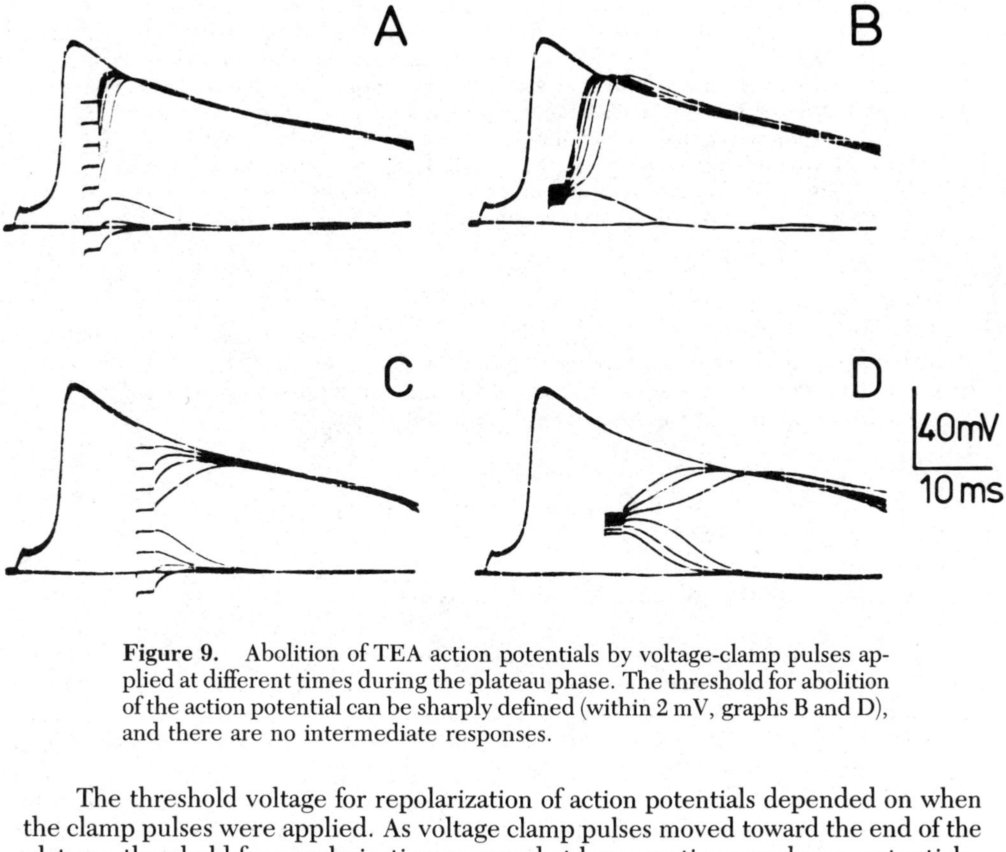

Figure 9. Abolition of TEA action potentials by voltage-clamp pulses applied at different times during the plateau phase. The threshold for abolition of the action potential can be sharply defined (within 2 mV, graphs B and D), and there are no intermediate responses.

The threshold voltage for repolarization of action potentials depended on when the clamp pulses were applied. As voltage clamp pulses moved toward the end of the plateau, threshold for repolarization occurred at less negative membrane potentials.

Two Phases of the Action Potential

The two phases of prolonged action potentials, spike and plateau, can be selectively abolished. To illustrate this behavior axons were perfused with TEA or NBA.

Figure 10A shows a control TEA action potential with the two phases, spike and plateau, already described. Superimposed traces show that action potentials developed at the end of a brief voltage-clamp pulse exhibited no spike; but, their plateau component superimposed on control records. These action potentials composed only of plateau were also seen when axons where perfused with only NBA (Fig. 10B).

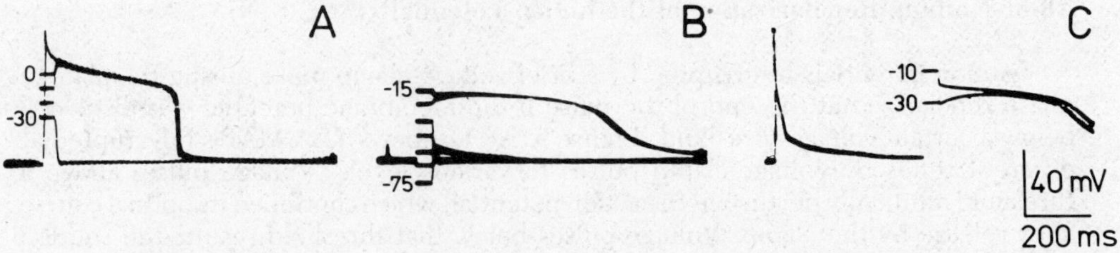

Figure 10. Two components of the action potential. Graph A shows an action potential obtained by perfusion of squid axons with TEA. The action potential with spike was obtained by stimulating with a current pulse. The other action potentials were developed at the end of a voltage-clamp pulse. Note that the plateau phase follows the same time course whether or not it is preceded by a spike. Graph B, an action potential from an axon perfused with only NBA, shows the plateau component without spike and the behavior of all-or-nothing repolarization when the clamp pulse is below the threshold level. Graph C, obtained after increasing the frequency of stimulation, shows only the spike component of an action potential. The mechanism underlying the plateau component is still developing as it can be demonstrated by a voltage-clamp pulse.

Conversely, at high frequencies of stimulation, the spike persisted, but the plateau was abolished (Fig. 10C). Even under these conditions, the slow inward current developed to a certain extent, as was demonstrated by voltage-clamp pulses (to −10 and −30 mV) that elicited a plateau at the end of the pulse (Fig. 10C).

Propagated Action Potentials

Interactions in Inhomogeneous Membrane Regions

Propagated action potentials were studied on a preparation developed to produce interactions between two regions of membrane with different properties. The preparation was a dissected axon consisting of a trunk and one axon branch, both of which were perfused with TEA, and the other branch, which remained perfused with normal SIS (Ramón and Moore, 1979).

When a single stimulus was applied to the SIS-perfused branch, interaction could be seen between the action potential generated in this branch and that propagated to the TEA-perfused branch. Figure 11 shows action potentials recorded in the trunk near the bifurcation (upper trace) and at the SIS-perfused branch (lower trace). When TEA perfusion of the trunk and a main branch was initiated, progressive effects of prolongation of action potentials occurred (upper traces in Fig. 11, A−F). As the action potential duration increased, a hump developed on the falling phase of action potentials in the TEA-free branch (Fig. 11, B−C, lower trace). This hump changed into an action potential of small amplitude (Fig. 11D, lower trace). With continued lengthening of the action potential at the trunk, the TEA-free branch developed two small action potentials (Fig. 11, E−F). The second one, of larger amplitude than the first one, reflected back to the axon trunk and produced a hump at the end of the repolarization phase (Fig. 11F). This reflection produced a third small action potential in the SIS-perfused axon branch (Fig. 11G). Later, a very complex interaction between

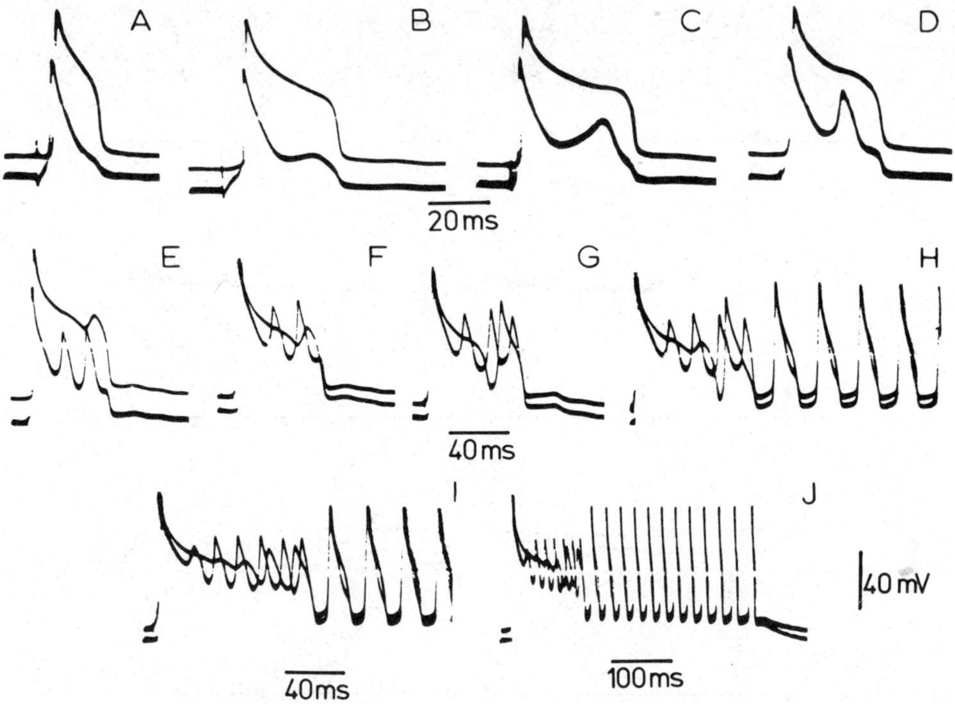

Figure 11. Action potentials recorded at two axon regions affected differently by internal perfusion with TEA. In all graphs, the upper trace is the recording from the axon trunk and the lower trace is from the axon branch TEA-free. A single stimulus is applied to the axon branch to elicit the propagated response. See text for further details (Modified from Ramón and Moore, 1979).

both axon regions occurred as spikes of different amplitude rode on the action potential recorded at the axon trunk. Finally, both axon regions synchronized their activities in a train of spikes that terminated spontaneously (Fig. 11, H–J). During the period of interactions between those axon regions, the speed of propagation of initial action potentials remained unchanged (about 10 m/sec), whereas that of reflected spikes varied (1.5 to 2.2 m/s) (see also Ramón and Moore, 1979).

Unidirectional Block

The effect of an asymmetric obstacle in the propagation of action potentials was studied on perfused squid axons. Axons were perfused with SIS and then placed between two plastic (Lucite™) plates of 1 cm in length and 520 μ in height. The plates were driven towards each other by a micromanipulator, and the space between them was covered with a microscope coverglass to prevent the axon from protruding up. In this way, the coverglass delimited a rectangular compartment (cross-section) whose dimensions were the height of the plates and a variable width. The axon accommodated to the compartment between the plates for the final shape illustrated in Figure 12.

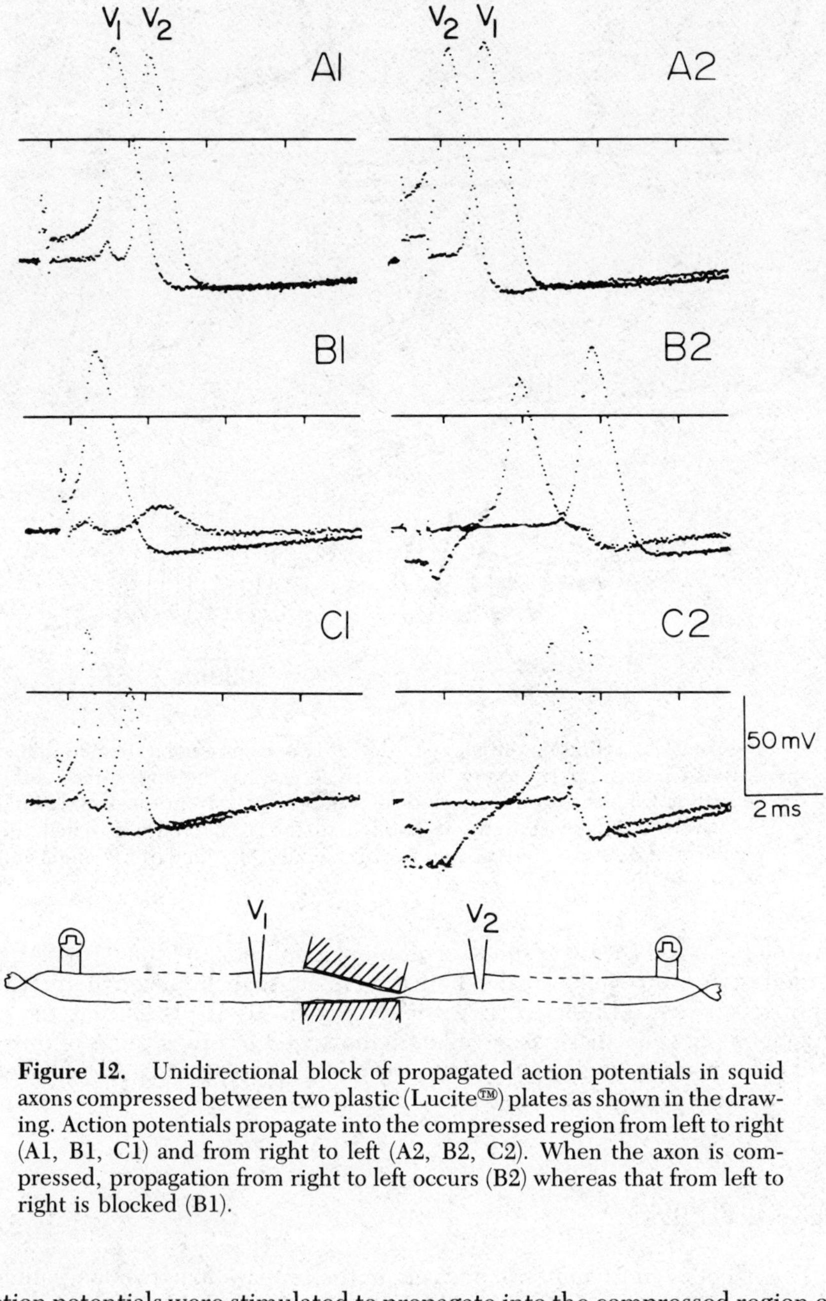

Figure 12. Unidirectional block of propagated action potentials in squid axons compressed between two plastic (Lucite™) plates as shown in the drawing. Action potentials propagate into the compressed region from left to right (A1, B1, C1) and from right to left (A2, B2, C2). When the axon is compressed, propagation from right to left occurs (B2) whereas that from left to right is blocked (B1).

Action potentials were stimulated to propagate into the compressed region of the axon from both sides. To assess propagation, microelectrode recordings were made at both sides of this region and were labeled V_1 and V_2 (Fig. 12). Panels A1 and A2 showed control records, with action potentials propagating from left to right on A1 and from right to left on A2. After the plates compressed the axon, recordings showed that propagation was occurring from right to left (Panel B2), but that from left to right (Panel B1) was blocked. When the compression was released, bidirectional propagation was reestablished (Fig. 12, C1–C2).

Discussion

Action potentials recorded from squid axons perfused internally with TEA (Tasaki and Hagiwara, 1957) resemble in shape those from cardiac muscle (Hoffman and Cranefield, 1960). Tasaki and Hagiwara (1957) conducted experiments such as those performed on cardiac muscle and suggested that similarities between axons and muscle were more than fortuitous. These similarities have been analyzed from time to time by different authors (Brady and Woodbury, 1960; FitzHugh, 1960; George and Johnson, 1961; Adelman et al., 1965; Bergman et al., 1968).

In this chapter, I describe experiments conducted to test the extent of similarities between squid axons perfused internally with TEA and cardiac muscle. The aim of these studies was to study the propagation of prolonged action potentials in a simple unidimensional structure, and not to analyze the membrane properties of cardiac muscle. Moreover, although there are obvious differences between axons and muscle (Vassalle, 1979), this chapter stresses the similarities rather than the differences.

Tetraethylammonium blocks potassium channels in squid axons (Armstrong and Binstock, 1965). Although TEA is thought to act selectively on potassium channels, it may also have some effects on sodium channels (Shoukimas and French, 1978). In the experiments reported here, however, the main result of internal perfusion of the axons with TEA (20 mM) was a marked reduction of potassium currents.

Squid axons perfused with solutions containing NaF (50 mM) have a steady-state sodium current that inactivates very slowly with a time constant of 1 to 3 sec at 16° C (Chandler and Meves, 1970c; see also Adelman and Senft, 1966). This component of the sodium current may involve a second open state of the sodium channel (Armstrong and Bezanilla, 1977). In axons perfused with normal internal solutions, the slow sodium current does not seem to have appreciable effects on action potentials (Baker et al., 1962b). Repolarization and post-hyperpolarization are completely dominated by a large increase in potassium conductance (Hodgkin and Huxley, 1952). On the other hand, when potassium currents are reduced by TEA, the absolute magnitude of both slow sodium and potassium currents becomes comparable during the plateau phase (Fig. 8).

Values for ionic conductances during the plateau phase of TEA action potentials were obtained by experiments in which the membrane potential control was turned on and off (Bezanilla et al., 1970). Results from these experiments are in agreement with voltage-clamp data and demonstrate that both sodium and potassium conductances remain higher during the plateau phase of action potentials than they are at rest. Furthermore, values for ionic conductances of these two components are similar.

Experiments in which axons were transiently voltage-clamped during the plateau, comparable to those performed on cardiac muscle (Vassalle, 1966; Goldman and Morad, 1977a; 1977b), produced similar results, including all-or-nothing repolarization with voltage-clamp pulses below the plateau level (Fig. 9) and lack of refractoriness after the action potential was prematurely repolarized (Gettes et al., 1972; Carmeliet, 1977).

Measurements of membrane resistance during the plateau phase of axon action potentials, however, produced results different from those in cardiac muscle. In all axons, the membrane resistance was always lower during the plateau than it was at resting levels. These results are similar to those of Armstrong and Binstock (1965; who also discussed reasons for discrepancies with results from Tasaki and Hagiwara, 1957), but different from those generally obtained in cardiac muscle (Fozzard and Sleator, 1967). Although there are reports of experiments in cardiac muscle in which plateau membrane resistance does not exceed resting values (Garnier et al., 1969; Vereecke and Carmeliet, 1971), our results suggest that axons and cardiac muscle have a different mechanism for bringing about repolarization of prolonged action potentials.

The cable properties of a tissue tend to linearize its input current-voltage relationships in a way that might lead to a region of very low slope conductance in the curve (Noble and Stein, 1966; Jack et al., 1975). To test if such a region would result in membrane resistance higher during the plateau phase of propagated action potentials than that at rest, I measured voltage changes in response to square-current pulses. These measurements did not show a plateau resistance higher than that of membrane action potentials but, in fact, membrane (input) resistance seemed unchanged. Thus, these results from PAP's support the conclusion that the mechanism producing the plateau of action potentials in cardiac muscle is somewhat different from that in axons (Noble and Tsien, 1972).

An explanation for the differences in repolarization between axons and cardiac muscle can be obtained by noticing that *(a)* in axons potassium currents are depressed, but TEA does not lower the potassium conductance below resting levels; and *(b)* the "slow" inward current of axons is of a different ionic nature than that postulated in cardiac muscle. Thus, in axons the plateau phase of action potentials is maintained by the slow sodium current, and repolarization seems to be produced when potassium current finally overcomes the slowly declining sodium current. This explanation of events leading to prolonged action potentials in axons perfused with TEA is remarkably similar to that proposed for cardiac muscle by Brady and Woodbury (1960). Recent data, however, has produced a much more complicated picture of events leading to cardiac muscle action potentials (McAllister et al., 1975; Beeler and Reuter, 1977).

In cardiac muscle, it has been proposed that action potentials are composed of two concomitant, but relatively independent, components (Trautwein and Dudel, 1954; Wright and Ogata, 1961; Paes de Carvalho et al., 1966; 1969). The behavior of action potentials from squid axons is clearly reminiscent of cardiac muscle, and voltage-clamp studies provide an explanation for this behavior. These two components, one (spike) mainly due to an increase in sodium conductance, and the other one (plateau) to both sodium and potassium conductances, can be affected independently (Fig. 10). Voltage-clamp pulses to values above −20 mV produce inactivation of the transient inward sodium current. Under these conditions, the conductances remaining are the slow sodium and potassium components. A brief voltage-clamp pulse that prevents the spike normally produced by the transient sodium conductance can still trigger these slow conductances to produce a plateau. This response takes the shape of an action potential without spike but with a plateau that follows a nearly normal course.

Alternatively, a fast repetitive rate of the stimulating current pulse produces action potentials without a plateau component. Because frequent stimulation does not provide enough time for the slow components to return to their resting values, only the transient inward sodium current is able to recover. Consequently, the plateau phase is abolished, and the initial spike of the action potential remains.

The behavior of those two conductance components also accounts for the all-or-nothing repolarization of action potentials. Hyperpolarizing voltage-clamp pulses that force the slow components to recover interrupt the action potential. But, if the voltage-clamp pulse does not reach a sufficiently negative potential or is not maintained long enough, the slow conductance parameters do not return to their resting values, and the plateau phase of the action potential follows a nearly normal course.

In cardiac muscle, the slow current component is thought to be caused by an inward movement of calcium and sodium ions (Coraboeuf, 1978). In squid axons, this current is due to sodium ions. But, if both calcium and sodium currents in cardiac muscle and delayed sodium currents in squid axons behave in approximately the same manner, as these experiments suggest, the resulting action potential would be similar. The shape of the action potential, or its propagation velocity, do not provide information about the ionic species carrying the inward current.

Having established that squid axons perfused with solutions containing TEA have prolonged action potentials similar to those from cardiac muscle, I studied two problems related to propagation. One of them was to observe interactions between two membrane regions with different membrane properties and action potential durations. The experiments demonstrated a number of interactions that took the form of spikes reflecting back and forth and leading to repetitive firing. Because similar interactions are to be expected between well-coupled cells, we have suggested that some cardiac arrhythmias could be due to these phenomena (Ramón and Moore, 1979).

The other propagation phenomenon that we have studied is the unidirectional block. Because axon geometrical parameters were changed only by compression, we concluded that changes in unidimensional properties are sufficient to produce unidirectional block. This type of propagation is a necessary condition for the presence of some cardiac arrhythmias.

In summary, voltage- and current-clamp experiments on squid axons perfused with solutions containing TEA show that these axons are useful to study properties of propagation of cardiac-like action potentials in unidimensional cable structures.

Acknowledgments

I wish to thank Dr. J.W. Moore for continuous support, and Drs. S.A. Simon, R.W. Joyner, and M. Lieberman for very useful discussions. Mr. E. Harris, Mrs. D. Crutchfield and Ms. E. Montaudouin-Daboll provided very capable technical and secretarial assistance. Thanks are also due to the Department of Physiology and Biophysics of the University of Iowa for the use of their facilities at the Marine Biological Laboratory, Woods Hole, Massachusetts. This work was supported by NIH Grants HL-22767 and NS-03437.

REFERENCES

Adelman WJ, Dyro FM, Senft J (1965) Long duration responses obtained from internally perfused axons. J Gen Physiol **48**:1–19

Armstrong CM (1975) Ionic pores, gates and gating currents. Q Rev Biophys **7**:179–210

Armstrong CM, Bezanilla F (1977) Inactivation of the sodium channel. II. Gating current experiments. J Gen Physiol **70**:567–590

Armstrong CM, Binstock L (1965) Anomalous rectification in the squid giant axon injected with tetraethylammonium chloride. J Gen Physiol **48**:859–872

Baker PF, Hodgkin AL, Shaw TI (1962a) Replacement of the axoplasm of giant nerve fibers with artificial solutions. J Physiol (Lond) **164**:330–337

Baker PF, Hodgkin AL, Shaw TI (1962b) The effects of changes in internal ionic concentrations on the electrical properties of perfused giant axons. J Physiol (Lond) **164**:355–374

Beeler GW, Reuter H (1977) Reconstruction of the action potential of ventricular myocardial fibers. J Physiol (Lond) **268**:177–260

Bergman C, Nonner W, Stampfli R (1968) Sustained spontaneous activity of Ranvier nodes induced by the combined actions of TEA and lack of calcium. Pfluegers Arch **302**:24–37

Bezanilla F, Rojas E, Taylor RE (1970) Sodium and potassium conductance changes during a membrane action potential. J Physiol (Lond) **211**:729–751

Brady AJ, Woodbury JW (1960) The sodium-potassium hypothesis as the basis of electrical activity in frog ventricle. J Physiol (Lond) **154**:385–407

Carmeliet E (1977) Repolarization and frequency in cardiac cells. J Physiol (Paris) **73**:903–923

Chandler WK, Meves H (1970a) Sodium and potassium currents in squid axons perfused with fluoride solutions. J Physiol (Lond) **211**:623–652

Chandler WK, Meves H (1970b) Evidence for two types of sodium conductance in axons perfused with sodium fluoride solution. J Physiol (Lond) **211**:653–678

Chandler WK, Meves H (1970c) Rate constants associated with changes in sodium conductance in axons perfused with sodium fluoride. J Physiol (Lond) **211**:679–705

Chandler WK, Meves H (1970d) Slow changes in membrane permeability and long-lasting action potentials in axons perfused with fluoride solutions. J Physiol (Lond) **211**:707–728

Coraboeuf E (1978) Ionic basis of electrical activity in cardiac tissues. Am J Physiol **234**: H101–H116

FitzHugh R (1960) Thresholds and plateaus in the Hodgkin-Huxley nerve equations. J Gen Physiol **43**:867–896

Fozzard HA, Sleator W (1967) Membrane ionic conductances during rest and activity in guinea-pig atrial muscle. Am J Physiol **212**:945–952

Garnier D, Rougier O, Gargouil YM, Coraboeuf E (1969) Analyse electrophysiologique du plateau des responses myocardiques; mise en evidence d'un courant lent entrant en absence d'ions bivalents. Pfluegers Arch **313**:321–342

George EP, Johnson EA (1961) Solutions of the Hodgkin-Huxley equations for squid axon treated with tetraethylammonium and in potassium-rich media. Aust J Exp Biol **39**:275–294

Gettes LS, Morehouse N, Surawicz B (1972) Effect of premature depolarization on the duration of action potentials in Purkinje and ventricular fibers of the moderator band of the pig heart. Circ Res **30**:55–66

Goldman Y, Morad M (1977a) Regenerative repolarization of the frog ventricular action potential: A time and voltage-dependent phenomenon. J Physiol (Lond) **268**:576–611

Goldman Y, Morad M (1977b) Ionic membrane conductance during the time course of the action potential. J Physiol (Lond) **268**:655–695

Hodgkin AL, Huxley AF (1952) A quantitative description of membrane current and its application to conduction and excitation in nerve. J Physiol (Lond) **117**:500–544

Hoffman BF, Cranefield PF (1960) Electrophysiology of the Heart. McGraw Hill Book Co., Inc. New York.

Jack JJB, Noble D, Tsien RW (1975) Electric current flow in excitable cells. Oxford, Clarendon Press

McAllister RE, Noble D, Tsien RW (1975) Reconstruction of the electrical activity of cardiac Purkinje fibres. J Physiol (Lond) **251**:1–59

Mobley BA, Page E (1972) The surface area of sheep cardiac Purkinje fibres. J Physiol (Lond) **220**:547–563

Noble D, Stein RB (1966) The threshold conditions for initiation of action potentials by excitable cells. J Physiol (Lond) **187**:129–162

Noble D, Tsien RW (1972) The repolarization process of heart cells. *In* Electrical Phenomena in the Heart, edited by WC DeMello, New York, Academic Press, pp 133–161

Oxford GS, Wu CH, Narahashi T (1978) Removal of sodium channel inactivation in squid giant axons by n-bromoacetamide. J Gen Physiol **71**:227–247

Paes de Carvalho A, Hoffman BF, Langan WB (1966) Two components of the cardiac action potential. Nature **211**:938–940

Paes de Carvalho A, Hoffman BF, Carvalho MP (1969) Two components of the cardiac action potential. I. Voltage-time course and the effect of acetylcholine on atrial and nodal cells of the rabbit heart. J Gen Physiol **54**:607–635

Ramón F, Moore JW (1979) Propagation of action potentials in squid giant axons. Repetitive firing at regions of membrane inhomogeneities. J Gen Physiol **73**:595–603

Shoukimas JJ, French RJ (1978) Blockage of peak and steady state sodium currents in squid axon by tetraethylammonium ions. Soc NeuroSci Abs **4**:237

Sommer JR, Johnson EA (1968) Cardiac muscle. A comparative study of Purkinje fibers and ventricular fibers. J Cell Biol **36**:497–526

Takenaka T, Yamagishi S (1969) Morphology and electrophysiological properties of squid giant axons perfused intracellularly with protease solution. J Gen Physiol **53**:81–96

Tasaki I, Hagiwara S (1957) Demonstration of two stable potential states in the squid giant axon under tetraethylammonium chloride. J Gen Physiol **40**:859–885
Trautwein W, Dudel J (1954) Aktionspotential und Mechanogramm des Katsenpapillarmuskels als Funktion der Temperatur. Pflüg Arch **260**:104–115
Vassalle M (1966) Analysis of cardiac pacemaker potential using a "voltage clamp" technique. Am J Physiol **210**:1335–1341
Vassalle M (1979) Electrogenesis of the plateau and pacemaker potential. Ann Rev Physiol **41**:425–440
Vereecke J, Carmeliet E (1971) Sr action potentials in cardiac Purkinje fibers. Pflug Arch **322**:60–82
Weidmann S (1951) Effect of current flow on the membrane potential of cardiac muscle. J Physiol (Lond) **115**:227–236
Wright E, Ogata M (1961) Action potential of amphibian single auricular muscle fiber: a dual response. Am J Physiol **201**:1101–1108
Wu CH, Narahashi T (1973) Mechanism of action of propranolol on squid axon membranes. J Pharmacol Exp Ther **184**:155–162

Discussion

LIEBERMAN: Strands 50 to 100 μm in diameter of cultured chick heart cells also have many of the conduction block characteristics that you have shown for the giant axon. For instance, a unidirectional block can be observed across segments of these thin strands where the number of cells in cross section is reduced and presumably is causing an increase in longitudinal resistance.

REUTER: If you had multiple branching in your preparations, it would certainly increase the complexity of your analysis and bring you closer to a model of what you get in cardiac muscle. Have you done any calculations or did you conduct any experiments in these more complex situations?

RAMÓN: No, I only have the calculations done according to the model of Cooley and Dodge for a single axon in which local changes in diameter have been created.

FOZZARD: In nerve, with a short action potential, the repolarizing current begins to flow quite early during the action potential. This early repolarizing current flow tends to slow the conduction of the action potential. In heart muscle, the repolarization is many milliseconds away from the depolarization, and this tendency is not manifest. Now, you have also separated depolarization from repolarization in the nerve by creating with TEA a prolonged plateau in the action potential. Does this speed conduction as compared with the normal situation in nerve?

RAMÓN: Conduction velocity in nerve, as in other excitable tissues, depends both on the local generation of currents and on the passive characteristics of the fiber lying ahead. As the upstroke of the action potential is almost entirely dominated by the sodium current and not by the potassium current, there is practically no difference in conduction velocity or upstroke velocity between a normal propagated action potential and a TEA action potential in a squid giant axon.

BROWN: I take it that what is generating the inward current during the prolonged plateau of the TEA action potential is this small, slowly inactivating sodium current that you have shown. Does this have the same reversal potential as the fast inactivating sodium current?

RAMÓN: Both the fast initial transient sodium current and the quasi steady-state slowly inactivating sodium current have the same equilibrium potential, but it is more difficult to measure the latter. Both these currents are equally sensitive to TTX or the lowering of external sodium.

CARMELIET: You showed that the sodium current was inactivated in two phases, a very fast one followed by a slow one. Does the recovery from inactivation present also two phases, or is it only slow?

RAMÓN: I don't know what the time constant of recovery of the slowly inactivated sodium current is. There are technical problems in doing this kind of determination because very long pulses are needed, and the axial wire polarizes. One never knows whether the results one gets are due to the polarization of the wire or to what is going on at the membrane.

BROWN: In the experiments where you looked at the time course of the potassium conductance changes by clamping to E_K, how can you be sure that the E_K is located where you say it is?

RAMÓN: It does not matter much if you go exactly to E_K or if you clamp the tissue to a potential that is only a few millivolts away from it. This was clearly shown by Benzanilla et al. (J Physiol **211**:729, 1970).

WEIDMANN: You showed that the slope resistance was measured by square pulses does not go up in the TEA-treated nerve action potential as much as it does in heart, where it goes beyond the level it had at rest (C. Haldimann, Arch Int. Pharmacodyn. Thér **146**:1–9, 1963). Do you explain this difference by the absence in nerve of the voltage-dependent drop of potassium conductance that exists in heart?

RAMÓN: Yes. The TEA action potential in squid nerve never shows a slope resistance higher than the resting value, and there is no sign of inward-going rectification.

JOHNSON: I would like to point out that it is not necessary to have a decrease in potassium conductance to have a decrease in slope conductance during the plateau. Kootsey and I made calculations a long time ago in which a cardiac action potential was generated by the interplay between a constant potassium ion conductance and a sodium ion conductance that was an instantaneous function of voltage. In a membrane action potential, there is no great perturbation of the plateau slope resistance. But an increased slope resistance during the plateau would be obtained when this action potential was made to propagate due to the interplay of these two conductances with cable properties. This type of problem was also shown in a communication of Paul George to the Physics Letters in 1960, although the specific point in tissue was not focused.

WEIDMANN: I presume you mean to say, that you can get an increased slope resistance in the plateau owing only to a voltage-dependent sodium current? This is what I originally thought was happening (Am J Physiol **183**:671 abstr 1955) before others convinced me that the potassium conductance decreased during the plateau of the action potential.

Chapter 7

Control of Conduction Velocity in Cardiac Purkinje Fibers

Harry A. Fozzard, David N. Levin, and Marc Walton

Conduction in heart muscle has been a challenging problem for a long time because of important differences between it and nerve (Fozzard, 1979). First, heart muscle is composed of independent cells, entirely bounded by sarcolemma, although it seems to function as a syncytium. Second, the measured membrane capacitance is so high that unreasonable values for excitatory inward currents seem to be required. Third, different parts of the heart have dramatically different conduction speeds, by a factor of 100, raising the possibility of different mechanisms of conduction. These problems, combined with the difficulty in making quantitative studies in this structurally complex tissue, have made conduction in heart muscle a fascinating and controversial subject. The problem is not only an intellectual one, but it has exceedingly important implications for clinical cardiology because of the role of conduction safety and speed in the genesis and control of arrhythmias.

This chapter will first review some of the principles of conduction to be expected from studies in nerve. We will then trace the progress made in sorting out the variables influencing conduction, drawing heavily on work from our laboratory over the last 20 years. The subject of electrotonic junctions and their role in permitting intercellular electrical coupling is described in detail by others in this volume (see Chapters 3–5). Special properties of slow conduction, as it may occur in the AV node and in diseased tissue, are also discussed elsewhere in this volume. Consequently, I will focus on "fast" conduction and discuss its properties in the cardiac Purkinje fiber, which is perhaps the best studied cardiac tissue for this question.

FORMAL RELATIONSHIPS BETWEEN CONDUCTION VELOCITY AND ITS DETERMINANTS

As in ancient Chinese and Indian philosophy, conduction is the consequence of two opposing forces, one tending to depolarize the cell membrane and the other opposing depolarization. A reasonable approach to conduction is to consider these two

Supported in part by USPHS HL 20592, HL 07381, and HD 07009.

forces separately. The force favoring depolarization, called the "source," is inward current, carried normally in atrial, ventricular, and Purkinje tissue by sodium ions (Na^+). The force opposing depolarization, called the "sink," is the charge stored on the membrane as capacity charge and the leakage of current out of the cell through the membrane or along the cell interior by any ion. A characteristic feature of conduction is that it occurs upon threshold stimulus and, after an initial acceleration, it propagates at a constant finite speed throughout uniform tissue.

The source, or Na^+ current, is a specific membrane conductance to Na^+, dependent on membrane voltage and time and an electrochemical gradient for Na^+ across the membrane. The sink is made up of both the membrane properties of leakage resistance and capacitance and the geometry of the tissue. Most quantitative studies in nerve and heart muscle have considered the simplest geometry permitting conduction—the cable—although extrapolations can be made to more complex geometries. Hermann (1899) proposed that, in the cable, propagation was by passive current flow from the excited to the unexcited region—local circuit current. This was supported for nerve by experiments of Hodgkin (1937), and eventually for heart by Barr et al. (1965). The first crucial attempt to develop a quantitative theoretical description of conduction was by Rushton (1937). The subject is also treated in detail by Jack et al (1975).

The simple cable model is illustrated in Figure 1A. It is a tube or cylinder of membrane separating the cytoplasm from the outside solution. The simple electrical analog is a membrane resistance (r_m, Ωcm) and capacitance (c_m, $\mu F/cm$) in parallel, connected to adjacent parts of the membrane through the resistance of the cytoplasm (r_i, Ω/cm) (outside resistance is assumed to be very low). Once the conducted action potential has reached constant velocity, membrane voltage (V, mV) has the same distribution in distance (x, cm) and time (t, sec), and

$$\frac{\delta^2 V}{\delta x^2} = \frac{1}{\theta^2} \cdot \frac{\delta^2 V}{\delta t^2} \tag{1}$$

where θ is conduction velocity (m/sec). This permits us to write the linear cable equation as

$$\frac{1}{r_i \theta^2} \cdot \frac{d^2V}{dt^2} = c_m \frac{dV}{dt} + \frac{V}{r_m} \tag{2}$$

A simplified solution leads to:

$$\tau_{\text{foot}} = 1/\text{r}_\text{i} \text{ ``}c_m\text{''}\ \theta^2 = (\lambda/\theta)^2/\text{``}\tau_m\text{''} \tag{3}$$

where τ_{foot} is the exponential time constant of the foot of the advancing action potential (Tasaki and Hagiwara, 1957), the cable length constant $\lambda = \sqrt{r_m/r_i}$, and the membrane time constant $\tau_m = r_m$"c_m." For nerve the "c_m" is truly the membrane capacitance. For Purkinje fibers it is much smaller, indicating that the capacitance that the upstroke of the action potential fills is only a part of the total membrane capacitance (Fozzard, 1966). In heart, this "c_m" is called c_{foot}, to distinguish it from c_m. For convenience, only the notation c_m is used in the following equations.

Another approach to the relationship between the variables is to rearrange Eq. 2:

$$\theta^2 = \frac{d^2V/dt^2}{r_i c_m\, dV/dt + r_i/r_m\, V} \tag{4a}$$

or,

$$\theta^2 = \lambda^2 \frac{d^2V/dt^2}{\tau_m\, dV/dt + V} \tag{4b}$$

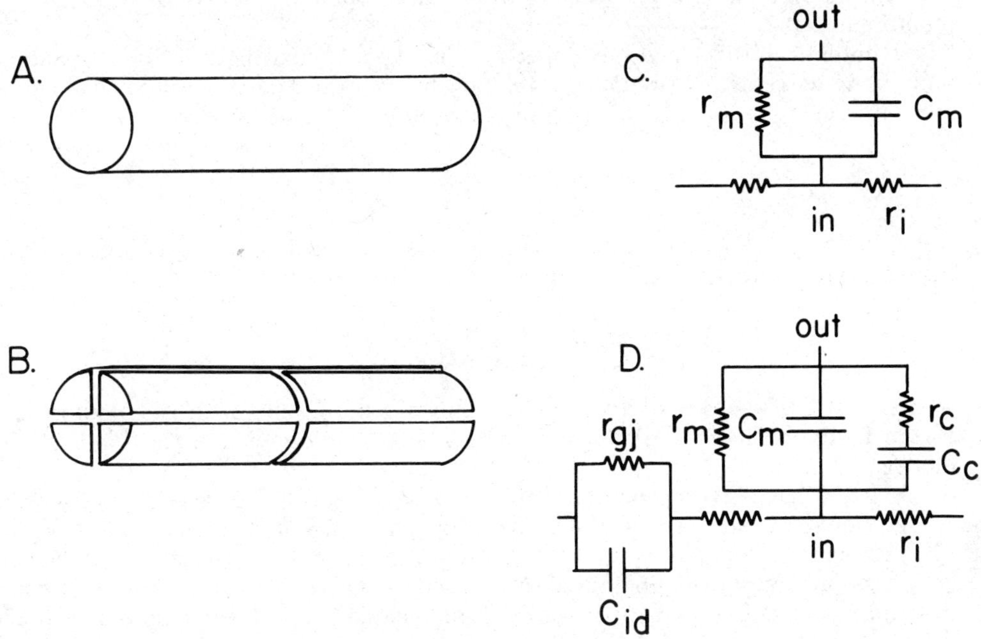

Figure 1. Simple cable and multiunit cable.

A, This is a representation of a simple cable with smooth surface and continuous interior. It is an accurate representation of a squid axon but is often used as an approximation for other tissues.

B, This is a schematic drawing of a cardiac Purkinje strand. It has four cells in cross section, with narrow intercellular clefts between. In addition, the cells are shown to have a finite length. Not illustrated is membrane folding in both the transverse and the longitudinal plane.

C, Analog circuit for the simple cable. A segment of the membrane is represented by a membrane resistance (r_m) and membrane capacitance (c_m). The segment is connected to adjacent membrane through a resistive core (r_i).

D, Analog circuit for the cardiac Purkinje strand. The membrane has an additional arm for current flow, containing a resistance (r_c) in series with membrane capacitance (C_c). In reality, the series r_c is distributed, rather than appearing as single values as in this diagram. The segment is connected to adjacent membrane by a resistive core, r_i, but at intercalated disks there is a gap junctional resistance (r_{gj}) and the capacitance of the apposed cell membranes (c_{id}) of the intercalated disk.

Now it is possible to suggest that θ is proportional to λ and inversely proportional to τ_m. It is also proportional to d^2V/dt^2 and inversely proportional to dV/dt. In conduction, current flows longitudinally from the excited region to an unexcited segment, and it is proportional to d^2V/dt^2. Part of the current that flows into a segment is used to discharge the capacitance of the segment, and it is lost from the total current available to flow into the next segment. This loss is equal to $c_m dV/dt$. Another way to write this is

$$i_i = \frac{1}{r_i\theta^2} \cdot \frac{d^2V}{dt^2} - c_m \frac{dV}{dt} \tag{5}$$

where using i_i in place of V/r_m makes the equation valid for the passive or the active membrane.

Hunter et al (1975) have developed a series of polynomial models of the excitatory membrane current that predict the relationship between passive properties, excitatory properties, and θ. In an appropriately modified form, they are

$$\theta = m \sqrt{\frac{2}{r_i c_m}} \sqrt{\frac{dV/dt_{max}}{V_{pk}}} \qquad (6a)$$

where $m = 1.1$—1.4, dV/dt_{max} is the maximal upstroke velocity, and V_{pk} is the peak action potential voltage;

$$\theta = m \sqrt{\frac{2}{r_i c_m}} \sqrt{\frac{-\hat{\imath}}{c_m} \Big/ V_{pk}} \qquad (6b)$$

where $m = 0.95$—1.3, and $\hat{\imath}$ is peak ionic current during the upstroke (Walton and Fozzard, unpublished). The value of m in these equations depends on the details of the models.

We now have several equations that describe θ in terms of passive properties (r_i, r_m, c_m, or c_{foot}) and in terms of active properties (d^2V/dt^2, dV/dt, i_i, and V_{pk}). The relation of the parameters of active properties to maximal sodium conductance (gNa), sodium equilibrium potential (E_{Na}), sodium current (i_{Na}), and the activation descriptors of Hodgkin and Huxley (1952) is much less clear. A few relations have been derived, such as the relation between dV/dt_{max} and i_{Na}, but the assumptions used are subject to criticism. Careful test of these relationships is required.

WILL THE CARDIAC ACTION POTENTIAL CONDUCT?

The large c_m measured in cable analysis of Purkinje strands led McAllister et al (1975) to use the very large value of 150 mS/cm^2 for gNa in their model of the Purkinje action potential. This is referenced to the crude surface area of the strand, ignoring clefts and membrane folding. It is similar to the value of 120 mS/cm^2 used by Hodgkin and Huxley (1952), but must discharge much more capacitance. McAllister et al (1975) suggested that even this high value was insufficient to provide upstroke velocity and θ comparable to experimental measurements.

The magnitude of gNa represents a question of the "source" size. But, for a conducted action potential, the Na^+ current never reaches its maximal value. As the wavefront approaches an unexcited segment, current flows into the segment from the excited region through the cytoplasm (i_{l_1}). This current divides into two important and one unimportant components. The important parts are i_{l_2}, which flows through the cytoplasm to the next segment, and i_c, which discharges the capacitance of the membrane. The unimportant part is i_i, the current that leaks out of the membrane. It is small because of the far lower effective resistance of the longitudinal and capacitance paths of the circuit. The capacitance current rapidly depolarizes the membrane (time constant, τ_{foot}, is about 0.1 msec) so that threshold for activation of the sodium current is passed long before the sodium current can activate. Maximal passive depolarization occurs shortly before the time dV/dt_{max} is achieved, which is at membrane potentials near 0 mV. As the Na^+ conductance rises, it finds the driving force on Na^+ rapidly diminishing. Consequently, the activation time for the Na^+ conductance may play an important role in conduction, in addition to gNa.

We have examined this relationship between activation, $\overline{gNa}$, and c_m in a model (Makielski and Fozzard, unpublished). We used the McAllister et al (1975) description of the Na^+ system for a membrane action potential and computed its conduction in a manner similar to Cooley and Dodge (1966). Using a $\overline{gNa}$ of 150 mS/cm^2 and a C_m of 10 μF/cm^2, we obtained a value for θ of 2.86 m/sec and a value for dV/dt_{max} of 480 V/sec. These are reasonable values for cardiac Purkinje strands, so the model of McAllister et al can apparently sustain reasonable conduction properties. Both θ and dV/dt_{max} were sensitive to the resting membrane potential (V_m). θ had a biphasic dependence on V_m, maximal at −81 mV and less with hyperpolarization or depolarization. With hyperpolarization, dV/dt_{max} rose monotonically, reaching levels of 680 V/S at −93 mV.

As mentioned previously, the $\overline{gNa}$ and C_m values of McAllister et al (1975) were referred to a smooth cable, but the actual membrane was quite redundant. If we assume that there is 1 μF/cm^2 of true membrane, then $\overline{gNa}$ is actually 15 mS/cm^2. We then calculated the conduction for a cable with a C_m = 4.3 μF (to correspond to the amount discharged by the action potential foot) and a $\overline{gNa}$ = 64.5 mS/cm^2 (to keep the ratio $\overline{gNa}/C_m$ = 15). With these parameters, θ rose to 3.3 m/sec without a change in dV/dt_{max}.

We also made calculations with a variation in the specific core resistivity, R_i, which showed that increasing R_i reduced θ and increased dV/dt_{max} (Fig. 2).

Although reassuring ourselves that the Na^+ system proposed by McAllister et al (1975) would produce θ and dV/dt_{max} typical of experimental results, we found the calculations to be insufficient because they were based on a model of the Purkinje strand as a simple cable. Because of the distributed resistance of the intercellular clefts, the appropriate value of c_m, that is to say, c_{foot}, would vary with θ.

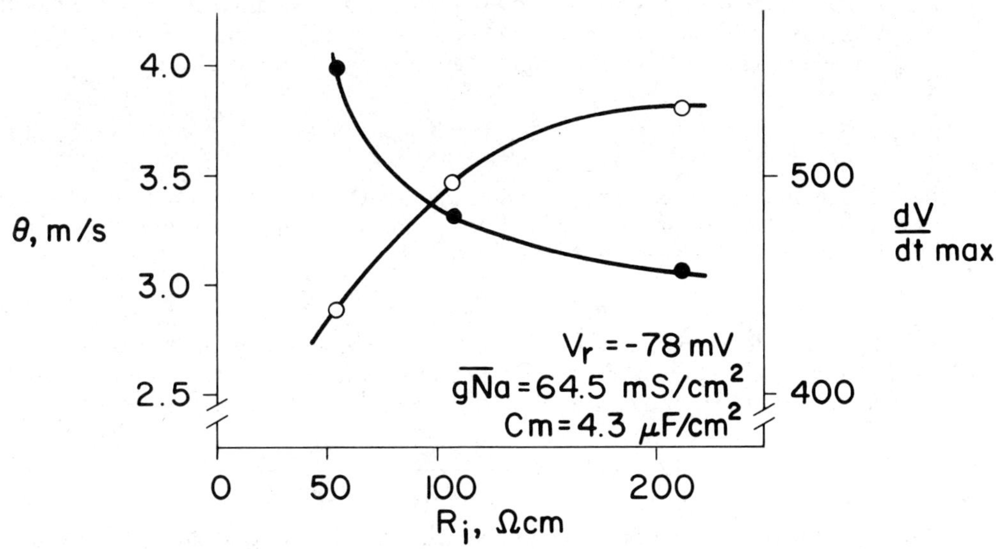

Figure 2. Relationship between core resistivity (R_i) and conduction velocity (θ) and maximal upstroke velocity (dV/dt_{max}). The points, solid (θ) and open (dV/dt_{max}), were obtained by computation of the conducted action potential in a simple cable using the McAllister et al (1975) equations and values indicated.

THE CLEFT PROBLEM

A serious problem is posed by the multicellular nature of the Purkinje strand. Narrow intercellular clefts exist that separate most of the membrane from the surface of the strand and the outside solution. The importance of these clefts to electrical studies was suggested by Weidmann (1952) in his early cable measurements and confirmed by Fozzard (1966) and Freygang and Trautwein (1970). The anatomic correlation was demonstrated by Sommer and Johnson (1968), and careful quantitative morphometrics of the sheep Purkinje strand were made by Mobley and Page (1972) and Hellam and Studt (1974).

The influence of the intercellular clefts on simple cable analysis was shown by Schoenberg et al (1975), who demonstrated the dependence of apparent r_m and c_m on strand diameter. The strands with larger diameter simply had more membrane facing clefts. Schoenberg et al (1975) also developed an equation for estimating voltage nonuniformity within a simple cleft,

$$V = V_f \frac{\cosh (x/\lambda_{cf})}{\cosh (a/\lambda_{cf})} \tag{7}$$

where V_f is the voltage at the mouth of the cleft, x is the position radially within the cleft ($x = 0$ at the center of the strand), a is the strand radius, and λ_{cf} is the length constant of the cleft. At the frequency of the propagating action potential, λ_{cf} is only about 8 μm, so that most of the membrane in a 100 μm diameter strand is not depolarized during the action potential upstroke. This agrees with the previous finding that C_{foot} is much less than C_m and was confirmed by Schoenberg et al (1975), who found that C_{foot} did not vary with strand diameter over 50 μm.

To investigate the importance of the clefts on passive electrical analysis and on θ, we had to develop equations for cables with clefts, which we did using a model based on the morphometric data available and a few assumptions (Levin and Fozzard, 1981). First, transverse current flow is related to an effective admittance Y:

$$Y = \frac{1}{R_m} + C_m p \tag{8}$$

where R_m is the unit membrane resistance, C_m is the unit membrane capacitance, and p is the Laplace transform variable ($|p| = 2\pi v$, where v is the frequency in Hz). The effective admittance per unit length (y_m) is

$$y_m = Y(L_e \phi_e^2 + L_i \phi_i^2 F) \tag{9}$$

where L_e and L_i denote lengths of surface and cleft membrane in the transverse plane if folding is ignored, ϕ_e and ϕ_i are folding factors of surface and cleft membrane, and F is the effective fraction of cleft membrane that conducts current. F is defined as

$$F = G \frac{\tanh (L/2\lambda_c)}{(L/2\lambda_c)} \tag{10}$$

where L is the folded length of cell sides facing the clefts, λ_c is $\phi_i \lambda_{cf}$, and G is a geometric variable related to the exact cleft network. If we examine the case of high frequency (>300 Hz),

$$y_m = L_e \phi_e^2 Y \left[1 + \frac{\phi_i}{\phi_e^2 L_e} \sqrt{\frac{2W}{R_e C_m p}} \right] \tag{11}$$

where W is width of the cleft, and R_e is the specific resistivity of the solution in the clefts. This is applicable at the frequency associated with the foot of the action potential.

Now, the specific capacitance associated with the action potential C_{foot} is

$$C_{foot} = C_m \phi_e^2 \left[1 + \frac{L_i \phi_i^2}{L_e \phi_e^2} F(k) \right] \tag{12}$$

where k is $1/\tau_{foot}$. For realistic values of k, we can simplify this equation. If it is combined with Eq. 3, we obtain

$$\theta^2 = \frac{2ka}{4R_iC_m\phi_e^2 \left[1 + \frac{\phi_i}{L_c \phi_e^2} \sqrt{\frac{2W}{R_eC_mk}} \right]} \tag{13}$$

This equation predicts θ to be 2.8 m/sec for a 150 μm strand, using average values for the passive membrane properties. The second part of the bracketed term represents the fractional contribution of the clefts to slowing of conduction. It has a typical value of 0.4. An estimate of what θ would be if clefts were not present (separated from the surface by an infinite resistance) is 3.3 m/sec, 18% faster.

It is also possible to estimate the effect of a capacitive element in the path for longitudinal current. Freygang and Trautwein (1970) found a time constant of 64 μsec in the longitudinal circuit, which they ascribed to capacitive coupling across the intercalated disk. It is relatively easy to modify Eq. 13 to include this circuit change. If this is done, and the measurements of Freygang and Trautwein are introduced, θ increases by 3%.

The validity of Eq. 13 could be tested experimentally by slowing conduction with tetrodotoxin or reduced Na_o^+. A change in R_i would also have a large effect on θ, but it is not easily controlled (DeMello, 1975; Weingart, 1977). Geometrical alterations would also be of great interest, but the need for morphometric analysis makes this approach difficult. We (Walton and Fozzard, unpublished) have, therefore, attempted experiments in which θ is changed by tetrodotoxin and low Na_o^+. The relation of interest is a modification of Eq. 12 and insertion of typical morphometric parameters, to yield

$$C_{foot} = 2.9 + 6.9 \sqrt{\tau_{foot}} \tag{14}$$

where the intercept is capacitance of the folded surface membrane only.

The most powerful approach to analysis of cleft properties is analysis in the frequency domain. It is possible to develop analytic equations for the cable appropriate to such an analysis, and this is likely to be a promising experimental approach (Levis, personal communication).

EFFECT OF DECREASE IN Na^+ CURRENT

The analytic expressions for the relationship between θ and parameters describing the passive cable properties (the sink) and the Na^+ current (the source) could be tested by systematic alteration in the parameters. It is difficult to alter an individual strand's geometry, and population studies of strands with varying geometric properties would require very time-consuming morphometric study. An example of the difficulty of this latter approach is seen in the puzzling result of Schoenberg et al (1975) that θ did not vary with apparent strand diameter. It is uncertain whether this results from an error in measuring the diameter or an error in our understanding of control of conduction. Change in R_i is difficult to achieve in a graded fashion. But, the Na^+ current can be altered systematically by reducing the Na^+ concentration in the perfusing solutions or by exposing the strands to tetrodotoxin.

The Na^+-reduction experiment is attractive, because it is possible to argue that this is equivalent to a proportional change in $\overline{gNa}$. There are two key assumptions in that equivalency. First, the Na^+ electrochemical driving force must not change. This requires that as Na_o^+ is reduced, there is a proportional fall in Na_i^+. Ellis (1977) showed that in sheep Purkinje fibers the Na_i^+, measured with glass ion-selective microelectrodes, did fall upon reduction of Na_o^+, and Sheu et al (1980), using liquid ion-exchanger microelectrodes, found little change in Na^+ electrochemical equilibrium potential with large changes in Na_o^+. The second assumption is that Na^+ movement in the channel is independent. This requires that the channel not show any saturation at normal Na_o^+ and that selectivity for Na^+ be very high.

We performed experiments replacing Na^+ with tetramethyl ammonium ion (TMA), recording at each condition passive cable properties, θ, C_{foot}, and the parameters of the inward current. With Na_o^+ reduced to 50%, 35%, 25%, and 20% of normal, the cable measurements of R_i, R_m, and C_m did not change significantly. θ fell gradually to 81% of normal at 50% Na_o^+ and 41% of normal at 25% Na_o^+. Conduction usually failed in 20% Na_o^+. The capacitance filled by the action potential foot (C_{foot}) rose in 25% Na_o^+ to double the control value.

The inward current parameters measured were dV/dt_{max}, voltage at which dV/dt_{max} occurred ($\overline{V}$), and the peak action potential voltage (V_{pk}). Each of these also fell as Na_o^+ was reduced, but with varying sensitivity, and all were fairly large just before conduction failure. Other measures could be extracted by use of Eq. 5, including peak inward current ($\hat{I}$), and upstroke power ($P = \int_o^{V_{pk}} I_i dV$). These latter measurements require normalization for surface area, if different fibers are to be compared. The total surface area is inappropriate, because with slower conduction more and more of the cleft membrane is recruited. The value for C_{foot} provides an approximation of this available membrane, so $\hat{I}$ and P are normalized to C_{foot}. In the normalized form, they fell with lowered Na_o^+ nonlinearly and faster then θ.

C_{foot} rose as expected with slower conduction, and in the direction predicted by Eq. 14. The ratio C_{foot}/C_m in control solutions was 0.211, similar to experimental values (Fozzard, 1966; Fozzard and Schoenberg, 1972). The relationship between C_{foot} and $\sqrt{\tau_{foot}}$ was apparently linear, as predicted by the equation, but the slopes varied and did not agree with the morphometrically predicted value. The reason for this deviation from prediction is not obvious, but it could have resulted from the presence of some clefts with wider diameter than the 40 nm assumed, greater folding factor than assumed, or smaller cell sizes.

The various models predicting the relationship between current parameters and θ could be reduced to some simple relationships that are a consequence of the cable and a constantly conducted action potential (Eq. 6). dV/dt_{max} is predicted to be linearly related to $\hat{I}/C_{foot}$, and this was confirmed by the experimental data. θ is proportional to $(dV/dt_{max}/V_{pk})^{1/2}$, and this also was confirmed by the experimental data. Consequently, the behavior of the models was not a result of their internal parameters, but of the cable itself.

Although important in demonstrating the relationship between experimental measures of inward current and θ, these results were disappointing. All of the measured variables decreased nonlinearly, although presumably the intrinsic ability to conduct was decreased linearly by the reduction in Na_o^+. None of these measurements could be considered a "safety factor." Reasoning that the power and energy of discharge of the membrane capacity ought to be factors crucial for conduction, we invented a possible "safety factor" ϕ_c.

$$\phi_c = \frac{P\,V_{pk}^2}{2\,C_{foot}} \qquad (15)$$

The factor declined linearly with decrease in Na_o^+ and reached zero when conduction failed. It has some of the features of a useful "safety factor," and may be helpful in future investigation.

SUMMARY

Progress has been made in a number of important areas for understanding and controlling conduction in heart muscle. We can characterize and study the gap junction that permits electrotonic coupling between separate cardiac cells. We are beginning to measure accurately the properties of inward Na^+ currents with improved voltage-clamp methods. We recognize that very slow conduction is a consequence of another inward current system with comparable very slow kinetics. We realize that the large membrane capacitance measured in cable analysis is due to a highly redundant surface membrane. This redundant membrane means that, along with increased charge storage capability, there is a greater area for inward current channels.

Several important areas resist solution. The complex geometry of cardiac muscle has made it difficult to determine the relationship between the geometry, the passive membrane properties, and conduction. We have developed analytic descriptions of the intercellular clefts and used them to predict conduction, with some success. Models that we and others have developed to describe the relationship of inward current to conduction all reduce to simple equations dependent on the cable and the assumption of constant conduction. These relationships may be of value in applying the results of voltage-clamp studies to conduction. They also demonstrate why θ and dV/dt_{max} do not always change in the same direction.

It remains for us to define properly the "safety factor" of conduction, if we are to apply these insights to abnormal or pathologic states. It is also apparent that electrical studies are heavily dependent on structural information. We can only obtain limited information from measurements that are independent of structural parameters. Full understanding of conduction will require close cooperation between these two areas of investigations.

REFERENCES

Barr L, Dewey MM, Berger W (1965) Propagation of action potentials and the structure of the nexus in cardiac muscle. J Gen Physiol **48**:797–823

Cooley JW, Dodge FA Jr (1966) Digital computer solutions for excitation and propagation of the nerve impulse. Biophys J **6**:583–599

DeMello WC (1975) Effect of intracellular injection of calcium and strontium on cell communication in heart. J Physiol **250**:231–245

Ellis D (1977) The effects of external cations and ouabain on the intracellular sodium activity of sheep heart Purkinje fibres. J Physiol (Lond) **273**:211–240

Fozzard HA (1966) Membrane capacity of the cardiac Purkinje fibre. J Physiol (Lond) **182**: 255–267

Fozzard HA (1979) Conduction of the action potential. *In* Handbook of Physiology, The Cardiovascular System I, edited by R.M. Berne and N. Sperelakis, Washington, D.C., American Physiological Society

Fozzard HA, Schoenberg M (1972) Strength-duration curves in cardiac Purkinje fibres: effects of liminal length and charge distribution. J Physiol (Lond) **226**:593–618

Freygang WH, Trautwein W (1970) The structural implications of the linear electrical properties of cardiac Purkinje strands. J Gen Physiol **55**:524–527

Hellam DC, Studt JW (1964) A core-conductor model of the cardiac Purkinje fibre based on structural analysis. J Physiol (Lond) **243**:637–660

Hermann L (1899) Zur Theorie der Erregungsleitung und der elektrischen Erregung. Pflüg Arch **75**:574–590

Hodgkin AL (1937) Evidence for electrical transmission in nerve. J Physiol (Lond) **90**:183–232

Hodgkin AL, Huxley AF (1952) A quantitative description of membrane current and its application to conduction and excitation in nerve. J Physiol (Lond) **117**:500–544

Hunter PJ, McNaughton PA, Noble D (1975) Analytical models of propagation in excitable cells. Prog Biophys Molec Biol **30**:99–144

Jack JJB, Noble D, Tsien RW (1975) Electric Current Flow in Excitable Cells. Oxford, Clarendon Press

Levin DN, Fozzard HA (1981) A cleft model for cardiac Purkinje strands. Biophys J **33**:383–408

McAllister RW, Noble D, Tsien RW (1975) Reconstruction of the electrical activity of cardiac Purkinje fibres. J Physiol **251**:1–59

Mobley BA, Page E (1972) The surface area of sheep cardiac Purkinje fibres. J Physiol (Lond) **220**:547–564

Rushton WA (1937) Initiation of the propagated disturbance. Proc Roy Soc B **124**:210–243

Schoenberg M, Dominguez G, Fozzard HA (1975) Effect of diameter on membrane capacity and conductance of sheep cardiac Purkinje fibres. J Gen Physiol **65**:441–458

Sheu, SS, Korth M, Lathrop DA, Fozzard HA (1980) Intra- and extracellular K^+ and Na^+ activities and resting membrane potential in sheep cardiac Purkinje strands. Circ Res **47**: 692–700

Sommer JR, Johnson EA (1968) Cardiac muscle: a comparative study of Purkinje fibers and ventricular fibers. J Cell Biol **36**:497–526

Tasaki I, Hagiwara S (1957) Capacity of muscle fiber membrane. Am J Physiol **188**:423–429

Weidmann, S (1952) The electrical constants of Purkinje fibres. J Physiol (Lond) **118**:348–360

Weingart R (1977) The actions of ouabain on intercellular coupling and conduction velocity in mammalian ventricular muscle. J Physiol (Lond) **264**:341–365

Discussion

I. COHEN: I must admit to being a bit confused about the MacAllister-Noble-Tsien (MNT) simulation. I have also performed a simulation with this model and found to my dismay that when I increased the external potassium concentration in the model, the current voltage relationships for both I_{K1} and I_{K2} did not cross over. To simulate the real world, we had to change the equations in the model. We published these changes in 1978, but unfortunately the *Journal of Physiology* printed the equations incorrectly. I would therefore like to know if you also changed the equations for I_{K1} and I_{K2} or if you actually used the MNT equations.

FOZZARD: After correcting the mistakes in the MNT formulation, we were still left with several things we must do. One was to avoid pacemaker properties, which was done by simply setting the I_{K2} variable to a constant. Second, to avoid the problem of changing extracellular potassium, we simply changed E_K. This was done in the computer by changing only the intracellular potassium and letting everything else be the same. We examined the possible consequences of this and found out that what it did to the potassium current did not make a difference in terms of the conduction of the action potential, because the potassium current does not change appreciably during the upstroke.

I. COHEN: Well, the importance of the potassium conductance is that it serves as background current for sodium current. One should expect differences in threshold current in high potassium when comparing a situation in which the voltage-current relationships cross over with one in which they do not.

FOZZARD: The importance of the leakage conductance, which is mainly potassium conductance in this case, is so trivial that it did not affect any of the results. We removed both voltage and time dependence of the potassium current, and found that it did not affect the upstroke of the action potential.

I. COHEN: Another problem I found with the MNT equations is that τ_m was found to be almost infinitely fast, whereas τ_h in effect was almost infinitely slow. In reality, we did not even need to simulate the action potential as we could analytically solve this by making the assumption that m always goes instantaneously to m_∞. In this condition, if you know the shape of the m_∞ curve, you do not need any characteristics for α_m and β_m at all. I wonder then if there might not be a very different solution if τ_m and τ_h where made to be closer in value. τ_m was 20 μsec at −20 mV; this seems awfully fast to me and is probably an overestimate considering whatever little voltage-clamp data there is. τ_h is also much slower in their model than seems appropriate.

FOZZARD: I appreciate your concern. m certainly did not behave as if it were an instantaneous variable in our simulation. What was especially sensitive to the activation time constant for the sodium channel (τ_m) was the voltage at which ionic current reverses from outward to inward. Actually, the fiber depolarized to the level of −20 to −15 mV before ionic current turned inward; that is, before an appreciable increase in sodium current occurred. We compared the MNT model data with Marc Walton's measurements in Purkinje fibers and obtained similar values for the current-reversal voltage. We also changed the activation time constant, slowing it by a factor of 4. We obtained a slower conduction velocity associated with a somewhat greater depolarization before the ionic current turned inward. The dependence of conduction velocity on membrane potentials still persisted in this situation. There is no doubt that conduction velocity was a function of the activation of m, but its biphasic dependence on membrane potential did not seem to be.

BONKE: You showed that when you impose a hyperpolarization in the model, a decrease in conduction velocity occurs concomitantly with an increase in the maximum upstroke velocity. Can you comment further on this point?

FOZZARD: It occurs in the model and is also observed in the experimental measurements that we previously reported (Dominguez and Fozzard, Circ Res **26**:565–574, 1970). This is actually a point that I do not readily understand, because it must involve the steady-state availability of Na^+ conductance, h, and the charge that must be displaced to reach threshold.

PAES DE CARVALHO: I wonder if the extra time spent at the foot of the action potential in a hyperpolarized situation before the voltage at which the maximum dV/dt is reached could contribute both to the higher upstroke velocity and to slower conduction. First, besides a more complete removal of inactivation, the m variable would have more time to develop before peak dV/dt is reached. Second, the longer foot observed below the current reversal voltage would slow down conduction.

FOZZARD: The time in the model was computed from the moment in which the membrane had depolarized by a tenth of a millivolt up to the moment when the net membrane current became inward. This latency had a biphasic character. It was shortest at the time of the highest conduction velocity and became longer in both directions as a function of resting membrane voltage. Perhaps in the hyperpolarized situation the long latency would allow more time for the sodium conductance to turn on and therefore contribute to the increase in upstroke velocity.

JOHNSON: Some calculations that we did many years ago in a simple cable showed that conduction velocity is relatively insensitive to $\bar{g}_{Na}$. It varied actually with the ¼ power of $\bar{g}_{Na}$, somewhat similar, therefore, to what Pickard found by some analytical argument. More recently, a figure of ⅛ power appeared in the literature.

FOZZARD: The models you mention predict either ¼ or ⅛ power depending on the assumptions they use in their calculations (Hunter et al, Prog Biophys Mol Biol **30**:99–144, 1975). They also suggest that conduction velocity depends on the square root of the membrane capacity. But, when we began to look at what the basis of the models were, we discovered that they depended heavily on assumptions. It should be noticed that it is not only the MNT model data that we are talking about, but also those of Hunter et al, Tasaki, etc. The MNT model, however, fitted well the experimental data of Marc Walton, where $\bar{g}_{Na}$ was reduced by reducing external sodium.

Chapter 8

Homogeneous and Nonhomogeneous Conduction of Impulses in Heart and Other Excitable Tissues

Antonio Paes de Carvalho, Teobaldo Antonio Saldeña, Eduardo Antonio Conde Garcia, Antonio Carlos Campos de Carvalho, Tetsuo Tashiro, and Marilene de Paula Carvalho

The mathematic analysis developed by Hodgkin and Rushton (1946) for cable-like cells has been used often by electrophysiologists to determine the passive constants of different types of myocardial tissue (Weidmann, 1952; Woodbury and Crill, 1961; Weidmann, 1970; Bonke, 1973a; 1973b; De Mello, 1977). Several authors have also used the Hodgkin and Huxley (1952) formulation of squid nerve propagated action potentials to study the passive behavior of the cardiac cell membrane during the spread of activity (Weidmann, 1970; Carmeliet and Willems, 1971; Clerc, 1976).

The phase-plane analysis of the Hodgkin-Huxley model, first applied by Jenerick (1963, 1964) to compute ionic currents during propagated action potentials of skeletal muscle, has also been applied to the heart (Paes de Carvalho et al., 1969; Paes de Carvalho, 1975). All these studies are based on two requirements. First, the mathematic description of current spread at any point of a syncytial bundle of heart muscle fibers should be identical to that of current spread along cable-like cells. Second, as a consequence, the propagation of activity should be homogeneous; that is, it should proceed with constant velocity and constant action potential shape. Both requirements implicitly assume that branching and convergence of cell bundles—as well as the local variations of fiber size and longitudinal resistance that must occur at a microscopic level—are of no consequence to the gross process of current flow in a homogeneous syncytial structure.

In this chapter we use phase-plane analysis to ascertain whether propagation in the heart is indeed a homogeneous process. We show that this technique reveals, in

This work was supported by grants from the Conselho de Pesquisas/UFRJ, Conselho de Desenvolvimento Científico e Tecnológico (SEPLAN/CNPq) and Financiadora de Estudos e Projetos (SEPLAN/FINEP). Antonio Paes de Carvalho and Marilene de Paula Carvalho are Career Investigators of SEPLAN/CNPq.

several instances, slight local microhesitations and microaccelerations. The validation of these conclusions is sought in the comparative analysis of homogeneous and non-homogeneous conduction in simpler cable-like cells such as squid nerve and frog skeletal muscle.

METHODS

Preparations, Solutions, and Drugs

Mammalian heart muscle preparations were obtained from rabbits (right and left atrium; ventricular papillary muscles; Purkinje fibers) or dogs (Purkinje fibers) and kept immersed in flowing Tyrode's solution, which was composed of 137 mM NaCl, 2.7 mM KCl, 2.7 mM $CaCl_2$, 12 mM $NaHCO_3$, 1.8 mM NaH_2PO_4, 0.5 mM $MgCl_2$, and 6 mM glucose. The bathing fluid was maintained at 35° C and was gassed with a mixture of 5% CO_2 in O_2.

Giant axons were obtained from the posterior nerve of the mantle of the Brazilian squid (*Loligo brasiliensis*; mantle length, 18 to 26 cm) captured at Cabo Frio, RJ, during the summer months. Unbranched axon segments 5 to 6 cm long and 300 to 450 μm in diameter were dissected free between the stellate ganglion and the first axon bifurcation. After its extremities were ligated, the axon was equilibrated in local sea water, the composition of which has been determined by Moreira da Silva (1974). The main ions of the sea water were 477 mM Na^+, 10 mM K^+, 54.4 mM Mg^{2+}, 10.4 mM Ca^{2+}, 556 mM Cl^-, 28 mM SO_4^{2-}, and 2.3 mM HCO_3^-. The bathing fluid was bubbled with air and was kept at 18° C (except in cooling experiments).

The gracilis muscle of the South American frog (*Leptodactilus ocellatus*) was dissected and kept immersed in normal frog-Ringer's solution. Preparations were studied at room temperature (approximately 23°C). Fibers at the free border of the muscle were selected for study and were stimulated individually or in small numbers to minimize movement. Some similar preparations were studied during superfusion with hypertonic Ringer's solution (Hodgkin and Horowicz, 1957; Caputo and Gimenez, 1967). In a few instances, single isolated fibers were dissected from the semitendinous muscle.

Drug additions or test alterations of ionic composition of the bathing fluid are indicated in the Results. In a group of experiments on giant axons and Purkinje fibers, a short (200 μm) central segment of the preparation was exposed to a high concentration of tetrodotoxin (1 to 4 μg/ml). A continuous stream of the TTX-containing solution was delivered through a micropipette (around 100 μm in tip diameter) positioned near the fiber, and both the general bath flow and the TTX solution flow were oriented perpendicularly relative to the fiber axis. The stream of TTX solution was visualized with the aid of indocyanine green (Cardiogreen, Hynson, Westcott & Dunning Inc.) to make sure that its flow remained unmixed so as to expose to the toxin only the desired axon segment.

Stimulation and Recording

All preparations were stimulated by brief rectangular pulses (0.1 to 1 msec, 1.5-fold threshold intensity applied at rates of 0.5 to 1.0 Hz). Stimuli, isolated from ground, were delivered through stainless steel or silver electrodes. Recording was effected through Ling-Gerard glass microelectrodes filled with 3 M *KCl*. The microelectrode resistance was around 20 MΩ, corresponding to a tip diameter of 0.15 to 0.3 μm (Oliveira Castro and Machado, 1969).

Measurements of microelectrode voltage (V) relative to a distant *Ag-AgCl* ground wire in the bath were taken with the help of a high-input impedance (higher than 10^{11} Ω) preamplifier provided with input capacity neutralization (WPI model M750). The first derivative ($\dot{V}$) of the voltage tracing was obtained by operational amplifiers compensated to yield minimal noise and tracing distortion. A calibrating ramp or triangular pulse was introduced between bath and ground to provide record calibration and to guide the compensating procedure (Paes de Carvalho et al, 1969). Both the ramp and the triangular calibration pulse represented displacements of 20 mV in 0.2 msec (100 V/sec) unless stated otherwise.

Records of V and $\dot{V}$ were kept both as a function of time (V,t and $\dot{V},t$ records) and in the phase plane, where V appeared in the abscissas and $\dot{V}$ in the ordinates ($\dot{V},V$ records). Tracings could be directly photographed from the screen of a double-beam oscilloscope (Tektonix 565), or V and $\dot{V}$ could be digitized in a PDP-12 DEC computer (12 K memory) and the average of eight successive cycles kept in digital tape for subsequent examination of time course and phase-plane analysis. Digitation rates of up to 20 μsec/point permitted many points to be placed even during the fastest upstrokes, and the simple-addition averaging procedure was effective in smoothing derivative noise without appreciable tracing distortion. Other information on the phase-plane recording of propagated action potentials can be found in Jenerick (1963; 1964), Paes de Carvalho et al. (1969), Paes de Carvalho (1975) and Paes de Carvalho et al. (1976).

Computer Simulation

Computer integration of the Cooley and Dodge (1966) model for a Hodgkin-Huxley axon was used to reproduce certain features of the squid data (Campos de Carvalho and Paes de Carvalho, 1980) and to support some of the conclusions drawn for cardiac muscle.

RESULTS

Homogeneous Propagation in Cable-like Cells

The propagation of action potentials in a long unbranched segment of squid giant axon is a very nearly homogeneous process; this is, a depolarization wave of constant shape travels at constant velocity along this cable-like cell. Conversely, the time course of action potentials recorded at any given point should also be constant anywhere along the axon segment where propagation is homogeneous. These concepts are features of the mathematic model of propagated action potentials (Hodgkin and Huxley, 1952) and can be easily shown also in the Cooley and Dodge (1966) model of propagation in a 6.25-cm long axon.

Figure 1 shows a series of superimposed V,t tracings obtained from this model at different points along the "axon." Except at the extremities ($x = 0$ where the "stimulus" was applied; and $x = 6$ where the "axon" was terminated by a segment of fixed membrane voltage equal to the resting potential), the time course of action potentials was indeed constant.

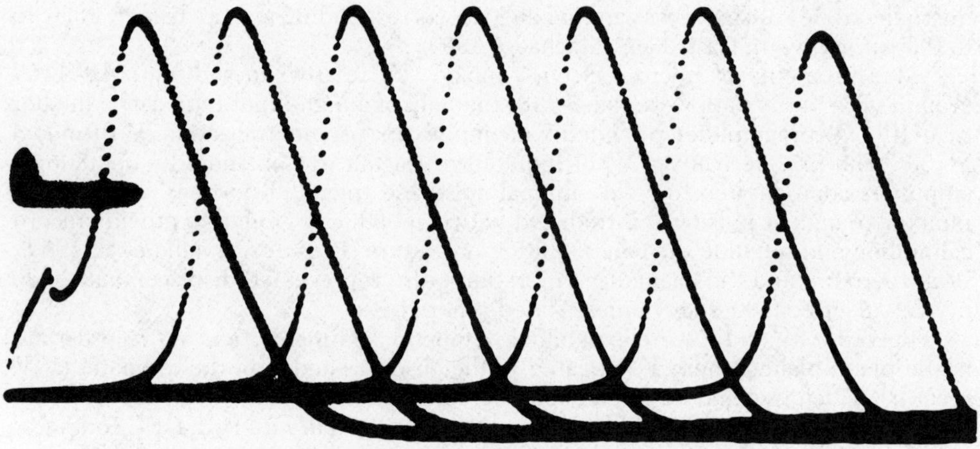

Figure 1. Transmembrane voltage computed as a function of time at 1-cm intervals along the Cooley-Dodge axon model during propagation of an action potential at 18°C. Stimulus characteristics: 10μA, 0.2 msec. Calibration bars: 10 mV (vertical) and 0.5 msec (horizontal). Integration unit intervals: time, 0.01 msec; distance, 0.05 cm. (From Campos de Carvalho, 1979; Campos de Carvalho and Paes de Carvalho, 1980).

Figure 2 shows the homogeneously propagated action potential yielded by the Cooley-Dodge model at position x = 3 cm. It also shows the corresponding phase-plane loop. The loop is inscribed clockwise, starting from resting voltage at the left of the record (see arrow). Loop slope and $\dot{V}$ amplitude can be measured at any point during activity. During the upstroke, the phase-plane record loops from the resting point to the peak of action potential (extreme right of tracing), passing through the point of maximal $\dot{V}$. This point divides the depolarization segment into an ascending and a descending limb (not to be confused with the ascending and descending limbs of the action potential itself). The smooth, undented appearance of the ascending and descending limbs of this trajectory, if maintained at successive recording sites, is the mark of homogeneous propagation.

The ascending limb of the phase-plane loop starts with a short linear segment that extends from the resting position (arrow) to the point where ionic current turns inward, some 15 to 17 mV to the right (see Fig. 6 for more information). This initial linear segment represents the exponential foot of the action potential. (In the phase-plane, a linear segment signifies that membrane voltage is coursing exponentially in time.) The initial loop slope, M_o, is a direct measure of the rate constant of the foot.

Note that the slope of the loop decreases *smoothly* and *monotonically* from its initial value M_o, and reaches zero at the point of maximal $\dot{V}$. From this point on, the slope becomes progressively more negative until a value of $\pm\infty$ is reached at the exact peak of the action potential (extreme right of the loop). Up to this point, no indentations and no positive slope larger than M_o are ever observed in the model. Indeed, none can occur during propagation in a homogeneous axon.

Figure 3A shows the superimposed tracings obtained from two sites along a real squid axon. The action potential time course seems identical in both sites, and the phase-plane loops are perfectly superimposable (except for the random noise of the $\dot{V}$ measurement). Conduction velocity was calculated to be 21.6 m/sec at 18° C. All the basic features of the phase-plane loop described above as characteristic of homoge-

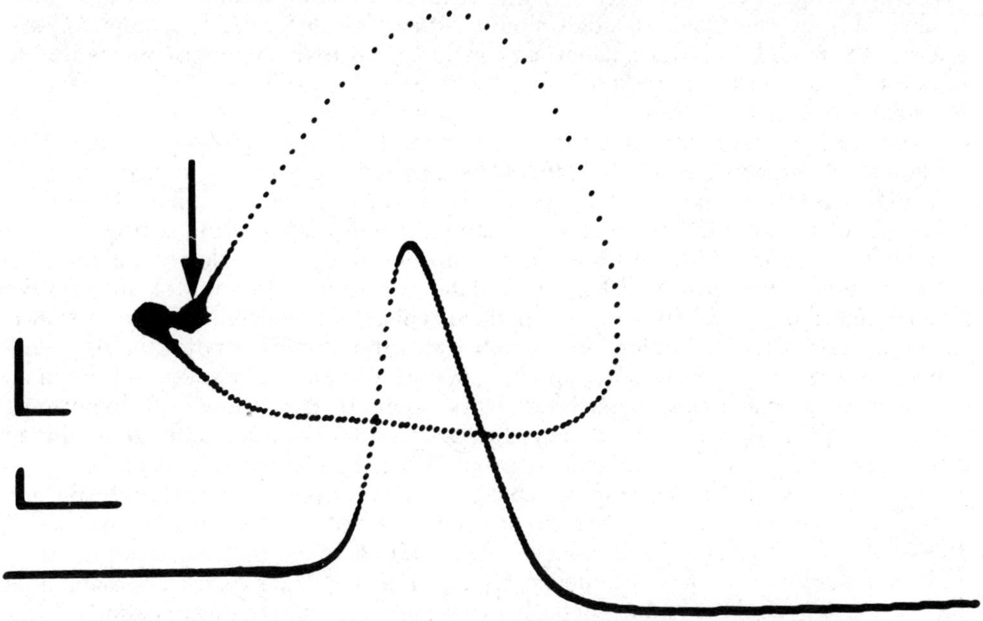

Figure 2. Transmembrane propagated action potential and corresponding phase-plane loop computed at the midpoint of the Cooley-Dodge axon model. *V*,*t* calibration (lower bars): 10 mV and 0.5 msec. $\dot{V}$,*V* calibration (upper bars): 100 v/sec (vertical) and 10 mV (horizontal). Same integration conditions as Fig. 1. (From Campos de Carvalho, 1979; Campos de Carvalho and Paes de Carvalho, 1980.)

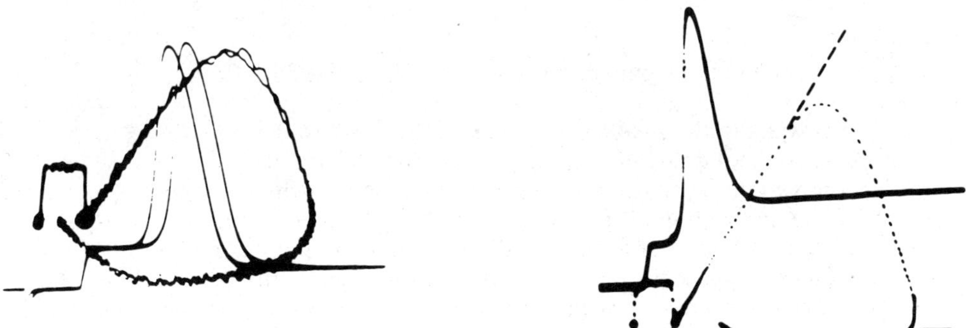

A B

Figure 3. *A*, superimposed propagated action potentials recorded from two different sites along a real squid axon in sea water at 18° C. Also shown superimposed are the corresponding phase-plane loops. The calibration ramp ascended 20 mV in 0.1 msec (200 v/sec). (From Saldeña, 1977). *B*, propagated action potential and corresponding phase-plane loop obtained from a skeletal muscle (m. gracilis) of the frog in normal Ringer's solution at room temperature (about 23° C). The calibration ramp ascended 20 mV in 0.2 msec (100 v/sec). (From Saldeña, 1977.)

neous propagation can be seen here. The real records are therefore well described qualitatively by the Cooley-Dodge model, although values for $\dot{V}_{max}$ and M_o are lower in the model. This discrepancy may be due partly to the higher resting potential of our axons and partly to the possible peculiarities concerning their rate constants, maximal conductance values, and ionic equilibrium potentials. Such quantitative differences do not hinder the qualitative concept that the same typical loop configuration for homogeneous conduction is yielded by both model and experiment in squid axon.

Figure 3B shows the simultaneous records of a propagated action potential and its phase-plane representation obtained at approximately 23° C from a frog skeletal muscle fiber in normal Ringer's solution. A constant conduction velocity of about 2.44 m/sec could be demonstrated by extracellular recordings. In spite of quantitative differences, the general smooth loop pattern typical of homogeneous conduction is again present. This illustration also demonstrates the important point that the existence of a T-tubule network does not alter significantly the smoothness and the main characteristics of a homogeneous conduction loop. In fact, the use of hypertonic solutions capable of severely reducing contraction does not modify the general loop pattern obtained from homogeneously propagating skeletal muscle fibers.

Phase-plane contours retain the same basic qualitative characteristics during any experimental maneuver that depresses or enhances conduction homogeneously along the whole fiber (Saldeña, 1977). The change of M_o observed in these experiments is in keeping with known fact and theory, which show that M_o is a close approximation for the constant K of the homogeneously propagated action potential equation (Hodgkin & Huxley, 1952; Paes de Carvalho et al, 1976). The K constant equals $r_i c\theta^2$, where r_i and c are the longitudinal internal resistance and surface membrane capacitance per unit length, and θ is the conduction velocity. A decrease of M_o is expected and actually observed whenever θ decreases during homogeneous conduction, as in low temperature, increased extracellular K^+, or exposure of the whole preparation to a low concentration of TTX.

Nonhomogeneous Propagation in Cable-like Cells

We investigated the phase-plane loop patterns in squid axons where conduction was made to be nonhomogeneous.

The left column of Figure 4 shows an experiment in which nonhomogeneity was created by the application of tetrodotoxin (TTX) in high concentration (1 μg/ml) to a short (~200μm) segment of axon according to the technique explained in Methods. The TTX pipette could be placed at any position along the fiber relative to the recording microelectrode. The control record before the TTX application shows a loop pattern characteristic of homogeneous conduction. When TTX was applied to the site of recording (position 0), the action potential diminished in amplitude and rate of rise. The shape of the phase-plane loop is clearly distorted except for its initial linear segment, which has the same length and slope M_o. This means that normal activity approaches the site of block unimpaired and establishes there a normal exponential action potential foot. But as soon as inward current is locally needed to continue depolarization, the loop fails to follow the original pattern and moves on to a lower $\dot{V}_{max}$ and a lower action potential amplitude, mostly contributed by surrounding segments. The point of departure between the two loops marks, therefore, the moment when inward current becomes discernible in the control situation (Campos de Carvalho and Paes de Carvalho, 1980).

The TTX application is then interrupted, and complete recovery is observed. The TTX pipette is next moved to the left so that the site of block precedes the site of

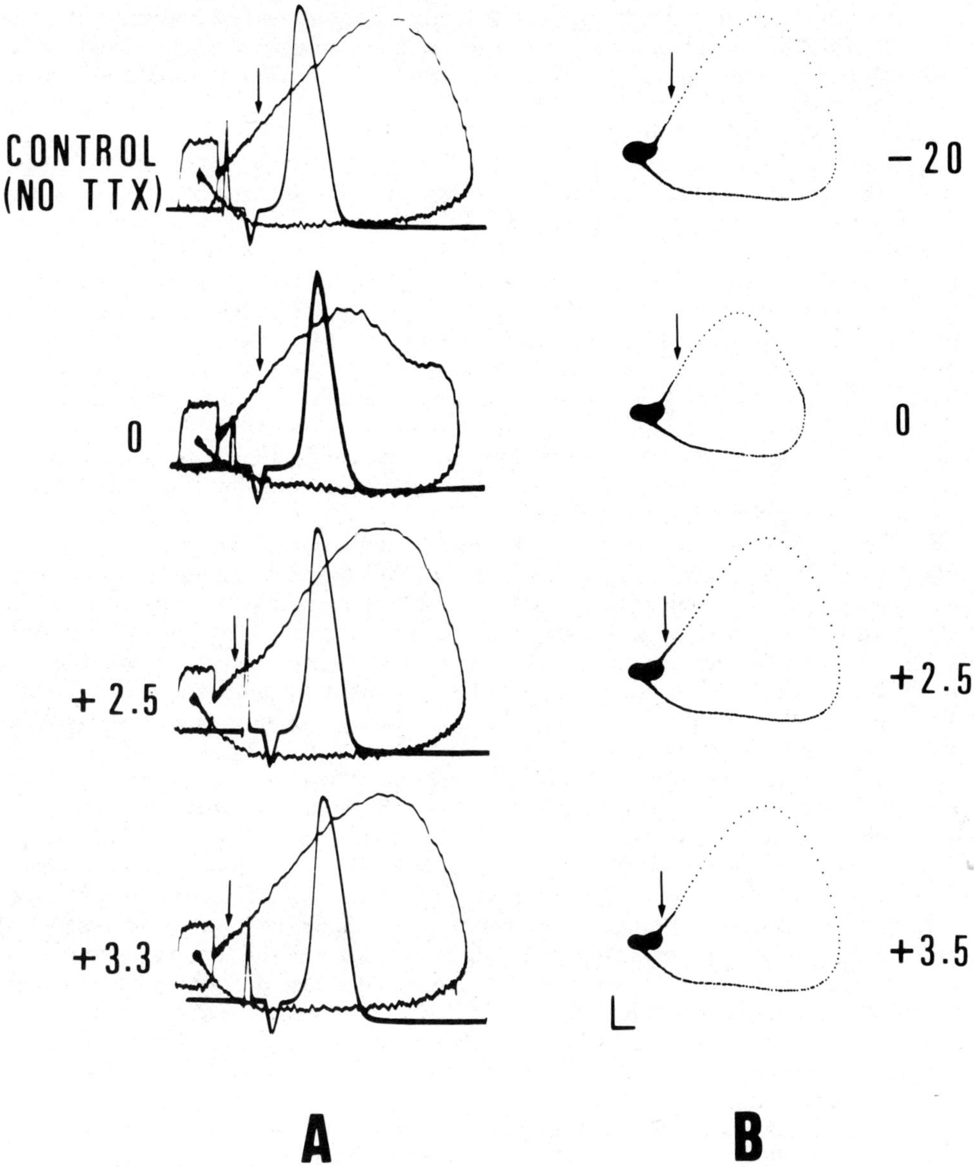

Figure 4. Comparison of nonhomogeneous conduction loops for real (left column) and model (right column) squid axons where a short segment was submitted to TTX poisoning. Numbers correspond to postion (in millimeters) of the recording electrode in the propagation pathways relative to the TTX-depressed site (200 μm in the real experiment). TTX-depression was mimicked in the Cooley-Dodge model by cutting $\overline{g_{Na}}$ to 10% of its control value in two successive length units (equivalent to 100 μm). Real squid data were obtained at 18.5° C in sea water (unpublished results of Saldeña, Ponce-Zumino, and Paes de Carvalho, 1978). Model data from Campos de Carvalho (1979). Triangular wave in squid records had an amplitude of 20 mV and a slope of 200 v/sec. Calibration of the model data corresponds to 100 v/sec (vertical) and 10 mV (horizontal). Arrows show end of initial linear segment of slope M_o.

recording in the path of propagation. The loop contour at a site 2.5 mm beyond the block is still altered but in a different way. It shows an obvious indentation in the ascending limb, the final slope of which is steeper than M_o. It should be noted, however, that *(1)* $\dot{V}_{max}$ has almost reached its control value and *(2)* the initial linear segment of slope M_o is now definitely shorter than it is in control or during the application of TTX at position O (see arrows). This means that while propagation moves up to the site of block unhindered, local current flow is already influencing the recording site beyond. When activity reaches the block and fails to provoke inward current there, conduction halts momentarily. From this moment onwards phase-plane loops recorded beyond the block will be altered. The first alteration will be an early interruption of their initial linear segment. The voltage at which this interruption occurs is closer to the resting potential in recording sites further removed from the blocked segment, as in these sites the foot of the action potential has progressed less at the time activity reaches the block (see position +3.3 mm). As points further away from the block are studied, the initial segment of unaltered slope M_o is shortened further and a loop contour characteristic of homogeneous conduction is progressively restored. In the present case, loops recorded 4.16 mm beyond the block (not shown) were virtually identical to control loops.

The real squid data of Figure 4 teach us that the initial linear segment of the phase-plane loop is a passive local expression of the advancing wavefront and, therefore, is not altered as long as propagation is unhindered and homogeneous up to the site of recording. Otherwise, this initial segment becomes shorter, even though its slope is unaltered. Findings such as these are entirely in keeping with expectation and have been reproduced in the Cooley-Dodge axon model (Campos de Carvalho and Paes de Carvalho, 1980). The data are shown in the right column of Figure 4 and the similarity of results is clear.

A second interesting example of nonhomogeneous conduction is what happens at a collision site in squid axon. Figure 5 shows records obtained in the middle of an axon during homogeneous propagation in either direction (panels A and B). Panel C is a superimposition of records A and B, to show that the phase loops are very nearly identical in both directions of propagation. Figure 5D shows the superimposition of tracings obtained during homogeneous conduction (smaller loop, identical to panel B) and during a collison provoked at the site of recording by the simultaneous stimulation of both ends of the axon. Notice that the phase-plane loops are perfectly coincident during the initial linear segment of slope M_o. M_o, however, is not the largest slope of the ascending limb of the collision loop. Notice also that $\dot{V}_{max}$ in the collision is larger and displaced to the right in the voltage axis. The peak amplitude of the action potential is also larger.

The results shown in Figure 5 are also expected from the Hodgkin-Huxley theory and can be qualitatively reproduced by the Cooley-Dodge axon model, as shown in Figure 6. There, too, the initial linear segment observed in the phase-plane loop of normal action potentials is unaltered in the collision. This is to be expected because the two exponential feet of the colliding action potentials are initially added to form an exponential of double amplitude constant but with the same rate constant M_o. Notice, however, that M_o is not the largest slope in the ascending limb of the collision loop, and that the voltage at which $\dot{V}_{max}$ occurs is displaced to the right.

Figure 6 also shows the model phase-plane loops of ionic (I_i), capacitive (I_c), and membrane (I_m) currents during homogeneous conduction (panel C) and a collision (panel D). A few points should be noticed in the current curves. First, I_c reproduces the loop contour of $\dot{V}$, as necessary by definition. Second, I_m and I_c depart appreciably only when I_i turns inward. This point (arrows) marks the end of the initial linear segment of the phase-plane loop in both cases. Third, peak I_i is actually smaller

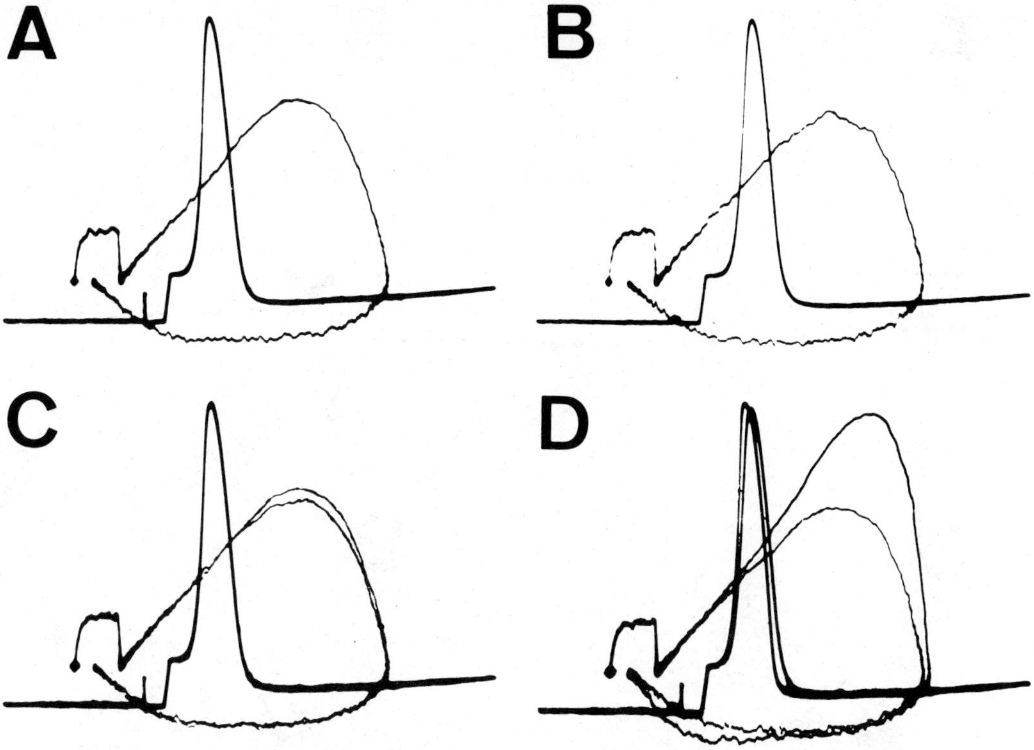

Figure 5. Collision experiment in a squid giant axon immersed in sea water at about 18.5° C. *A* and *B* are control records of action potentials and corresponding phase-plane loops obtained by stimulating the axon at each end separately. *C* shows the superimposition of records *A* and *B*. In *D*, record *B* appears superimposed with the record of a collision obtained by simultaneous stimulation of both extremities of the axon. Horizontal calibration bar in center of figure represents 1 msec for the *V,t* records. Calibration ramp has a 20 mV amplitude and a 200 v/sec slope. (From Tashiro, 1980).

during collision. Therefore, the larger peak I_c (or $\dot{V}_{max}$) of the collision action potential is due to a larger contribution of I_m caused by the longitudinal flow of current from the two wavefronts that converge onto the recording site. This is then a situation in which an increase in $\dot{V}_{max}$ clearly does not reflect an increase in peak I_i.

In the two situations above—local TTX block and collision—the loop segment of slope M_o remains undisturbed as long as the propagation of the approaching wavefront is undisturbed. This point becomes clear in the TTX experiment, where the initial linear segment recorded at points beyond the block is terminated as soon as the propagating action potential reaches the site of block upstream.

One is now left to wonder about the effect of a localized increase of longitudinal resistance (r_i) of the axon, for which no phase-plane modeling is yet available. Consider first the time course of voltage of the subthreshold foot of the action potential just beyond the site of increased r_i. It is intuitive that it will follow the time course of voltage before the block with a delay imposed by the product $r_i c$, where r_i is locally increased due to the added longitudinal resistance at the discontinuity. One can therefore guess at the effect of a local increase of r_i on M_o, provided one knows what happens to M_o just before this particular site.

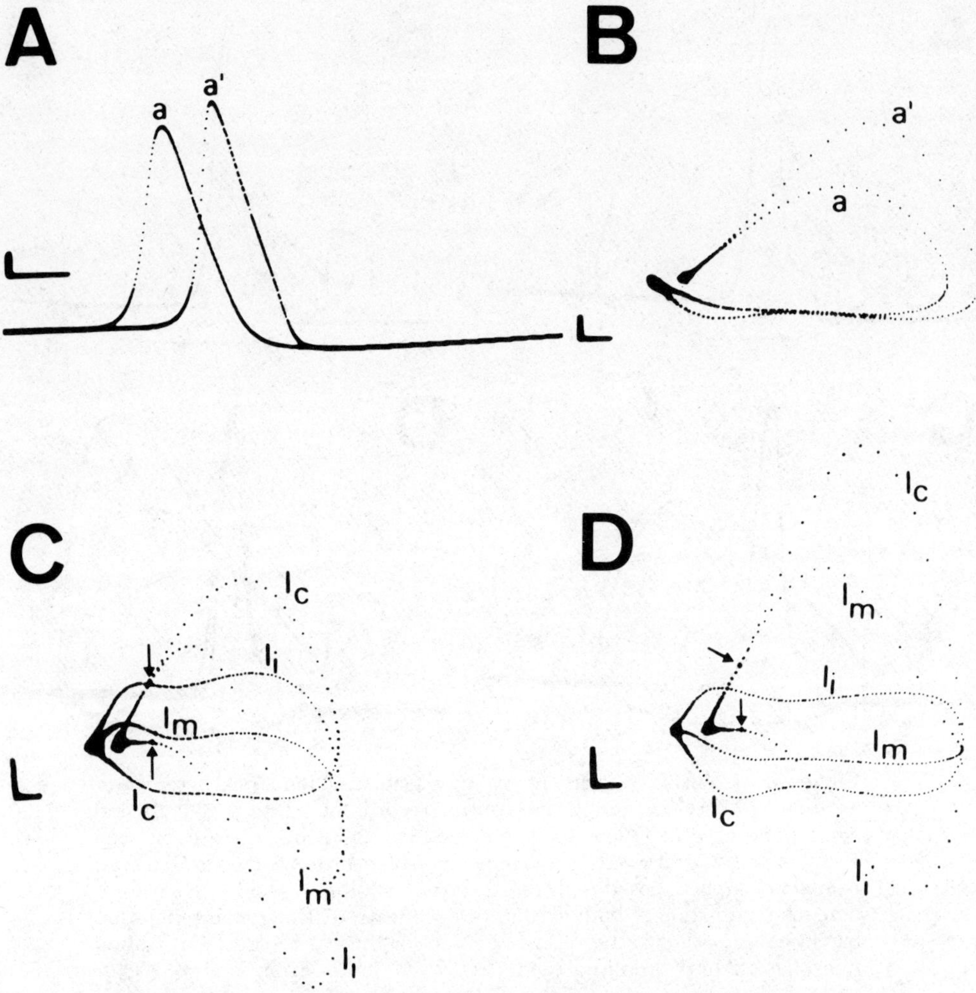

Figure 6. Collision in the Cooley-Dodge model. *A*, homogeneously propagated (a) and collision (a′) action potentials obtained in the midpoint of the axon model. *B*, corresponding phase-plane loops (a, a′). *C*, ionic (I_i), capacitive (I_c) and membrane (I_m) currents computed for the homogeneous action potential, displayed in the phase-plane (membrane voltage in abscissae). *D*, equivalent data for the collision action potential. Calibration bars: 100 $\mu A/cm^2$ (vertical) and 10 mV (horizontal). (From Tashiro, 1980.)

When a propagating action potential meets with a sealed end (infinite r_i), it will rise faster to its peak, and $\dot{V}_{max}$ should be noticeably greater. The longitudinal flow of current will be "reflected" back at the sealed end. As a result of this phenomenon, the exponential rise of the foot of the action potential at the sealed end will have the same rate constant M_o but twice the amplitude constant. This situation is therefore similar to what happens at a collision where the initial loop segment of slope M_o is identical to that found in homogeneous propagation. Also as in collision, the phase-plane loop should curve upwards at the ionic current reversal voltage and form a slope higher than M_o. Preliminary modeling of this situation shows the prediction to be true. The same is hinted at by Goldstein and Rall (1974).

Now, if r_i is increased locally but is not infinite, the situation will be intermediate between that of homogeneous conduction and that found at a sealed end. In other words, M_o just before the r_i discontinuity will remain unchanged. It is also intutitive that some fraction of the longitudinal current will be able to flow through the site of increased r_i and passively depolarize the capacitance of membrane areas beyond. Therefore, as the r_ic product for passive depolarization of the segment beyond the discontinuity is increased, it is fair to assume that the foot of the action potential recorded in that segment will follow an exponential rise with a lower rate constant. This would be translated into phase-plane representation as a lower slope for the initial linear segment of the loop.

Considering the discussion above, it seems safe to state that only two conditions compatible with geometrical reality in an unbranched squid axon may yield a decrease of the initial loop slope M_o in a given site of recording: *(1)* a decrease in M_o in the fiber segment that immediately precedes the site of recording and *(2)* a discrete, localized increase in r_i. In the second condition, if the fiber beyond the discontinuity is homogeneous, normal homogeneous propagation and loop configuration will be mostly resumed within 1 to 2 space constants.

If the data interpretation and the predictions advanced above are true, it should be possible to decide about the homogeneity of propagation in a cable-like cell by studying phase-plane contours at different sites. It should also be possible to obtain information on the cause of nonhomogeneous conduction by the use of this same type of analysis. Phase-plane recording of propagated action potentials can be equally useful in the study of conduction in such complex structures as heart muscle, as will be shown below.

Variability of Phase-Plane Contours in Heart Muscle

Paes de Carvalho et al. (1969) pointed out that in the heart, phase-plane contours of the action potential upstroke vary from one region to another. Loop configurations were found to vary also within a presumably homogeneous region. Loop contours that we now recognize as characteristic of homogeneous propagation could occur side by side with contours in which the ascending limb was distorted. The finding of loop slopes higher than M_o was not uncommon.

Garcia (1975) examined phase loops of a large number of intracellular records taken at random from rabbit atria (231 cells) and dog Purkinje fibers (210 cells). Figure 7 shows samples of the different types of patterns he found for the ascending limb (patterns A1-A9). Patterns A1 and A8 are very nearly compatible with homogeneous conduction. They represent together only 23% of all records in either type of preparation. This percentage increases to 31% if types A5 and A6, in which M_o is the largest slope, are added to this class. On the other hand, pattern A2, in which M_o is clearly not the largest slope, accounts for 48% of the records in dog Purkinje fibers and 50% in rabbit atrium, although the increase in slope beyond the initial linear segment is variable and also much less obvious in Purkinje fibers than it is in atrium (Garcia, 1975; Saldeña, 1977). To these loop patterns one can add type A4, also clearly pointing to nonhomogeneous conduction. This represents an additional 11% in Purkinje and 18% in atrial fibers, the alterations in slope being again less noticeable in Purkinje fibers. Patterns A3 and A7 are negligibly rare (less than 3%). From these observations one is led to conclude that propagation in a large percentage of cases shows signs of nonhomogeneity.

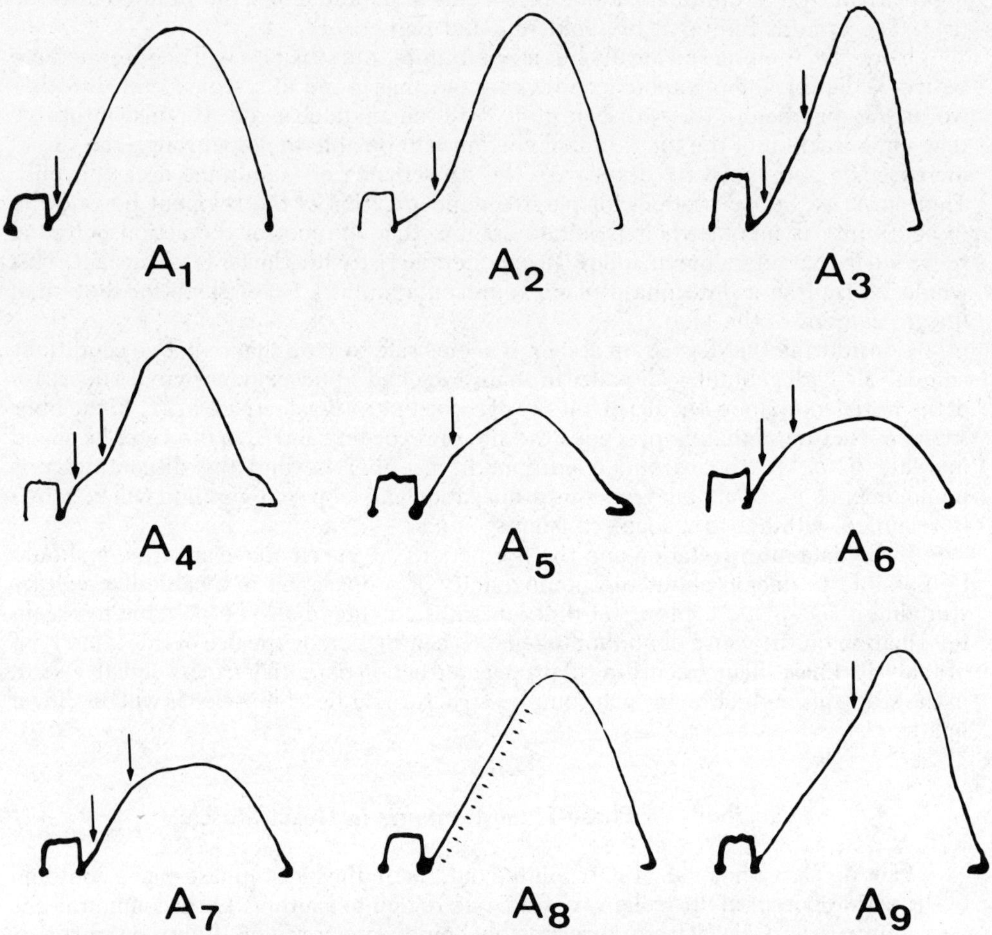

Figure 7. Phase-plane patterns of intracellular action potential upstrokes recorded from mammalian hearts by Garcia (1975). Vertical arrows indicate discrepancies of the ascending phase of the loops relative to contour expected of a homogeneously conducted action potential. In A8, arrows call attention to the long linear segment. Rectangular calibration at left side of loops: 20 mV (horizontal) and 100 v/sec (vertical).

We later realized that the patterns demonstrated by Garcia suffered from the criticism that simple intracellular records referred to a distant bath ground reproduce not only the transmembrane voltage but add to it the extracellular voltage of the interstitial space surrounding the fiber. The influence of this interference will depend on the mass and nearness of tissue involved in the genesis of the extracellular potential and on the timing of activity in contributing bundles. Accordingly, the extracellular voltage can be large or small and can have a sharp synchronous time course or be multiphasic and asynchronous (Masuda and Paes de Carvalho, 1975). It is therefore reasonable to assume that such interference may distort the phase-plane record. It is also reasonable to expect the interference to be less conspicuous in Purkinje fibers.

To circumvent these possible errors, we performed another series of experiments in which the extracellular contribution could be measured and eliminated. The experiment involved two steps. First, the intracellular voltage and its first time derivative were recorded. Each of eight successive, identical cycles were digitized on line, averaged for improved signal to noise ratio, and the averages of V and $\dot{V}$ stored. Next, the microelectrode was carefully withdrawn so that its tip remained in the immediate vicinity of the cell from which the intracellular voltage has been recorded. The extracellular voltage and its first time derivative were obtained and treated in the same manner outlined above. The V and $\dot{V}$ records were subsequently examined and subtracted off-line, allowing the determination of a true transmembrane voltage and dV/dt for each cell under study. Columns A and B in Figure 8 show the data from two atrial cells studied in this fashion. In either column, the upper record displays the stored raw data for intracellular ($V,\dot{V}$) and extracellular ($S,\dot{S}$) measurements. The middle record shows the phase-plane plot obtained from the intracellular record alone. In the lower record, the subtracted transmembrane records are presented, together with their phase-plane displays. A slight time shift of the action potential relative to stimulus did sometimes occur in the few minutes that elapsed between the intracellular and extracellular recordings of a given cell. In this case, the extracellular record pair was displaced in time so that the desired synchrony was reestablished. Such time corrections were 280 and 180 μsec for columns A and B, respectively. In some other records no time correction was necessary.

In Figure 8A the phase-plane loop of the intracellular voltage is quite clearly of the A2 type. The extracellular voltage is represented by a simple biphasic potential (S), as expected from synchronous conduction. Note that the derivative of this biphasic potential ($\dot{S}$) shows a sizable negative peak that is synchronous with the peak of $\dot{V}$. When the transmembrane voltage difference is calculated, it is seen that *(1)* the resulting transmembrane $(\dot{V} - \dot{S})_{max}$ is higher than the original intracellular $\dot{V}_{max}$ by an amount equal to the amplitude of the negative $\dot{S}$ peak; and *(2)* both the initial linear segment and the inflection seen near the end of the descending limb of the loop are unaltered by the subtraction of the extracellular S and $\dot{S}$, except that the initial segment is made more linear due to the disappearance of small irregularities. These observations are entirely expected when the extracellular record is mostly generated by a small, synchronous bundle of which the studied cell is part. Figure 8A shows, therefore, that the finding of phase loops of type A2 (slopes steeper than M_o during the upstroke) cannot be explained away by extracellular interference at a synchronous wavefront. The extracellular interference alters directly the intracellularly measured $\dot{V}_{max}$, so that true transmembrane value $\dot{V} - \dot{S}_{max}$ is larger and the phase loop more peaked than that observed for the raw data. The same finding is pointed out by Spach (Chapter 9).

Figure 8B illustrates the case of a cell for which the extracellular record shows a multiphasic extracellular potential due to the combination of two simple biphasic waves. The first is due to the very wavefront of which the recorded action potential is part. The second is due to a slightly delayed wave of larger amplitude generated by another mass of tissue nearby. Irregularities of the loop contour of intracellular voltage can be seen clearly in the ascending and descending limbs. The calculated transmembrane loop is free of most of these irregularities. A clearly linear initial segment is now followed by a slightly steeper segment, and a higher derivative peak is observed. Also, the indentation present in the descending limb has been eliminated. The study of this cell teaches us that asynchronous activation of adjacent cell masses can indeed generate different types of irregularities in the phase-plane loop. But even in these more complex cases, the transmembrane data still yield A2 loop contours if present in the original data.

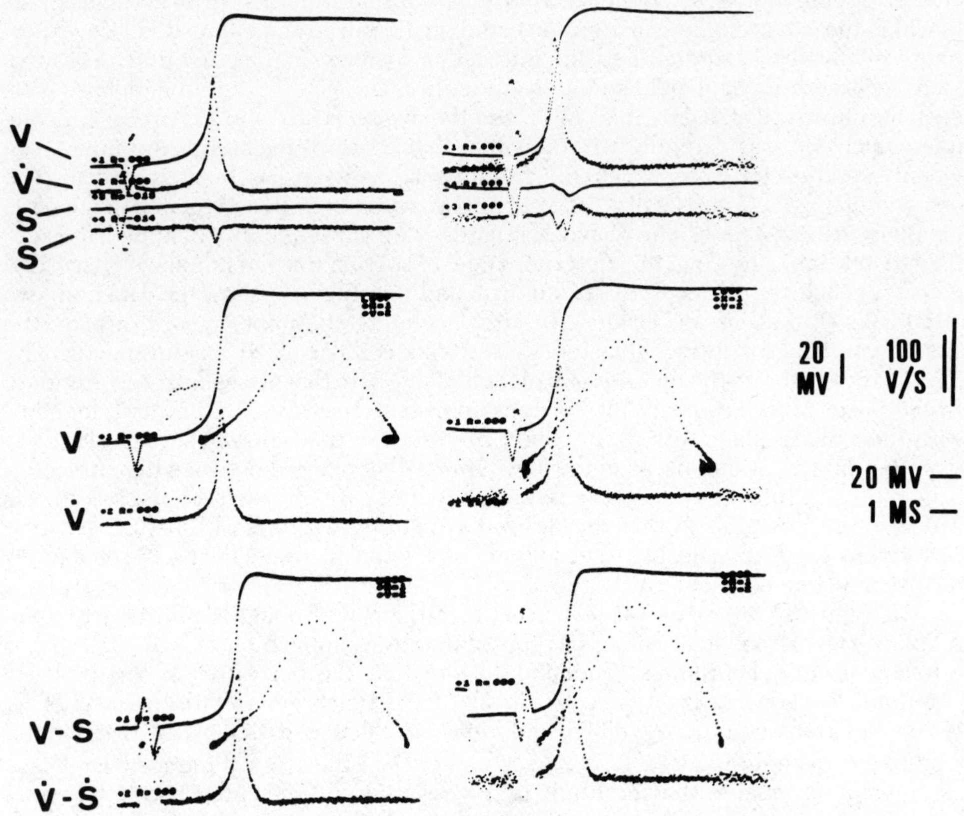

Figure 8. Determination of transmembrane voltage and dV/dt as a function of time and in the phase-plane for two atrial cells of the rabbit (columns A and B). In each column, the upper record is the original intracellular $(V,\dot{V})$ and extracellular $(S,\dot{S})$ data; the middle record shows the original intracellular V and $\dot{V}$ as a function of time and in the phase-plane; the lower record shows the same displays for the calculated transmembrane voltage $(V-S$ and $\dot{V}-\dot{S})$. Calibrations for voltage, time and derivatives are located at the right side of the illustration.

We can therefore conclude that all phase-plane loops of intracellular voltage are more or less flattened in the region of $\dot{V}_{max}$ depending on the amplitude of the negative peak of the derivative of extracellular voltage. This distortion was found to be minimal or nonexistent in many cases where the amplitude of the extracellular potential was very small (below 1 mV peak-to-peak). A second conclusion is that the appearance of an initial segment in the ascending limb followed by an upward inflection towards a slope higher than M_o is indeed a common finding in the heart. This phenomenon is not abolished by the subtraction of extracellular voltage. The termination of the initial linear segment is always in the range of 20 to 30 mV above resting potential. In Garcia's analysis of intracellular voltage, the voltage at which the slope changed from M_o was 20 ± 0.6 mV (average ± SEM) for dog Purkinje fibers and 25 ± 0.5 mV for rabbit atrium. As pointed out above, the upward inflection of the ascending limb (type A2, Fig. 7) is much less marked in Purkinje fibers, where the slope increase is mostly below 10%. In atrium, the slope after the inflection in type A2 records ranges from slight to nearly two times M_o.

In light of the above comments, we suggest that intracellular voltage patterns A2 and A8 in Figure 7 are approximately correct representatives of transmembrane findings. Possibly the same can be said of pattern A4, although we did not find it in any of the subtraction experiments. As to the other patterns, we tend to regard them as distorted by small irregularities that could be eliminated by determining transmembrane instead of intracellular recordings. It can be seen that these other patterns (A1, A3, A5–7, and A9 in Fig. 7) might convert to type A8 patterns after subtraction of irregularities due to extracellular interference. If this contention is correct, Garcia's statistical findings can be rewritten as follows:

Type A2 = atrium: 50%; Purkinje fiber: 48%
Type A4 = atrium: 18%; Purkinje fiber: 11%
Type A8 = atrium: 32%; Purkinje fiber: 41%

We shall now restrict our interpretation to records of types A2 and A8, both of which we deem to represent existing transmembrane loop contours. Type A8 is very obviously the same pattern previously associated with homogeneous propagation whereas type A2 is certainly characteristic of nonhomogeneous conduction. It remains to be seen what this nonhomogeneity represents.

Significance of A2 Loop Patterns as Revealed by Local Blockade Induced by Tetrodotoxin in Purkinje Fibers

It is possible to use Purkinje fibers to perform the same experiment of localized application of tetrodotoxin described above for squid axons (see Fig. 4 and related text). In fact, these experiments were first performed by Garcia (1975) on Purkinje fibers, and their repetition in squid nerve was prompted by the need for an exact interpretation of the Purkinje fiber data. Figure 9 illustrates typical results obtained by applying a narrow band (less than 200 μm) of TTX in Tyrode's solution to the site where intracellular voltage was recorded. Figure 9B shows the effect of this experiment on a loop contour of type A8. Notice that the initial linear segment of the loop is not disturbed up to a voltage of about 20 mV above resting potential. From then on, the TTX effect is noticeable as a decrease in $\dot{V}_{max}$ and action potential amplitude. The original contour is readily recovered upon termination of the TTX application. By analogy with the squid observations and modeling, we interpret the point of transition between no TTX effect and noticeable TTX effect as the point at which ionic current turns inward in the control record. Figure 9A illustrates the effect on a loop contour of the A2 type. Here again the initial linear segment is untouched by TTX. The toxin effect becomes noticeable only at the point of upward inflection of the ascending limb, some 20 mV above resting potential. We submit this finding as evidence that in A2 type records the upward inflection of the ascending limb corresponds to the voltage at which ionic current turns inward.

When discussing the squid axon data, we stated that no spatially homogeneous condition can yield a phase-plane loop different from type A8 for homogeneous conduction (except for a negligible upward inflection caused by introducing gating currents into the axon model, as shown by Saldeña in 1977). We are then led to conclude that the control loop in Figure 9A, as well as other instances of type A2 contour, do indeed represent nonhomogeneous conduction. It can be seen from the linear initial segment that the flow of local currents to the impaled cell rises exponentially in time. Then, as activity is triggered and ionic current turns inward, the loop inflects upward as if local active currents were excessive for the set of passive cable characteristics that generated the initial linear segment of the loop. As pointed out above in the section on nonhomogeneous conduction in cable-like structures, such a

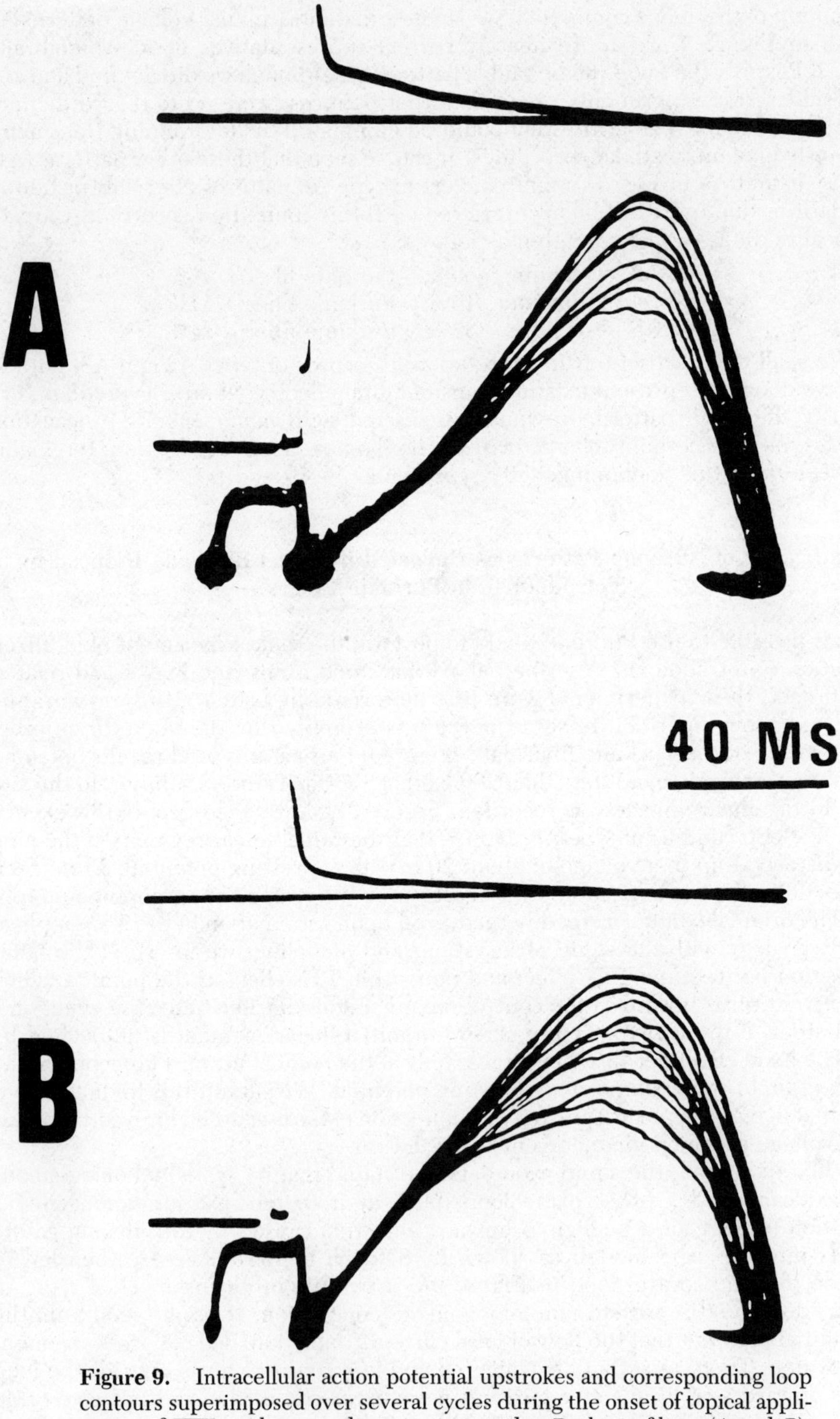

Figure 9. Intracellular action potential upstrokes and corresponding loop contours superimposed over several cycles during the onset of topical application of TTX to the recording site in two dog Purkinje fibers (*A* and *B*). Calibration ramp rises 20 mV in 0.2 msec (100 v/sec). (From Garcia, 1975.)

phase-plane configuration can be generated by one of the following conditions: *(1)* a local increase of r_i in the next fiber segment along the propagation pathway; *(2)* a local increase of the r_ic product just prior to the site of recording; or *(3)* a combination of both previous conditions. In the case of condition 1, M_o should be unchanged and $\dot{V}_{max}$ increased relative to homogeneous propagation. In condition 2, M_o and $\dot{V}_{max}$ should be smaller, although $\dot{V}_{max}$ is expected to resume full amplitude shortly afterwards.

The question now is which of the causes stated above actually underlie A2 type phase-plane loops in cardiac muscle.

The Relationship between Loop Contour and Direction of Propagation in Rabbit Atrium

Garcia (1975) observed that the loop contour at a given cell often changed markedly when the site of stimulation of the preparation was changed. Figure 10, which illustrates some of his typical results with intracellular potentials, shows records obtained from three cells in the rabbit atrium. Each row (A, B, and C) corresponds to one cell. Records at the left are control samples. Records in the middle column were obtained during the same impalements a few cycles after the site of stimulation was changed. Records at the right are the return to control stimulation. Loop contour changes immediately upon change of stimulus site; no adaptation or progressive change was ever seen.

Figure 10 deserves careful consideration. First, all records are of A2 or A8 types. We assume them to be good approximations of true transmembrane loop contours. Second, in all three cells, the control configuration happened to be compatible with homogeneous propagation. Third, in the three cells the displacement of stimulus site caused a change from one type of loop contour to another. Fourth, in all three cells, M_o is diminished when the A2 contour is present. Fifth, $\dot{V}_{max}$ is always increased concomitantly with the appearance of an A2 contour. Sixth, the voltage at which $\dot{V}_{max}$ is observed is displaced to the right in A2 contours.

The features associated with the change to the A2 contour vary in intensity in different records but were observed in all of Garcia's tracings except one in which $\dot{V}_{max}$ was smaller. Such features were associated with the geometry of intercellular connections, which differs according to the direction upon which the cell is invaded by the propagating wavefront (Garcia, 1975; Paes de Carvalho et al., 1976). A local increase in r_i due to a decreased junctional area in a given direction of spread would for instance explain a lower postjunctional M_o. The simultaneous observation of a higher $\dot{V}_{max}$ could, on the other hand, be explained by a local increase in r_i at the next cell junction. Finally, the displacement to the right of the voltage at which $\dot{V}_{max}$ is achieved would be expected from the increased input and output resistances. In this situation, the local ionic current would be mostly engaged in discharging the local capacitance. The $\dot{V}$ curve would then follow more closely the i_i curve, the peak of which occurs at voltages higher than that of $\dot{V}_{max}$ in a homogeneous propagating action potential (see Fig. 6C for the squid axon model). If all this is true, one would also expect to find a few cases where a cell showed an increased input r_i and a small output r_i in a given propagation direction. In this case, one would see a loop with a smaller M_o but with the same or smaller $\dot{V}_{max}$ relative to homogeneous propagation.

To lend support to this hypothesis, we performed experiments in which the loop contour was observed first when a cell was invaded along the longitudinal preferential direction of the muscle bundles and then, by changing the stimulus site, when invasion

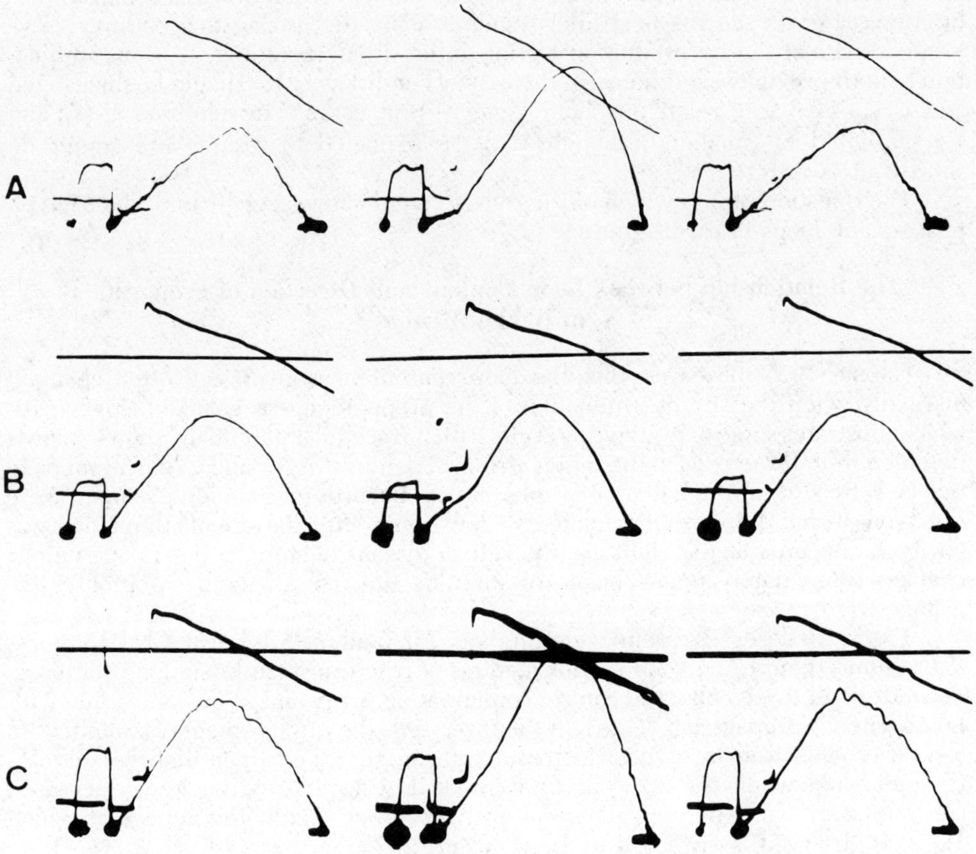

Figure 10. Change of upstroke loop configuration with direction of propagation in three atrial muscle cells (A, B and C). Left column: control stimulation at first site; middle column: change to second stimulation site; right column: return to first stimulation site. All records show intracellular voltage as a function of time and in the phase-plane. Calibration ramp ascended 20 mV in 0.2 msec (100 v/sec). (From Garcia, 1975).

proceeded transversely (perpendicularly) to this preferential axis. The results of such experiments are shown in Figure 11. The preparation was the rabbit left atrial roof, and transmembrane loop contours free of extracellular contamination were obtained with the same technique outlined for the experiment of Figure 8. The results reproduce all the qualitative findings of Figure 10, even though in the two cells for which results are shown the differences in M_o between longitudinal and transverse conduction were only around 10%. It is thus conceivable that with transverse propagation the increased r_i can be represented by more sparse cell connections between adjacent cell bundles. Obviously, a more exact morphologic analysis of cell arrangement and connections in rabbit atrium is necessary before a quantitative treatment of our data can be advanced with any degree of reality. We are then left to wonder to what extent Garcia's type A2 findings are due to propagation in directions other than the preferential direction of fiber bundles.

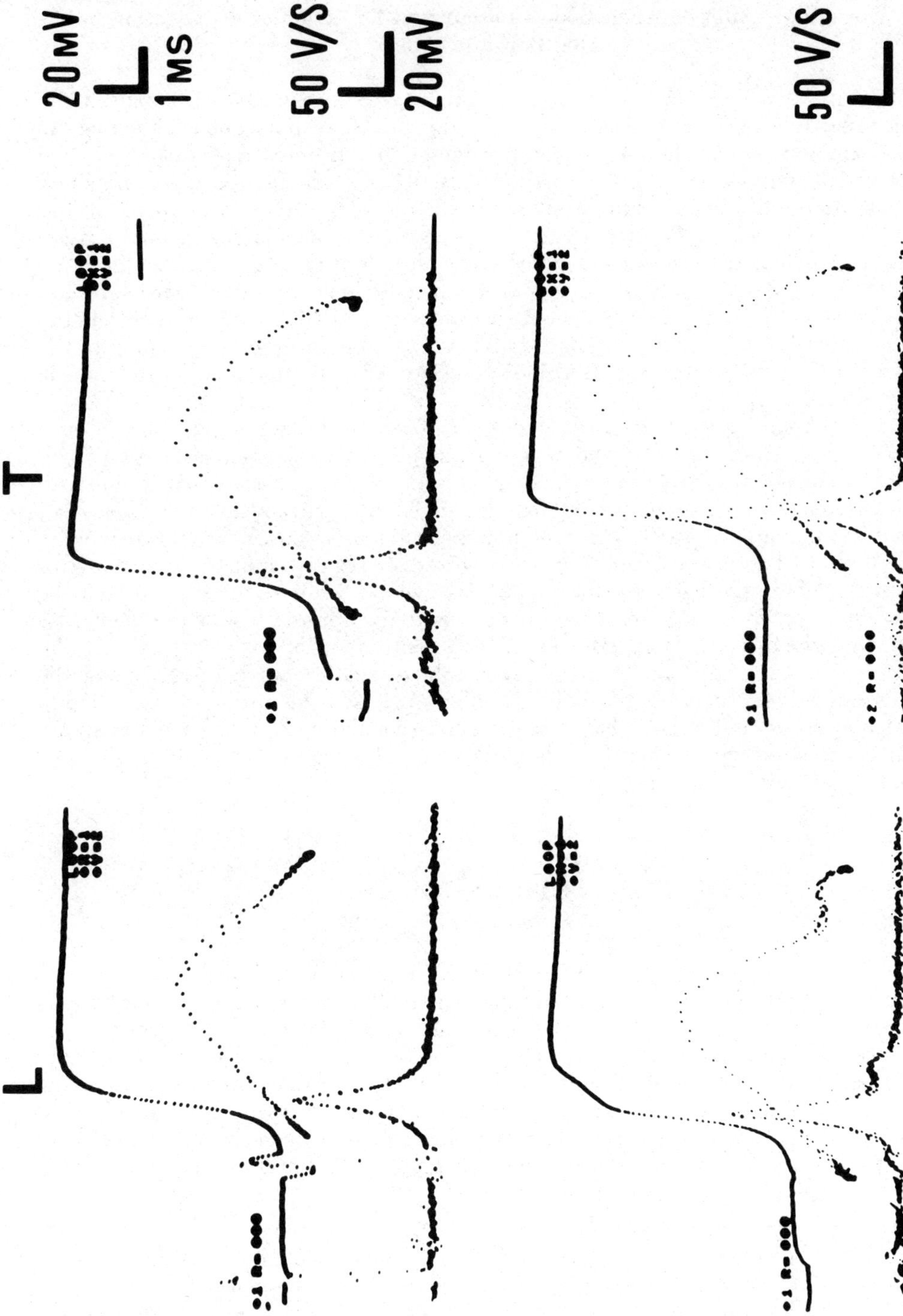

Figure 11. Transmembrane voltage and its first time derivative observed as a function of time and in the phase-plane for two rabbit left atrial cells (A and B) under longitudinal (L) and transverse (T) spread of activity.

The Relationship between Loop Contour and Direction of Propagation in Dog Purkinje Fibers

Figure 12 shows data obtained by Saldeña (1977) in which he explored the directional differences of loop contour in long dog Purkinje fibers (about 1 cm long, up to 900 μm in diameter) driven alternately from either extremity. As Garcia (1975) had observed, an important percentage of the recorded loops were of type A2, even though the difference between M_o and the subsequent larger slope of the ascending limb was much less noticeable in Purkinje fibers than it was in atrium. No relationship between direction and loop pattern could be detected for all cells in a Purkinje fiber. A direction of spread that yielded an A2 contour in one cell could yield an A8 contour in another and vice-versa (Fig. 12). When A2 and A8 contours were obtained from a given cell, the A2 contour showed a lower M_o and a higher $\dot{V}_{max}$, both differences being of the order of 10%. Other cells (Fig. 12A) showed A8 (or A2) contours in both directions of propagation.

In light of the arguments presented so far, we suggest that propagation in a thick Purkinje fiber is not necessarily homogeneous along its course, or at least not homogeneous in many of the cell strands it contains. It is tempting to associate this finding with the randomness of the geometry of cells and their couplings in any given Purkinje fiber (Sommer and Johnson, 1968). This randomness would often cause a situation in which a cell's input and output resistance for a given direction of propagation may be above or below that of the average value for the fiber as a whole, whereas the situation may be quite different when the stimulus is moved over to the opposite end of the fiber. This type of slight directional differences in loop contours of a single cell can also be encountered in atrium and ventricle when the excitatory wave travels along the preferential direction of fiber bundles in different senses. No attention was called to this point above as it seems that A2 contours associated with transverse spread are often more strikingly deviant from homogeneous propagation than the phenomena pointed out here for Purkinje fibers.

DISCUSSION

The phase-plane data presented in this chapter show that the time course of propagated transmembrane action potentials from different regions of the heart differs appreciably from the pattern expected of homogeneously conducted action potentials. The skeletal muscle data also show to our satisfaction that the observed differences are not due to peculiarities of striated muscle membrane arrangement, in which the T-tubular system is thought to play a role in determining the passive equivalent circuit (Falk and Fatt, 1964). In fact, except for recordings obtained near the motor end plate, loop patterns of the upstroke of propagated action potentials in skeletal muscle adhere

---

Figure 12. Upstroke loops of intracellular action potentials recorded from two cells (A and B) in a dog Purkinje fiber. The fiber was stimulated alternately at each extremity during four cycles (1,2,3,4). Arrows show direction of propagation for the records in the left (1,3) and right (2,4) columns. Calibration ramp ascended 20 mV in 0.2 ms (100 v/s). Horizontal bar in center of illustration represents 2 msec for V,t records. (From Saldeña, 1977.)

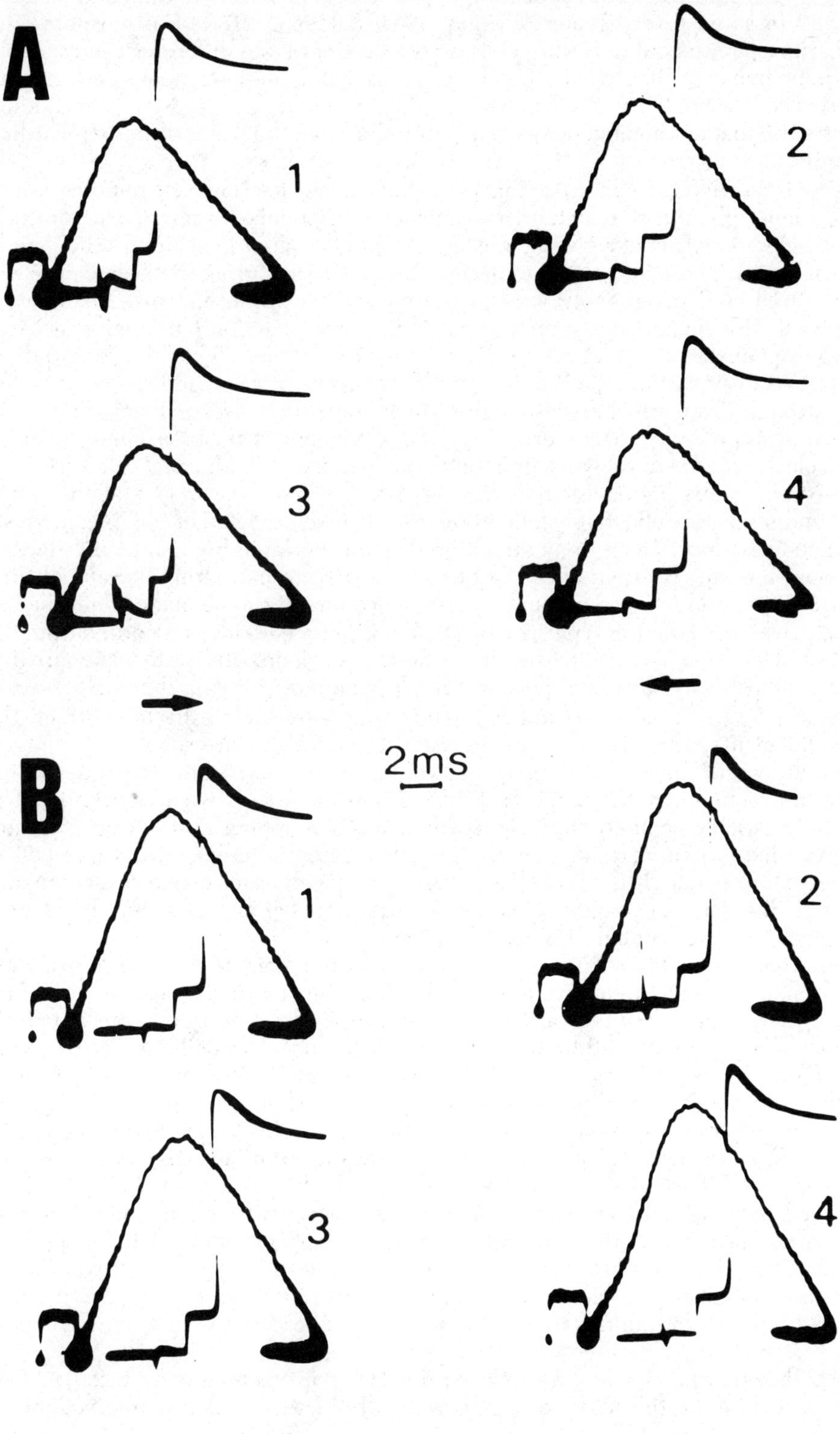
A
1
2
3
4
2ms
B
1
2
3
4

closely to the pattern of both predicted by the Hodgkin-Huxley model and actually observed in squid axons (Jenerick, 1963; 1964; Saldeña, 1977). Furthermore, the peculiarities pointed out in cardiac cells cannot be ascribed to differences in excitable membrane behavior, because both homogeneous and nonhomogeneous patterns can be observed in a single site just by changing the direction of propagation. This finding suggests also that nonhomogeneous loop patterns are not the result of faulty recording techniques.

One is then left to face the fact that propagation along heart muscle bundles is not a homogeneous phenomenon at a microscopic level. Evidence for microhesitations (or microaccelerations) along a given pathway are found as often in atrium as they are in Purkinje fibers. These microhesitations may become large during transverse propagation in atrial (and presumably ventricular) muscle, as Spach and his collaborators (Chapter 9) also suggest based on V,t and $\dot{V},t$ records of action potential upstrokes. This concept deviates, at a microscopic level, from the previous belief that longitudinal propagation in a heart muscle bundle is a homogeneous process; and it deviates even more strongly from the belief that the much slower transverse propagation is a homogeneous process too (Draper and Mya Tu, 1959; Sano et al., 1959; Clerc, 1976). It is thus clearly unsafe to rely on action potential homogeneity for exact calculations in myocardium unless one is assured, through phase-plane recording, that the waveshape under scrutiny effectively follows the time course expected of a homogeneously conducted response. Even in an apparently simple Purkinje fiber, microhesitations may cause the time constant of the foot to deviate 10% or more from its value during homogeneous conduction. The same cautionary comment can be made about the use of $\dot{V}_{max}$, which is larger in type A2 loops than it is in type A8 loops recorded from the same cell. Here, too, it is useful to evaluate phase-plane loop patterns to make sure that changes in pathway during experimental interventions are not the real cause of changes in $\dot{V}_{max}$. To this we add the need to measure (or ideally to subtract) the extracellular interference whenever precise values of $\dot{V}_{max}$ are sought.

Granting that microhesitations actually occur, it is fair to assume, as pointed out in the Results section, that they happen at some geometric or resistive discontinuity. The extremely variable geometry and contact area of cell couplings in the heart indicates that microhesitations may happen as the action potential crosses from one cell to another. More strikingly deviant A2 loops associated with transverse propagation may be due to difficulty of current flow across the presumably much less abundant lateral connections among parallel bundles (see Chapter 1).

Microhesitations in a Purkinje fiber are slight but suggest that the propagation wavefront in this structure may not be entirely flat at any particular cross section. This is hardly surprising when the variable cell and coupling geometry in a Purkinje fiber are considered (Sommer and Johnson, 1968). The finding of a smaller M_o is expected, for instance, if a cell process is invaded prior to the main cell input. If it is invaded shortly after, some degree of collision or restriction of current spread is expected within the cell, resulting in a variable degree of increase in $\dot{V}_{max}$. Soon afterwards, the wave fuses again into a synchronous homogeneous front, and A8 contours can be observed in cells located further along the fiber. This effect could not be obtained in a linear cell array, because an A2 contour generated at a resistive junction would take two to three space constants of unhindered propagation to change back to a smooth A8 contour. This would require that the resistive couplings be separated by over 5 to 10 mm to accommodate the finding that about half of the contours are type A8. A closer spacing of the discontinuities in a linear array would lead to the finding of A2 loops only.

On the other hand, when transverse propagation in atrium is considered, all loop patterns seem to be the A2 type. Compared with the A2 loops of nonhomogeneous longitudinal propagation in Purkinje fibers, these loops exhibit a more marked difference between the initial slope M_o and the slope observed after the ionic current reversal voltage. Their M_o is always lower, and $\dot{V}_{max}$ is almost always higher, with its voltage often displaced toward more depolarized values than those observed for homogeneous propagation in the same cell.

This suggests to us that atrial cells are transversely coupled through junctions that exhibit a higher resistance (or a more restricted contact area relative to the post-junctional cell membrane area) than do longitudinal junctions. The data also suggest that such lateral cell junctions are always less than 0.3 λ away from the site of recording, and that within this range there are no highly pervious parallel paths through which a cell can "see" the approach of a homogeneously propagated wavefront. This last contention is based on the observation that transverse propagation is always associated with A2-type loops in which the inflection point at the end of the initial linear segment occurs in the neighborhood of the ionic current reversal voltage. We presume this to be the case for the middle column of Figure 10, although propagation direction was not rigorously controlled in those experiments (Garcia, 1975). It seems therefore plausible to state that during transverse conduction the wavefront hesitates slightly as it crosses sideways from one bundle of cells to another. These lateral junctions should be less than 300 μm apart if one admits that λ in rabbit atrium is around 1 mm in the longitudinal direction (Bonke, 1973a).

It is possible to estimate the amount of time spent in a microhesitation. This can be done by comparing the A2 and A8 loop patterns obtained from a given cell during propagation in different directions (as in Figs. 10, 11, and 12). Time is implicit in the phase-plane, and the time difference (Δt) between any two points of the loop is given by

$$\Delta t_{2-1} = \int_1^2 \frac{dV}{\dot{V}}$$

The expression can be integrated once $\dot{V}$ is known as a function of V. Graphically, the task is easy for any linear segment of slope M, when

$$\Delta t_{2-1} = \frac{1}{M} \ln \frac{V_2 - V_x}{V_1 - V_x}$$

where V_1 and V_2 are the voltages of any two points of the linear segment, and V_x is the voltage at which the straight line crosses the voltage axis. At the particular case when $M = 0$

$$\Delta t_{2-1} = \frac{V_2 - V_1}{\dot{V}}$$

With these relationships, any loop can be graphically approached by connecting linear segments, and the time spent in different loop sectors can be computed.

In Purkinje fibers, the study of microhesitations with the method described above shows local delays of 50 to 100 μsec relative to homogeneous propagation. This may indicate that a given cell process can be reached by local current flow that much sooner than the main cell input. This slight asynchrony seems to be readily mended as the wavefront fuses again in a single homogeneous movement.

We may now estimate the time loss in a microhesitation during transverse propagation. Table 1 shows time measurements obtained from the phase-plane loops of Figure 10, where we presume the middle column to be representative of transverse conduction. It can be seen that nonhomogeneous conduction loops of the A2 type are

Table 1
Differences in Time Course Between Action Potentials of a Same Cell during Propagation in Two Different Directions (Homogeneous and Nonhomogeneous Conduction).

Time Differences during Upstroke[1] (in μsec)	Cell #10A	Cell #10B	Cell #10C
Δ Time to threshold[2]	1,360	650	100
Δ Time to $\dot{V}_{max}$[3]	1,380	660	120
Δ Time to peak[4]	910	620	−370

[1]Calculated from phase plane loops of intracellular action potentials in rabbit atrium as the difference nonhomogeneous *less* homogeneous conduction records.
[2]Difference in time elapsed at the action potential foot, from 1 mV depolarization to the ionic current reversal voltage.
[3]Difference in time from 1 mV depolarization to the voltage where $\dot{V}_{max}$ is reached.
[4]Difference in time from 1 mV depolarization to 1 mV below action potential peak voltage.

always associated with a time loss at the foot of the action potential, up to the voltage where $\dot{V}_{max}$ is reached. During the final lap of the upstroke, the A2 loop is actually faster, as its $\dot{V}$ values are all higher in that voltage range. Some of the time loss is regained at the end of the upstroke because of this effect, as seen in cells 10A and 10C. In the first, the action potential peak is still almost a millisecond behind in the A2 loop. But in cell 10C, where the time loss at the foot was slight and the difference in $\dot{V}_{max}$ quite important, the acceleration of the final part of the upstroke makes the peak appear earlier in the A2 loop. A question is whether an actual acceleration of overall conduction can be obtained through this mechanism. We do not think this is the case, as the firing of the next cell along a given path probably occurs well before the action potential peak of the cell in cause. Nevertheless, a microhesitation clearly occurs at the foot of all action potentials in the middle column of Figure 10. These delays should influence conduction time, and we wonder how much they have contributed to the decrease in overall conduction velocity observed by several authors during transverse spread (Draper and Mya Tu, 1959; Sano et al., 1959; Clerc, 1976; Spach, Chapter 9).

The observation of loop contours compatible with homogeneous propagation lends additional support to Weidmann's original views on the low electrical resistance of cell coupling in the heart (Weidmann, 1952, 1970; see also Chapter 3). The finding of type A2 loops suggests, however, that the effective coupling resistance, which depends also on cell geometry and junctional area, is often increased to the point of creating at cell boundaries microhesitations that may be capable of influencing overall conduction velocity appreciably. The concept of slow conduction associated with high longitudinal resistance is implicit in the cable treatment of propagated action potential in squid axon (Hodgkin and Huxley, 1952). Lieberman et al. (1973) have proposed that this might represent an important mechanism for slowing conduction in the slender fibers of tissues such as sinoatrial (SA) and atrioventricular (AV) node. They went on to model the possible role of a localized increase in r_i at cell junctions and concluded that this could indeed represent an important factor in slowing conduction, even though they still had to introduce a decrease of the active ionic currents to achieve the very low velocity values observed in SA and AV nodes. Nevertheless, their contention concerning junctional r_i is very much in agreement with our interpretation of the phase-plane data presented above. A different but related model reported by Heppner and Plonsey (1970) also points out the possibility of propagation delays at cell abutments. More recently, Clapham et al. (1980) showed in cultured embryonic chick heart cells that the progressive establishment of electrical coupling between two myospheres that are pushed together leads first to delayed excitation and then to progressive shortening of time loss at the junction.

Finally, we would like to speculate on how conduction in cardiac muscle would be affected in metabolically depressed areas. Besides the progressive decrease in resting potential, which slows propagation through its effect on the state of inactivation of the fast sodium channel, cell coupling may be affected (see Chapters 4 and 5). If so, one would expect, first, that the more difficult transverse communication between adjacent bundles would be hindered, resulting in longitudinal dissociation. Second, conduction along cell bundles would be increasingly slowed, as longer microhesitations produced by an increased coupling resistance combine with further degrees of inactivation. Garcia and Paes de Carvalho (1977) have shown that normal atrial tissue kept in Tyrode's solution containing 10.8 mM Ca^{2+} at 29° C and subjected to high frequencies of stimulation (over 3 Hz) showed, in extracellular tracings, a progressive deterioration of wavefront synchronization typical of a longitudinal dissociation. This excitatory asynchronism was furthered by epinephrine and caffeine and was reversed by D-600. These pharmacologic responses are suggestive of an involvement of Ca^{2+} loading and decreased cell coupling between cells. We wonder if similar phenomena can happen in more physiologic media in the presence of metabolic inhibition and consequent hindrance of calcium-pumping activity. We thus suggest that partial cell uncoupling may provide just the right conditions for the appearance of reentrant rhythms in diseased myocardium. Such a mechanism seems to deserve more attention as a source of disturbances of the cardiac rhythm.

REFERENCES

Bonke FIM (1973a) Passive electrical properties of atrial fibers of the rabbit heart. Pflüg Arch **339**:1–15

Bonke FIM (1973b) Electrotonic spread in the sinoatrial node of the rabbit heart. Pflüg Arch **339**:17–23

Campos de Carvalho AC (1979) Modelo de propagação de potenciais de açao através de um segmento não-uniforme do axônio gigante da lula; uma análise pela técnica do plano de fase. M.Sc. thesis presented to the Instituto de Biofísica, Universidade Federal do Rio de Janeiro, Brazil

Campos de Carvalho AC, Paes de Carvalho A (1980) Phase-plane analysis of uniform and non-uniform propagation of activity in a model of squid giant axon. An Acad Brasil Ciênc **52**:893–902

Caputo C, Gimenez M (1967) Effects of external calcium deprivation on single muscle fibers. J Gen Physiol **255**:335–346

Carmeliet E, Willems J (1971) The frequency dependent character of the membrane capacity in cardiac Purkinje fibers. J Physiol (Lond) **213**:85–93

Clapham DE, Shrier A, Dehaan RL (1980) Junctional resistance and action potential delay between embryonic heart cell aggregates. J Gen Physiol **75**:633–654

Clerc L (1976) Directional differences of impulse spread in trabecular muscle from mammalian heart. J Physiol (Lond) **255**:335–346

Cooley JW, Dodge FA (1966) Digital computer solutions for excitation and propagation of the nerve impulse. Biophys J **6**:583–599

DeMello WC (1977) Passive electrical properties of the atrioventricular node. Pflüg Arch **371**:135–139

Draper MH, Mya Tu MH (1959) A comparison of conduction velocity in cardiac tissues of various mammals. Q J Exp Physiol **44**:91–109

Falk G, Fatt P (1964) Linear electrical properties of striated muscle fibers observed with intracellular electrodes. Proc Roy Soc B **160**:69–123

Garcia EAC (1975) Importância do acoplamento intercelular para a propagação da atividade elétrica miocárdica. PhD. thesis presented to the Instituto de Biofísica, Universidade Federal do Rio de Janeiro
Garcia EAC, Paes de Carvalho A (1977) Efeitos da estimulação sobre a resistência longitudinal no miocárdio. Arq Brasil Cardiol **30** (supl 1):7–22
Goldstein SS, Rall W (1974) Changes of action potential shape and velocity for changing core conductor geometry. Biophys J **14**:731–757
Heppner DB, Plonsey R (1970) Simulation of electrical interaction of cardiac cells. Biophys J **10**:1057–1075
Hodgkin AL, Horowicz P (1957) The differential action of hypertonic solution on the twitch and action potential of a muscle fiber. J Physiol (Lond) **136**:17P
Hodgkin AL, Huxley, AF (1952) A quantitative description of membrane current and its application to conduction and excitation in nerve. J Physiol (Lond) **117**:500–544
Hodgkin AL, Rushton WAH (1946) The electrical constants of a crustacean nerve fiber. Proc Roy Soc B **133**:444–479
Jenerick H (1963) Phase plane trajectories of the muscle spike potential. Biophys J **3**:363–377
Jenerick H (1964) An analysis of the striated muscle fiber action current. Biophys J **4**:77–91
Lieberman M, Kootsey JM, Johnson EA, Sawanobori T (1973) Slow conduction in cardiac muscle. A biophysical model. Biophys J **13**:37–55
Masuda MO, Paes de Carvalho A (1975) Sinoatrial transmission and atrial invasion during normal rhythm in rabbit heart. Circ Res **37**:414–421
Moreira da Silva P (1974) Curso de oceanografia de pesca. Fundação de Estudos do Mar, Rio de Janeiro, Brazil
Oliveira Castro GM, Machado RD (1969) Control of glass microelectrodes for intracellular recordings. Experientia **25**:556–558
Paes de Carvalho A (1975) Phase plane determination of membrane currents in propagated action potentials: possibilities and difficulties. *In* Concepts of Membranes in Regulation and Excitation, edited by M. Rocha e Silva, G. Suarez-Kurtz, New York, Raven Press, pp 85–96
Paes de Carvalho A, Garcia EAC, Saldeña TA (1976) Phase plane analysis of propagated electrical activity in muscle cells. Pontificiae Academiae Scientiarum Scripta Varia **40**: 153–172, Vatican Academy of Sciences, Vatican
Paes de Carvalho A, Hoffman BF, Paula Carvalho M (1969) Two components of the cardiac action potential: I. Voltage time course and the effect of acetylcholine on atrial and nodal cells of the rabbit heart. J Gen Physiol **54**:607–635
Saldeña TA (1977) Estudo comparativo da morfologia do potencial de ação transmembrana observado no plano de fase. PhD thesis presented to Instituto de Biofísica, Universidade Federal do Rio de Janeiro
Sano T, Takayama N, Shimamoto T (1959) Directional difference of conduction velocity in the cardiac ventricular syncytium studied by microelectrodes. Circ Res **7**:262–267
Sommer JR, Johnson EA (1968) Cardiac muscle. A comparative study of Purkinje fibers and ventricular fibers. J Cell Biol **36**:497–526
Tashiro T (1980) Colisão de potenciais de ação analisada no plano de fase. M.Sc. thesis presented to Instituto de Biofísica, Universidade Federal do Rio de Janeiro.
Weidmann S (1952) The electrical constants of Purkinje fibers. J Physiol (Lond) **118**:348–360
Weidmann S (1970) Electrical constants of trabecular muscle from mammalian heart. J Physiol (Lond) **210**:1041–1054
Woodbury JW, Crill WE (1961) On the problem of impulse conduction in the atrium. *In* Nervous Inhibition, edited by E. Florey, Oxford, Pergamon Press, pp 124–135

Discussion

REUTER: What would the phase-plane plot look like in the case of a membrane action potential?

PAES DE CARVALHO: If the membrane action potential is generated by a nearly threshold stimulus, I would expect that the initial slope would not be the fastest positive slope during the upstroke. The phase-plane display would begin with a lower slope and then increase the slope in the voltage range at which $\bar{g}_{Na}$ rises faster. This is obtained when modeling phase-plane displays of membrane action potentials in the Hodgkin-Huxley model for squid nerve (Saldeña, PhD Thesis, Rio de Janeiro, 1977) and should be the same for cardiac action potential models.

Chapter 9

The Electrical Representation of Cardiac Muscle Based on Discontinuities of Axial Resistivity at a Microscopic and Macroscopic Level

A Basis for Saltatory Propagation in Cardiac Muscle

Madison S. Spach

We have found increasing evidence to support the theory that cardiac muscle is structured to propagate electrical activity in a saltatory or discontinuous fashion owing to recurrent discontinuities of effective axial (intracellular) resistivity that affect the membrane currents (Spach et al., 1981). Although we have prepared such a model (Kootsey et al., to be submitted for publication) at present there is no appropriate model or simulation in the literature. Therefore, in the absence of a quantitative model in the literature, I will present a qualitative analysis of the effects of recurrent discontinuities of axial resistivity at both the microscopic and the macroscopic level, and I will show selected experiments that test the theoretical choice between two models that could represent cardiac muscle electrically at both levels. One model is consistent with the changes in core conductor geometry (with continuous properties of axial resistivity); the other, with discontinuities of axial resistivity. For the latter model, I will use the term "$\bar{R}_a$ hypothesis" to emphasize that the anatomical complexities contributing to the effective axial resistivity $\bar{R}_a$ (cellular geometry, packing, and the resistance, distribution, and quantitative extent of the cell-to-cell connections)—at a microscopic and macroscopic level—have an important influence on the propagation of depolarization in normal and abnormal cardiac muscle.

Theoretical studies have shown that in an otherwise continuously uniform structure the shape of propagating action potentials can change at sites that represent a change in core conductor geometry (Goldstein and Rall, 1974). Such changes in action potential shape due to alterations in geometry result from a change in the effective cross-sectional area of the core conductor (for example, a change due to branching). In turn, this changes the current load at the site of the geometric discontinuity due to the change in the magnitude of the capacitance to be discharged for depolarization

This work was supported in part by USPHS Grant HL11307.

to occur downstream. In 1960, Hayashi used this interpretation (that is, fiber branching) to account for a slight but definite change he noted in the configuration of the depolarization phase of the same cell in canine ventricular muscle when he modified the direction of impulse conduction (Hayashi et al., 1960; Kanno, 1970). In a paper kindly forwarded to us recently by Professor Paes de Carvalho, he and his associates found in their phase-plane analysis of propagated action potentials that shape changes occurred when propagation originated at different sites in atrial muscle (Paes de Carvalho et al., 1976). They could not account for these changes on the basis of a uniform cable model and pointed out that this result was not consistent with the use of continuous cable theory in the analysis of propagation in cardiac muscle. They indicated that cellular branching was the likely explanation.

The mechanism associated with changes in core conductor geometry also has been considered generally to account for propagation failure, as well as for changes in the shape of action potentials, associated with structural discontinuities at a macroscopic level in cardiac muscle. For example, it is the basis for the "funnel hypothesis" of Mendez et al. (1970) and for a model of the atrioventricular (A-V) node that produces action potential shape changes similar to those that are actually measured (Van Cappelle and Janse, 1976). Further, it has been used to explain propagation failure when a (depressed) action potential propagates from a narrow isthmus of muscle into a region of larger muscle volume in atrial muscle (De La Fuente et al., 1971).

As I will show, our results in cardiac muscle cannot be explained by any model of propagation in which the cytoplasm is continuous, even if it is assumed to divide, splitting the intracellular current. Instead, I will focus on the role of discontinuities of *effective* axial resistivity and provide evidence for changes in current load on the membrane of individual cells or groups of cells due to discontinuities of axial resistivity at a microscopic and macroscopic level, rather than to apparent geometric discontinuities related to changing core conductor geometry (with constant axial resistivity). The results of the analysis at a microscopic level have been published recently (Spach et al., 1981). Because the results of that paper are important in considering the nature of propagation at a microscopic level in cardiac muscle, portions are repeated here (with some additions) before going on to generalize the idea to discontinuities of propagation at a macroscopic level.

THE PROBLEM

In a continuously uniform structure, the propagation velocity of action potentials can be altered only in two ways: by changing the membrane properties or by changing the axial resistance in the direction of propagation. The first mechanism has been studied extensively in cardiac muscle. For example, changes in propagation velocity have been produced through modulation of membrane properties (presumably the fast sodium current mechanism) by changing the outside potassium concentration (Dominguez and Fozzard, 1970). A correlation between propagation velocity and the fast sodium mechanism had been suggested previously by the theoretical analysis of Pickard (1966). The general nature of the relationship is a positive correlation between propagation velocity and maximum sodium current, large sodium currents producing high velocities.

It is generally concluded that when the propagation velocity is varied by changing the time course of the membrane permeabilities, the shape of the action potential is also changed. For example, when the propagation velocity is decreased by stimulation at a more depolarized transmembrane potential, the maximum rate of rise of the action potential also decreases (Singer et al., 1967; Sano et al., 1967). The time constant of the foot of the action potential also has been reported to be larger when the propagation velocity is low (Abe and Tomita, 1968; Dominguez and Fozzard, 1970). The exact functional dependence of these shape changes on propagation velocity have not been determined experimentally in cardiac muscle, but it has been assumed that the relationships are the same as they are in nerve and skeletal muscle (Fozzard, 1979).

The second mechanism of variation of the propagation velocity, with axial resistance, has received little experimental study in cardiac muscle. Lieberman et al. (1973) attributed propagation velocity changes in cultured strands of chick embryonic heart muscle to decreased electrical coupling between cells. Others have suggested that the coupling might be changed through variations in intracellular resistivity (Hauswirth, 1969; Sperelakis et al., 1970) or in the number and distribution of cell junctions (Woodbury and Crill, 1961; DeFelice and Challice, 1969; Martinez-Palomo et al., 1970). Variations in propagation velocity with direction have been observed in cardiac muscle (Sano et al., 1959; Draper and Mya-Tu, 1959). Clerc (1976) also found variations in velocity with direction and attributed the variation of propagation velocity to directional differences in cell-to-cell connections. He also concluded from his measurements that the shape of the action potential did not change with direction or velocity and considered this result to be an agreement with theoretical predictions of the relationship between velocity and axial resistance.

In our studies, we varied the propagation velocity in both of the ways discussed above, looking carefully for shape changes in the upstroke of the action potential as the velocity was varied. We found shape changes in both circumstances—whether the velocity was varied through premature action potentials or through changes in the direction of propagation. The variations were, however, in exactly the opposite direction in the two cases. When the velocity was decreased in a Purkinje strand by premature stimulation, the maximum rate of rise of the action potential decreased, and the time constant of the foot increased, as expected from continuous cable theory. On the other hand, when the velocity was decreased by changing the direction of propagation with respect to the fiber orientation, the maximum rate of rise increased, and the time constant of the foot decreased!

Both of these cases were studied carefully, looking for an explanation for this apparently anomalous propagation that would be consistent with the known morphology of cardiac muscle. We were unable to find a satisfactory explanation on the basis of the commonly-used continuous cable theory. But when we viewed propagation in cardiac muscle as being, under many circumstances, a kind of saltatory propagation (that is, proceeding in steps, discontinuous), the observed changes in action potential shape with direction and velocity could be accounted for. This chapter considers the implications of such a mechanism for the propagation of action potentials in cardiac muscle at both a microscopic and macroscopic level.

METHODS

Propagation at a Microscopic Level

The in vitro methods, described in detail elsewhere (Spach et al., 1981), will be summarized briefly here. Preparations included the crista terminalis and surrounding tissue for the atrium, papillary muscle from the right ventricle, and Purkinje strands on the surface of the left ventricular septum. All measurements were made at a constant temperature of 35° C. The concentration of the perfusate was 128 mM NaCl, 4.69 mM KCl, 1.18 mM $MgSO_4$, 0.41 mM NaH_2PO_4, 20.1 mM $NaHCO_3$, 2.23 mM $CaCl_2$, and 11.1 mM dextrose. The solutions were gassed in a reservoir with a mixture of 95% O_2 and 5% CO_2 and perfused through the tissue bath (15 cm in diameter) at a rate of 100 ml/min.

The intracellular potentials were recorded with conventional glass microelectrodes filled with 3 M KCl. The extracellular electrodes were made of flexible tungsten wire, 50 μm in diameter, and insulated except at the tip. Each extracellular electrode was connected to one input of an AC-coupled differential amplifier, having a frequency-response flat between 0.1 and 30,000 Hz. The separate reference electrodes for each extracellular or intracellular electrode were positioned 7 cm away from the recording site.

A pacemaker stimulus 0.5 to 1.0 msec in duration and 1.5 to 2.0 times the threshold was applied to the surface of the preparation by a unipolar electrode. A PDP-11/20 computer system (Barr et al., 1976) controlled the rate at 1 stimulus per second and synchronized the pacing stimuli with the data recording. The computer stored the data and displayed the waveforms on a Tektronix 4002 display unit. A dissecting microscope equipped with a Nikon F250 35-mm camera was used to document the positions of the stimulus and recording electrodes.

The transmembrane potential (V_m) was calculated by subracting the extracellular potential from the intracellular potential. It was important to position the extracellular electrode very close to the impalement site because slight changes in the distance between the electrode and the site caused prominent changes in the waveforms. Care was taken to impale cells only at the surface of the preparation.

Changes in propagation velocity at one site were studied by analyzing the records (intracelluar and extracellular) associated with the impalement of a single cell, thus keeping constant many parameters that could not be measured. The propagation velocity at the impalement site was varied either by stimulating prematurely (to modulate the fast sodium-current mechanism) or by changing the direction of propagation. We were able to achieve successful recording conditions in each of nine atrial and six ventricular preparations.

Because the analysis depended critically on the shapes of the recorded waveforms, particular care was taken to ensure that the stimulus current did not interfere with the recorded waveforms. Three precautions were taken. *(1)* Each stimulus site was located several millimeters from the impaled cell (several resting space constants [Woodbury and Crill, 1961; Weidmann, 1970]). *(2)* An interval of constant resting potential was allowed between the stimulus artifact and the recorded waveform. *(3)* Propagation was initiated within 200 μm of each stimulus electrode, as determined by extracellular activation mapping. Any irregularities in propagation within the immediate vicinity (radius of 1.5 mm) of the impalement site, such as may be caused by connective tissue divisions, were grounds for moving the observation site. Such irregularities show up in the extracellular waveforms as notches (Spach et al., 1979).

Membrane Effects

To study the situation where velocity changes through modulation of the fast sodium-current mechanism, we chose small, functionally single Purkinje strands on the left ventricular septal surface (diameter, 125 to 250 μm). In these strands, the activation wavefront remains perpendicular to the long axis of the cells, even for premature action potentials. Three extracellular electrodes were spaced along the strands for velocity measurements, and the stimulus electrode was positioned 10 mm away from the nearest recording electrode, a distance of many space constants (Weidmann, 1952). Action potentials that propagate at different velocities were initiated by premature stimuli introduced before the fibers were completely repolarized. A premature stimulus was injected after every 15th regular stimulus that occurred at a constant rate of 1/sec.

Directional Effects

Two to six stimulating electrodes were located around the impalement site. The propagation velocity was greatest when the wavefront proceeded down the long axis of the cells, smallest along the perpendicular axis, and varied continuously and monotonically along intermediate axes. The interval between stimuli was kept constant at 1000 msec, but the site of stimulation was changed randomly between the stimulus electrodes every 10 to 15 beats to change the direction of propagation. Five extracellular recording electrodes were positioned around the impalement site. The microelectrode was then advanced into the tissue within 50 μm of the extracellular electrode tip at that site. If there was any change in the extracellular waveform, the microelectrode was withdrawn until the waveforms returned to the control state. If they did not recover, another site was chosen for study. To get a value for the propagation velocity for each direction of propagation, we recorded a detailed activation sequence for each stimulus site after we completed the intracellular measurement.

Data Analysis

Isochrone maps were constructed from the extracellular recordings, taking the time of the peak negative derivative (intrinsic deflection) as the instant of excitation. Conduction velocity then was calculated as the distance traveled normal to the isochrone per unit of time.

Transmembrane potential waveforms were calculated by taking the difference between the recorded intracellular and extracellular potentials. The maximum rate of rise ($\dot{V}_{max}$) was obtained from the recorded intracellular or calculated transmembrane potential by numerical differentiation. The waveforms of each activation sequence were analyzed also to ensure that the proper extracellular potential was recorded. If the extracellular electrode was not sufficiently close to the impalement site (horizontally as well as vertically), the intra-extracellular waveforms were misaligned in time. In the atrium, the large anisotropy of propagation produced drastic changes in the extracellular potential as the electrode position shifted away from the region of fast propagation. In this situation, the potential dropped as much as 80% in 100 μm.

The time constant of the foot of the action potential (τ_{foot}) was calculated graphically by plotting the first 8 mV of depolarization on semilogarithmic paper and fitting a straight line by eye. After the experiments were concluded, histologic studies verified the fiber orientation.

Propagation at a Macroscopic Level

The same in vitro methods noted above were used to study propagation at a macroscopic level in the dog atrium. The macroscopic anatomical discontinuities studied were those that could be identified easily by eye. They included sites of branching where pectinate muscles arise from the crista terminalis and the junction sites where two separate muscle bundles interconnect. Detailed isochrone maps were made from the extracellular waveforms recorded at 30 to 100 sites within the area of conduction velocity change; that is, in muscle bundles forming the visible anatomical discontinuity. From a practical standpoint, it was impossible to detect and to analyze adequately the velocity changes at these sites by means of intracellular measurements. Therefore, the analysis was performed by using extracellular, rather than intracellular, potentials as suggested recently for detailed study of propagation in cardiac muscle (Spach et al., 1979). They not only provided a means to detect the presence of the macroscopic discontinuities of propagation, but they provided a way to study the mechanism associated with changes in axial resistance per unit length at these sites.

Once an area of velocity change was identified in relation to an anatomical discontinuity, 10 to 18 extracellular recording electrodes were positioned along and across the muscle bundles that formed the junctional area. Two to four stimulus electrodes were then positioned to produce propagation into the branch or junction site from different directions. Propagation of normal action potentials was measured while the stimulus site was varied randomly and the stimulus rate remained constant at 1/sec. Action potentials that propagated at different velocities were initiated at each stimulus site by the following procedures: *(1)* The extracellular potassium concentration was elevated by using a high-potassium solution that was identical to the regular perfusing solution, except that the KCl concentration was 15 mM. The KCl solution was introduced so that the concentration increased gradually over 30 min. The concentration at the preparation was measured from samples withdrawn through a previously positioned cannula as the solution flowed across the preparation. *(2)* Under conditions of normal extracellular potassium concentration (4.69 mM), a premature stimulus was injected after every 15th regular stimulus, which occurred at a constant interstimulus interval of 800 to 1000 msec. The location of the stimulus was shifted randomly from one stimulus electrode to another for each interval of delay between the prior normal stimulus and the premature stimulus. The refractory period of each muscle bundle that formed the anatomical discontinuity was measured in the usual way; that is, the time interval at which a 1-msec additional delay just produced propagation to a distant recording site located 2 to 3 cm from the stimulus electrode.

RESULTS

Propagation at a Microscopic Level

Membrane Effects

When the resting potential or take-off potential (Peon et al., 1978) in Purkinje strands was made more negative by delaying the premature stimulus, both the velocity of propagation (θ) and the maximum rate of rise ($\dot{V}_{max}$) increased, as well as the peak-to-peak amplitude of the extracellular potential. The increase in $\dot{V}_{max}$ appeared to be linearly related to the propagation velocity. Such an increase in $\dot{V}_{max}$ with velocity is consistent with similar observations in Purkinje fibers (Dominguez and Fozzard, 1970) and in the atrium (Sano et al., 1967) when the resting potential and velocity were changed by altering the extracellular potassium concentration.

We plotted the time constant of the foot of the action potential (τ_{foot}) for a single impalement as a function of θ and $\dot{V}_{max}$. As the premature action potential was delayed longer and longer, τ_{foot} decreased approximately linearly as both θ and $\dot{V}_{max}$ increased (correlation coefficient = −0.99, $P < 0.01$). A rectangular hyperbolic relationship between τ_{foot} and θ was predicted by Tasaki and Hagiwara (1957) on the basis of continuous, one-dimensional cable theory. It is not clear whether the difference between our results and their theoretical prediction is due to insufficient accuracy of the measurement or to inappropriate assumptions for our tissue in the theoretical calculation. There is, however, agreement in the *direction* of change in τ_{foot} as θ increases. The same direction of change in τ_{foot} with θ was found by Dominguez and Fozzard (1970) as they changed the extracellular potassium concentration from 4.0 to 7.0 mM.

Thus, we found that when we observed the relationship between propagation velocity and the maximum rate of rise or time constant of the foot of the action potential by modulating the membrane properties, keeping the relationship between the direction of propagation and the cell geometry constant, both variables changed in the direction predicted theoretically and observed previously.

Directional Effects

A typical result for atrial muscle is shown in Figure 1. Two activation sequences from the crista terminalis are shown. The crista terminalis is a large, flat muscle in which the parallel orientation of the fibers underneath the endocardium along the longitudinal axis is very apparent. Both activation sequences were initiated by point stimuli from an extracellular electrode (stimulus symbol). Note that the two sequences are very similar in appearance, although they were initiated at different sites on the muscle, displaced both longitudinally and transversely. In both cases, there was rapid propagation in the longitudinal direction (along the axis of the fibers) and slow propagation in the transverse direction (perpendicular to the long axis of the fibers). In nine crista terminalis experiments, the maximum velocities fell in the narrow range between 0.9 and 1.2 m/sec and the minimum velocities ranged between 0.05 and 0.12 m/sec. These low values are within the range of velocities observed by Cranefield et al. (1972) for very slow conduction of "slow response" action potentials.

In the right-hand part of Figure 1, typical intracellular and extracellular waveforms are shown from a single impalement for the two situations of high velocity (parallel propagation) and low velocity (transverse propagation). Note that the intracellular potential rises *faster* when the velocity is low; that is, $\dot{V}_{max}$ is higher and τ_{foot} is lower, the exact opposite of the effects seen with premature action potentials.

In the following paragraphs, some of the possible explanations of this apparently anomalous result and some of its implications will be considered.

In nerve and muscle, the speed of propagation of action potentials has been associated with the peak magnitude of the sodium current (Hodgkin and Katz, 1949). Weidmann (1955) pointed out the connection between $\dot{V}_{max}$ and the magnitude of the fast sodium current, making it possible to estimate this current in cardiac cells. Thus, θ and $\dot{V}_{max}$ became closely associated quite early, even though the connection was not made in a quantitative theory until relatively recently (Hunter et al., 1975). So close has been this association that some workers have measured only $\dot{V}_{max}$ and considered it an indirect measure of propagation velocity. The few instances in which both θ and $\dot{V}_{max}$ were measured supported the relationship between high velocity and high $\dot{V}_{max}$. For example, atrial fibers with higher $\dot{V}_{max}$ values have been thought to have special membrane properties producing large sodium currents and thus fast conduction (Wagner et al., 1966). Some investigators have considered that there are "specialized" cells that are organized into a narrow

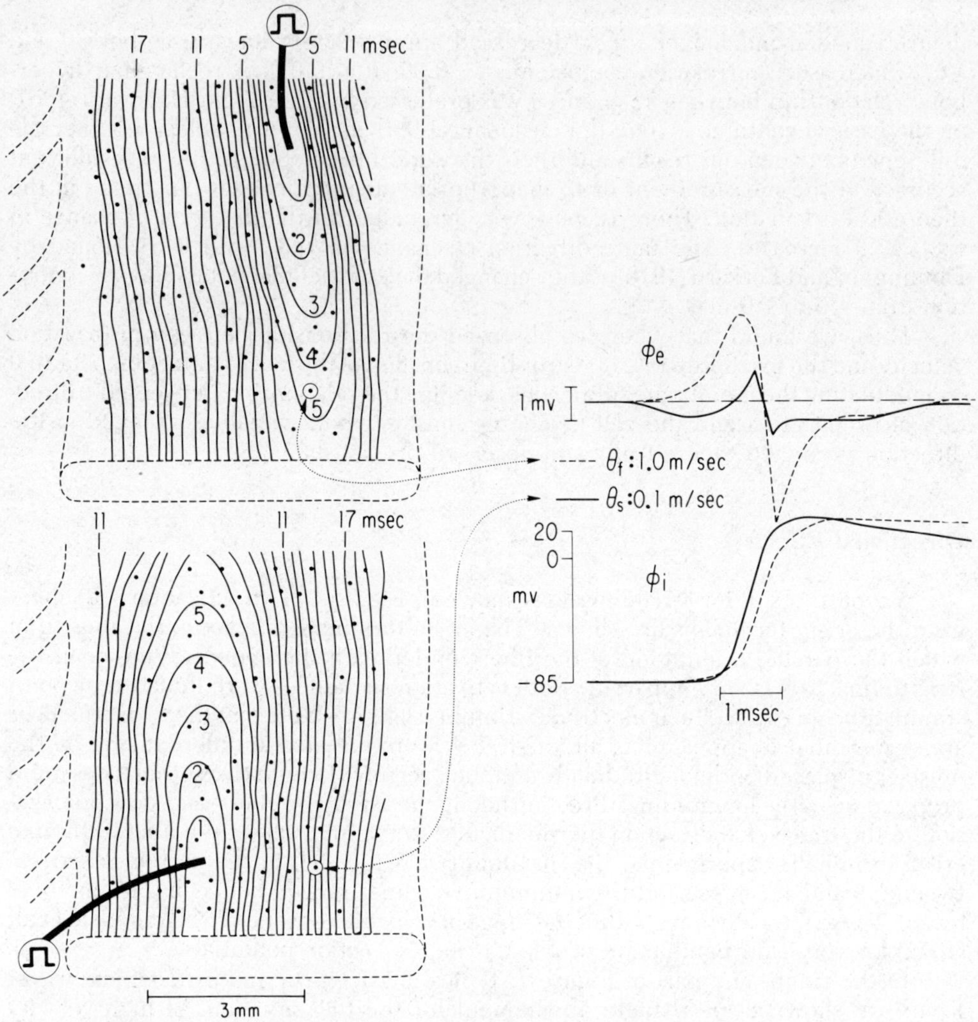

Figure 1. *Effects of the Direction of Propagation on the Action Potential in the Crista Terminalis*. The activation sequences for two stimulus sites are shown on the left. The points on the outline of the preparation indicate the locations of the extracellular recordings from which the activation maps were constructed; the solid lines represent isochrones drawn for each millisecond. The intracellular (ϕ_i) and extracellular (ϕ_e) potential waveforms on the right were measured at the indicated site when excitation proceeded in the longitudinal and transverse directions. (From Spach et al. [1981], by permission of the American Heart Association, Inc.).

tract of fixed position in specific atrial muscle bundles. Indeed, it is now widely accepted that within selected atrial muscle bundles (for example, the crista terminalis) "specialized" fibers are organized into a specialized, narrow tract that produces preferential rapid conduction within the muscle bundle (James, 1963; Wagner et al., 1966; Hogan and Davis, 1968). Also, decremental conduction and unidirectional block are generally attributed to action potentials propagating into an area where membrane properties are changing toward increased refractoriness—implying a reduction in fast sodium current.

Is it possible that the marked differences in propagation velocity we observed in the crista terminalis were caused by differences in membrane properties, possibly a narrow specialized tract?

Two aspects of the results of Figure 1 demonstrate that the difference in velocity cannot be accounted for by differences in membrane properties or a specialized tract. First, comparing the upper and lower excitation sequences in Figure 1, note that the pattern of propagation is determined by the site of the stimulus electrode and the fiber orientation. We stimulated at many other sites across the muscle bundle and always found the same result: there was rapid conduction from the stimulus site along the long axis of the fibers and slow conduction in a transverse direction. Such propagation patterns can be generated only by a muscle that is anisotropic but has uniform properties (including membrane properties) along any one axis. If the rapid propagation demonstrated in our experiments was produced by a single tract of fixed location (Joyner et al., 1975), the pattern of propagation would have changed markedly with the stimulus site—whether the tract differed in membrane properties or in resistive connections. Thus, our recorded sequences provide definitive proof that the preferential conduction (fast or slow) was not caused by a specialized tract of fixed location.

Second, we observed a higher speed of depolarization (higher $\dot{V}_{max}$ and lower τ_{foot}) when the velocity was low, the opposite of what would be predicted if the velocity difference were due to a tract with specialized membrane properties. The velocity at the site of cell impalement changed without a change in the membrane resting potential, which remained at a high negative value (−85 mV).

Interestingly, propagation velocities as low as 0.05 m/sec can be observed in normal atrial muscle during ordinary excitation. Similar low velocities are routine in the A-V node (Hoffman et al., 1959) and in depressed tissue (Cranefield et al., 1971). The very low propagation velocities we observed were achieved without the low resting potential, small amplitude, or slow rate of rise associated with equally slow propagation caused by "slow response" action potentials (Paes de Carvalho et al., 1969; Cranefield et al., 1972). The more slowly propagating action potentials that we recorded originated from resting potentials around −85 mV and had fast upstrokes (even faster than the fast propagating action potentials).

The question naturally arises as to how the depolarization shape varies between the upper and lower velocity limits. In a preparation with different propagation velocities along the two major axes, the apparent velocity will vary monotonically and continuously as the direction of measurement is varied continuously from one major axis to the other. Thus, intermediate propagation velocities can be studied by choosing the direction of measurement at various angles to the orientation of the fiber. In the crista terminalis, however, we found the ratio between the propagation velocities along the two major axes to be about 10; the variation with angle was so steep that the study of intermediate velocities was not practical. In a previous study, we had found a lower ratio of velocities in anisotropic propagation in ventricular muscle (Spach et al., 1979). Thus, we studied the depolarization shape associated with different velocities in papillary muscle preparations from the right ventricle. In six successful experiments, the maximum velocity of each preparation occurred within the narrow range of 0.47 to 0.52 m/sec (parallel propagation), and the minimum velocity varied between 0.14 and 0.20 m/sec (transverse propagation).

Figure 2 shows the intracellular and extracellular potentials at the impalement site for each of four velocities produced by changing the direction of propagation from four different stimulus sites and for a collision in ventricular muscle. The collision was included with the other measurements because it represents an approximation to zero velocity; that is, there is no propagation away from the recording site. The presence of a collision was verified by the extracellular waveform; positive waveforms have been

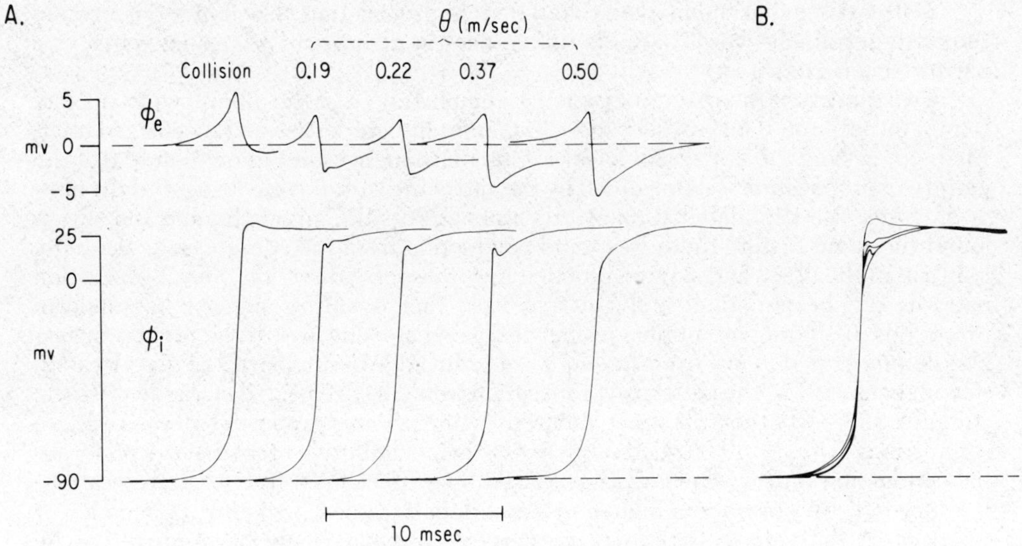

Figure 2. *Intracellular and Extracellular Potential Waveforms Associated with Different Velocities and with a Collision in the Papillary Muscle*. The different velocities (θ) were produced by changes in the direction of propagation from multiple stimulus sites. The intracellular potential waveforms (ϕ_i) in panel A were superimposed for comparison of the shapes in panel B. (From Spach et al. [1981], by permission of the American Heart Association, Inc.).

shown to be characteristic of collisions (Spach et al., 1971). It can be seen in Figure 2 that there was a change in the shape of the upstroke with velocity. As the velocity decreased, the τ_{foot} changed and the peak amplitude increased, with the largest amplitude associated with the collision. Also, when propagation occurred in a direction other than the long axis of the fibers, the action potentials frequently had irregular notches immediately after the peak of the upstroke.

The transmembrane potentials (V_m) were calculated by subtracting the measured intracellular and extracellular potentials. The amplitude and rate of rise were greater in V_m than they were in the intracellular potential, ϕ_i. Whenever there was a notch in the intracellular potential, the notch persisted in V_m as well. Arlock (1979) observed similar differences between transmembrane and intracellular potentials, and he also observed notches. He attributed these notches to the proximity of the stimulating electrode to the recording site and to the influence of the extracellular potentials. We observed notches even in V_m, and we found no proximity effect. The presence or absence of notches was not correlated with the position of the electrodes, but rather with the direction of propagation with respect to the fiber orientation.

From continuous one-dimensional cable theory, Hodgkin (1954) concluded that the shape of the transmembrane potential as a function of time should not change "if the velocity is altered by factors which change the current distribution in the fiber without affecting the membrane." Clerc (1976) applied this conclusion to anisotropic propagation in cardiac muscle. He assumed that the change in velocity with direction could be represented by a change in longitudinal resistance in the direction of propagation, and he concluded, from this argument, that the shape of the action potential should not change as the velocity was varied by varying the direction of propagation. He interpreted his measurements in calf ventricular muscle to agree with his theoretical conclusion.

The prediction of no change in the shape of the upstroke was based on the application of cable theory (Hodgkin, 1954) written in terms of the *transmembrane* potential. Therefore, it was not sufficient to examine the intracellular potential for shape changes; it was critical to know whether V_m changed as the direction of propagation was varied. The values of $\dot{V}_{max}$ and τ_{foot} from the ventricular impalement (Table 1) demonstrated a monotonic decrease in $\dot{V}_{max}$ and an increase in τ_{foot} as the velocity was increased. Note that τ_{foot} varied with velocity in the opposite direction as compared with the changes that occurred when the velocity was altered by modulation of the membrane properties. But, the direction of variation of τ_{foot} with $\dot{V}_{max}$ was the same in both cases (that is, τ_{foot} decreased as $\dot{V}_{max}$ increased). The changes in the upstroke in Table 1 are not in agreement with the theoretical prediction or the experimental conclusion of Clerc (1976) that the shape should not change with the direction of propagation.

Table 1
Action Potential Characteristics for Different Propagation Velocities, Corresponding to Different Directions of Propagation in Ventricle Muscle

Velocity (m/sec)	Amplitude of Upstroke (mV)		$\dot{V}_{max}$ (V/sec)		τ_{foot} (μsec)	
	V_m	ϕ_i	V_m	ϕ_i	V_m	ϕ_i
0.19	110	106	171	155	669	668
0.22	110	106	166	149	758	771
0.37	109	105	152	141	891	1008
0.50	104	100	124	114	921	1086

Sample values from one ventricular impalement (Fig. 2). The resting transmembrane potential (−90 mV) was the same for all action potentials.

The variation of propagation velocity with direction in cardiac muscle has been assumed to be caused by different axial resistances in different directions (Joyner et al., 1975; Clerc, 1976). Although this assumption may account for the dependence of velocity on direction, it does not explain our observation of shape changes in the action potential. Is it possible that the reduced velocity transverse to the long fiber axis is due to a tortuous path of propagation? In a structure consisting of packed, elongated cells interconnected at their ends, the macroscopic velocity would be reduced because of the zigzag path of propagation on the microscopic scale. This picture of microscopic propagation might account for directional differences in propagation velocity, but it is not consistent with our observation of shape changes with velocity. The zigzag path is analogous to propagation down a folded, one-dimensional cable: the apparent velocity would be reduced, but the transmembrane potential of each membrane element would have the same time course.

There is evidence in our data that the reduction in velocity is due to increased axial resistance. In a previous paper (Spach et al., 1979), we showed that the amplitude of the extracellular potential waveform is quantitatively related to the axial current in the direction of propagation in anisotropic muscle. That is, the extracellular potential increases as the axial (intracellular) current increases. In the case of propagation velocity reduction with premature action potentials, the extracellular potential and the rate of depolarization decreased together. This is in agreement with the previous theoretical prediction on the basis of propagation in a uniform cable structure and modulated membrane properties (Spach et al., 1972). When the velocity was changed through the direction of propagation, however, the amplitude of the extracellular potential and the rate of depolarization changed in opposite directions (Figs. 1 and 2).

When the velocity decreased, the extracellular potential also decreased, but the rate of depolarization increased. Thus, the decrease in the extracellular potential is consistent with a decrease in the axial current when propagation is slowed by changing the direction of propagation. The correlation of reduced velocity and decreased axial current is also consistent with the conclusion of Clerc that the cause of slowing is increased axial resistance in the direction of propagation (Clerc, 1976).

$\bar{R}_a$ Hypothesis

What is the origin of the shape changes that occur when the propagation velocity is altered by changing the axial resistance? Clearly, there is a problem in accounting for these changes because past applications of cable theory have predicted that they should not occur. Because the physical laws on which the cable analysis is based are not in question, one of the assumptions made in applying the analysis to cardiac muscle must be in error. Which assumption might be modified or eliminated so that as the propagation velocity changes with direction, the time course of membrane currents and permeabilities is changed?

Initially, assume that propagation along any axis in anisotropic muscle can be treated as one-dimensional propagation. Although this assumption is not true for propagation in general, it is reasonable at a macroscopic level when the excitation wavefronts are parallel over several millimeters and when the direction of propagation is taken perpendicular to the wavefronts.

Further, let us assume, temporarily, that the action potential propagates along a continuous structure, uniform in any given direction. This is clearly an oversimplification because the descriptive parameters for this "continuous" structure represent complex microscopic effects as being uniformly distributed on a macroscopic level. *Intracellular current*, for example, will involve many cells and cell-to-cell connections. As the direction of propagation is changed in anisotropic muscle, the pathway for intracellular current flow will also change and be different; a different direction in the cell orientation and different cell-to-cell couplings. Our velocity is also a macroscopic variable that represents the speed along a given axis averaged over many cells.

The resistance to current flow in the direction of propagation depends on the intracellular and extracellular resistivities, the size and shape of the cells, the relative volumes of intracellular and extracellular space (cell packing), and the resistance, number, and distribution of the cell-to-cell couplings. We use the term *effective* axial resistivity ($\bar{R}_a$) to include the effects of all of these (Spach et al., 1979).

Hodgkin pointed out (1954) that, in a continuous one-dimensional structure, there is a fixed relationship between the transmembrane current and the shape of the action potential that, for a propagating action potential, involves the velocity and the axial resistance. In particular, if the action potential shape remains constant, the velocity is inversely related to the square root of the axial resistance. The action potential can be made to propagate as rapidly or as slowly as is desired by choosing the appropriate axial resistance; the shape of the action potential remains constant whereas the spatial distribution of transmembrane potential and the axial current change. As will be shown, when these conditions are met, the axial current increases steadily as the axial resistance is decreased (and the velocity is increased). Therefore, we looked at the relationship between axial current and axial resistance implied by our data (on the basis of the continuous cable approximation discussed above).

In a continuous one-dimensional electrical cable, the axial or longitudinal current i_a is related to the transmembrane potential by

$$i_a = \frac{1}{r_a} \frac{\partial V_m}{\partial x} \tag{1}$$

where r_a is the axial resistance per unit of length. Substituting into Eq. 1 the definition of velocity $\theta = dx/dt$, the axial current is

$$i_a = \frac{k'}{\bar{R}_a \theta} \frac{\partial V_m}{\partial t} \tag{2}$$

The effective axial resistivity $\bar{R}_a$ has been substituted in Eq. 2 for the axial resistance r_a per unit length. The proportionality of r_a and $\bar{R}_a$ is included in the constant k'. Taking the specific instant when the rate of depolarization is maximum, the maximum axial current I_a^{max} is

$$I_a^{max} = \frac{k'}{\bar{R}_a \theta} \dot{V}_{max} \tag{3}$$

When the membrane properties are kept constant in a continuous cable, the product of the axial resistance and the square of velocity is also constant (Hodgkin and Huxley, 1952), so that

$$\bar{R}_a \theta^2 = k \tag{4}$$

where the membrane constant k includes the effects of the membrane properties and the cell size. By combining Eqs. 3 and 4, we have the following relationship between I_a^{max} and $\bar{R}_a$:

$$I_a^{max} = \frac{K}{\sqrt{\bar{R}_a}} \dot{V}_{max} \tag{5}$$

where K is a new constant (related to k and k′). In the calculations that follow, based on Eqs. 4 and 5, the measured values of θ and $\dot{V}_{max}$ were used and the values of the constants k and K were selected arbitrarily [values were selected to make the resulting numbers comparable to those from previous calculations (Spach et al., 1979)].

According to Eq. 5, if the shape of the action potential does not change with $\bar{R}_a$, the maximum axial current I_a^{max} is inversely proportional to the square root of $\bar{R}_a$. This relationship is shown as the broken line in Figure 3. Note that I_a^{max} decreases steadily as $\bar{R}_a$ increases and that I_a^{max} changes slowly with $\bar{R}_a$ for large values of the resistivity. When $\bar{R}_a$ is small, however, both the value and the rate of change in I_a^{max} are large.

Our observation was that $\dot{V}_{max}$ was not constant, but that it varied with the propagation velocity as the direction of propagation was changed. This, in turn, implies a different relationship between I_a^{max} and $\bar{R}_a$. To see what this relationship was, we first plotted the values of $\dot{V}_{max}$ from the experiment summarized in Table 1 and Figure 2 as a function of θ and fitted the points with the empirical function shown in Figure 4A. Next, we calculated the relative values of $\bar{R}_a$ for each velocity value, using Eq. 4; these are plotted in Figure 4B, showing the relationship between $\dot{V}_{max}$ and $\bar{R}_a$. (Note that both curves are steepest at high velocities: $\dot{V}_{max}$ changes most rapidly with velocity at high velocity and with resistance at low resistance.) I_a^{max} was

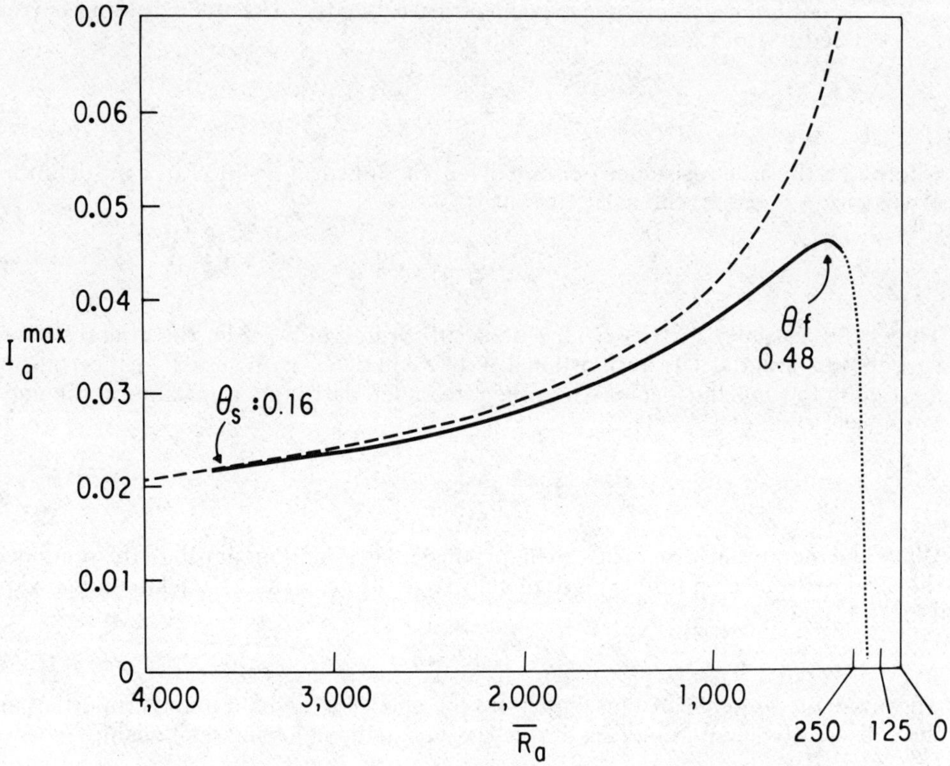

Figure 3. *Maximum Axial Current I_a^{max} as a Function of Effective Axial Resistivity*, $\bar{R}_a$. The dashed curve represents I_a^{max} calculated from Eq. 5 with the assumption of constant $\dot{V}_{max}$. In the solid curve, I_a^{max} was calculated from the curve fitted to the measured values of $\dot{V}_{max}$ (see Fig. 4) by Eq. 5. The dotted region represents an extension of the solid curve beyond the measured values by extrapolating the fitted curve of Figure 4. The units along both axes are arbitrary (vertical axis = μA, horizontal axis = Ω·cm). Note the reversed direction of the values on the horizontal axis. (From Spach et al. [1981], by permission of the American Heart Association, Inc.)

then plotted as a function of $\bar{R}_a$ (Fig. 3, solid curve with dotted extension). For this, the value of $\bar{R}_a$ was inserted directly into Eq. 5; the associated $\dot{V}_{max}$ value was obtained from Figure 4B.

Note three important aspects of the relationship (derived from our measurements) between I_a^{max} and $\bar{R}_a$: *(1)* The maximum axial current decreased gradually as $\bar{R}_a$ increased when $\bar{R}_a$ was large. This is the region of low propagation velocity; that is, the region transverse to the long cell axis. *(2)* The axial current reached a peak at low values of $\bar{R}_a$ and decreased sharply were $\bar{R}_a$ to decrease further. Note that the maximum propagation velocity (in the direction of the long axis of the cell) occurred at the peak of the I_a^{max} curve. *(3)* The curve derived from our measurements follows the inverse square-root relationship ($\dot{V}_{max}$ = constant) at high values of $\bar{R}_a$ and deviates from it more and more as $\bar{R}_a$ decreases.

What aspect of propagation could be responsible for this relationship? Considering the known morphology of cardiac muscle—individual, elongated cells coupled electrically through junctional complexes—perhaps we are seeing the effects of the

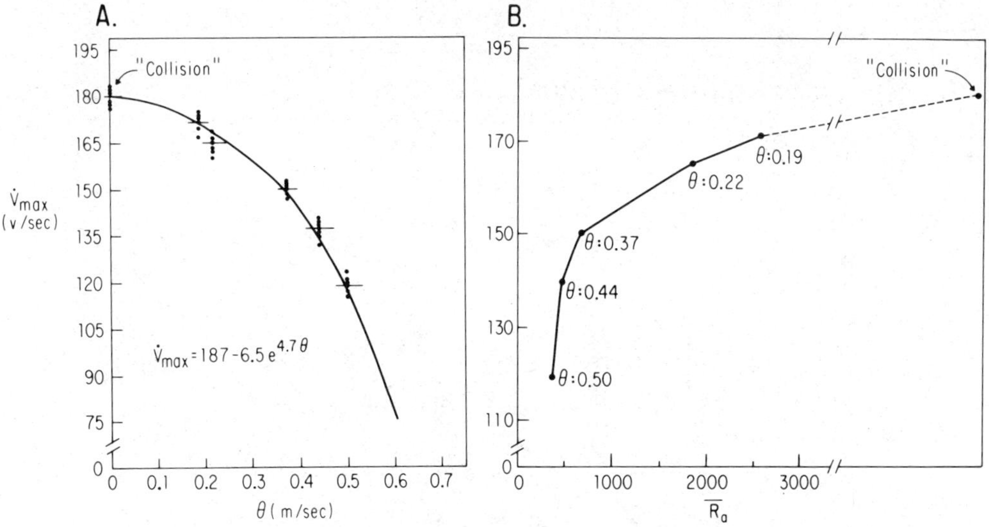

Figure 4. *The Relationship of $\dot{V}_{max}$ to Propagation Velocity (Measured) and to Effective Axial Resistivity, $\bar{R}_a$ (Calculated From Measured Velocity).* A: $\dot{V}_{max}$ is plotted as a function of velocity, recorded from one impalement in a ventricular propagation (Fig. 2). The "crosses" are made up of a vertical line of points representing $\dot{V}_{max}$ measurements of several action potentials with the same velocity and a horizontal bar to indicate the average $\dot{V}_{max}$ value of the group of points. The solid line is an empirical fit to the data points; the equation for the curve is given in the figure. B: The same data as in panel A are plotted as a function of $\bar{R}_a$ calculated from the velocity from Eq. 4. (From Spach et al. [1981], by permission of the American Heart Association, Inc.)

nondistributed nature of the effective axial resistivity $\bar{R}_a$. It is well known that propagation in a discontinuous structure (such as myelinated nerve) depends on geometric, cytoplasmic, and membrane properties in a way different from that in a continuous structure (such as unmyelinated nerve). Brill et al. (1977), simulating propagation in myelinated fibers, found that as the internodal distance increased, the propagation velocity increased to a maximum, and then decreased gradually for larger internodal distances. It can be seen in their Figure 2A that in the range where the propagation velocity increased with internode distance, $\dot{V}_{max}$ decreased, and τ_{foot} increased as the velocity increased—the same dependence we observed in cardiac muscle.

In considering the nature of the effective axial resistivity $\bar{R}_a$ in cardiac muscle, however, it is clear that the features of myelinated nerve fibers that cause saltatory propagation are not analogous to those responsible for the changes in the depolarization shape related to $\bar{R}_a$ in cardiac muscle. Changing the direction of propagation in cardiac muscle changes the length of cytoplasm through which the current must pass from one cell junction to another. This is schematically represented in Figure 5A. When propagation occurs in the direction of the long axis of the cells, the current traverses the entire cell length before encountering a junction. In the transverse direction, the current passes through a junction every cell width, so that there are more junctions per unit of length in the intracellular current pathway. In models of myelinated nerve (Fig. 5B), the node length is kept constant when the internode

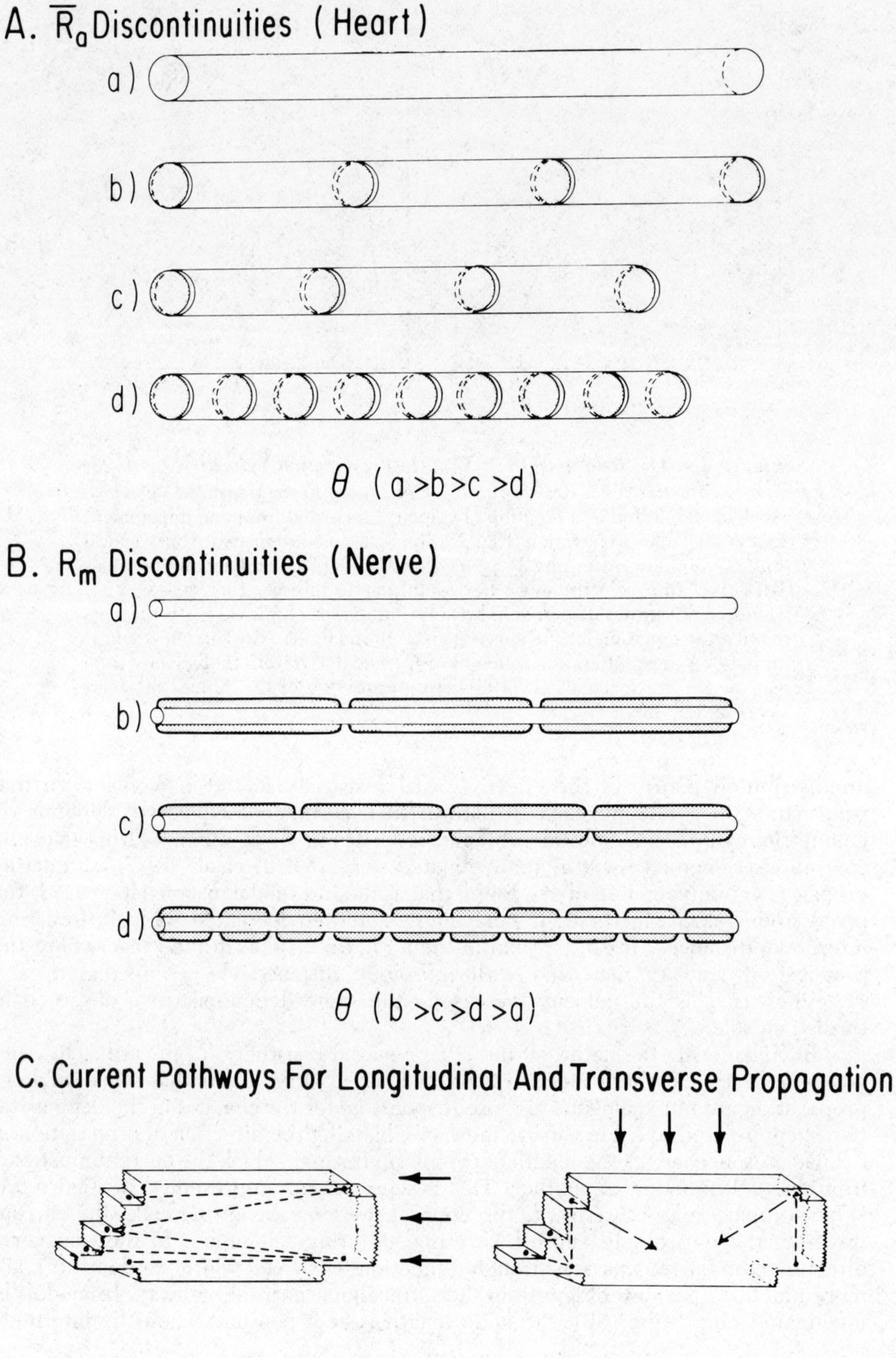
A. $\overline{R}_a$ Discontinuities (Heart)
a)
b)
c)
d)
θ (a>b>c>d)
B. R_m Discontinuities (Nerve)
a)
b)
c)
d)
θ (b>c>d>a)
C. Current Pathways For Longitudinal And Transverse Propagation

distance is varied; patches of active membrane of fixed area are coupled by different lengths of passive cable. But, in cardiac muscle, the total area of active membrane remains constant as the distance between the junctions is varied.

A decreased velocity with increased effective axial resistivity in the transverse direction is consistent with such a discontinuous structure for cardiac muscle. If a substantial part of the resistance to intracellular current were in the cellular junctions (Chapman and Fry, 1978), it would mean that the effective axial resistance would be greater in the transverse direction where more junctions would be encountered per unit of length. Although a one-dimensional representation of more frequent discontinuities of axial resistivity represented by the cell-to-cell connections accounts for the increasing axial resistance per unit of length and the decreasing velocity with more frequent connections (Fig. 5A), the changes in the intracellular current pathway in the real tissue must be considerably more complex when the direction of propagation changes. This is schematically represented in Figure 5C, which illustrates the change in the distance between the cellular couplings when the direction of propagation changes, as well as changes in the pattern of current flow (it may not be appropriate to ignore voltage gradients in the cytoplasm).

Note that it is not necessary to have side-to-side couplings between cardiac cells for propagation to occur in the transverse direction. Corbin and Scher (1977) and Geselowitz (1980) have suggested that the current flow within a single cell is longitudinal for all directions of propagation. But, as pointed out by Muir (1965), because of the irregular arrangement of the cell-to-cell connections, current flow within a single cell should occur both longitudinally and transversely. Further, cardiac cells are not long, uniform cells, but their borders "jut in and out in rectangular steps of irregular width and length, and the steps of one fiber interlock more or less closely with those of its neighbors" (Sommer and Johnson, 1979). Thus, it is likely that intracellular current can spread in any direction, even though all of the junctions are oriented in a fixed direction with respect to the long cell axis (Muir, 1957; 1965). The pattern of spread of the current through the tissue is further illustrated schematically in Figure 7A for a wavefront propagating in the longitudinal and transverse direction.

The second effect of the discontinuous structure consistent with our results is the presence of notches immediately following the depolarization phase of the action potential. The presence of notches suggests that propagation is, indeed, saltatory or discontinuous in that direction. Notches might be expected when the intracellular current has to pass through localized regions (cell junctions) of high resistance relative to the cytoplasm. Such junctions would separate the active membrane into patches, loosely coupled with each other. The peak after a notch would be caused by the firing of the next patch, after a short delay for charging its capacitance. Heppner and Plonsey (1970) showed such notches in their simulations of propagation across the single

---

Figure 5. *Comparison of the Recurrent Discontinuities in Cardiac Muscle and Myelinated Nerve*. A: A schematic one-dimensional representation of cardiac muscle for different directions of propagation. (a) Continuous cable (previously assumed to represent cardiac muscle); (b) in the direction of the long axis of the cells (widely-spaced couplings); (c) in the transverse direction (short distances between couplings); (d) intermediate direction with intermediate spacing between couplings. B: Similar representation for nerves including unmyelinated (a) and myelinated (b–d) with several node spacings. C: Schematic drawing of longitudinal and transverse current pathways through a cardiac cell. The cell is foreshortened in the horizontal direction. The cell shape is similar to those reported by Muir (1965).

junction between cardiac cells, as did Lieberman et al. (1973) during the repolarization phase with longer delays. Indeed, such notches were observed (Fig. 2) when propagation was in the transverse direction, but not in the longitudinal direction. Given the observed propagation velocity in the transverse direction and the timing between peaks on either side of the notches, the distance between discontinuities related to the notch can be estimated to be about 100 μm. Recent studies by Sommer and Dolber (1982) provide a morphologic explanation for such widely-spaced discontinuities. The intercellular connections in a trabeculum of ventricular muscle of about 1-mm diameter were similar to those previously described for a single (approximately 100-μm diameter) Purkinje strand (Johnson and Sommer, 1967). Sommer and Dolber showed that the trabeculum was composed of several strands; the strands were connected side-by-side, but at relatively widely spaced intervals—spacing approximately equal to the diameter of the strand. Propagation transversely, then, would be quite different from propagation in a longitudinal direction. Longitudinally, propagation would be more or less continuous, similar to that of unmyelinated nerve. Transversely, each strand would fire more or less as a unit, with a delay between the firing of such units because of the high resistance of the relatively small and infrequent connections between them.

Does the recognition of the discontinuous structure of cardiac muscle help us to understand the relationship we observed between $\dot{V}_{max}$ and velocity (Fig. 4A)? A qualitative argument shows that the introduction of discontinuities of axial resistivity can produce results that change in the right direction. A specific set of membrane properties will produce the largest $\dot{V}_{max}$ when the membrane is in the form of an isopotential patch (Van Capelle and Janse, 1976). When the membrane is distributed in the form of a cable, each piece of membrane (as it is depolarizing) has to supply charging current for the next piece of membrane downstream, slowing its own depolarization. It is reasonable, then, that $\dot{V}_{max}$ might be larger for transverse propagation than it is for longitudinal propagation. In the transverse direction, the membrane is divided into relatively isolated patches by frequent high-resistance cell junctions, whereas in the longitudinal direction, the membrane distribution more closely approximates a continuous cable. During transverse propagation, then, activity would seem to hesitate momentarily before moving on to the next unit along the path. The action potential would be expected to be closer to a membrane action potential; that is, more similar to a collision.

Predicted Abnormal Propagation

Assuming that cardiac muscle is best described as a structure with recurrent discontinuities of axial resistivity, we can predict an unexpected kind of propagation that would not be possible in a continuous structure. Uniform propagation occurs if a patch of membrane can, once its permeability mechanism is triggered, supply enough current to depolarize itself and to supply the necessary current to charge the capacitance of the neighboring tissue that has yet to depolarize. The terms "safety ratio" and "safety factor" have been used (Schmitt and Schmitt, 1940; FitzHugh, 1969) to compare the maximum current a cell can supply with the current required to bring it to threshold; if the ratio is greater than one, propagation can occur, and if it is less than one, stable propagation cannot occur.

Uniform propagation was observed along the solid line in Figure 3. The part of the curve near and to the right of the peak (low $\bar{R}_a$ values) is probably a region of propagation where the safety factor is low. Two aspects of our results indicate the possibility of a low safety factor in this region: $\dot{V}_{max}$ is low there, and the effective axial resistance is also low—implying that the cells or regions of membrane are tightly coupled for the flow of current. The amount of axial current in a given direction is determined by the source characteristics of a patch of membrane (described in terms of permeabilities and equilibrium potentials) and by the impedance (or loading) of the surrounding tissue. The combination of low $\dot{V}_{max}$ and low $\bar{R}_a$ is, therefore, consistent with a large current load on the membrane and a low safety factor.

If propagation along the axis with low $\bar{R}_a$ does indeed have a lower safety factor than does that along the axis with high $\bar{R}_a$, then propagation in a sheet of cardiac muscle should fail first in the direction of low $\bar{R}_a$ as the ability of the membrane to supply depolarizing current is reduced. We tested this prediction in a crista terminalis preparation, where the normal ratio of longitudinal propagation velocity to transverse propagation velocity is large. If the safety factors differ with $\bar{R}_a$ as proposed, the difference should be most apparent when the velocity ratio is large. We reduced the maximum membrane current during depolarization by stimulating prematurely, activating the fast sodium mechanism before it was completely reactivated late in repolarization. We eliminated other causes of altered propagation (for example, a change in $\bar{R}_a$ in a given direction) by comparing recordings from normal and premature beats initiated at a single stimulus site.

We recorded a full sequence of responses in seven preparations. Eleven to 18 extracellular electrodes were arranged in a cross-shaped pattern (Fig. 6). Normal stimuli were applied at intervals of 500 msec, and a single premature stimulus was inserted after every 15th normal stimulus. A typical set of recordings is shown in Figure 6. A premature stimulus with a long delay (290 msec) produced a normal propagation pattern of high velocity in the longitudinal direction and low velocity in the transverse direction.

Starting the premature stimulus in the absolute refractory period and increasing the delay, the earliest distant extracellular potential occurred at a delay of 130 msec (Fig. 6, upper right). The activity being recorded was clearly decremental because it was recorded only by the closest extracellular electrode in the longitudinal direction.

As the premature stimulus was delayed to 134 and 145 msec, the decremental propagation in the longitudinal direction grew in strength and was observed at greater distances. Nothing could be seen in the transverse direction, even at 145 msec.

By 155 msec, stable propagation was evident in the transverse direction whereas longitudinal propagation was still decremental. Note the shape of the extracellular potentials from the longitudinal electrodes numbered 1 through 4. At electrode 1, the potential was sharp and biphasic, indicating an action potential approaching and leaving the recording site. Electrode 3, on the other hand, showed a positive uniphasic potential, indicating that the propagation terminated near that site. To see if the propagation in the longitudinal direction was truly decremental, we calculated the propagation velocity between various pairs of electrodes. The resulting values were 0.38 m/sec (electrodes 0 to 1), 0.24 m/sec (electrodes 1 and 2), and 0.11 m/sec (electrodes 2 and 3). At the same time, the action potential propagated in both transverse directions at about 0.05 m/sec.

Note the later waveforms on electrodes 1 through 4 at a stimulus delay of 155 msec. The waveforms are biphasic, evidence of a propagating wavefront, and their sequence in time indicates propagation toward the stimulus electrode (from electrode 4 toward electrode 1). Such a wavefront could not have originated from the original longitudinal propagation, because it decremented to extinction. Thus, the reverse wavefront must have been the result of the original transverse wavefront and is further evidence that the slow transverse propagation was not decremental.

The pattern of propagation shown in Figure 6 (155 msec) represents reentry; the exact pathway of the reentrant beat was not known, but the path could not have been

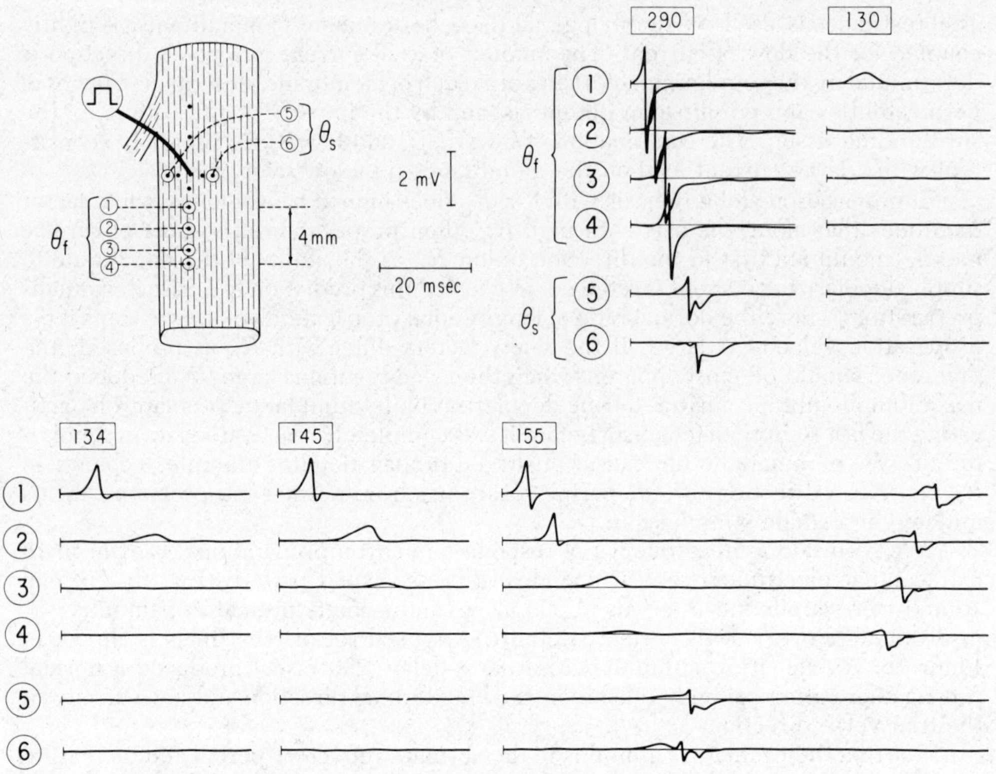

Figure 6. *Simultaneous Decremental and Nondecremental Propagation of Early Premature Action Potentials*. The drawing at the upper left shows the locations of the stimulating electrode (pacer symbol) and the recording electrodes (solid dots) on the crista terminalis preparation. The waveforms were recorded from the extracellular electrodes at the numbered locations. The numbers in the boxes represent the delay time (in msec) between the prior normal stimulus and the premature stimulus. (From Spach et al., [1981], by permission of the American Heart Association, Inc.).

very long because of the time delays observed. We observed simultaneous decremental and nondecremental propagation along the two axes in all seven preparations studied; reentry of the form shown was observed in six of these seven studies.

How could we be sure that the patterns of propagation (including decremental conduction and reentry) illustrated in Figure 6 were not due to nonuniform membrane properties? We made the following checks:

(1) Refractory periods were measured at multiple sites in the entire area of extracellular recording. If the refractory periods differed by more than 7 msec throughout the recording area, another region was selected for study.

(2) The stimulus electrode and a few of the recording electrodes were moved to other sites within the initial measurement area, and a portion of the sequence of premature beats was repeated. In all seven preparations and for all sites tested, the pattern of simultaneous decremental and nondecremental propagation was observed for some range of delay of the premature stimulus. The unusual conduction patterns were clearly related to the direction of fiber orientation and not to small differences in

refractory period. In the experiment shown in Figure 6, for example, the measured refractory periods were 151 msec at the stimulus site and 144 msec at electrode 4, a variation in the opposite direction required to explain the decremental conduction.

I emphasize, however, that the predicted patterns of propagation for premature action potentials described above depend on the presence of recurrent discontinuities of axial (intracellular) resistance. If the medium of propagation had been continuous, propagation would have had to fail in both directions simultaneously because, in that case, varying $\bar{R}_a$ would scale only the variation of V_m with distance and not the variation with time.

Propagation at a Macroscopic Level

The above concept of saltatory or discontinuous propagation at a microscopic level was generalized to the premise that it would also occur at a macroscopic level when an action potential propagates into a region that represents an abrupt change in the distribution of the cell-to-cell connections; that is, an abrupt change in the effective axial resistivity, $\bar{R}_a$.

The mechanism by which the velocity of propagation is altered by changing the axial resistance at a macroscopic level also has received little experimental study in cardiac muscle. In a one-dimensional cylinder, a change in the axial resistance per unit of length, r_a, alters the space constant λ ($\lambda = \sqrt{r_m/r_a}$, where r_m is the membrane slope resistance times the length, and r_a is the sum of the internal and external resistances per unit of length.) But, r_a is determined both by the cross-sectional area of the cylinder and by the axial resistivity according to the following relationship:

$$r_a = \frac{\bar{R}_a}{\pi a^2} \tag{7}$$

where $\bar{R}_a$ is the effective axial (internal) resistivity, and a is the radius of the cylinder.

Both mechanisms indicated by Eq. 7 have been considered to be the cause of changes in r_a that, in turn, are associated with changes in action potential shape and in the velocity of propagation in nerve and cardiac muscle:

(1) Change in radius. In previous analyses of this mechanism, the core resistivity has been considered to have continuous and uniform electrical properties (Lieberman et al., 1973; Goldstein and Rall, 1974). Although this mechanism (changing core conductor geometry) has been considered primarily for unmyelinated nerves (Joyner et al., 1978), it has been considered also to affect the propagation of action potentials in cardiac muscle at a macroscopic level. Most notably, it has been used to account for propagation failure across the Purkinje muscle junctions (that is, the "funnel" hypothesis of Mendez et al., [1970]), for action potential shape changes and propagation failure in a model of the A-V node by Van Capelle and Janse (1976), and for conduction block when (depressed) action potentials propagate from a long narrow isthmus of atrial muscle into a region of larger muscle volume (De La Fuente et al., 1971).

(2) Change in axial resistivity. In cardiac muscle, alterations in the velocity of propagation due to differences in axial resistivity have been considered to be caused by differences in the distribution of the cell-to-cell connections in the direction of propagation (Clerc, 1976), in the quantitative extent of the cellular connections (Martinez-Palomo et al., 1970), and in the resistance of the cell couplings (Lieberman et al., 1973). In a recent paper, Sharp and Joyner (1980) simulated propagating action

potentials in a continuous cable, except there was a short segment that had a higher specific axial resistivity than the rest of the one-dimensional cable. A change in action potential shape and a delay in propagation occurred across the region of elevated resistance. They likened the short segment of elevated resistance to the paucity of intercellular connections in the transitional cells of the Purkinje ventricular muscle junctions (Martinez-Palomo et al., 1970). They pointed out the similarity of this mechanism to the one involved in the "funnel" hypothesis of Mendez et al. (1970); that is, a change in current load seen by the propagating action potential.

The essential question is this: which one of these two mechanisms exists in cardiac muscle when the velocity of propagation is altered by changes in the axial resistance per unit of length, r_a, in the direction of propagation? Is this a structural difference without an electrical distinction?

Directional Effects of Branching in Cardiac Muscle

Figure 7 illustrates schematically two models that can be examined at a macroscopic level to determine whether cardiac muscle is best represented electrically as changes in core conductor geometry or as a structure with macroscopic discontinuities of effective axial resistivity, $\bar{R}_a$. A schematic representation of microscopic discontinuities of $\bar{R}_a$ that affect the cell-to-cell current-spread of a propagating wavefront in anisotropic cardiac muscle is shown in panel A (Fig. 7). The difference in cell orientation with respect to the direction of the propagating wavefront is consistent with a low value of $\bar{R}_a$ along the long axis of the cells and a high value of $\bar{R}_a$ in the transverse direction.

Microscopic $\bar{R}_a$ discontinuities can result in the directional differences of axial resistivity in relation to the orientation of the cells (see Fig. 7A). Provided the junction represents a change in distribution of the cellular couplings in the direction of propagation, they should produce an abrupt change in axial resistivity and a change in the safety factor of propagation at the site where two muscles join. This is illustrated in panel B. When an action potential propagates into branch site 1, it should encounter a region of abrupt transition from low to high values of $\bar{R}_a$, due to the change of the distribution of the cell couplings. But, when an action potential propagates into branch site 2, there should be little or no change in the orientation of the cells in the direction of propagation (no change in $\bar{R}_a$) as the action potential enters the branch; in other words, propagation should not be altered. On the other hand, when the action potential enters branch site 3, a mirror image of branch site 2, the action potential should encounter an area of increased axial resistivity as it turns to enter the side branch. That is, the direction of propagation would change from the longitudinal axis of the fibers to the transverse axis of the fibers as the action potential enters branch site 3 (arrows), but at branch site 2 the action potential would continue to propagate along the same axis of the fibers.

A model based on changes in core conductor geometry with constant properties of axial resistivity is illustrated in panel C (Fig. 7) for the same macroscopic geometric discontinuities of panel B. With propagation into branch site 1, there should be no change in the safety factor of propagation because the diameter of the parent branch is equal to the sum of the diameters of the two distal branches (Goldstein and Rall, 1974). Further, an action potential propagating into branch site 2 and 3 (panel C) should undergo the same change in propagation at both branch sites; that is, changes in action potential shape, propagation velocity, and safety factor at branch sites are dimensionless for this model (Goldstein and Rall, 1974). For example, as the action potential

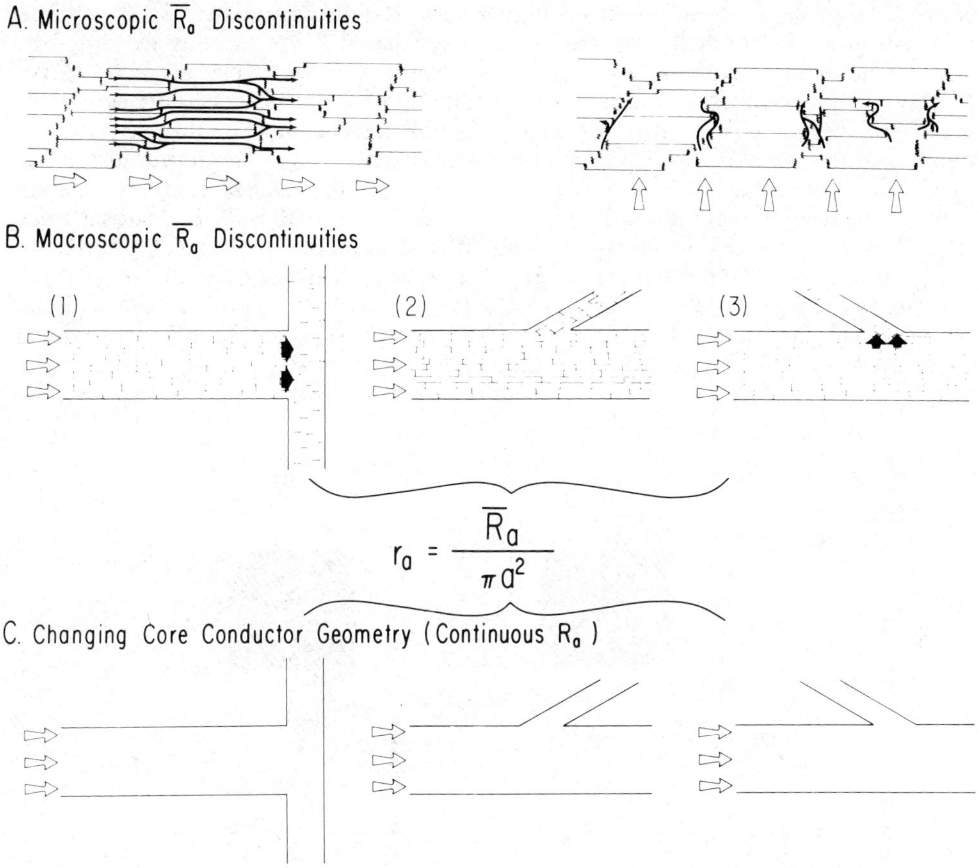

Figure 7. *Electrical Representation of Cardiac Muscle: Classical Core Conductor Model or a Model Based on $\overline{R}_a$ Discontinuities?* A. Schematic representation at a microscopic level of differences in the intracellular current pathway when the direction of propagation of a wavefront is along the longitudinal axis of the cells versus the transverse axis of the cells. Such a model of intracellular current flow (lines with arrows) results in a much shorter length of cytoplasm between the cellular connections when the action potential propagates in the transverse direction (small Δx) versus the longitudinal direction (large Δx). B. Schematic representation of a macroscopic model of cardiac muscle based on macroscopic discontinuities of effective axial resistivity $\overline{R}_a$ (arrows) at branching sites due to changes in the orientation of cellular couplings (that is, fiber orientation) in the direction of propagation. C. Schematic representation of a macroscopic model of cardiac muscle based on changes in core conductor geometry with continuous properties of the core conductor resistivity R_a. The equation in the figure is to identify the differences in the two ways by which it is possible for r_a (resistance per unit of length) to change in cardiac muscle.

enters branch sites 2 and 3, the velocity of propagation should decrease to the same lower value as compared with the larger parent branch (the velocity should vary approximately as the square root of the diameter [Hodgkin, 1954; Pickard, 1966]).

Assuming that branch sites produced by cardiac muscle can be represented by changes in cellular coupling in the direction of propagation, we can predict changes that should not occur if the branching electrically represents changes in core conductor geometry. For example, with normal propagation there should be directionally dependent differences in both the velocity of propagation and the amplitude of the extracellular potential (which reflects the magnitude of the axial current in the direction of propagation) when the action potential enters the small branch at sites 2 and 3 (Fig. 7B). We proceeded to test this prediction at branch sites in atrial muscle.

A typical result is shown in Figure 8A. The schematic drawing represents a branch site produced by a pectinate muscle and the crista terminalis. The extracellular potential was recorded on the initial part of the branch (solid dot). When propagation occurred in the left-to-right direction (stimulator 1), there was a large biphasic extracellular waveform, which was similar in amplitude to the waveforms recorded on the

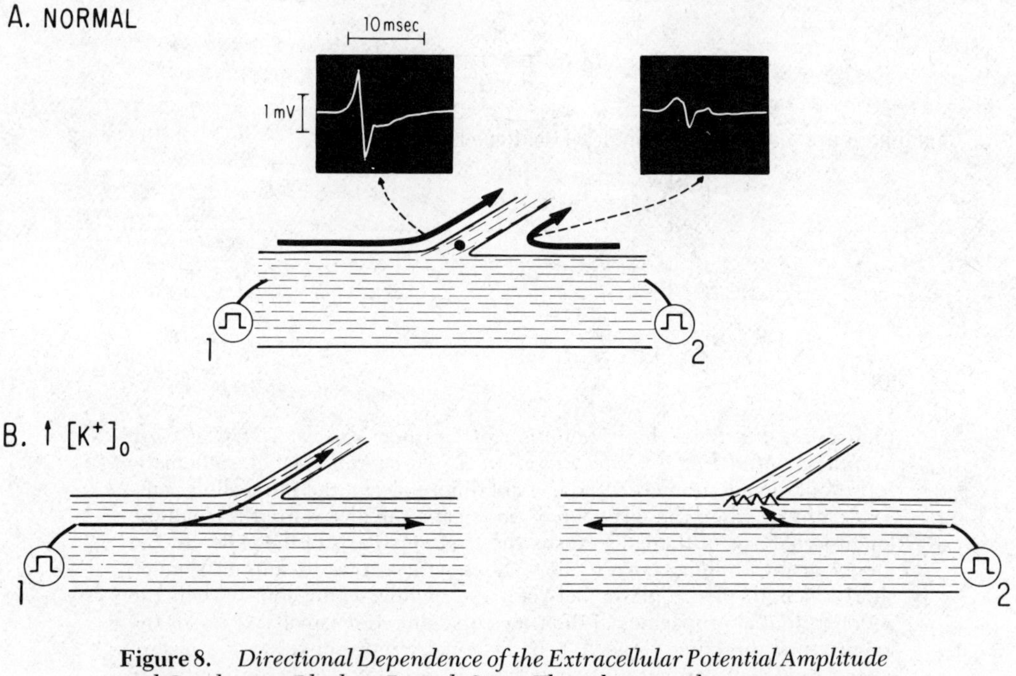

Figure 8. *Directional Dependence of the Extracellular Potential Amplitude and Conduction Block at Branch Sites.* The schematic drawing represents the crista terminalis with a small pectinate muscle branch connected at the designated angle. In panel A, the extracellular potential waveforms are shown that were recorded at a proximal position (solid dot) in the small branch. In panel B, the patterns of propagation are shown (solid lines with arrows) that occurred reproducibly for an interval of 3 min, during which the extracellular potassium concentration was 9.5 mEq/liter. The stimulus was delivered at a frequency of 1/sec while the stimulus site was alternated between stimulators 1 and 2 every 8 to 10 beats.

larger parent branch (crista terminalis). But when propagation proceeded from right-to-left (stimulator 2), there was a marked decrease in the amplitude of the extracellular potential. Measured excitation sequences demonstrated that the propagation velocity along the crista terminalis (0.95 m/sec) remained the same when excitation entered the smaller pectinate muscle from a left-to-right direction. But when propagation occurred from stimulator 2, the velocity decreased from 0.90 to 0.12 m/sec in the region where the wavefront turned to enter the pectinate muscle branch.

The above differences should not occur in a structure with changes in core conductor geometry and constant axial resistivity (Fig. 7C), because the changes in axial current flow at branch sites are dimensionless in that model (Goldstein and Rall, 1974). Histologic studies showed that the fiber orientation at such branch sites remained the same in a left-to-right direction along the edge of the crista terminalis into the pectinate muscle. Thus, the changes in the extracellular potentials and in the velocity of propagation in the right-to-left direction are consistent with changes in axial current due to changes in $\bar{R}_a$; that is, changes in the fiber orientation in the direction of propagation at the branch site.

It is generally agreed that a change in the safety factor of propagation (or a change in current load) occurs at sites that represent a change in axial resistance per unit of length (Lieberman et al. 1973, Goldstein and Rall, 1974; Sharp and Joyner, 1980). If there is a directional difference in $\bar{R}_a$ as suggested, then propagation into the same branch site should fail first when it arrives from a direction that represents a change in $\bar{R}_a$ (a change in fiber orientation). This would provide a critical test of the question as to whether branch sites in cardiac muscle are best represented electrically as regions of change in $\bar{R}_a$ or by changes in core conductor geometry (in which, changes in the safety factor at branches are dimensionless).

Figure 8B illustrates the propagation patterns found when the active membrane properties were modulated by elevating the extracellular potassium concentration to 9.5 mEq/liter. Although the action potential continued to propagate into the branch from the direction that resulted in little or no change in fiber orientation at the branch site (stimulator 1), it failed to propagate into the branch from the opposite direction (stimulator 2). The pattern of unidirectional-propagation failure at the branch site shown in panel B was reproduced randomly for an interval of 3 min at the high extracellular potassium concentration (stimulus rate = 1/sec).

Effects of the Junction of Two Separate Muscles

We further tested the idea that propagation failure should occur at sites that represent an abrupt change in the distribution of the cellular couplings by studying propagation across the junction of two separate muscle bundles. Eight to ten extracellular electrodes were positioned along the muscle bundles that formed the junction. A typical result in the adult dog atrium is shown in Figure 9. The schematic drawing at the top shows the anatomical arrangement of the connections between two atrial muscle bundles (arch of crista terminalis and taenia sagittalis), and the tracings below show the waveforms at the location of four recording sites (dots). Normally, action potentials propagated from one branch to the other with only slight delay in either direction. When the potassium concentration was elevated to 9.0 mEq/liter, however, propagation ceased to occur into the distal branch from either direction. Bidirectional block at the junction site of two mutually perpendicular muscle bundles was commonly encountered throughout the atrium when the extracellular potassium concentration was elevated. The change in fiber orientation from either direction of propagation was seen easily through the dissecting microscope (confirmed histologically) at these

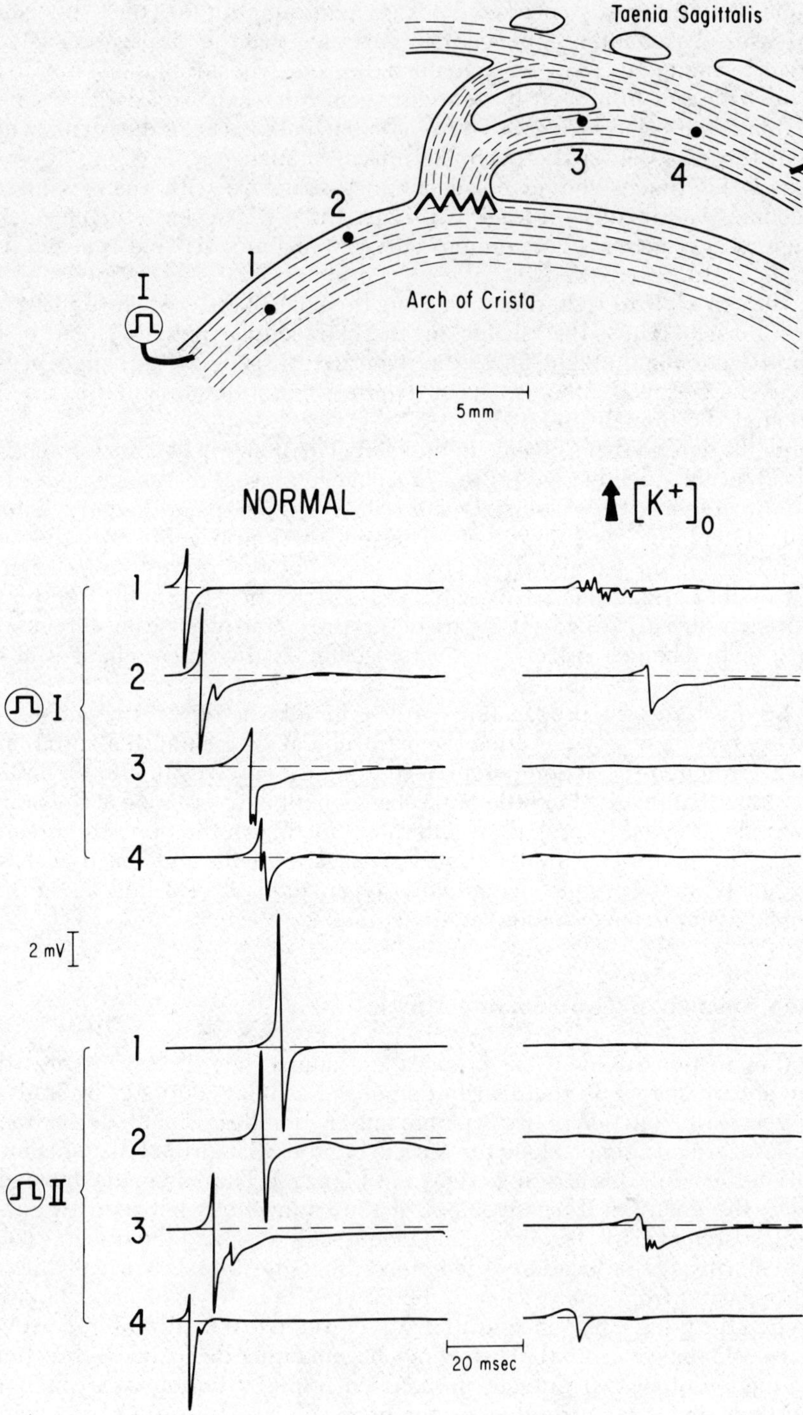
Taenia Sagittalis
II
3
4
2
1
I
Arch of Crista
5 mm
NORMAL
[K+]0
1
2
3
4
I
2 mV
1
2
3
4
II
20 msec

junction sites. Interestingly, conduction block can occur at these localized sites, resulting in the disappearance of action potentials distally, whereas uniform propagation can occur in the distal muscle if it is stimulated directly.

Events During Reentrant Propagation

Allessie et al. (1976) demonstrated circus movement of the impulse within a small (15 × 15 mm) segment of rabbit left atrium by applying an appropriately located and properly timed premature stimulus. The premature action potential conducted in one direction and failed in another. They considered the unidirectional block, which set the stage for circus movement, to be caused solely by spatial nonuniformity of the recovery of excitability, which was consistent with their refractory period measurements. They proposed the "leading circle" concept (Allessie et al., 1977) to emphasize that no insulated barrier is required to provide an anatomical loop around which the impulse has to propagate to induce reentry. Our results, however, suggest that in addition to the classical requirement of nonuniform recovery of excitability (Han and Moe, 1964; Allessie et al., 1976), the anatomical arrangement of the muscle bundles and the distribution of the muscle junctions (that is, the macroscopic discontinuities of effective axial resistivity) within such a small area also should be an important determinant of reentrant propagation.

We attempted to mimic the conditions of Allessie et al. (1976) in their atrial experiments by studying the details of propagation on the endocardial surface of the right atrial appendage of the dog. It was easy to produce repetitive reentrant propagation when the stimulus electrode was positioned at selected positions, a finding similar to that of Allessie et al. (1976). As yet, we have not been successful in mapping a complete sequence of excitation through all of the small muscle bundles comprised by regions as small as 10 × 10 mm during reentrant beats. We have found evidence, however, of several mechanisms that cause "unidirectional" block during the initial reentrant beat that sets the stage for a train of reentrant beats. These mechanisms include *(1)* spatially different refractory periods (Allessie et al., 1976), *(2)* decremental conduction due to anisotropic cellular coupling at a microscopic level (see Fig. 6), and *(3)* macroscopic discontinuities of effective axial resistivity represented by the pectinate muscle junctions.

An example of bidirectional conduction block due to the combined effects of spatially different refractory periods and to a macroscopic discontinuity of $\bar{R}_a$ is shown in Figure 10. The schematic drawing shows the anatomical configuration of the pectinate muscles within a small area. The stimulation site (pacer symbol) was varied between the two major muscle bundles while extracellular waveforms were monitored

---

Figure 9. *Bidirectional Conduction Block at the Junction of Two Separate Muscle Bundles*. The schematic drawing at the top shows the anatomical configuration of two prominent atrial muscle bundles (arch of the crista terminalis and the taenia sagittalis) that were mutually perpendicular. Five electrodes were positioned on each muscle that formed the junction site. The four waveforms shown were recorded at the positions designated by the solid dots. The stimulus rate remained constant at 1/sec, whereas the stimulus site was randomly changed between stimulators I and II. The waveforms recorded when extracellular potassium concentration $[K^+]_o$ was normal are shown on the left side of the figure. The waveforms recorded when $[K^+]_o$ was high (9.0 mEq/liter) are shown on the right.

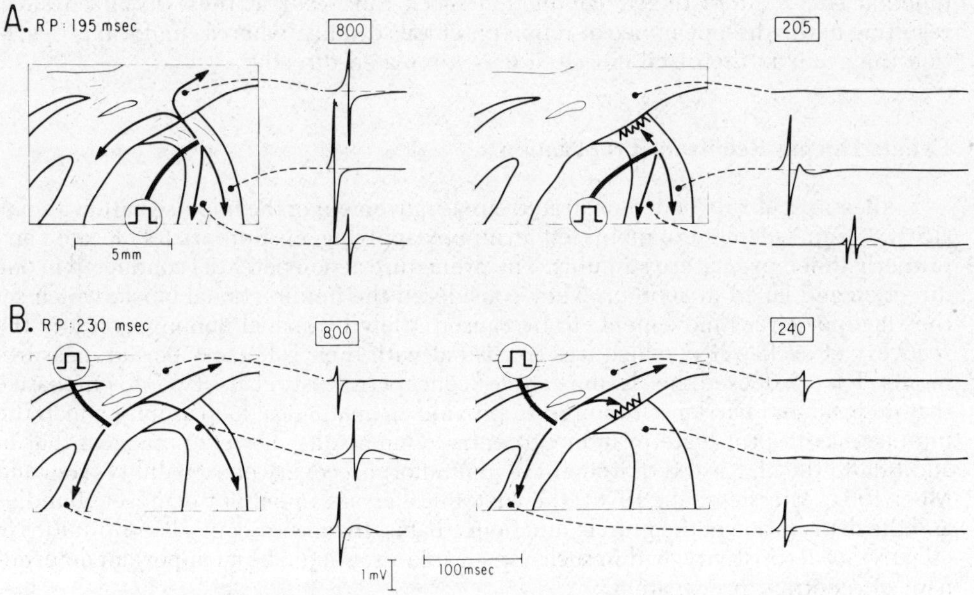

Figure 10. *Combination of Mechanisms in the Production of Bidirectional Conduction Block of Premature Action Potentials at the Same Muscle Junction*. The schematic drawing of the preparation represents the configuration of the pectinate muscle bundles in a small area of the right atrium. Selected waveforms are shown for the designated recording positions. The numbers in the boxes represent the time (in msec) between the prior normal stimulus and the premature stimulus. The refractory periods (RP) are indicated for each stimulus site. The "sawtooth" symbol at the muscle junction (right side of figure) indicates the location of propagation failure of the premature action potentials.

at 10 positions. Selective waveforms are shown, along with a representation of the general direction of propagation from each stimulus site (solid lines with arrows). Regularly spaced stimuli were delivered with an interstimulus interval of 800 msec, and a premature stimulus was injected after every 15th beat. The refractory periods were determined by stimulating at three positions on each muscle in an area within 2 mm of the muscle junction. As shown in the panels on the left side of Figure 10, propagation occurred bidirectionally with little delay across the muscle junction for normal action potentials (interstimulus interval = 800 msec). But, with an early premature stimulus, propagation failed to traverse the muscle junction from either direction, although it continued along the longitudinal axis of each bundle being stimulated. As shown, the refractory period (RP) at stimulus site A was 35 msec shorter than it was in the muscle on the other side of the junction site (RP of muscle A = 195 msec, RP of muscle B = 230 msec). The failure of propagation shown in panel A for a premature stimulus interval of 205 msec can be explained on the basis of the marked and spatially abrupt difference in the refractory periods across the junction of the two bundles. On the other hand, propagation failure across the junction from muscle B for the premature beat with a delay interval of 240 msec cannot be explained on this basis because the marked difference in the refractory periods occurred in the opposite direction. The localized propagation failure in that direction, however, was quite consistent with conduction block produced by macroscopic discontinuities of $\bar{R}_a$, as noted at other muscle junctions during modulation of the membrane properties by elevating the extracellular potassium concentration.

The results of Figure 10 demonstrate that the mechanism of bidirectional-conduction block at a single muscle junction can depend on the direction of propagation; in other words, in one direction the propagation failure can be accounted for by the abrupt increase in the duration of the refractory period across the muscle junction, and in the opposite direction the mechanism of the conduction block is consistent with a macroscopic discontinuity in effective axial resistivity, $\bar{R}_a$. Interestingly, such large differences in refractory periods can occur over apparent distances as small as 100 to 200 μm. We found similar prominent differences at many muscle junctions in the atrium, and the spatially abrupt changes in refractory periods coincided in each case with the junction site of two mutually perpendicular muscle bundles.

DISCUSSION

Propagation at a Microscopic Level

Several aspects of the propagation of excitation in cardiac muscle at a microscopic level are inconsistent with the electrical representation of the tissue as a continuous structure. In a continuous structure, the propagation velocity can be reduced in two ways: the axial resistance can be increased or the membrane ionic properties altered. In the former case, the theory of propagation in continuous media predicts no change in the shape of the action potential, and in the latter case, the rate of depolarization should be slowed with the velocity. Recording transmembrane action potentials at a single site as excitation arrived from different directions and at different velocities, we found that the shape of the depolarization phase of the action potential did change. Furthermore, $\dot{V}_{max}$ and τ_{foot} varied in the opposite direction with velocity from what would be expected if the velocity change was caused by altered or modulated membrane properties. We also observed notches immediately following the upstroke of the action potential when excitation propagated in a direction at an angle to the long axis of the fibers. Such notches would not be expected in a continuous, uniform structure, but would be produced by patches of membrane coupled by relatively high resistance junctions.

The discontinuous propagation of excitation between cardiac cells coupled through cell junctions can be thought of as a form of saltatory propagation. The term *saltatory* is used to indicate that propagation literally would be "jumping" or proceeding by steps (i.e., discontinuous) with slight hesitations at the recurrent sites of reduced conductivity. The defining characteristic of a discontinuous spatial derivative of the transmembrane potential, originally described for myelinated nerve (FitzHugh, 1962), would also apply to cardiac muscle (Heppner and Plonsey, 1970). We have found the term saltatory a useful descriptor to emphasize the electrical representation of cardiac muscle as recurrent discontinuities of axial resistivity, rather than as geometric discontinuities in the form of changing core conductor geometry. The features of myelinated nerve fibers that cause saltatory propagation are not analogous, however, to those responsible for such propagation in cardiac muscle. The discontinuities in the two tissues are physically and electrically quite different. In myelinated nerve, the node length is usually considered constant when the internode distance is varied; patches of active membrane of fixed area are coupled by different lengths of passive cable. In cardiac muscle, the discontinuities consist of local reductions in the intracellular conductivity where the cells are coupled. Future work will be necessary to distinguish the effects of discontinuities produced by the cell-to-cell connections versus the side-by-side connections of the unit bundles of Sommer (1982).

The results suggest that in an anisotropic preparation of cardiac muscle with a specified set of membrane properties, the maximum velocity should occur within an optimal range of $\dot{V}_{max}$ values. That is, within a narrow range of low values of the effective axial resistivity, $\bar{R}_a$, there should be an optimal current load on the cell membrane that results in an optimal value of $\dot{V}_{max}$ at maximum velocity (along the longitudinal axis of the cells). Any further reduction in $\bar{R}_a$ would result in a sharp decrease in axial current and the approach of propagation failure (Fig. 3). It is intriguing that the same relationship between the rate of rise of the action potential and the peak velocity of propagation can be seen in the results of the simulation of propagation in myelinated nerve by Brill et al. (1977). As the internodal distance increased, the propagation velocity increased to a maximum, then gradually decreased for larger internodal distances, whereas the rate of depolarization decreased monotonically as the internodal distance increased.

The results at a microscopic level, which demand the inclusion of discontinuities for their explanation, cannot be reconciled by cell branching. Strictly speaking, cardiac cells do not branch (Muir, 1965; Sommer and Johnson, 1979), but they appear to do so where one cell joins with two or more. Branching in cardiac muscle, thus, must be thought of in terms of a network of cell junctions, rather than branching cytoplasm. From theoretical studies on branched models with continuous cytoplasm, small delays are produced at branching sites (Lieberman et al., 1973; Goldstein and Rall, 1974; Joyner et al., 1978), but the amount of slowing observed would require a degree of branching not consistent with the known morphology of cardiac cells. In the phase-plane studies of Paes de Carvalho et al. (1976), they found shape changes in the action potential when propagation was initiated at different sites. They emphasized that this was inconsistent with a uniform cable model and suggested that cellular branching might be a possible explanation. As noted, our results cannot be accounted for by any model of propagation in which the cytoplasm is continuous.

Knowing that cardiac cells are elongated structures coupled electrically through cell junctions, the directional difference in propagation velocity is reasonable because the distribution of the cell junctions should vary with direction. The reduced velocity in the transverse direction then would be caused by increased intracellular (axial) resistivity in that direction. When this explanation for directional-velocity differences is combined with the presence of recurrent discontinuities of axial resistivity, an unexpected corollary results. Propagation at a microscopic level in each of two perpendicular directions responds differently to the same change in membrane properties. Propagation can become decremental and stop in one direction while it continues as uniform propagation in the other. In fact, uniform propagation ceases and becomes decremental first in the direction having the highest velocity, as the membrane activity is depressed. Thus, the "safety factor" is lower when the velocity is high and vice versa. The words "optimal" and "preferential" often have been applied to regions of fast conduction, implying that conditions are advantageous and that propagation is safer there. This is true in a continuous structure if the velocity is changed by modifying the membrane properties. But, the introduction of recurrent discontinuities of axial resistivity and modification of the propagation velocity by changing the intracellular resistance reverse the relationship of velocity and safety factor. For these conditions during premature beats and depression states, slow propagation in the direction transverse to the main axis of the fibers is safer than is fast propagation along the axis of the fibers.

Discontinuities of Propagation at a Macroscopic Level: Implications for Reentry

When the above electrical representation of cardiac muscle at a microscopic level is generalized to a macroscopic level, it is not surprising that we find inconsistencies with many current theories of conduction abnormalities. The macroscopic discontinuities of propagation occurred at locations where there were associated anatomical (geometrical) discontinuities; for example, at branch sites and at the junctions of separate muscle bundles. Although these anatomical discontinuities represented easily visible changes in the gross geometry of the muscular structures involved, the associated discontinuities of propagation could not be accounted for by representing these sites electrically as changes in core conductor geometry with continuous properties of axial resistivity. But, the changes in velocity, as well as the associated changes in the extracellular potentials, were accounted for at these sites by macroscopic discontinuities of effective axial resistivity due to abrupt changes in the distribution of the cellular couplings in the direction of propagation.

The primary requirement for producing reentry in cardiac muscle has been considered to be spatially nonuniform membrane properties; that is nonuniform recovery of excitability (Allessie et al., 1976). We have demonstrated that reentry can occur within a small area having uniform membrane properties (Fig. 6). Directional block can be produced by directional differences in cell couplings, so the pattern of propagation during reentry is related to the cell orientation, not to regional differences in membrane properties. The effects on propagation produced by directional differences in cellular coupling at a microscopic level are recapitulated at a macroscopic level owing to resultant discontinuities of effective axial resistivity. The results show that branch sites and the junctions of separate muscle bundles represent areas in which the fiber orientation changes in the direction of propagation. In turn, they result in localized areas where the safety factor is low, as shown by the failure of propagation at these sites during premature beats and during elevation of the extracellular potassium concentration.

Our results at a microscopic and macroscopic level indicate that reentry is likely to occur as a function of more than the single mechanism of spatially different refractory periods. In proposing the "leading circle" concept, Allessie et al. (1977) indicated that the reentrant propagation in the left atrium they measured was due to spatial differences in refractory periods without a gross obstacle for the impulse to circulate around; that is, there was no inexcitable central obstacle. But our results show that the sites where muscle bundles branch and join together represent macroscopic discontinuities of axial resistivity. Although these electrical discontinuities present no significant barrier to the propagation of normal or moderately depressed action potentials, they can be the sole basis for propagation failure during early premature beats and depressed states. In the pectinate muscle area of the atrium, we found that the anatomical arrangement of the small interconnecting muscle bundles provided multiple discrete and separate "pathways" for propagation within a very small area (1 cm^2), and that the muscle junctions represented sites of conduction block during reentrant beats.

The results at a microscopic and macroscopic level suggest that the occurrence of reentry in a given region of the heart depends on the specific combination of several mechanisms, which are related to both the spatial differences in the membrane properties and to anatomical complexities. The anatomical complexities include *(a)* anisotropic cellular coupling at a microscopic level (saltatory or discontinuous propagation), *(b)* macroscopic discontinuities of effective axial resistivity represented by branching sites and the junctions of muscle bundles, and *(c)* the geometric arrangement of muscle bundles and their connection sites. Thus, reentry is a function of the specific combination of several mechanisms, any one of which can act independently or in combination with the others depending on the state of the membrane properties and the anatomical complexities involved within the area comprised by the reentrant pathway.

Acknowledgment

I would like to gratefully acknowledge valuable discussions with Dr. J.M. Kootsey, Dr. E.A. Johnson, and Dr. R. Plonsey.

REFERENCES

Abe Y, Tomita T (1968) Cable properties of smooth muscle. J Physiol (Lond) **196**:87–100

Allessie MA, Bonke FIM, Schopman FJG (1976) Circus movement in rabbit atrial muscle as a mechanism of tachycardia. II. The role of nonuniform recovery of excitability in the occurrence of unidirectional block, as studied with multiple microelectrodes. Circ Res **39**:168–177

Allessie MA, Bonke FIM, Schopman FJG (1977) Circus movement in rabbit atrial muscle as a mechanism of tachycardia. III. The "Leading Circle" Concept: A new model of circus movement in cardiac tissue without the involvement of an anatomical obstacle. Circ Res 41:9–18

Arlock P (1979) The influence of the surface electrogram on the rising phase of the mammalian cardiac action potential. Pflüg Arch **380**:139–144

Barr RC, Herman-Giddens GS, Spach MS, Warren RB, Gallie TM (1976) The design of a real-time computer system for examining the electrical activity of the heart. Comput Biomed Res **9**:445–469

Brill MH, Waxman SG, Moore JW, Joyner RW (1977) Conduction velocity and spike configuration in myelinated fibres: computed dependence on internode distance. J Neurol Neurosurg Psych **40**:769–774

Chapman RA, Fry CH (1978) An analysis of the cable properties of frog ventricular myocardium. J Physiol (Lond) **283**:263–282

Clerc L (1976) Directional differences of impulse spread in trabecular muscle from mammalian heart. J Physiol (Lond) **255**:335–346

Corbin LV III, Scher AM (1977) The canine heart as an electrocardiac generator. Dependence on cardiac cell orientation. Circ Res **41**:58–67

Cranefield PF, Klein HO, Hoffman BF (1971) Conduction of the cardiac impulse. I. Delay, block, and one-way block in depressed Purkinje fibers. Circ Res **28**:199–219

Cranefield PF, Wit AL, Hoffman BF (1972) Conduction of the cardiac impulse. III. Characteristics of very slow conduction. J Gen Physiol **59**:227–246

DeFelice LJ, Challice CE (1969) Anatomical and ultrastructural study of the electrophysiological atrioventricular node of the rabbit. Circ Res **24**:457–474

De La Fuente D, Sasyniuk B, Moe GK (1971) Conduction through a narrow isthmus in isolated canine atrial tissue: A model of the WPW syndrome. Circulation **44**:803–809

Dominguez G, Fozzard HA (1970) Influence of extracellular K^+ concentration on cable properties and excitability of sheep cardiac Purkinje fibers. Circ Res **26**:565–574

Draper MH, Mya-Tu M (1959) A comparison of the conduction velocity in cardiac tissues of various mammals. Quart J Exptl Physiol **44**:91–109

FitzHugh R (1962) Computation of impulse initiation and saltatory conduction in a myelinated nerve fiber. Biophys J **2**:11–21

FitzHugh R (1969) Mathematical models of excitation and propagation in nerve. *In* Biological Engineering, edited by HP Schwan, New York, McGraw-Hill, pp. 1–85

Fozzard HA (1979) Conduction of the action potential. *In* Handbook of Physiology, Section 2, Vol I. The Heart, edited by RM Berne, N Sperelakis, SR Geiger. Bethesda, American Physiological Society, pp 335–356

Geselowitz DB (1980) Representation of electric sources in anisotropic cardiac muscle. *In* IEEE 1980 Frontiers of Engineering in Health Care, Engineering in Medicine and Biology Society, pp 6–8
Goldstein SS, Rall W (1974) Changes of action potential shape and velocity for changing core conductor geometry. Biophys J **14**:731–757
Han J, Moe GK (1964) Nonuniform recovery of excitability in ventricular muscle. Circ Res **14**:44–60
Hauswirth O (1969) Effects of halothane on single atrial, ventricular, and Purkinje fibers. Circ Res **24**:745–750
Hayashi H, Yamagishi S, Kanno T (1960) Conducting pathway dependency of the rate of rise of the cardiac action potential. Nippon Seirigaku Zasshi **22**:692 (abstract)
Heppner DB, Plonsey R (1970) Simulation of electrical interaction of cardiac cells. Biophys J **10**:1057–1075
Hodgkin AL (1954) A note on conduction velocity. J Physiol (Lond) **125**:221–224
Hodgkin AL, Huxley AF (1952) A quantitative description of membrane current and its application to conduction and excitation in nerve. J Physiol (Lond) **117**:500–544
Hodgkin AL, Katz B (1949) The effect of sodium ions on the electrical activity of the giant axon of the squid. J Physiol (Lond) **108**:37–77
Hoffman BF, Paes de Carvalho A, de Mello WC, Cranefield PF (1959) Electrical activity of single fibers of the atrioventricular node. Circ Res **7**:11–18
Hogan PM, Davis LD (1968) Evidence for specialized fibers in the canine right atrium. Circ Res **23**:387–396
Hunter PJ, McNaughton PA, Noble D (1975) Analytical models of propagation in excitable cells. Prog Biophys Molec Biol **30**:99–144
James TN (1963) The connecting pathways between the sinus node and A-V node and between the right and left atrium in the human heart. Am Heart J **66**:498–508
Johnson EA, Sommer JR (1967) A strand of cardiac muscle: Its ultrastructure and the electrophysiologic implications of its geometry. J Cell Biol **33**:103–129
Joyner RW, Ramón F, Moore JW (1975) Simulation of action potential propagation in an inhomogeneous sheet of coupled excitable cells. Circ Res **36**:654–661
Joyner RW, Westerfield M, Moore JW, Stockbridge N (1978) A numerical method to model excitable cells. Biophys J 22:155–170
Kanno T (1970) The heterogenous structure of the specialized tissue in the heart as a factor in atrioventricular conduction delay. Jap J Physiol **20**:417–434
Kootsey JM, Johnson EA, Spach MS, Geselowitz DB (To be submitted) A theoretical study of the depolarization waveform and propagation velocity.
Lieberman M, Kootsey, JM, Johnson EA, Sawanobori T (1973) Slow conduction in cardiac muscle. A biophysical model. Biophys J **13**:37–55
Martinez-Palomo A, Alanis J, Benitez D (1970) Transitional cardiac cells of the conductive system of the dog heart. Distinguishing morphological and electrophysiological features. J Cell Biol **47**:1–17
Mendez C, Mueller WJ, Urguiaga X (1970) Propagation of impulses across the Purkinje fiber-muscle junctions in the dog heart. Circ Res **26**:135–150
Muir AR (1957) An electron microscope study of the embryology of the intercalated disc in the heart of the rabbit. J Biophys Biochem Cytol **3**:193–201
Muir AR (1965) Further observations on the cellular structure of cardiac muscle. J Anat (Lond) **99**:27–46
Paes de Carvalho A, Hoffman BF, de Paula Carvalho M (1969) Two components of the cardiac action potential. I. Voltage-time course and the effect of acetylcholine on atrial and nodal cells of the rabbit heart. J Gen Physiol **54**:607–635
Paes de Carvalho A, Garcia EAC, Saldeña TA (1976) Phase-plane analysis of propagated electrical activity in muscle cells. Pontificiae Academiae Scientiarum Scripta Varia **40**:153–174
Peon J, Ferrier GR, Moe GK (1978) The relationship of excitability to conduction velocity in canine Purkinje tissue. Circ Res **43**:125–135
Pickard WF (1966) On the propagation of the nervous impulse down medullated and unmedullated fibers. J Theoret Biol **11**:30–45
Sano T, Takayama N, Shimamoto T (1959) Directional difference of conduction velocity in the cardiac ventricular syncytium studied by microelectrodes. Circ Res **7**:262–267

Sano T, Iida Y, Yamagishi S (1967) Changes in the spread of excitation from the sinus node induced by alterations in extracellular potassium. *In* Electrophysiology and Ultrastructure of the Heart, edited by T Sano, V Mizuhira, K Matsuda. New York, Grune & Stratton, Inc., pp 127–142

Schmitt FO, Schmitt OH (1940) Partial excitation and variable conduction in the squid giant axon. J Physiol (Lond) **98**:26–46

Sharp GH, Joyner RW (1980) Simulated propagation of cardiac action potentials. Biophys J **31**:403–423

Singer DW, Lazzara R, Hoffman BF (1967) Interrelationships between automaticity and conduction in Purkinje fibers. Circ Res **21**:537–558

Sommer JR, Dolber PC (1982) Cardiac muscle: Ultrastructure of its cells and bundles. *In* Normal and Abnormal Conduction of the Heart Beat, edited by A Paes de Carvalho, BF Hoffman, M Lieberman. Mt. Kisco, New York, Futura Publishing Co

Sommer JR, Johnson EA (1979) Ultrastructure of cardiac muscle. *In*Handbook of Physiology, Section 2, Vol. I. The Heart, edited by RM Berne, N Sperelakis, SR Geiger. Bethesda, American Physiological Society, pp. 113–186

Spach MS, Barr RC, Serwer GS, Johnson EA, Kootsey JM (1971) Collision of excitation waves in the dog Purkinje system. Circ Res **29**:499–511

Spach MS, Barr RC, Serwer GA, Kootsey JM, Johnson EA (1972) Extracellular potentials related to intracellular action potentials in the dog Purkinje system. Circ Res **30**:505–519

Spach MS, Miller WT III, Geselowitz DB, Barr RC, Kootsey JM, Johnson EA (1981) The discontinuous nature of propagation in normal canine cardiac muscle. Evidence for recurrent discontinuities of intracellular resistance that affect the membrane currents. Circ Res **48**: 39–54

Spach MS, Miller WT III, Miller-Jones E, Warren RB, Barr RC (1979) Extracellular potentials related to intracellular action potentials during impulse conduction in anisotropic canine cardiac muscle. Circ Res **45**:188–204

Sperelakis N, Mayer G, MacDonald R (1970) Velocity of propagation in vertebrate cardiac muscles as functions of toxicity and $[K^+]_o$. Am J Physiol **219**:952–963

Tasaki I, Hagiwara S (1957) Capacity of muscle fiber membrane. Am J Physiol **188**:423–429

Van Capelle FJL, Janse MJ (1976) Influence of geometry on the shape of the propagated action potential. *In* The Conduction System of the Heart, edited by HJJ Wellens, KI Lie, MJ Janse. Philadelphia, Lea & Febiger, pp. 316–335

Wagner ML, Lazzara R, Weiss RM, Hoffman BF (1966) Specialized conducting fibers in the interatrial band. Circ Res **18**:502–518

Weidmann S (1952) The electrical constants of Purkinje fibres. J Physiol (Lond) **118**:348–360

Weidmann S (1955) The effect of the cardiac membrane potential on the rapid availability of the sodium-carrying system. J Physiol (Lond) **127**:213–224

Weidmann S (1970) Electrical constants of trabecular muscle from mammalian heart. J Physiol (Lond) **210**:1041–1054

Woodbury JW, Crill WE (1961) On the problem of impulse conduction in the atrium. *In* Nervous Inhibition, edited by E Florey. New York, Pergamon Press, pp 124–135

Discussion

PAES DE CARVALHO: I agree with you that the finding of a higher upstroke velocity associated with the lower conduction velocity in transverse spread points towards some sort of anatomical discontinuity along the pathway. This is very much in keeping with the phase-plane data I showed just previously. As we pointed out, we are probably dealing with a situation in which both the input and the output resistance of the cell (or the cell group involved in the recording) is larger in the transverse direction than it is in the longitudinal direction. This would explain the finding of a higher maximal rate of rise during transverse spread as more of the ionic inward current would be involved in local depolarization, and less would be drained forward to the resting region ahead. It would also explain the lower initial slope of the phase-plane record because the longitudinal currents of the advancing wavefront would find difficulty in depolarizing a cell through an increased coupling resistance. On the other hand, one has to consider the possibility of collision occurring at a grosser level when the wavefront propagates transversely, invading zig-zag fashion muscle fascicles that have only sparse lateral connections. According to Dr. Sommer, the connections between fascicles running side by side may be 1 to 1.5 mm apart, so that a fascicle could be invaded transversely at two points almost simultaneously, and propagation wavefronts would tend to collide somewhere between these points. Although we do not favor this hypothesis to explain the increased $\dot{V}_{max}$ in transverse spread, would you care to comment on these two possibilities?

SPACH: Our data point more in the direction of discontinuities in longitudinal resistance along the path of transverse propagation than they do in the direction of the findings being explained solely by a collision of wavefronts. The situation seems to be closer to a membrane action potential than it is to a collision. A collision is actually a little more than a membrane action potential caused by reinforcement of the local depolarization by current flowing from adjacent segments. Collisions can be detected with extracellular electrodes, and indeed in the complex geometrical structure of the atrium we did detect them often enough. Mapping, however, showed that such collisions were occurring at a macroscopic level and not at a microscopic level. These macroscopic collisions cannot therefore explain the finding that all cells show increased upstroke velocity with transverse propagation.

CRANEFIELD: You showed that when propagation is critical block happens more easily in one direction than it does in another. In my experience wherever you have block you have abnormal action potential shapes in the neighborhood. Did you record action potentials in the situation where you have propagation blockade? When you have normal action potentials, you should not get this much heterogeneity.

SPACH: You are correct. This is not observed with normal action potentials, only with the somewhat depressed action potentials obtained in the present case with early extrasystolic stimulation. One interesting aspect of the data is that we are getting slow propagation caused by discontinuities in axial resistance along the transverse path with conduction velocities that were only to be seen previously in the atrioventricular node. Also we show that this slow transverse propagation is less likely to block in critical conditions.

Chapter 10

The Sodium Current in Heart Muscle

Arthur M. Brown, Kai S. Lee and Trevor Powell

The sodium (Na) current in heart muscle is responsible for the rapid upstroke of the cardiac action potential and for the propagation of the cardiac impulse. Until recently, its time course and magnitude have been unknown, and it has been assumed that Na channels in heart muscle are similar to those in axons (Beeler and Reuter, 1977). In fact, this may be the case for aggregates of embryonic chick heart cells (Ebihara et al., 1980). On the other hand, for adult heart muscle, there are numerous results indicating that the Na channel may be different. For example, we confirmed the results of other investigators (for references, see Trautwein, 1973) that the blocking dose of tetrodotoxin (TTX) is two to three times greater than that in axons (Lee, et al., 1979), whereas the blocking dose of the local anesthetic lidocaine is two to three times smaller (Brown et al., 1980). The TTX result may be due to the temperature dependence of the off-rate constant for binding, but the lidocaine result suggests a more fundamental difference. Moreover, the time required for reactivation of Na channels is much greater than the time required for their inactivation (Gettes and Reuter, 1974), an observation that is not consistent with any simple closed-opened-inactivated reaction for a single set of channels.

The major obstacle to the study of Na currents in cardiac muscle has been the syncytial nature of the tissue. Another limitation has been the inability to alter the intracellular ionic composition. We have overcome these obstacles by enzymatic dispersion of the heart into its single cell constituents and by using a suction pipette method for voltage-clamp and internal perfusion. The details of the methods and their limitations have been presented elsewhere (Lee et al., 1979; Brown et al., 1981a; 1981b). In this report, the principal results of our work will be considered with some emphasis on problems introduced by enzymatic dispersion.

The first important result is that cells prepared according to Powell and Twist (1976) had an average resting potential of −30 mV, measured with two suction pipettes, although values of −80 mV were sometimes obtained. Our average values were not as negative as those found by Powell et al. (1980) and might be attributed to the fact that extracellular Ca at 5 to 10 mM, which is a prerequisite for obtaining steady recorded potentials of about −80 mV with glass microelectrodes, cannot be used with suction pipettes. Nevertheless, the cells could be polarized to −90 mV by about 5 ×

Support by N.I.H. Grant #HL-25145

10^{-10} A, indicative of a large input resistance. A brief depolarizing current could then produce an action potential with an amplitude of 120 mV, a duration of 180 msec, a plateau of 50 msec, and a maximum rate of rise ($\dot{V}_{max}$) of 230 V/sec^{-1}, as shown in Figure 1.

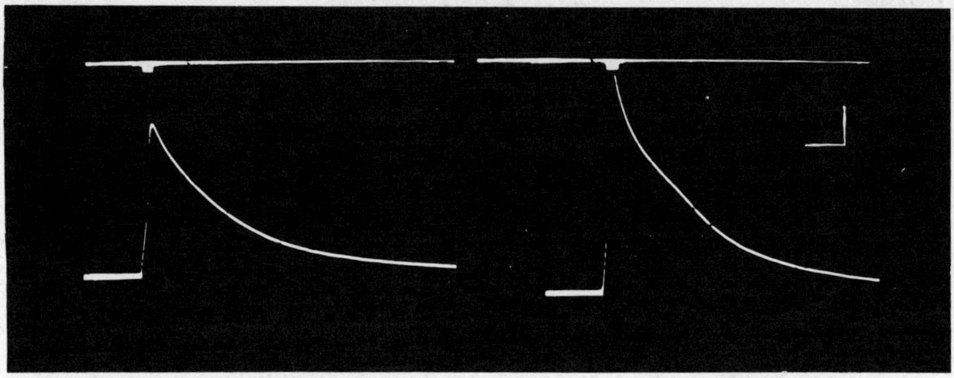

Figure 1. Action potentials recorded using one or two suction pipettes from the same heart cell at 20° C. Measured resting potentials were −90 mV, and the action potential recorded by one suction pipette is shown to the left. Current trace is at the very top. Differences of this magnitude between the two recording techniques were observed when currents of up to 10 nA were required to maintain the membrane potential at −90 mV. Normally, holding currents were less than 1 nA, and action potentials recorded by two suction pipettes were 5 to 10% greater in amplitude than those measured with one pipette. Calibration, 20 mV; 20 msec.

The electrical constants of a single cell in normal extracellular Krebs solution and K_2PO_4 internal solution are shown in Table 1. These values were similar to the results obtained in intact tissue. The length constant (λ) was calculated from voltage measurements made at two different points in the same cell and had a value of 500 μm, which could be compared with an effective length (L) of 50 μm. The true length of 100 μm was halved because the cell was aspirated into two suction pipettes placed at either end (Fig. 2). In studies of sodium currents (I_{Na}), cesium was substituted for potassium in the internal and external solutions, which raised the membrane resistance (R_m) and doubled λ. At peak Na chord conductance (gNa), R_m could be reduced as much as 100-fold so that λ was reduced 10-fold. This gives an L/λ ratio, in the worst case, of 0.3 to 0.5, which, in theory, should cause inadequate spatial control of voltage.

Even in this circumstance, however, voltage control was judged to be adequate using the following criteria: (*a*) absence of abominable notches on the current trace, (*b*)

Table 1
Cable Parameters of a Single Adult Rat Cardiac Myocyte

R_{in} (MΩ)	C_{in} (pF)	C_m^* (μF cm^{-2})	R_m ($10^3 \times$ Ωcm^2)
44.5 ± 4.6	400 ± 42	5 ± 0.5	2.8 ± 0.3

*Calculated from input resistance and membrane time constant, assuming a cell surface area of 8000 μm^2 (Page & McCallister, 1973).

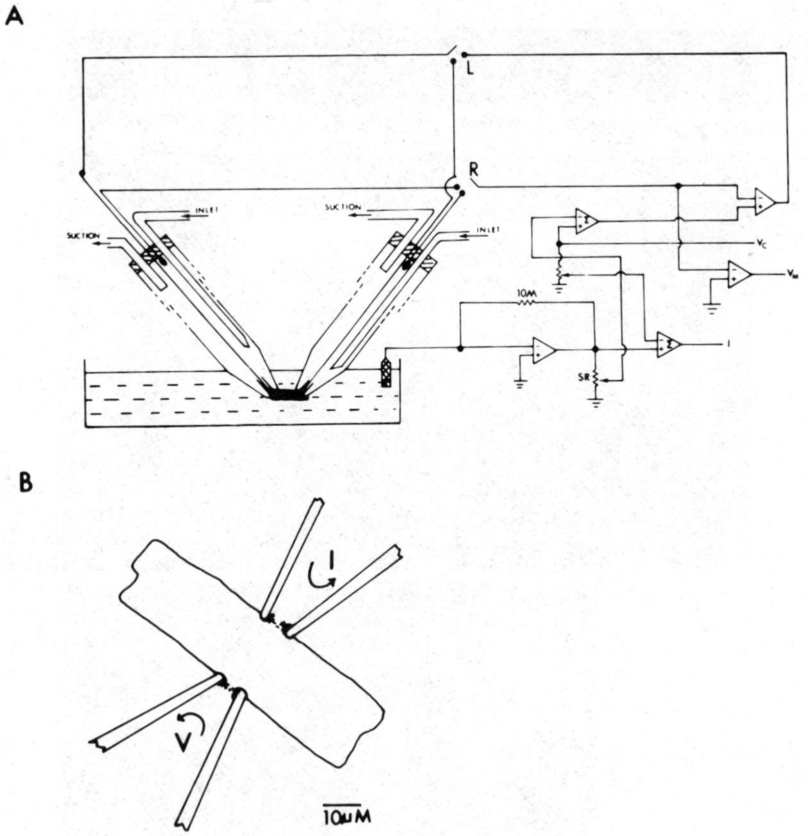

Figure 2. A. Recording system for two suction pipettes on a single ventricular muscle cell. Either pipette can be used to record voltage, or inject current, or both by using the switches L and R in the circuit diagram. V_m and V_c are membrane potential and command voltage, respectively, I is current, and SR is series resistance compensation (Hodgkin et al., 1952). The clamp amplifier had a gain of at least 1000 and a frequency response flat to 10 kHz. B. A voltage-recording pipette (V) and current-injecting pipette (I) applied centrally across a cell. Arrows indicate direction of flow for internal solution.

an envelope for tail currents that was similar in time course to the transient current during a single voltage step, and (*c*) current-voltage (I-V) plots that were similar in shape in extracellular sodium (Na_o) solutions varying from 50% to 12.5% of normal or in doses of TTX that partially block Na.

Spatial control of voltage may be inadequate when only a single suction pipette is used to both measure voltage and apply current (Lee et al., 1979; Undrovinas et al., 1980). In this case the voltage drop across the pipette tip cannot be compensated for, and voltage control may be poor. In our studies, temporal resolution was limited by the capacitative current transient, which had a time constant of about 300 μsec. A series resistance of 750 kΩ was the main cause of this transient. Although compensation was useful in reducing the series resistance, its application was limited because of a tendency to produce ringing in the currents.

The sodium currents recorded by the double-suction pipette method are shown in Figure 3. Potassium currents (I_K) were suppressed by substituting cesium, and

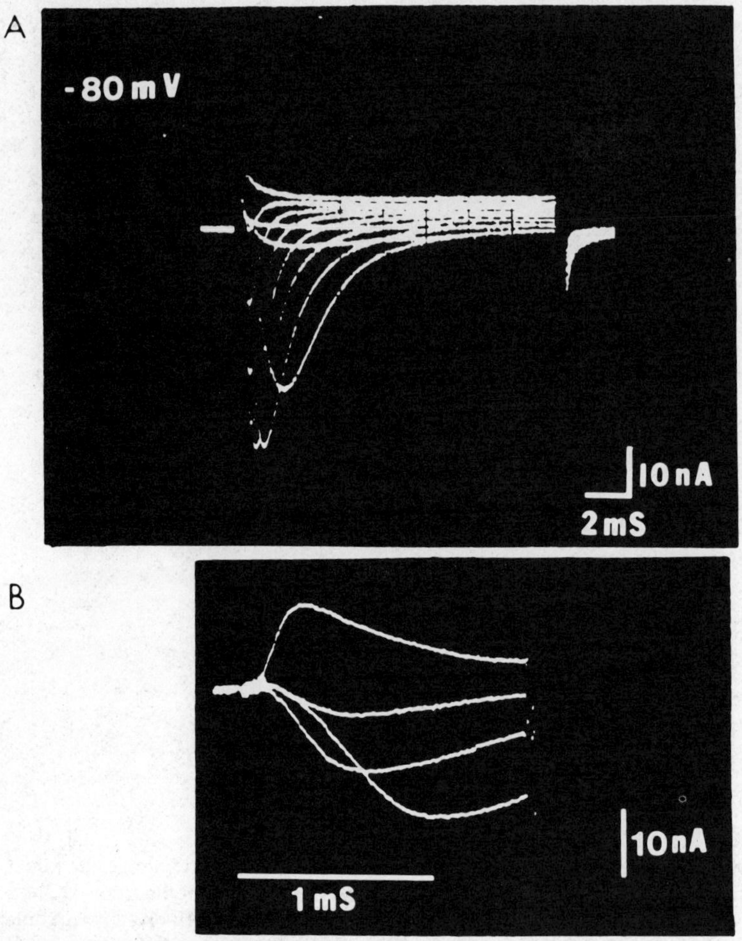

Figure 3. A. Sodium currents recorded under voltage clamp in Ca-free, K-free, and Cl-free external solution with 72.5 mM Na, and internal perfusion solution containing 16 mM Na. The currents were not corrected for capacitative and leakage currents. Holding potential was −80 mV, and clamp potentials were from −60 to +30 mV in 10 mV steps. B. Sodium currents with linear components of capacitative and leakage currents subtracted. Currents produced at clamped potentials of −10, 0, 10, and 40 mV, from a holding potential of −80 mV. Na current was preceded by a 100-μsec zero-current interval, which was obscured by the capacitative current transient in nonsubtracted records.

calcium currents (I_{Ca}) were suppressed by substituting manganese or cobalt for calcium. The product of peak I_{Na} and membrane capacitance (C_m) were consistent with measured values of ($\dot{V}_{max}$) (230 V/sec^{-1}). The reversal potential changed in a Nernstian manner when intracellular sodium (Na_i) or Na_o was altered, indicating a high selectivity for Na ions. This result has a considerable practical value because membrane potential measurements made with a suction pipette are prone to fluctuations caused by leaks in the suction line. Because E_{Na} can be controlled, it provides a valuable reference potential.

Instantaneous I-V curves were linear and g_{Na} could be treated as a chord conductance. The g_{Na}-V relationship is shown in Figure 4, where $\bar{g}_{Na}$ was 25 mS cm^{-2} in 100% Na_o. In its steepest portion, g_{Na} changed e-fold for a 4- to 6-mV change in potential, a finding consistent with four to six electronic charges moving through the membrane field. The rising phase of I_{Na} began after delay and had an inflection; it could be fitted with an m^3 model in Hodgkin-Huxley terms. The falling phase could be fitted either by an exponential function with a small persistent current or by two exponentials, the slower one having a time constant three times greater than the faster process, which was in turn five to ten times slower than τ_m. It is unlikely that the double exponential time course of inactivation was an artefact caused by series resistance because the latter tended to remove the slower process (Meves, 1978). Both inactivation processes were eliminated by TTX, but the relative sensitivity was not examined. There are two possible explanations for these kinetic features: two populations of channels or one population with two inactivated states.

The relationships between voltage, steady-state activation (m_∞), and steady-state inactivation (h_∞) are shown in Figure 5. The h_∞-V relationship was obtained using prepulse durations of 40 to 60 msec, which may not have inactivated all of the more slowly inactivating channels. There was, however, substantial overlap between the two parameters, so that a persistent inward Na current during the plateau of the action potential could have been possible cause.

Reactivation of I_{Na}, examined at −90 to −70 mV, was greatly prolonged and thus confirmed the earlier report of Gettes and Reuter (1974). We also confirmed the large micromolar doses of TTX and the smaller micromolar doses of lidocaine necessary to block I_{Na}.

For lidocaine, use-dependence was not a prominent feature, and only about 70% of the tonic block was relieved by hyperpolarization. Recovery from inactivation was, however, prolonged (Lee et al., 1981).

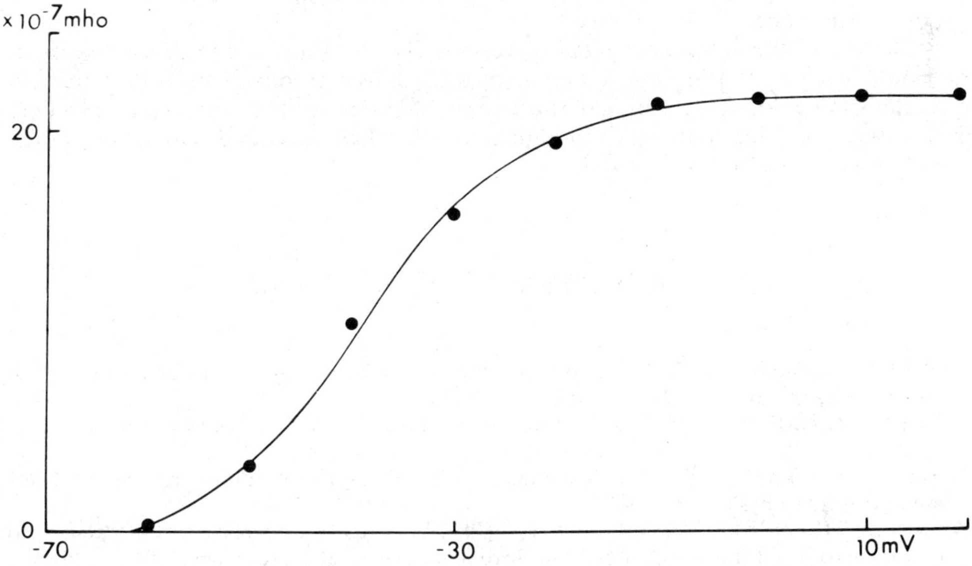

Figure 4. Variations of chord conductance (gNa) with membrane potential. gNa changed e-fold for a 6-mV potential change and gNa was 25 mS·cm^{-2} in 100% extracellular Na, assuming a cell surface area of 8,000 μm^2.

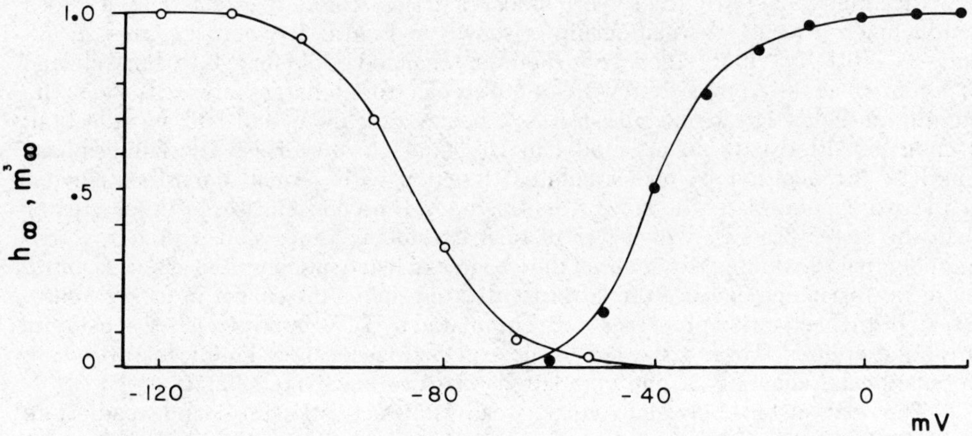

Figure 5. Relationships between steady-state activation (m_∞) and voltage (V), and between steady-state inactivation (h_∞) and V. The $m_\infty{}^3$-V relationship is denoted by closed circles (●); the h_∞-V relationship, by open circles (○). Overlap is within the potential range of −40 to −70 mV.

To summarize, the Na channels of cells obtained by enzymatic dispersion of adult rat heart muscle differ from those of axon and embryonic chick heart muscle. Assuming similar unit conductances, the density of Na channels is reduced by 25 to 50%. A significant amount of persistent or slowly inactivating current is present, although it now appears that this is true in squid giant axon as well. Reactivation is very prolonged at potentials near the resting membrane potential, and this cannot be explained by the two inactivation processes apparent in the kinetics of I_{Na}, which points to a third process that appears to be involved.

Pharmacologic differences are also present. The most important, from a therapeutic point of view, is the large element of tonic block produced by lidocaine (and quinidine). Further optimization of therapy should be possible if Na-channel blockers with a strong use-dependence and a high affinity for the inactivated state produced by depolarization can be synthesized.

REFERENCES

Beeler GW, Reuter W (1977) Reconstruction of the action potentials of ventricular myocardial fibres. J Physiol **268**:177–210

Brown AM, Lee KS, Powell T (1981a) Sodium current in single rat heart muscle cells. J Physiol (in press)

Brown AM, Lee KS, Powell T (1981b) Voltage-clamp and internal perfusion in single rat heart muscle cells. J Physiol (in press)

Brown AM, Hume JR, Giles WR, Lee KS (1980) Voltage-clamp analysis of lidocaine- and quinidine-induced depression of sodium current in isolated rat ventricular cells. (Proc Physiol Soc, p 68p, June 7, 1980) (in press)

Ebihara L, Shigeto N, Lieberman M, Johnson EA (1980) The initial inward current in spherical clusters of chick embryonic heart cells. J Gen Physiol **73**:437–456

Gettes LS, Reuter H (1974) Slow recovery from inactivation of inward current in mammalian myocardial fibers. J Physiol **240**:703–724

Hodgkin AL, Huxley AF, Katz B (1952) Measurements of current voltage relations in the membrane of giant axon of *Loligo*. J Physiol **116**:424–448
Lee KS, Weeks TA, Kao RL, Akaike N, Brown AM (1979) Sodium current in single heart muscle cells. Nature **278**:269–271
Lee KS, Hume JR, Giles W, Brown AM (1981) Lidocaine- and quinidine-induced depression of sodium current in isolated ventricular cells. Nature (in press)
Meves H (1978) Inactivation of the sodium permeability in squid giant nerve fibers. Prog Biophys Molec Biol **33**:207–330
Page E, McCallister LP (1973) Studies of the intercalated disc of rat left ventricular myocardial cells. J Ultrastruct Res **43**:388–411
Powell T, Terrar DA, Twist VW (1980) Electrical properties of individual cells isolated from adult rat ventricular myocardium. J Physiol **302**:131–153
Powell T, Twist VW (1976) A rapid technique for the isolation and purification of adult cardiac muscle cells having respiratory control and a tolerance to calcium. Biochem Biophys Res Com **72**:327–333
Trautwein W (1973) Membrane currents in cardiac muscle fibers. Physiol Rev **23**:793–835
Undrovinas AI, Yushmanova AV, Hering S, Rosenshtraukh, LV (1980) Voltage clamp method on single cardiac cells from adult rat heart. Experientia **36**:572–574

Discussion

WEIDMANN: You reported that you were unable to restore full inward current under lidocaine by hyperpolarizing to −140 mV. I must confess that I previously overemphasized the ability of hyperpolarization to restore fully the fast inward current under local anesthetics (J Physiol *129*:568–582, 1955). There always was a shift of the curve relating peak dV/dt to resting potential along the voltage axis towards more negative potentials; but there never was complete restoration with hyperpolarization.

CARMELIET: In the same experiment with lidocaine, were the hyperpolarizing pulses of long duration or of short duration?

BROWN: The duration of hyperpolarizing pulses was 100 msec. We should repeat these experiments with longer duration pulses.

REUTER: From the position of your m_∞ and h_∞ curves in the voltage axis, you should expect a very large window current. Have you seen a hump in the steady-state current-voltage relationship that might correspond to this window current?

BROWN: We have not examined the steady-state I-V relationship because the steady currents are small; a hump would be expected, however.

PAES DE CARVALHO: I noticed that your h_∞ curve has a tail going all the way to −20 mV. In experiments with rabbit atrium in which the resting potential is sitting at −45 or −50 mV, the inactivation of the fast sodium channel seems to us to be already complete, as no TTX sensitivity to the slow-response action potential elicited from this voltage level can be noticed. Is this a peculiarity of the rat as compared to the rabbit or do you think you may have already some slow current channel activation at that voltage level?

BROWN: In our preparation, there appears to be some sodium channels with slower inactivation characteristics. Similar observations have been made in squid giant axon. The number of sodium channels that show this particular inactivation property may change from preparation to preparation. These channels were blocked by TTX in our hands. Their contribution to the slow response action potential might be too small to be detected using TTX sensitivity of the action potential as an indicator.

FOZZARD: Do your data permit you to make an estimate about the value of $\bar{g}_{Na}$?

BROWN: Yes. It is about 25 mS/cm^2 in 100% sodium.

JOHNSON: With respect to Fozzard's question on g_{Na}, we got a very similar figure, about 23 mS/cm^2, in experiments in which we did a complete voltage-clamping analysis of fast current in tissue culture preparations.

PAES DE CARVALHO: A preliminary phase-plane estimate of peak g_{Na} during propagated action potentials in rabbit atrium yielded in our hands a value of 15.8 mS/μF (Paes de Carvalho A (1975) *In* Concepts of Membranes in Regulation and Excitation, edited by M. Rocha e Silva, G.S. Kurtz, New York, Raven Press, pp 85−96). Action potentials studied in this fashion rose from a resting voltage of nearly −80 mV and h_∞ may have been lower than 1. Also, C_m in atrium is probably higher than 1 $\mu F/cm^2$. Our values are therefore compatible with a $\bar{g}_{Na}$ above 20 mS/cm^2.

Chapter 11

Block of Cardiac Sodium Channels by Tetrodotoxin and Lidocaine: Sodium Current and $\dot{V}_{max}$ Experiments

Bruce P. Bean, Charles J. Cohen and Richard W. Tsien

Sodium channels in heart are vital for rapid impulse propagation and are also a primary target for the antiarrhythmic actions of lidocaine and other drugs. These channels have been difficult to study by the voltage-clamp method because of technical difficulties inherent in the structure of most cardiac preparations. Until very recently, information about cardiac sodium channels has come by two indirect routes: by extrapolation from nerve axons or skeletal muscle, where sodium channels are easier to study, or by use of the maximal upstroke velocity of the cardiac action potential ($\dot{V}_{max}$). Although recognizing that the information was indirect, cardiac physiologists have been comforted by the rather good agreement between these two sources. After all, the pioneering work of Weidmann (1955a) had shown an S-shaped relation between $\dot{V}_{max}$ and membrane potential, much the same as that found for the sodium current (I_{Na}) (Hodgkin and Huxley, 1952b). Similarities between heart and nerve were also striking upon examination of the various effects of sodium (Weidmann, 1955a; Hodgkin and Huxley, 1952a), calcium (Weidmann, 1955b; Frankenhaeuser and Hodgkin, 1957), and cocaine and other drugs (Weidmann, 1955b; see Hille, 1978 for review of literature in nerve and skeletal muscle).

So it has been widely believed that cardiac sodium channels are virtually identical to those in nerve. This view has received its strongest challenge from experiments using tetrodotoxin (TTX). While nanomolar concentrations of TTX inhibit I_{Na} in most nerve and skeletal muscle fibers, micromolar concentrations are needed to block the rapid impulse in mammalian heart (see for example, Dudel et al., 1967; Carmeliet and Vereecke, 1969; Coraboeuf et al., 1979). By itself, this difference in sensitivity might indicate nothing more than a trivial variation in the chemical groups that interact with the toxin. But the recent work of Reuter and colleagues (Baer et al. (1976) and Reuter et al. (1978)) suggests a more profound difference between heart and other excitable tissues. Measuring $\dot{V}_{max}$ in guinea pig ventricular muscle, they reported that the binding of TTX was both voltage- and frequency-dependent: the reduction of $\dot{V}_{max}$ was enhanced by steady depolarization or by increasing the frequency of action potential stimulation. This is in contrast to nerve, where TTX appears to act as a simple plug in the outer mouth of the sodium channel, and where the effectiveness of toxin seems to be unaffected by steady depolarization (Ulbricht and Wagner, 1975) or by the frequency of stimulation (Courtney, 1974).

These results leave cardiac physiologists with a difficult choice. One possibility is that cardiac sodium channels are genuinely and significantly different from those in other tissues. If so, the many extrapolations that have been made from nerve to heart would need reexamination. On the other hand, it is also possible that $\dot{V}_{max}$ is a misleading indicator of how cardiac sodium channels really behave. If this is the case, we would be forced to reevaluate the large body of data that has been gathered using $\dot{V}_{max}$, including much work on the action of antiarrhythmic drugs. Finally, it is conceivable that both sources of information have serious limitations.

Although $\dot{V}_{max}$ has been used for many years as an index of the availability of sodium channels, its use as anything more than a qualitative indicator of sodium current has never had a firm theoretical basis. In nerve, mathematical reconstructions of action potentials using voltage-clamp data show that $\dot{V}_{max}$ is expected to be nonlinearly related to the available sodium conductance, g_{Na} (Frankenhaeuser and Huxley, 1964; Khodorov and Timin, 1975; Hunter et al., 1975; Cohen and Strichartz, 1977), and a nonlinear relationship has been demonstrated experimentally in nerve (Ulbricht and Wagner, 1975) and skeletal muscle (Colquhoun et al., 1974). A recent controversy about whether $\dot{V}_{max}$ ought to be linearly related to g_{Na} for cardiac action potentials (see Cohen and Strichartz, 1977; Hondeghem, 1978; Strichartz and Cohen, 1978; Walton and Fozzard, 1978) has led to the conclusion that too little is known about sodium currents in heart to settle the issue theoretically.

In light of the controversy about $\dot{V}_{max}$ and the interest in any unusual properties of cardiac sodium channels, it is particularly timely that recent advances have been made in methods for studying cardiac sodium currents under voltage clamp (Colatsky and Tsien, 1979b; Lee et al., 1979; Ebihara et al., 1980). In this article, we describe work that we have done using a two-microelectrode method for studying sodium currents in short pieces of rabbit Purkinje fiber; the favorable geometry and cable properties of this preparation (Colatsky and Tsien, 1979a) allow sodium currents to be measured under good voltage control (Colatsky and Tsien, 1979b; Colatsky, 1980). Our experiments show that cardiac sodium channels have unique pharmacological properties, as suggested by $\dot{V}_{max}$ experiments, but they also demonstrate that $\dot{V}_{max}$ measurements can be very misleading and that much of the data gathered with this technique may need to be reinterpreted.

RESULTS

Does TTX Block Show Steady-State Voltage Dependence?

Figure 1 shows the results of a voltage-clamp experiment designed to be similar to the $\dot{V}_{max}$ experiment by Baer et al. (1976) that originally suggested voltage-dependent binding of TTX. Baer et al. determined dose-response curves for the reduction of $\dot{V}_{max}$ by TTX at two membrane potentials: at a negative resting potential, the concentration required for half-maximal reduction of $\dot{V}_{max}$ was 14 μM, but when the membrane was depolarized by 18 mV, only 1.2 μM was needed. In Figure 1, dose-response curves for the block of I_{Na} by TTX were determined in the same preparation at two membrane potentials separated by 15 mV. The upper set of symbols shows the block of I_{Na} when I_{Na} was elicited by a depolarizing step to −44

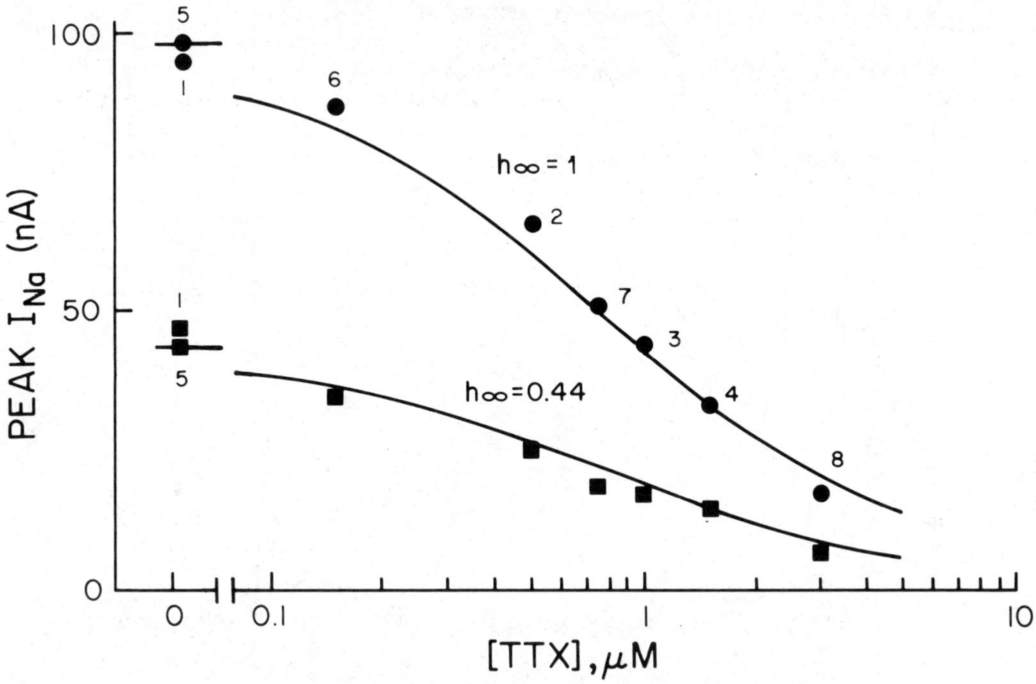

Figure 1. Concentration-dependence of TTX block at membrane potentials giving different degrees of sodium channel inactivation. I_{Na} was evoked by a test pulse to −44 mV following 45 sec at −104 mV (●) or −89 mV (■). Numbers indicate sequence of solutions. Upper curve is a least-squares fit, using the expression $I_{Na} = \hat{I}_{Na}/(1+[TTX]/K_D)$, where $\hat{I}_{Na}$ = 98.7 nA, K_D = 0.82 μM. Lower curve is the same expression, scaled by 0.44 to allow for I_{Na} inactivation. Preparation C44-1, 10 mM Na_o, 18° C. Reproduced from Cohen et al. (1981).

mV from a holding potential of −104 mV. The symbols are numbered to indicate the sequence of drug concentrations; the point labeled 5 was taken in the absence of TTX as a check against progressive run-down. The lower set of symbols show I_{Na} during the same sequence of bathing solutions, but with I_{Na} evoked from a less negative holding potential (−89 mV). In the absence of TTX, I_{Na} was smaller at −89 mV than it was at −105 mV because of inactivation of some of the sodium channels. The important aspect of Figure 1 is that both sets of points are fit by a 1:1 binding curve that corresponds to half-maximal inhibition by 0.82 μM TTX. In other words, the dissociation constant for the toxin-receptor complex, or K_D, is the same at both membrane potentials: block by TTX is not voltage-dependent. Thus, the voltage-clamp result is at odds with the earlier V_{max} experiments. The discrepancy led us to use the voltage-clamp technique to determine experimentally if the different results could be accounted for by V_{max} being an indirect, nonlinear measure of available g_{Na}. The term "available g_{Na}" refers to those sodium channels that are neither blocked by drug nor inactivated, but which are ready to open following membrane depolarization. In the terminology of Hodgkin and Huxley (1952b), this conductance could be written as $\bar{g}_{Na} \cdot h_o$, but in this paper we shall refer to "available g_{Na}" or simply "g_{Na}."

$\dot{V}_{max}$ as a Measure of g_{Na}

We directly examined the relationship between $\dot{V}_{max}$ and g_{Na} by using TTX to vary g_{Na}. If $\dot{V}_{max}$ were a linear measure of available g_{Na}, a reduction of g_{Na} (and I_{Na}) by a given concentration of TTX should result in the same reduction of $\dot{V}_{max}$. Figure 2 compares the effects of 3 μM TTX on $\dot{V}_{max}$ and I_{Na}. For the $\dot{V}_{max}$

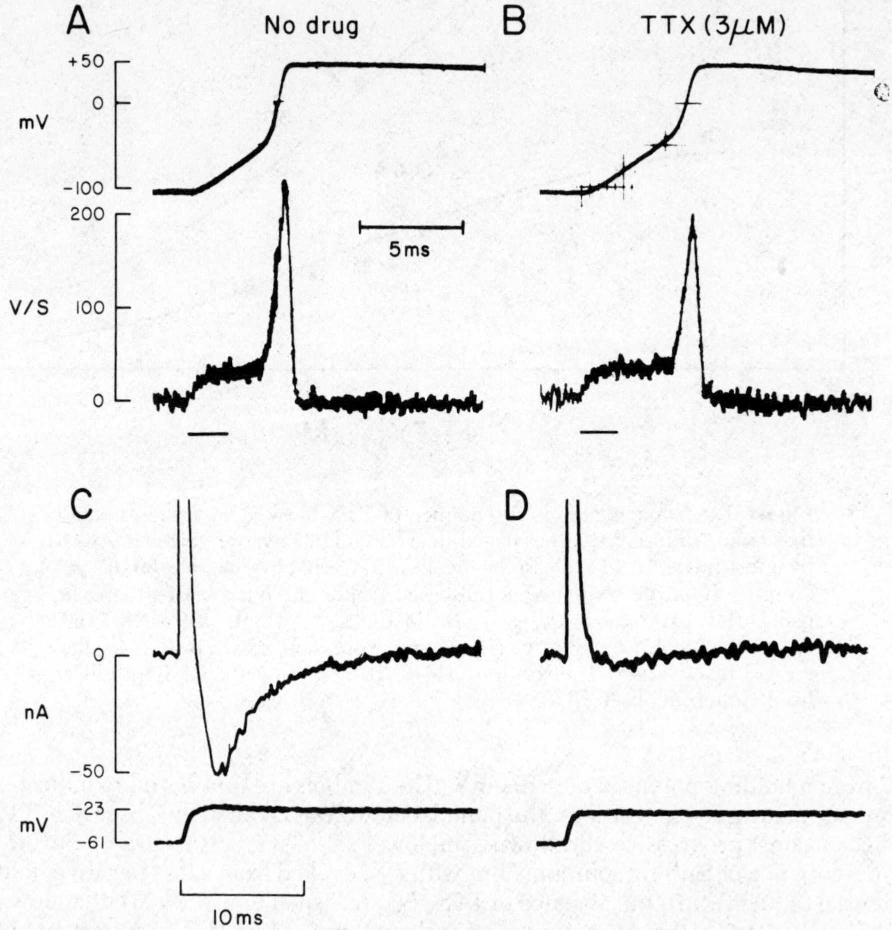

Figure 2. Comparison of TTX effects on $\dot{V}_{max}$ and I_{Na}. *Upper panels*: Membrane potential (V) and its first time derivative ($\dot{V}$). Action potential upstrokes were initiated by a pulse of depolarizing current (bar), applied intracellularly after the membrane potential had been clamped at −104 mV for more than 20 sec. Records were obtained before drug application (A) or after 6.5 min of exposure to 3 μM TTX (B). After washout of TTX, $\dot{V}_{max}$ recovered completely, and in this fiber actually attained a value 17% greater than that before toxin exposure. Preparation C64-1. *Lower panels*: Sodium currents obtained under voltage clamp before drug application (C) or after 3.5 min of exposure to 3 μM TTX (D). The membrane potential was held at −61 mV for 25 sec prior to a test pulse to −23 mV. Preparation C66-4. Both experiments were performed at 17.5° C in 155 mM Na, 1.8 mM Ca, and 3.6 mM Mn.

measurements shown in panels A and B of Figure 2, the preparation was held at a negative potential (−105 mV) under voltage-clamp, then released from voltage-clamp and stimulated with a brief pulse of depolarizing current. The resulting action potential (top trace) was differentiated electronically, and the upstroke velocity (dV/dt) was recorded on the same time scale (bottom trace). The peak value of dV/dt, or $\dot{V}_{max}$, was 231 V/sec in the control (Fig. 2A); 3 μM TTX (Fig. 2B) reduced $\dot{V}_{max}$ to 194 V/sec, or 84% of control. The lower panels of Fig. 2 illustrate the effect of 3 μM TTX on I_{Na}, in a different fiber. 3 μM TTX reduced I_{Na} to 13% of control, a much greater reduction than was seen with $\dot{V}_{max}$. In a total of five experiments of this type, 3 μM TTX reduced I_{Na} to 0.15 ± 0.02 (mean ± SEM) of control; in four upstroke-velocity experiments, 3 μM TTX reduced $\dot{V}_{max}$ to 0.67 ± 0.03 of control. Thus, $\dot{V}_{max}$ is much less sensitive to TTX than is I_{Na}, or, to put it another way, $\dot{V}_{max}$ is a very nonlinear measure of g_{Na}.

Figure 3 shows how $\dot{V}_{max}$ and g_{Na} responded to a wide range of TTX concentrations. Plotted are dose-response curves for the block of I_{Na} and $\dot{V}_{max}$, determined in two different fibers. Triangles show the reduction of $\dot{V}_{max}$ by various concentrations of TTX; the data points are fit by a dose-response curve corresponding to a $K_{0.5}$ *of* 8.4 μM. This value is not very different from the $K_{0.5}$ of 14 μM found by Baer et al. (1976) for action potentials elicited at 37° C from a negative holding potential in guinea pig ventricle. The filled circles in Figure 3 show the reduction of I_{Na} by

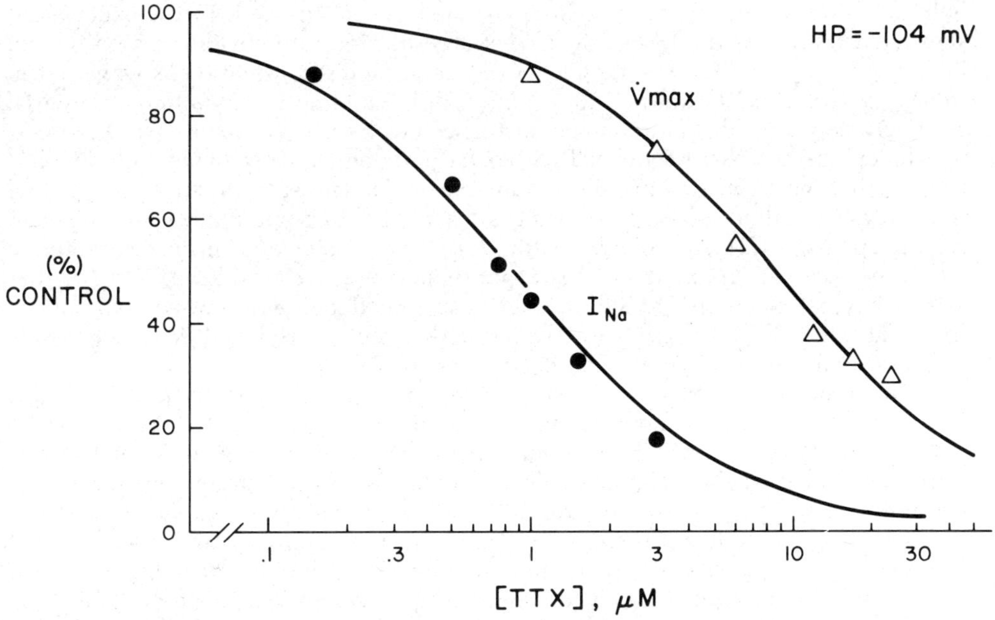

Figure 3. Concentration-dependence of TTX effect on $\dot{V}_{max}$ and I_{Na}. Filled circles are the sodium currents normalized to the current in the absence of drug. These are the same experimental points as shown in the upper curve of Figure 1, for which K_D = 0.82 μM. Open triangles are the relative values of $\dot{V}_{max}$ for the same preparation used in the upper half of Figure 2. The curve through these points is a least-squares fit to the equation (relative $\dot{V}_{max}$) = $(1+[TTX]/K_{0.5})^{-1}$, where $K_{0.5}$ = 8.4 μM. Both I_{Na} and $\dot{V}_{max}$ measurements were preceded by rest periods ⩾ 25 sec at −104 mV. I_{Na} measured in 10 mM Na, $\dot{V}_{max}$ measured in 155 mM Na.

TTX; the data points and the 1:1 binding curve (K_D = 0.82 μM) are the same as the upper set of symbols in Figure 1. The results show that the relative insensitivity of $\dot{V}_{max}$ holds for a broad range of toxin concentrations. For example, $\dot{V}_{max}$ was reduced to about 30% of control by 24 μM TTX, while only about 3% of the sodium channels were not blocked. An interesting feature of Figure 3 is how well the $\dot{V}_{max}$ data are fit by a 1:1 binding curve, despite the fact that the midpoint of the curve ($K_{0.5}$) is about ten times higher than the true K_D for the channel-toxin interaction. This feature of the $\dot{V}_{max}$ dose-response curve, which was also seen by Baer et al. (1976), illustrates that fits by 1:1 binding curves cannot always be interpreted in terms of a simple molecular interaction. But, fortuitous as it may be, the fact that the $\dot{V}_{max}$ curve is well-fit by this empirical 1:1 binding curve is convenient in using such dose-response curves to describe the dependence of $\dot{V}_{max}$ on g_{Na}.

In Figure 4, the results from Figure 3 are replotted as relative $\dot{V}_{max}$ versus relative g_{Na}. The solid curve may be contrasted with the 45° line that corresponds to the ideal of a linear dependence of $\dot{V}_{max}$ on g_{Na}. The curve (from Fig. 3) falls within error limits of the crossed symbol, which represents the collected results from several experiments using 3 μM TTX, already mentioned above.

This agreement is a reassuring check on the two methods we used to reduce I_{Na} to manageable size. It would be ideal to study I_{Na} under exactly the same conditions of high extracellular sodium (Na_o) and negative holding potential used in $\dot{V}_{max}$ experiments. This is not possible with our preparation; establishing good voltage control requires that I_{Na} be kept small, either with low Na_o or with depolarized holding potentials so that most sodium channels are inactivated. In the experiment shown in Figure 2, C and D (and the collected results indicated by the crossed symbol in Figure 4), 3 μM TTX was applied in the same high Na_o solution as was used in the $\dot{V}_{max}$ experiment, and I_{Na} was kept small by holding the membrane potential relatively depolarized. The rationale for this comes from experiments like Figure 1, which demonstrate that fractional TTX block is not detectably changed with depolarizations that inactivate most of the sodium channels. The smooth curve in Figure 4 represents the other approach, of using the same holding potential (−104 mV) and relying on Na_o as a means of attenuating I_{Na} for the voltage-clamp measurements. Here, the argument is based on other experiments that have established that Na_o has little, if any, influence on TTX affinity. The near coincidence of the crossed symbol and the solid curve is consistent with the view that neither reduced Na_o nor steady depolarization seriously alters the effectiveness of TTX.

The dashed curve in Figure 4 shows the empirical relationship between $\dot{V}_{max}$ and available g_{Na} in the node of Ranvier, as determined in TTX experiments by Ulbricht and Wagner (1975). Similar nonlinearity has been reported in skeletal muscle (Colquhoun et al., 1974; Pappone, 1980). Although theoretical arguments have been presented that $\dot{V}_{max}$ is a more faithful measure of available g_{Na} in heart (Hondeghem, 1978; Walton and Fozzard, 1979), our results show that, in rabbit Purkinje fibers at least, $\dot{V}_{max}$ can be an even more nonlinear index than it is in other tissues. Some consequences of the nonlinear relationship between $\dot{V}_{max}$ and available g_{Na} are: *(1)* the availability curve of $\dot{V}_{max}$ versus membrane potential will be shifted in the depolarizing direction relative to the true g_{Na} inactivation curve; *(2)* the time course of reactivation measured by $\dot{V}_{max}$ will be distorted and nonexponential, even if the underlying recovery of g_{Na} is exponential; and *(3)* drugs that have large effects on g_{Na} may reduce $\dot{V}_{max}$ only slightly. We think it is likely that a similar nonlinearity exists between $\dot{V}_{max}$ and g_{Na} in other cardiac preparations, although there is little doubt that the degree of nonlinearity may vary depending on factors such as channel kinetics, muscle geometry, and stimulation parameters.

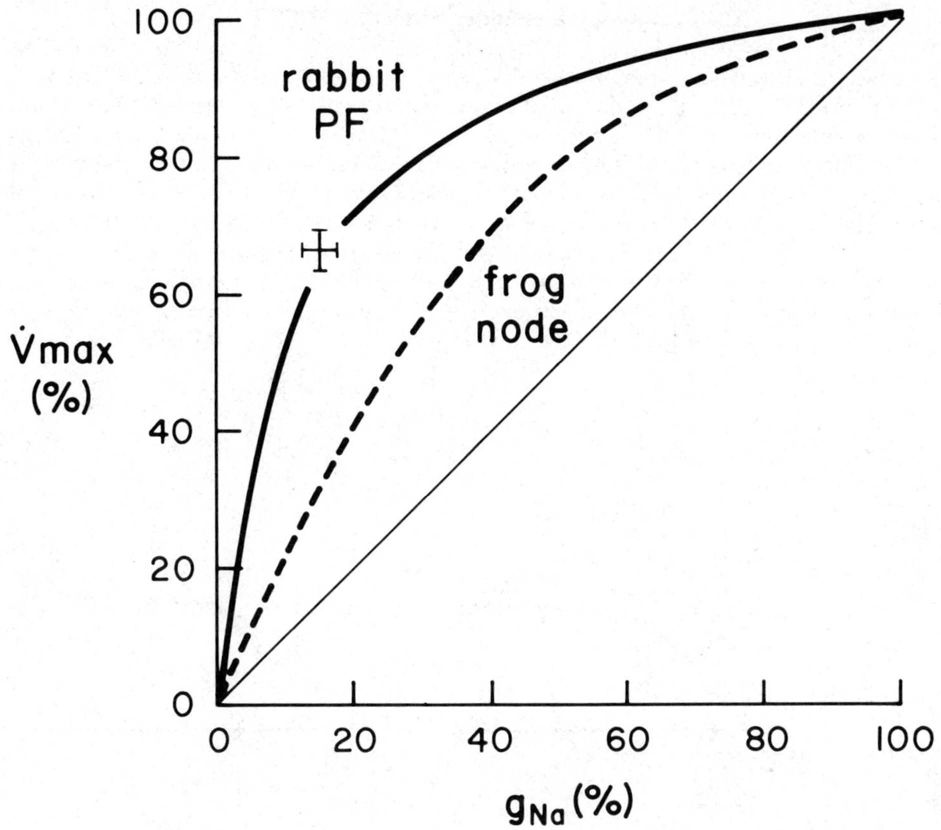

Figure 4. The relationship between normalized $\dot{V}_{max}$ and normalized g_{Na}. The straight line at 45° represents a linear relationship between $\dot{V}_{max}$ and g_{Na}. The solid curve is based on the dose-response relationships for TTX shown in Figure 3:

$$\dot{V}_{max}/\hat{\dot{V}}_{max} = [1 + [TTX]/10\ K_D]^{-1}$$
$$= [1 + (\hat{I}_{Na} - I_{Na})/10\ I_{Na}]^{-1} = 10g_{rel}/(1+9g_{rel})$$

where $g_{rel} \equiv (g_{Na}, \text{TTX})/(g_{Na}, \text{no TTX})$. For simplicity, the curve is drawn to correspond to an exactly tenfold difference in the concentrations required for 50% block of $\dot{V}_{max}$ and g_{Na}, almost identical to the ratio $K_{0.5}/K_K(=8.4/0.82=10.2)$ found between the least-squares fits to the dose-response curves in Figure 3. The crossed error bars represent collected results from a total of 5 experiments studying I_{Na} and 4 experiments measuring $\dot{V}_{max}$, all in 155 mM Na_o. The bars show ± 1 SEM. The dashed curve is the relationship between $\dot{V}_{max}/\hat{\dot{V}}_{max}$ and g_{rel} found in frog node of Ranvier by Ulbricht and Wagner (1975):

$$\dot{V}_{max}/\hat{\dot{V}}_{max} = [1+.267([TTX]/K_D)^{1.22}]^{-1}$$
$$= (1+.267[(1-g_{rel})/g_{rel}]^{1.22})^{-1}.$$

Frequency-Dependent Block by TTX

In addition to voltage-dependence, $\dot{V}_{max}$ experiments have suggested that TTX block of cardiac sodium channels can be modulated by the frequency of stimulation (Robinson and Sleator, 1977; Reuter et al., 1978; Mary-Rabine et al., 1979). In this case, we have confirmed the earlier result under voltage-clamp. Figure 5 shows an example of "use-dependent" or "frequency-dependent" block by TTX. Trains of 50-msec pulses to −40 mV were applied at 2.5 Hz after a long rest period at −91 mV. In the absence of drug, I_{Na} changed very little from pulse to pulse (Fig. 5C); the first and tenth sodium currents in the train were almost exactly the same (Fig. 5A). In the presence of 2 μM TTX, the same pattern of depolarizations resulted in a prominent decline in I_{Na} from one pulse to the next (panels B, C). After 10 to 15 pulses, the

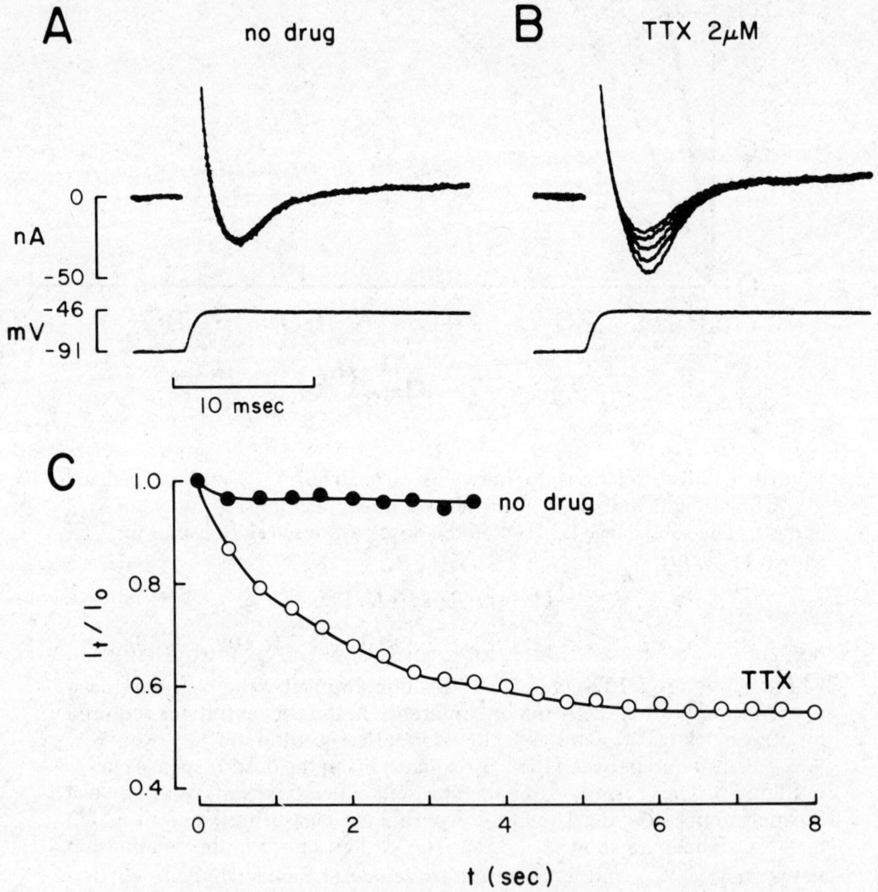

Figure 5. Use-dependent effect of TTX. Membrane currents during trains of 50-msec pulses from −91 to −46 mV at 2.5 Hz following a rest period of 11 sec. A, records taken with no TTX, 20 mM Na, during pulses 1 and 10 of the train. B, records in 2 μM TTX, 35 mM Na, during pulses 1, 2, 4, 8, and 16. C, sodium current amplitudes from the same runs, plotted as a fraction of the first I_{Na} of each train. Preparation T92-1, 18° C. Reproduced from Cohen et al. (1981).

decline leveled off with I_{Na} at 0.55 of its amplitude during the first pulse following the rest period. It is important to add that the use-dependent block seen with TTX was in addition to a substantial tonic block seen with very infrequent pulses (see Fig. 1). This tonic block is masked in Fig. 5 because the external sodium concentration was raised in the TTX solution to maintain I_{Na} at a size that could be conveniently measured.

Why is frequency-dependent block seen in the presence of TTX but not in the absence of drug? In the absence of drug, the interpretation is as follows: before the first pulse in the train, channels are mostly in a resting state, available to be activated by a depolarizing pulse. During the first depolarizing pulse of 50 msec, channels open transiently, for the first 10 msec or so, and then become inactivated. On repolarization of the membrane during the interval between the first and second pulses, the channels return from the inactivated state to the resting state and once more become available for activation by a depolarization. In the absence of toxin, reactivation proceeds with a time constant of about 100 msec and thus is nearly complete during the 350-msec recovery interval between pulses. Consequently, I_{Na} during the second pulse is only very slightly decreased relative to that during the first pulse, and so on for subsequent pulses. This interpretation suggests that when TTX is present, the progressive decline in I_{Na} must be caused by incomplete reactivation of channels during the recovery intervals, as if 350 msec is not long enough for complete reactivation when TTX is present. Thus, TTX must slow the time course of channel reactivation.

Figure 6 looks directly at how TTX affects the time course of sodium channel reactivation. Channels were inactivated by a 5-sec conditioning pulse to −34 mV, and then the membrane potential was returned to −83 mV for a variable length of time, following which a pulse to −34 mV was given to assay the amount of reactivation that had occurred during the recovery period. In each run, with or without drug, the test pulse currents were normalized with respect to a test pulse following a long rest at −83 mV, to emphasize the rates of reactivation rather than tonic block by the drug. In the absence of toxin, reactivation was fairly rapid and occurred nearly exponentially ($\tau \cong 140$ msec). TTX affected the recovery in a dose-dependent manner. In 1 μM TTX, about 60% of the sodium current reprimed with the same exponential time course as it did in the absence of drug, but the recovery of the remaining 40% barely began within a period of 1 sec. When the TTX concentration was increased to 10 μM, the slowly recovering component of current increased to about 80%. Figure 6B plots the data in 6A and additional points from the same experiment to show the complete time course of recovery. In both 1 μM and 10 μM TTX, the slow recovery phase shows a similar exponential time course, $\tau = 4.4$ sec. Thus, TTX slows the rate of recovery not by simply lengthening the time constant for reactivation, but by introducing a new slowly reactivating fraction of channels, in addition to the remaining fraction of channels that reactivate normally. After a long depolarizing conditioning pulse, as in Figure 6, sodium channels appear to be in two groups: channels that are in the normal inactivated state, which reactivate normally, and channels in a condition we call "extra block," which reactivate very slowly. From a variety of experiments aimed at understanding how channels enter and recover from the condition of extra block, we have concluded that this condition represents channels that are both inactivated *and* toxin-bound, and that the slow recovery of these channels occurs because they must first unbind toxin before they can reactivate (Cohen, et al., 1981).

The slowly reactivating state induced by TTX, and the associated phenomenon of frequency-dependent block, are features of TTX action that are unique to cardiac sodium channels. As mentioned previously, TTX block in nerve is not modulated by frequency. But, the effect of tertiary amine local anesthetics on $\dot{V}_{max}$ or I_{Na} is modulated by frequency, and the basis of this effect is also thought to be the formation of a slowly reactivating pool of channels that are in a drug-bound, inactivated state

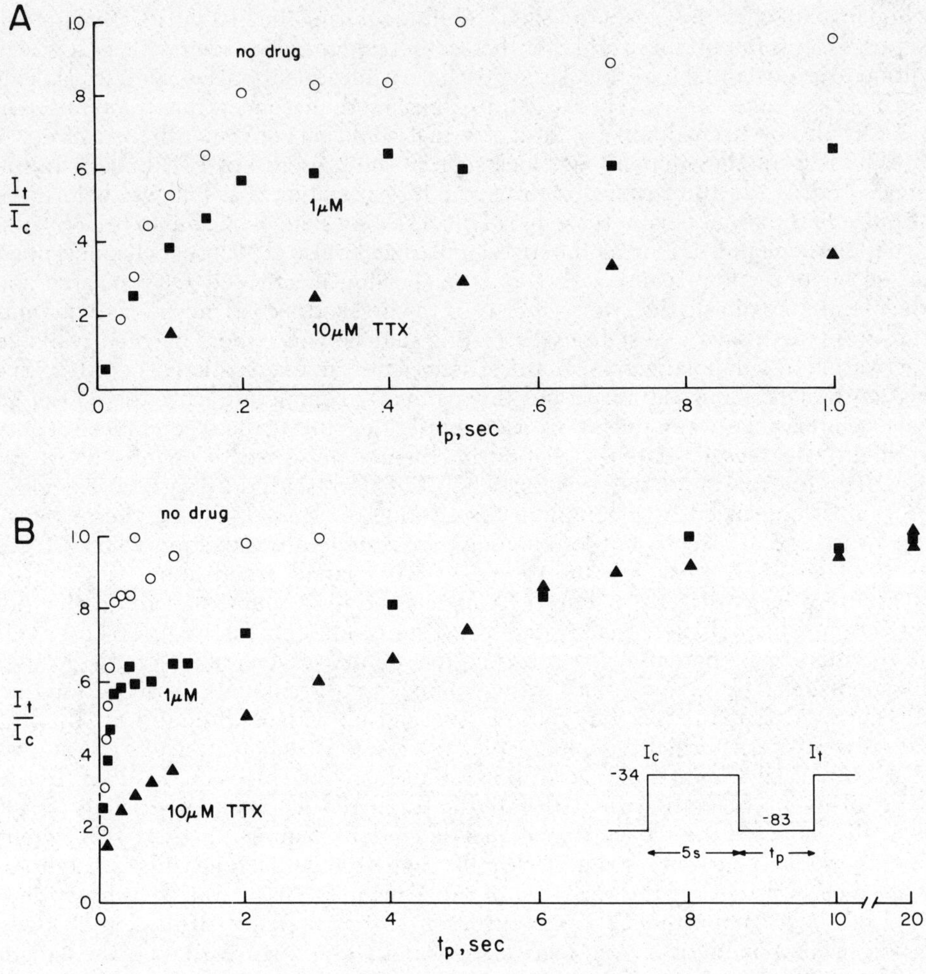

Figure 6. Effect of TTX on I_{Na} repriming as studied by a two-pulse procedure. Results plotted on expanded (A) and slow (B) time bases. Sodium currents were evoked by a test pulse at a varying interval (t_p) following a 5-sec conditioning pulse. Sodium current during the test depolarization (I_t) was normalized by I_{Na} during the immediately preceding conditioning pulse (I_c). Records taken during consecutive runs at 0 TTX, 10 mM Na_o (0), 1 μM TTX, 10 mM Na_o (■), and 10 μM TTX, 80 mM Na_o (▲). Preparation C43-1, 18° C. Reproduced from Cohen et al. (1981).

(Hille, 1977; Hondeghem and Katzung, 1977). However, TTX binding in cardiac muscle is different in an important way from the models that have been given for local anesthetic binding. A key aspect of these models is the hypothesis that the drug binds much more strongly to the inactivated state than it does to the resting state. This gives rise to a voltage-dependence for drug binding. When the membrane potential is changed, the distribution of channels between the resting state and the inactivated state is changed; at very negative potentials, most channels are in the resting state, and binding of drug will occur according to the K_D for resting channels; at less negative potentials, many channels are in the inactivated state, and the effective K_D for drug binding will be much lower, because it reflects binding of toxin to inactivated as well as resting channels. In Figure 1, where TTX was applied at two membrane potentials, depolarizing the membrane to −89 mV in the absence of TTX caused about half the current to be inactivated, but the K_D for toxin binding was unaffected. Thus, the lack of voltage-dependent block in Figure 1 shows that the binding of toxin to an inactivated channel is governed by the same K_D as for binding to a resting channel, unlike what is believed for local anesthetics. TTX block of these sodium channels is an intermediate case between TTX block in nerve (neither use-dependent nor voltage-dependent) and local anesthetic block in nerve (both use-dependent and voltage-dependent).

Figure 7 shows a simple kinetic interpretation of how TTX binding can give rise to use-dependent block. In this scheme, sodium channels in the absence of toxin are considered to be either in a resting state (*R*) or an inactivated state (*I*), and they undergo transitions between these states according to voltage-dependent Hodgkin-Huxley parameters, α_h and β_h, so that at negative potentials most channels are in *R* and at depolarized potentials most channels are in *I*. For large enough depolarizations, channels will transiently open on the way from *R* to *I*; opening of the channels serves as a measure of the fraction of channels available in the *R* state, but for simplicity the open state is not explicitly included in the scheme. Both *R* and *I* can bind TTX, and they have the same equilibrium dissociation constant, K_D (where $T/K_D = k/\ell$), consistent with Figure 1. However, the individual rate constants for binding and unbinding of toxin are ω times faster for *R* than they are for *I*, so that the approach to equilibrium is much faster for *R*. The toxin-blocked states *RT* and *IT* are connected by rate constants similar in voltage-dependence to α_h and β_h but scaled ν-fold. The factor ν must be less than one to account for the slow repriming of channels in the toxin-bound, inactivated state *IT*. In practice, we think that ν is near zero, so that channels in *IT* must first unbind toxin to form *I* before repriming.

The lower panels of Figure 7 give a specific example of how the kinetic scheme accounts for use-dependent block. For numerical simplicity, we consider a limiting case where $\nu = 0$ and $\omega \gg 1$. Also, the analysis is restricted to a sequence of two depolarizations, which might be thought of as the first two pulses in a train. The analysis is performed for a concentration of toxin equal to 9 times the K_D value. Fig. 7A shows the equilibrium distribution of channels at a negative holding potential where inactivation is completely removed: 0.1 of the channels are in *R* and 0.9 are in *RT*. Figure 7B shows the distribution following a long depolarization to a potential where inactivation is complete: channels reach equilibrium with 0.1 in *I* and 0.9 in *IT*. There is no *net* binding or unbinding of toxin by the end of the depolarization, because 0.9 of the channels are toxin bound at A or B, but channels originally in *RT* must sequentially unbind and then rebind toxin to reach *IT*. Figure 7C illustrates the effect of following the depolarization with a repolarization of, say, 1 sec. This is long enough for toxin-free channels to completely recover from inactivation, and it is long enough for the *R* to *RT* transition to nearly reach equilibrium, but the *IT* to *I* transition, which is much slower, barely begins. Thus, channels that are in *I* at the beginning of the repolarization distribute to equilibrium between *R* and *RT*, whereas channels in *IT* remain there. At the end of the 1-sec repolarization, then, there will be 0.01 channels in *R*, 0.09 channels in *RT*, and 0.9 in *IT*. The current during a second pulse will be proportional to the 0.01 fraction of channels in *R*, a reduction by a factor of 10 from the current during the first pulse, which was proportional to the 0.1 fraction originally in *R*.

In the example shown in Figure 7, with a concentration of toxin equal to 9 times the K_D, I_{Na} is reduced to 0.1 of control even with infrequent pulses from a negative holding potential. The formation of the slowly reactivating state *IT* could lead to a

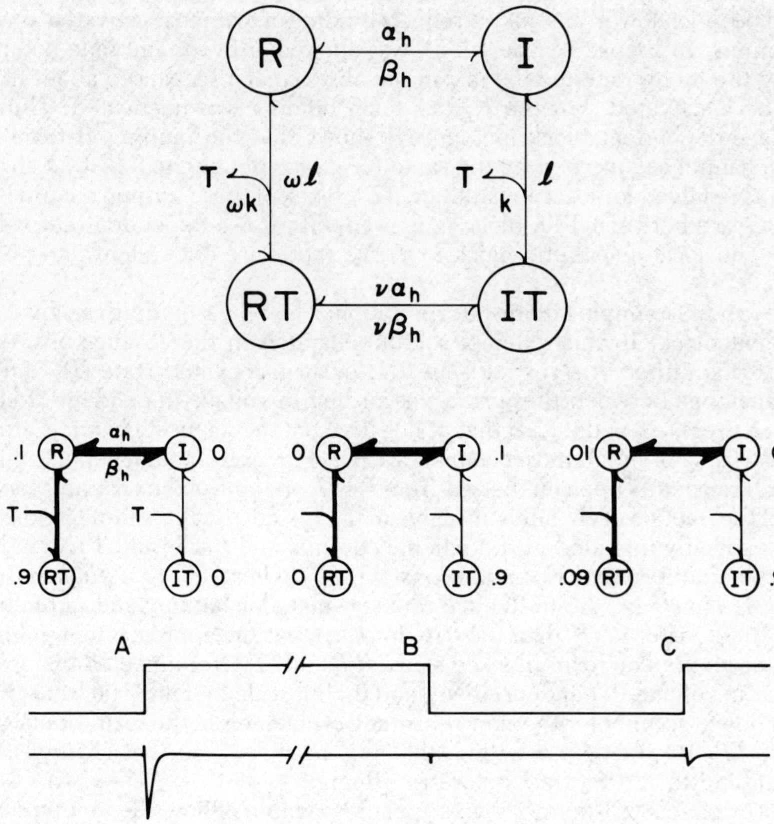

Figure 7. A simple scheme for interpreting kinetic aspects of TTX block. Extra block is accounted for as a long-lasting perturbation away from the equilibrium distribution among channel states. In upper panel, κ and ℓ are forward and backward rate coefficients in units of sec^{-1}, and ω and ν are dimensionless coefficients that determine the relative speed of reactions. The model assumes that toxin binding and inactivation are independent at equilibrium because no such interaction could be detected experimentally (compare with Reuter et al. 1978, p. 138, and Hille, 1978, Fig. 11). In the lower panels (A–C), the relative speed of reactions is indicated schematically by the thickness of the arrows. For further details, see text. Reproduced from Cohen et al. (1981).

further reduction by a factor of ten during subsequent pulses. Because Figure 7 treats a limiting case, the extra reduction by a factor of ten is the maximum extra reduction that can be obtained with any pattern or train of pulses with this concentration of TTX. It is a fundamental feature of kinetic models like that in Figure 7, where the equilibrium binding of drug is the same for both resting and inactivated states, that the degree of extra use-dependent block cannot exceed the degree of tonic block seen with infrequent pulses. In the next section, this property of TTX use-dependence will be contrasted with the use-dependent that is produced by lidocaine.

What does a scheme like that in Figure 7 imply about the molecular interaction between TTX and the sodium channel? Gating of the channel between the resting and inactivated states does not affect the equilibrium binding of the TTX molecule, but it does change the rate constants for the interaction: in effect, the channel-TTX interaction is catalyzed when the channel is in the resting state. A possible interpretation is that the configuration of the TTX receptor is the same in both states of the channel, but that TTX molecules have more ready access to the receptor when the channels are in the resting state. From another perspective, binding of TTX to the receptor greatly modifies the gating properties of the channel, because the slow repriming of IT requires that the transition between RT and IT be slowed relative to that between R and I. Thus, TTX alters the rate of channel gating, and channel gating alters the rate of TTX binding and unbinding. Mutual interactions between channel gating and drug binding have been described, in a variety of specific forms, for a number of molecules that bind to ionic channels (see Hille, 1977; 1978). This property suggests that the action of many drugs will not be understood on the molecular level until the gating of the target channels is understood in molecular terms.

The scheme in Figure 7 captures the main features of TTX block and, in particular, shows how there can be use-dependent block without voltage-dependence of steady-state TTX binding. However, the scheme is deliberately oversimplified for the purpose of clarity. Experiments aimed at understanding, in detail, the kinetics of TTX binding and unbinding have led us to believe that there are actually two distinct inactivated states of the channel, and that only one of these reactivates slowly when it is toxin-bound. Also, the lower panels of Figure 7 imply that the formation of the slowly reactivating state IT takes place only by the binding of toxin to the inactivated state I. Experiments show, however, that for pulses that are large enough to elicit I_{Na} there are two separate phases in the formation of IT, a fast phase that parallels channel activation, and then a slower phase that appears to correspond to the binding of toxin by inactivated channels. A more complete kinetic hypothesis, which explicitly includes the open state and two inactivated states, has been presented elsewhere (Cohen et al., 1981).

Is Lidocaine Block Voltage- or Use-Dependent?

We have already referred to actions of tertiary amine local anesthetics on sodium channels. Such antiarrhythmic drugs reduce $\dot{V}_{max}$ of the cardiac action potential, and the degree of reduction can be modulated by the resting membrane potential (Weidmann, 1955b) and by the frequency of stimulation (Johnson and McKinnon, 1957; Heistracher, 1971). In nerve and skeletal muscle, interactions between local anesthetics like lidocaine and sodium channels have been investigated in considerable detail (see Hille, 1977, 1978; Schwarz et al., 1977). Because block of these channels is modulated by frequency and membrane potential in a manner that is qualitatively similar to $\dot{V}_{max}$ measurements in cardiac preparations, it has been attractive to think that the receptor for local anesthetic molecules in heart is the same as it is in nerve and skeletal muscle.

Our studies with TTX indicate that this viewpoint must be reevaluated with voltage-clamp measurements. We have begun to study the effect of lidocaine on I_{Na} to reexamine the following points: *(1)* Is the binding of lidocaine to cardiac sodium channels truly voltage-dependent? Availability curves determined with $\dot{V}_{max}$ are shifted in the hyperpolarizing direction by the drug (for examples, see Chen et al., 1975; Weld and Bigger, 1975) but as the TTX results indicate, $\dot{V}_{max}$ measurements can be misleading on this point. *(2)* Do clinical doses of lidocaine have little effect on cardiac sodium channels at slow stimulation rates, as $\dot{V}_{max}$ measurements suggest, or is the effect of lidocaine on g_{Na} simply underestimated because $\dot{V}_{max}$ is an insensitive index? *(3)* Why does cardiac tissue respond to lower concentrations of lidocaine than nerve or skeletal muscle do? Does this reflect a fundamental difference in the sodium channel structure of these tissues, as was found for the TTX receptor? Some of these questions have also been addressed by Brown and his coworkers (see chapter 10), who used single dialyzed cells obtained from rat ventricle. There are similarities between our results and theirs, but there are also important differences.

Figure 8 shows the effect of lidocaine on sodium currents in a rabbit Purkinje fiber under two conditions: after a long resting period at a negative potential (−105 mV), and then during a train of stimulating voltage clamp pulses. The three panels in Figure 8A show, superimposed, I_{Na} during the first and the twelfth voltage clamp pulses in a train of 500-msec pulses given at 1 Hz. In the absence of drug (left panel), the first and twelfth currents were just about the same size. With 20 μM lidocaine present (middle panel), the first pulse in the train elicited a current that was almost unchanged from the control. Subsequent currents during the train became, however,

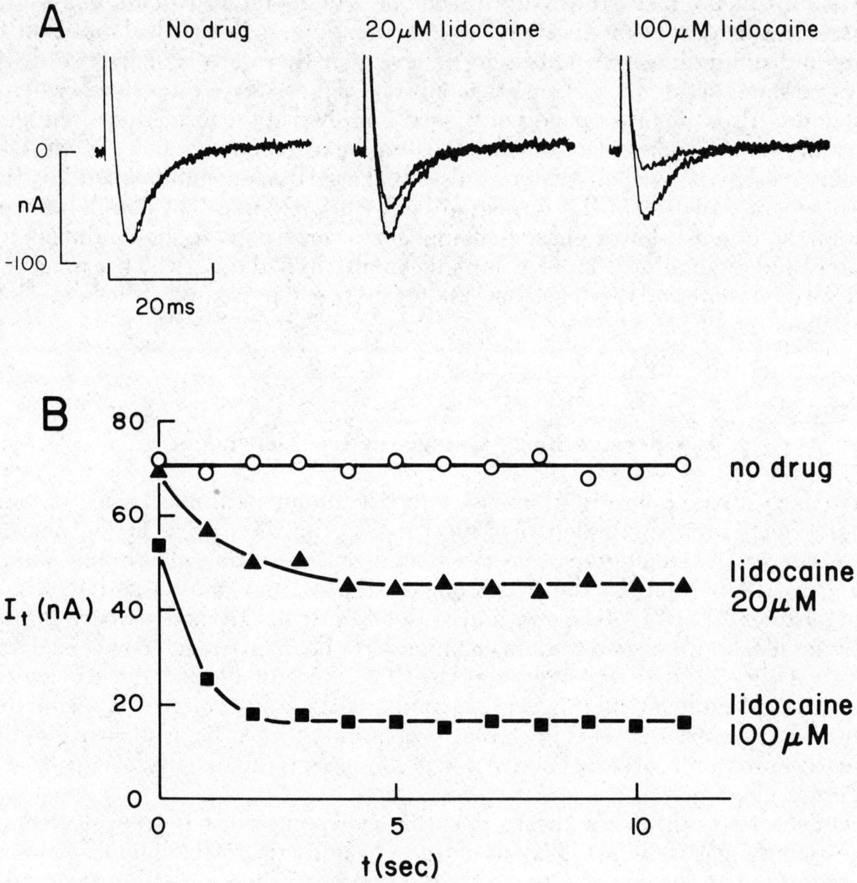

Figure 8. Use-dependent effect of lidocaine. I_{Na} measured during trains of 500-msec pulses from −105 to −35 mV at 1.0 Hz. A: the membrane currents measured on the 1st and 12th pulses in (from left to right) 0, 20, and 100 μM lidocaine. The rest period before each train was long enough for effects of previous trains to be removed. B: peak sodium current amplitudes measured for each of the pulses. The decrease in current magnitude has been fitted by an exponential curve, with τ = 1.3 sec in 20 μM lidocaine and τ = 0.7 sec in 100 μM lidocaine. Preparation C74-3. 10 mM Na, pH 7.0, 17° C.

progressively smaller and by the twelfth pulse, I_{Na} was reduced to 63% of its size with no drug present. In 100 μM lidocaine (right panel), the first pulse elicited a current reduced to 75% of control, and the current during the twelfth pulse was down to 22%. Figure 8B shows the time course of the use-dependent effect during the trains of pulses. With the 500-msec pulses, the development of the use-dependent block during a train was quite rapid in both concentrations of lidocaine and was faster in 100 μM lidocaine ($\tau = 0.7$ sec) than it was in 20 μM lidocaine ($\tau = 1.3$ sec).

The most interesting aspect of Figure 8 is that 20 μM lidocaine, at the high end of the spectrum of clinical concentrations, had almost no effect on I_{Na} during the first depolarization following a rest period, whereas it markedly reduced I_{Na} during stimulation at a moderate frequency. Moreover, the reduction of I_{Na} was apparent even during the second pulse of the train (Figure 8B). Our results with lidocaine are different from those of Lee et al. (1980), who found very little use-dependence in single rat ventricular cells.

It is interesting to compare the use-dependent block seen with lidocaine with that induced by TTX. The most dramatic difference is that lidocaine can induce substantial use-dependence with almost no tonic or resting block, whereas with TTX, use-dependent block is always accompanied by resting block. This difference is related to another difference between the drugs, which is that although TTX binding is not voltage-dependent, lidocaine binding is extremely voltage-dependent. Performing experiments like that in Figure 1 with lidocaine has shown that the apparent K_D for block of I_{Na} by lidocaine is much smaller at more depolarized membrane potentials, where more channels are in the inactivated state. Preliminary analysis suggests that the K_D for binding to the resting state is about 500 μM but that the K_D for binding to the inactivated state is only about 10 μM (Bean et al., 1981).

Figure 9 shows a simple kinetic scheme for lidocaine binding to the sodium channel that is useful for interpreting use-dependent block. Like Figure 7, it considers four states of sodium channel: the resting (*R*) and inactivated (*I*) states, and the corresponding lidocaine-bound states. Unlike Figure 7, however, Figure 9 postulates that drug binds much more strongly to an inactivated channel than to a resting channel, just as in the models for local anesthetic action given by Hille (1977) and Hondeghem and Katzung (1977). As in their models, and as in Figure 7, the drug-bound, inactivated state *IL* is a slowly-reactivating state, the state that underlies the use-dependent phenomena. Because this state reactivates slowly, the *IL* to *RL* transition could be much slower than the *R* to *I* transition; for simplicity, it is made zero in Figure 9. The lower panels of Figure 9 show a simulation of block by ~ 10 μM lidocaine. At rest at a negative potential, channels are in the *R* state; very few resting channels are toxin-bound because the effective K_D for binding of drug to *R* is about 500 μM. For simplicity, Figure 9A shows no binding with 10 μM lidocaine. During a long depolarization, that completely inactivates the channels (Figure 9B), channels end in an equilibrium between *I* and *IL*, which is governed by the K_D for binding to the inactivated state. With the K_D of 10 μM postulated in Figure 9, this results in 0.5 of the channels being in *I* and 0.5 in *IL*. Figure 9C shows the effect of following the long depolarization by repolarization of a duration that is long compared with normal reactivation of the *I* channels ($\tau \sim 100$ msec) and short compared with unbinding of drug and reactivation of the *IL* channels ($\tau \sim 2$ sec), so that, to a first approximation, the channels in *I* return to *R*, whereas the channels in *IL* do not reactivate at all. If a second depolarization is given at this time, I_{Na} will be reduced to one-half of its value after a long resting period. Thus, the difference in the binding affinity between the *R* and *I* states leads to substantial use-dependent block in the absence of significant tonic block, in agreement with the experimental result in Figure 8 and in contrast to the result obtained with TTX.

Figure 9 is deliberately over-simplified for clarity. It ignores the very important issue of differences in the binding characteristics of the protonated and unprotonated forms of lidocaine (see Schwarz et al. [1977]). Also, although Figure 9 shows no transition between the *IL* and *RL* states, this is still an open question experimentally.

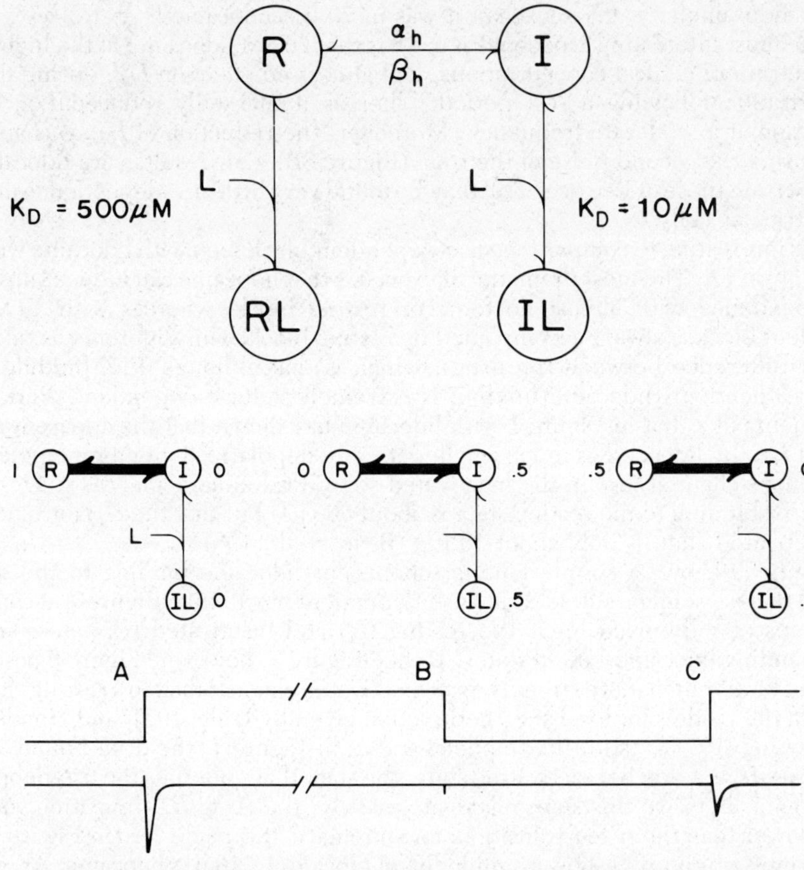

Figure 9. A model to account for frequency-dependent block with lidocaine. The additional block seen with increased rates of stimulation corresponds to accumulation of channels in state *IL*. Note that this model differs from that in Figure 7, in that the dissociation constants for *IL* and *RL* are unequal. The notation of this figure follows that of Figure 7. For further details, see text.

Figure 9 is a limiting case of the "modulated receptor" model given by Hille (1977; 1978) and Hondeghem and Katzung (1977) for local anesthetic action in nerve. So far, the picture that is emerging from lidocaine binding to rabbit Purkinje fiber sodium channels is strikingly similar to the particular modulated receptor model used by Schwarz et al. (1977) to describe lidocaine binding to sodium channels in frog skeletal muscle. This may seem surprising because it is well known that concentrations of lidocaine that are clinically useful in heart are much lower than are those used for local anesthesia in nerve. But, cardiac muscle differs from nerve in having a relatively long action potential; because sodium channels are inactivated during the plateau, the strong interaction of the drug with inactivated channels is heavily weighted.

CONCLUSION

Our voltage-clamp results show that rabbit Purkinje fibers respond to TTX in a way that is dramatically different from nerve and skeletal muscle, suggesting that cardiac sodium channels are different from those in other excitable membranes. In addition, because the rate of interaction of TTX with Purkinje fiber sodium channels depends on whether the channels are resting or inactivated, the difference in TTX action on the various membranes may be related to fundamental properties of channel gating. It is intriguing to speculate that the difference between cardiac and other sodium channels may extend to other kinetic and pharmacological properties of the channels. The action of low doses of lidocaine on cardiac sodium channels is, however, much the same as it is in skeletal muscle and nerve.

Probably the most unsettling aspect of our work is the demonstration that $\dot{V}_{max}$ is a highly nonlinear measure of available g_{Na}, even more nonlinear than it is in nerve. The nonlinearity can lead to $\dot{V}_{max}$ results that are qualitatively as well as quantitatively misleading, as illustrated by the issue of whether TTX binding to cardiac sodium channels is voltage-dependent. In the future, voltage-clamp experiments will be necessary to answer detailed questions about sodium-channel function and pharmacology, but $\dot{V}_{max}$ measurements will continue to be useful for pilot experiments in preparations that cannot be voltage-clamped.

REFERENCES

Baer M, Best PM, Reuter H (1976) Voltage-dependent action of tetrodotoxin in mammalian cardiac muscle. Nature **263**:344–345

Bean BP, Cohen CJ, Tsien RW (1981) Lidocaine binding to resting and inactivated cardiac sodium channels. Biophys J **33**:208a

Carmeliet E, Vereecke J (1969) Adrenaline and the plateau phase of the cardiac action potential. Pflüg Arch **313**:300–315

Chen C-M, Gettes LS, Katzung BG (1975) Effect of lidocaine and quinidine on steady-state characteristics and recovery kinetics of $(dV/dt)_{max}$ in guinea pig ventricular myocardium. Circ Res **37**:320–329

Cohen CJ, Bean BP, Colatsky TJ, Tsien RW (1981) Tetrodotoxin block of sodium channels in rabbit Purkinje fibers: Interactions between toxin binding and channel gating. J Gen Physiol **78**:383–411

Cohen IS, Strichartz GR (1977) On the voltage-dependent action of tetrodotoxin. Biophys J **17**:275–279

Colatsky TJ (1980) Voltage clamp measurements of sodium channel properties in rabbit cardiac Purkinje fibres. J Physiol **305**:215–234

Colatsky TJ, Tsien RW (1979a) Electrical properties associated with wide intercellular clefts in rabbit Purkinje fibers. J Physiol **290**:227–252

Colatsky TJ, Tsien RW (1979b) Sodium channels in rabbit Purkinje fibers. Nature **278**:265–268

Colquhoun D, Rang HP, Ritchie JM (1974) The binding of tetrodotoxin and α-bungarotoxin to normal and denervated mammalian muscle. J Physiol **204**:199–226

Coraboeuf E, Deroubaix E, Coulombe A (1979) Effect of tetrodotoxin on action potentials of the conducting system in the dog heart. Am J Physiol **237**:H561–H567

Courtney K (1974) Frequency-dependent inhibition of sodium currents in frog myelinated nerve by GEA 968, a new lidocaine derivative. Doctoral dissertation, Univ. of Washington, Seattle, Wash. University Microfilms, Ann Arbor, No. 74-29,343

Dudel J, Peper K, Rudel R, Trautwein W (1967) The effect of tetrodotoxin on the membrane current in cardiac muscle (Purkinje fibers). Pflüg Arch **295**:213–226

Ebihara L, Shigeto N, Lieberman M, Johnson EA (1980) The initial inward current in spherical clusters of chick embryonic heart cells. J Gen Physiol **75**:437–456

Frankenhaeuser B, Hodgkin AL (1957) The action of calcium on the electrical properties of squid axons. J Physiol **137**:218–244

Frankenhaeuser B, Huxley AF (1964) The action potential in the myelinated nerve fiber of *Xenopus laevis* as computed on the basis of voltage clamp data. J Physiol **171**:302–315

Heistracher P (1971) Mechanism of action of antifibrillatory drugs. Naunyn Schmiedebergs Arch Pharmacol **269**:199–212

Hille B (1977) Local anesthetics: hydrophilic and hydrophobic pathways for the drug:receptor reaction. J Gen Physiol **69**:497–515

Hille B (1978) Local anesthetic action on inactivation of the Na channel in nerve and skeletal muscle: Possible mechanisms for antiarrhythmic agents. *In* Biophysical Aspects of Cardiac Muscle, edited by M. Morad, New York, Academic Press, pp 55–74

Hodgkin AL, Huxley AF (1952a) Currents carried by sodium and potassium ions through the membrane of the giant axon of *Loligo*. J Physiol **116**:449–472

Hodgkin AL, Huxley AF (1952b) The dual effect of membrane potential on sodium conductance in the giant axon of *Loligo*. J Physiol **116**:497–506

Hondeghem LM (1978) Validity of $\dot{V}_{max}$ as a measure of the sodium current in cardiac and nervous tissues. Biophys J **23**:147–152

Hondeghem LM, Katzung BG (1977) Time- and voltage-dependent interactions of anti-arrhythmic drugs with cardiac sodium channels. Biochim Biophys Acta **472**:373–398

Hunter PJ, McNaughton PA, Noble D (1975) Analytical models of propagation in excitable cells. Prog Biophys Mol Biol **30**:99–144

Johnson EA, McKinnon MG (1957) The differential effect of quinidine and pyrilamine on the myocardial action potential at various rates of stimulation. J Pharmacol Exp Ther **120**:460–468

Khodorov BI, Timin EN (1975) Nerve impulse propagation along non-uniform fibres. Prog Biophys Molec Biol **30**:145–184

Lee KS, Hume JR, Giles W, Brown AM (1981) Sodium current depression by lidocaine and quinidine in isolated ventricular cells. Nature **291**:325–327

Lee KS, Weeks TA, Kao RL, Akaike N, Brown AM (1979) Sodium current in single heart muscle cells. Nature **278**:269–271

Mary-Rabine L, Hoffman BF, Rosen MR (1979) Participation of slow inward current in the Purkinje fiber action potential overshoot. Am J Physiol **237**:H204–H212

Pappone PA (1980) Voltage-clamp experiments in normal and denervated mammalian skeletal muscle fibres. J Physiol **306**:337–410

Reuter H, Baer M, Best PM (1978) Voltage dependence of TTX action in mammalian cardiac muscle. *In* Biophysical Aspects of Cardiac Muscle, edited by M Morad, New York, Academic Press, pp 129–142

Robinson RB, Sleator WW (1977) Tetrodotoxin effects in mammalian cardiac muscle: Frequency and calcium dependence. Proc Int Union Physiol Sci XIII: 632

Schwarz W, Palade PT, Hille B (1977) Local anesthetics: Effect of pH on use-dependent block of sodium channels in frog muscle. Biophys J **20**:343–368

Strichartz G, Cohen I (1978) $\dot{V}_{max}$ as a measure of $\bar{g}_{Na}$ in nerve and cardiac membranes. Biophys J **23**:153–156

Ulbricht W, Wagner H-W (1975) The influence of pH on equilibrium effects of tetrodotoxin on myelinated nerve fibres of *Rana esculenta*. J Physiol (Lond) **252**:159–184

Walton M, Fozzard HA (1979) The relation of $\dot{V}_{max}$ to I_{Na}, $\bar{g}_{Na}$, and h_∞ in a model of the cardiac Purkinje fiber. Biophys J **25**:407–420

Weidmann S (1955a) The effect of the cardiac membrane potential on the rapid availability of the sodium carrying system. J Physiol **127**:213–224

Weidmann S (1955b) The effects of calcium ions and local anesthetics on electrical properties of Purkinje fibres. J Physiol **129**:568–582

Weld FM, Bigger JT Jr (1975) Effect of lidocaine on the early inward transient current in sheep Purkinje fibers. Circ Res **37**:630–639

Discussion

I. COHEN: You suggested that the use of maximum dV/dt to obtain h_∞ curves in the heart has to be reevaluated carefully. I fully agree with your conclusion but I think your own studies have to be evaluated carefully as well. Your experiments are conducted at 18° C. The calculations that David Attwell, Gary Strichartz, and I have done recently suggest that at this temperature the nonlinearity of the relationship between maximum dV/dt and peak g_{Na} is most marked. If the temperature is raised by 20° C to get to the physiologic range, I would expect most of the nonlinearity to disappear. Therefore, before we can conclude that peak dV/dt is a nonlinear indicator of peak g_{Na} we might as well try to repeat the experiments in the same temperature range in which most of the h_∞ determinations are made.

C. COHEN: I agree that it would be a mistake to extrapolate our data on the nonlinearity of the relationship between peak dV/dt and peak g_{Na} to all other experimental conditions.

REUTER: How do you account for the nonlinearity of the relationship between peak dV/dt and I_{Na}? Ira Cohen has shown that in our model (Beeler and Reuter, J Physiol *268*:177, 1977) linearity is expected due to the rather large difference between τ_m and τ_h. On the other hand, in the Hodgkin-Huxley axon, the nonlinearity is related to a rather small difference between τ_m and τ_h. What is your explanation?

C. COHEN: I presume that the nonlinearity is due to large values of τ_m. The rate of sodium channel inactivation in rabbit Purkinje fibers is much slower than that observed in rabbit motor neurons, which have been studied by Chiu and his colleagues (Chiu et al., J Physiol *292*:149, 1979; Chiu et al., Nature *279*:327, 1979). Channel activation may likewise be slower. Unfortunately, we cannot determine τ_m in our preparations with our current techniques.

WEIDMANN: I was astonished to see the poor proportionality between maximum dV/dt and peak I_{Na}. I always knew there was no strict proportionality, but I never expected a curve so far off. My question then is, would we be better off measuring the upstroke velocity of a collision action potential instead of a propagated action potential? Would that lead closer to proportionality between maximal upstroke velocity and peak inward sodium current? How much local circuit current has to be deleted in a collision?

C. COHEN: In the case of the peak dV/dt measurements that I showed, the situation was as nearly as possible that of a membrane action potential. The fiber was very short and was stimulated intracellularly through our current passing electrode. Our results are similar to what has been found for upstroke velocity measurements using uniformly propagated action potentials. We have no personal experience with collision action potentials.

PAES DE CARVALHO: Concerning the question posed by Dr. Weidmann, peak dV/dt measurements in a collision action potential will be of very little use as an indicator of sodium current. In a collision action potential, the two advancing wavefronts make a huge contribution to local current in the central patch of membrane. Because of this, the collision action potential depolarizes much faster than a normally propagated action potential does. We can show by modeling, however, that the peak inward ionic current during this fast collision upstroke is actually much smaller than it is in a normal propagation! The reason for this is that τ_m is large enough to prevent the development of full activation within the short time in which maximum dV/dt is reached.

I. COHEN: Another point is related to your h_∞ curve. It seems that $h_\infty = 0.50$ corresponds to a voltage of −85 mV. This is a very negative curve that does not correspond to the experimental conditions in which most people work. Such a negatively displaced curve would yield an inappropriate relationship between τ_h and voltage. How do you explain the very negative position of your availability curve?

C. COHEN: The position of the h_∞ curve that we obtain in low sodium solutions at 17° C may not be quite the same as that found at 37° C in Tyrode's solution or in other preparations. The intracellular concentrations of calcium and protons are likely higher than normal under our conditions, and studies in nerve have demonstrated that both of these species have effects on surface potentials. I think that the position of our h_∞ curves is not at all unreasonable if a shift of about 5 mV in the midpoint is allowed for; that is, if the midpoint is at −80 mV instead of −85 mV. Myocardial cells would then have about 90% of their sodium channels available for opening after diastole.

I. COHEN: Still we cannot think of your inactivation curve as representing the normal situation, because an action potential can be readily obtained from a resting level of −70 mV, whereas your h_∞ curve shows almost complete inactivation at −70 mV. Your curve must indeed be negatively shifted appreciably.

C. COHEN: Our h_∞ curves may seem anomalous because their midpoint is much more negative than that of availability curves determined with $\dot{V}_{max}$ measurements. However, our results with TTX predict this discrepancy. Recall that the apparent K_D for TTX binding determined by $\dot{V}_{max}$ measurements differed from the true K_D by a factor of 10. This means that $\dot{V}_{max}$ will be reduced by half only when about 90% of the sodium channels are blocked by TTX or, equivalently, inactivated by depolarization. Because our h_∞ curves typically have their midpoint at about −85 mV and a slope factor of 5, our results with TTX predict that availability curves determined with $\dot{V}_{max}$ will be shifted to more positive potentials by 13 mV; they will have the same slope factor of 5, but the midpoint will be at −72 mV. The predicted availability curve is not unlike those typically found in Tyrode's solution at 37° C.

I. COHEN: I think that although you have demonstrated in your preparations that the voltage-clamp control is quite good, you have not yet simulated the amount of time necessary to achieve constant voltage. Considering the voltage ramp used and the time taken to charge the capacity through the series resistance, times of the order of 2 to 3 msec have elapsed before the clamp voltage is actually settled across the membrane. I would certainly appreciate seeing a simulation of the effects of these parameters before conclusions can be made on the amplitude of your peak Na^+ currents.

C. COHEN: We are making a point of working at fairly negative test potentials and at 10 mM Na^+. The peak of the *I-V* curve is located at about −35 mV, which is typically the test voltage to which we clamp for inward current measurements. The time to peak inward current at this voltage is about 4 or 5 msec, counting from the instant at which the test pulse is applied. The time constant for charging the membrane capacity is often 500 to 800 μsec. Therefore, the voltage step is practically complete in about 2 msec, well before the peak of I_{Na}. Considering that our overshoot is only a few millivolts, we should get a fairly accurate measure of peak inward current.

FOZZARD: I certainly agree very much with Dr. Ira Cohen about the peculiar implications of this very negative h_∞ curve in terms of the behavior of the tissue. I also agree with him that modeling of the sodium currents upon the application of a test clamp pulse is important. Mark Schoenberg and I (Biophys J 25:217−234, 1979) developed such a model for the sheep Purkinje fiber using such parameters as we could find. This model showed dramatic distortions for sodium current measurements. We also applied the numbers that were available for rabbit Purkinje fibers and found almost no distortions for the peak sodium current, although we did find some distortion in the determination of the activation time constant. So, in a sense, clamping the rabbit Purkinje fiber has been modeled if the anatomical parameters are correct.

I. COHEN: Can we be sure that your data on lidocaine can be extrapolated to the case of a healthy normal preparation in normal Tyrode's at 37° C?

C. COHEN: The amount of use-dependence seen with lidocaine will be sensitive to a number of factors, particularly bath pH. Also, the binding constant for lidocaine to inactivated channels may vary some with species or temperature. We believe, though, that the general features that we see are quite representative of what may go on in other species or other experimental conditions, even if it turns out that at 37° C the binding constant may be 5 μM or 20 μM instead of 10 μM. These differences do not change the general features of the mechanism by which this drug is acting.

REUTER: Charles Cohen's experiments with lidocaine reproduce our findings obtained with peak dV/dt measurements, insofar as he finds at 18° C the same shift in the h_∞ curve that we found at 37° C.

LIEBERMAN: I would like to raise the possibility that nonspecific TTX binding may account for some of the differences in TTX-binding from preparations of nerve, skeletal muscle, and cardiac muscle. For example, there is a considerable amount of a collagen around the fiber bundles in your preparations. Recently, TTX receptors have been demonstrated in a variety of nonmuscle cell types, particularly fibroblasts (Pouysségur et al., Nature *286*:162–164, 1980). In addition, Sperelakis attempted to use TTX to follow the development of the sodium channel in the chick embryo heart and observed that TTX binding decreased with age despite evidence that sodium channels increase with development (see Developmental and Physiological Correlates of Cardiac Muscle, edited by Lieberman and Sano, New York, Raven Press, 1975, pg. 223). These results could be accounted for by TTX binding to inactivated sodium channels, as well as the negatively charged cardiac jelly. Consequently, I am interested in knowing how you have taken into account the nonspecific binding of TTX.

C. COHEN: I am aware of the fact that there are reports of apparent sodium channels in nonexcitable cells. These reports are based on the findings that sodium fluxes in these other cells seem to be TTX-sensitive. I am, however, unaware that TTX, even in the micromolar range, affects any channels other than sodium channels. I should add that in our studies the only significant current we are looking at are sodium currents, and we seem to get a good fit to a 1/1 binding curve.

PAPPANO: I have been puzzled by the properties of sodium channels in mammalian heart muscle for a long time. There are data from embryonic chick hearts that show that a 50% reduction of peak dV/dt occurs at 10^{-8}M TTX (Iijima and Pappano, Circ Res *44*:358, 1979). In the frog ventricle, Hagiwara and Nakajima (J Gen Physiol *49*:793, 1966) found something in the same order of magnitude, as did Connor et al. (Biophys J *15*:1047, 1975) in the frog atria. I would like to ask, how do you account for this big difference between mammalian heart muscle and other vertebrate heart muscle?

C. COHEN: This is certainly an interesting question. It is quite obvious that the sodium channels of frog and chick hearts are much closer to nerve and skeletal muscle in their sensitivity to TTX than they are to mammalian heart muscle. I have no explanation at the molecular level for this difference.

Chapter 12

Inward Going Rectification in Sheep Cardiac Purkinje Fibers

Edward Carmeliet

Inward rectification is a general characteristic of potassium (K) channels in frog skeletal muscle (Katz, 1949), heart cells (see McAllister and Noble, 1966), and egg cell membranes (Hagiwara and Takahashi, 1974). In heart cells, inward going rectification plays an important role in the genesis of the plateau and the long duration of the cardiac action potential. According to an analysis by McAllister and Noble (1966), the conductance of the inward rectifier is dependent on two factors, ($E_m - E_K$) and extracellular potassium (K_o); the conductance increases in an instantaneous way for negative values of ($E_m - E_K$) and decreases for positive values; the conductance is higher the greater the extracellular K concentration is.

The experimental results to be reported in this paper show that *(1)* slow time-dependent conductance changes occur in the inward rectifier channel, *(2)* the conductance of the channel and the relative importance of the rapid and slow conductance changes depend on K_o; and *(3)* the inward rectifier conductance is inhibited by extracellular sodium (Na_o) or extracellular cesium (Cs_o); the Cs block being a potential-dependent phenomenon. A model is presented in which the inward rectifier is activated when, under the influence of the electric field, binding or access of external K to a certain site in the membrane occurs. At low K_o, activation is predominantly slow; at higher K_o, activation occurs in two phases, a rapid "instantaneous" one and a slow one; the higher the K_o, the more important the rapid phase. By interfering with the access of K to the site in the membrane, external Na and Cs exert a blocking effect on the inward rectifier. Part of the results have been published in communication form (Carmeliet, 1979a; 1979b).

METHODS

The two-microelectrode voltage-clamp technique was applied to small segments (< 1 mm) of sheep cardiac Purkinje fibers. The current-passing electrode was beveled and contained 2 M K citrate, 1 M KCl (resistance, 2 to 3 MΩ); the voltage recording electrode was the classical type (3 M KCl, 10 MΩ).

The composition of normal Tyrode's solution was 150 mM NaCl, 5.4 mM KCl, 3.6 mM $CaCl_2$, 0.5 mM $MgCl_2$, 10 mM Tris-Cl, and 100% O_2. A Na-free, K-free solution was made by substituting 150 mM Tris-Cl, Tris-acetylglycinate, or choline Cl for NaCl and omitting the KCl (atropine 1 mg/liter was added to the choline Cl solution). Solutions containing a variable amount of K or Na were made by substituting KCl or NaCl for Tris-Cl. The effect of Cs was studied in Na-free solutions by adding CsCl in variable concentrations (0.05 to 20 mM).

RESULTS

Induction of Inward Going Rectification

The starting point of my investigation was an unpublished observation by Hecht and Weidmann (cited by Carmeliet, 1961) that sheep cardiac Purkinje fibers show two stable resting potentials in a K-free, Na-free solution (for other conditions in which two stable-state potentials exist, see Wiggins and Cranefield, 1976; Gadsby and Cranefield, 1977). A resting potential of about −100 mV was obtained when the solution was first made Na-free and afterwards K-free; a low level of about −50 mV was obtained when the reverse sequence was followed. When the appropriate current was passed, the potential shifted from one level to the other (Carmeliet, 1961). In a first stage, it was confirmed that the shift from one level to the other could be brought about by clamping the membrane potential to a given level for a certain duration.

From a hypothetical point of view, two stable states for E_m can originate in different ways. By definition, the steady-state current-voltage relation (CVR) should intersect with the voltage axis at the two resting potentials, and the slope should be positive. At the resting potential, net current, indeed, must be zero; that is, outward and inward currents must be in balance. In Figure 1, a number of theoretical possibilities are represented in a schematic way. Because of the particular experimental condition of a Na-free, K-free solution, the number of currents that play a role is restricted; passive inward as well as active outward Na currents, and the pacemaker current are excluded (Deck and Trautwein, 1964; McAllister and Noble, 1966).

In Figure 1A the membrane is characterized by a single CVR that intersects the voltage axis at three different levels, of which two have a positive slope (stable levels) and one has a negative slope (unstable level). This relationship predicts an instantaneous shift from one stable level to the other if a voltage step of sufficient amplitude is applied. Experiments with voltage clamps of variable durations to different levels of membrane potential show, however, that clamps of 1 to 30 sec (depending on the potential and on the preparation) are needed to cause a stable shift from one level to the other.

A second possible way to explain the shift between both stable levels is presented in Figure 1B. Construction of the CVR is based on the existence of an inward and outward K rectifier, on an inward Ca background current and an important Cl background current. Cl ions are assumed to be passively distributed; the chloride CVR, which is assumed to be linear, thus crosses the voltage axis at the resting potential. Hyperpolarizing or depolarizing voltage steps that result in a shift from one level to the other are supposed to result in a change of intracellular Cl concentration so that E_{Cl} becomes equal to E_m. The results obtained with clamps of variable duration and to different levels exclude this possibility. The current flowing during the clamp is too small to result in any marked change of intracellular Cl concentration. Furthermore, a shift between the two stable states is also possible in Cl-free medium.

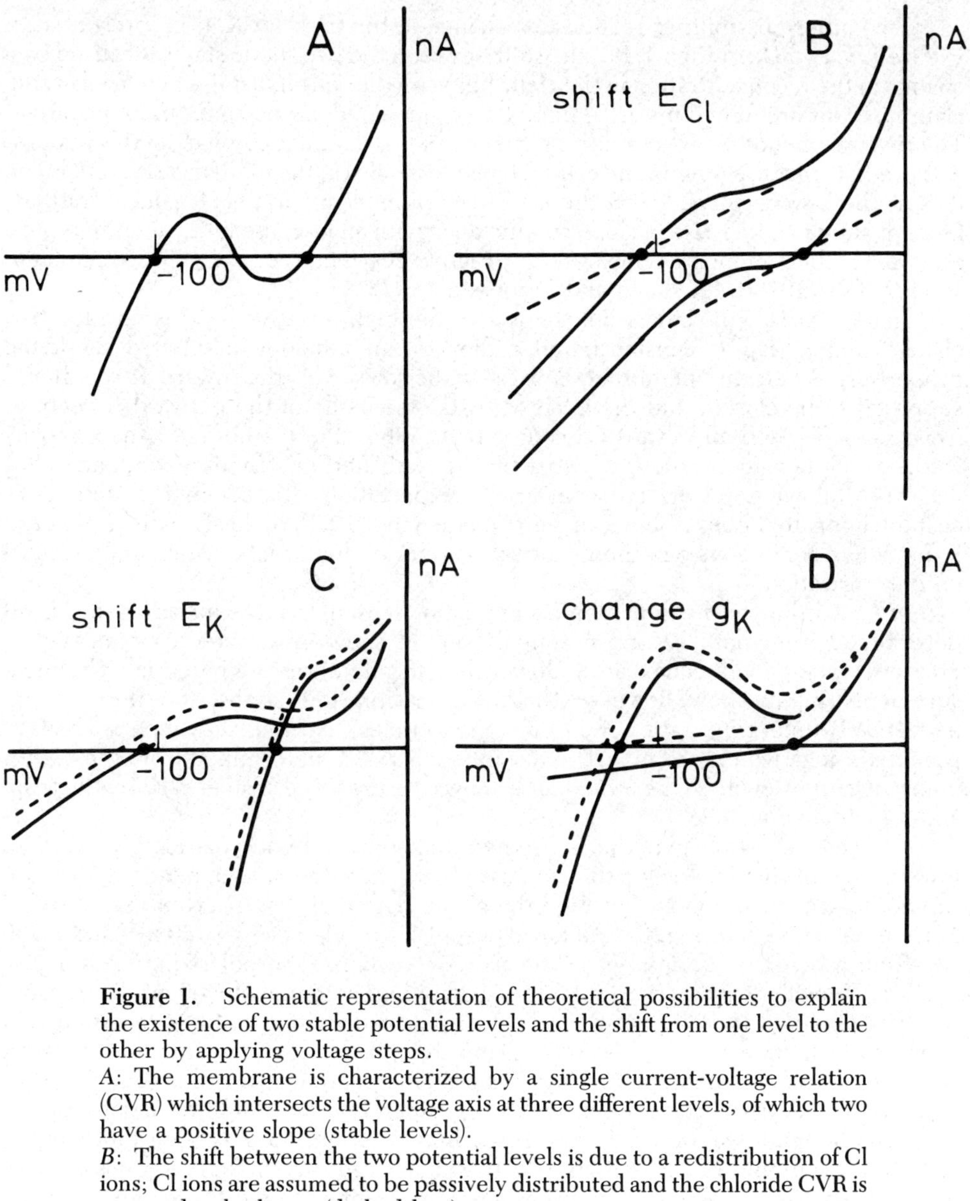

Figure 1. Schematic representation of theoretical possibilities to explain the existence of two stable potential levels and the shift from one level to the other by applying voltage steps.
A: The membrane is characterized by a single current-voltage relation (CVR) which intersects the voltage axis at three different levels, of which two have a positive slope (stable levels).
B: The shift between the two potential levels is due to a redistribution of Cl ions; Cl ions are assumed to be passively distributed and the chloride CVR is assumed to be linear (dashed line).
C: The shift in membrane potential is caused by a decrease in the K concentration in the clefts between cells during hyperpolarizing clamps and an increase in K during depolarizing clamps.
D: At the depolarized level, the K inward rectifier is supposed to be closed; during a hyperpolarizing clamp K conductance increases, owing to the movement of K ions to a critical site in the membrane. Dashed lines in C and D represent the potassium CVR.

Two other possibilities related to a change in the CVR for K are represented in Figure 1, C and D. In Figure 1C, the shift between the two stable states is caused by a change in the K concentration in the clefts between the cells. During a hyperpolarizing clamp, K ions are forced inwards, depletion occurs, and E_K becomes more negative. The reverse phenomena occur during a depolarizing clamp. A corollary of this hypothesis predicts that the membrane conductance is smaller at the high negative level than it is at the low negative level: the CVR determined in variable K concentrations, indeed, shows an increase in slope conductance with an increase in K_o and the typical cross-over phenomenon as illustrated in Figure 1C (Dudel et al., 1967; McGuigan, 1974; Noble, 1976; McDonald and Trautwein, 1978).

In Figure 1D, the shift from the low to the high negative level is not due to a change in E_K (E_K is constant), but rather to an induction of inward rectifying properties. When the membrane is fixed at the low level, the inward K rectifier is supposed to be closed, and the CVR consists essentially of the outward K rectifier (reversal at E_K)and an inward Ca component. When the membrane is hyperpolarized, K conductance in the inward rectifier is activated in a time-dependent way.

The following results are contrary to expectations, based on the depletion-accumulation hypothesis, but can be explained by the hypothesis, which assumes induction of conductance in the K inward rectifier on hyperpolarization and removal on depolarization

(1) According to the depletion-accumulation hypothesis, the instantaneous CVR determined from both resting potentials should show inward rectification with a greater slope or conductance at the lower (less negative) resting potential. The measurements (Fig. 2) show, however, that inward rectification is absent in the instantaneous CVR determined from −60 mV (open circles) and that the slope is small at potentials negative to −80 mV. The instantaneous CVR determined from the higher (more negative) level, on the other hand, shows the presence of an inward rectification and a high conductance.

(2) The depletion hypothesis predicts that during hyperpolarizing clamps an inward current should develop that decreases with time; the time-dependent decrease should be greater the more negative the clamp potential (Baumgarten et al., 1977). Such an effect is seen (Fig. 3, left) for hyperpolarizing clamps to −120 mV and −130 mV from a holding potential of −110 mV. But, when hyperpolarizing clamps to a similar range of potentials are applied from a holding potential of −60 mV, a different result is obtained (Fig. 3, right): at −110 mV, an inward current is recorded that decreases with time, but at −130 mV, the inward current increases with time. This last result is contrary to the depletion hypothesis. An apparent reversal potential is thus obtained at −120 mV. This level probably corresponds to the equilibrium potential for K ions (although K was omitted from the bathing solution, the K concentration in the clefts may be around 1 mM). Both the decreasing inward current for potentials positive to −120 mV as well as the increasing inward current negative to this level can be interpreted as increasing K currents. The rise in membrane conductance was further confirmed by measuring the slope conductance during hyperpolarizing clamps by superimposing small hyperpolarizing steps of 5 mV (not shown). The reason depletion is not seen at the start of a hyperpolarizing clamp from −60 mV to very negative potentials is related to the absence of an open, conductive K channel.

The decreasing outward currents during depolarizing clamps from a holding potential of −110 mV to −50 mV and −40 mV can be interpreted as a decreasing outward K current caused by closing of the inward rectifier. But, because the K channel is open at the start of the clamp, simultaneous accumulation phenomena will interfere. The picture is further complicated by possible activation of the positive dynamic current (compare currents at −40 mV for the two holding potentials).

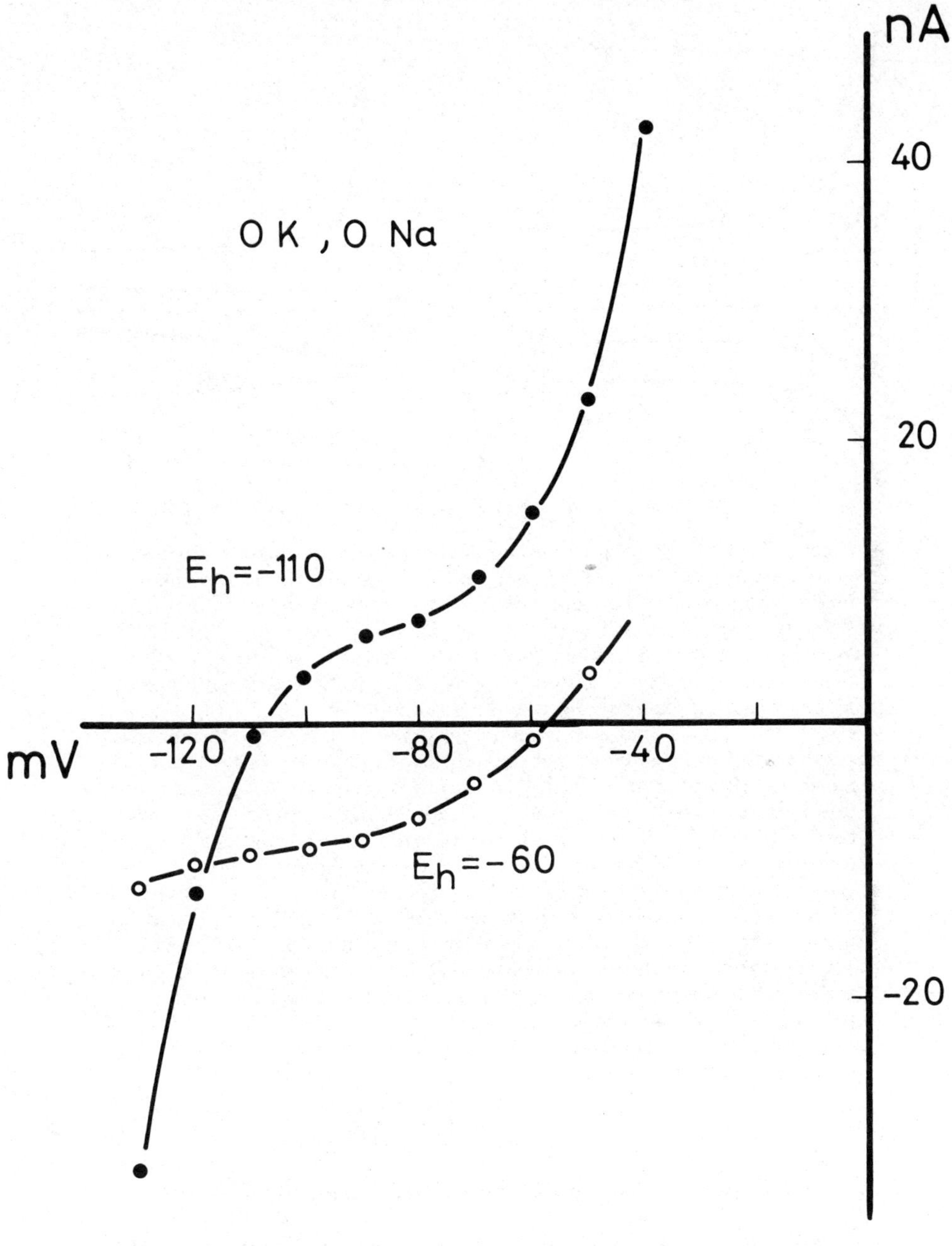

Figure 2. Instantaneous current-voltage relation in K-free, Na-free solution determined from a holding potential (E_h) of −110 mV (full circles) and from a holding potential (E_h) of −60 mV (open circles). The CVR shows the presence of inward rectification when the holding potential is −110 mV, whereas the CVR determined from the holding potential of −60 mV is linear and has a small slope in the region of potentials negative to −80 mV.

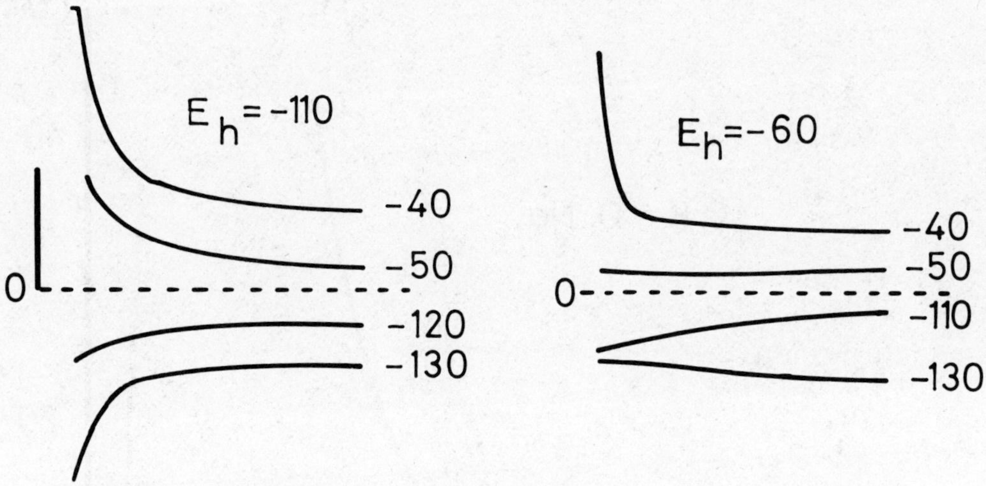

Figure 3. Illustration of the time-dependent current changes during potential clamps to different levels (−40 to −130 mV) from two different holding potentials (−110 and −60 mV). Same preparation as in Fig. 2. Hyperpolarizing clamps from a holding potential of −110 to −120 mV and −130 mV result in an inward current that decreases with time; the time-dependency is probably caused by K depletion in the extracellular clefts. Hyperpolarizing clamps from a holding potential of −60 mV to the same range of potentials (that is, a much larger gradient than in the former case) result in an inward current that decreases with time at −110 mV but that increases with time at −130 mV (apparent reversal potential −120 mV); this behavior cannot be explained by depletion but suggests an induction of a K conductance during hyperpolarization; depletion is absent because the K inward rectifier is closed at the start of the hyperpolarizing clamp. During depolarizing clamps from a holding potential of −110 mV, a decreasing outward current is observed, which can be interpreted in part as a decreasing K outward current caused by closing of the K inward rectifier. These currents, however, are contaminated by simultaneously occurring accumulation phenomena and activation of a positive dynamic current (compare currents at −40 mV in both recordings; note, however, that the full extent of the outward current was not recorded in the left part of the figure). Current calibration: 20 nA.

Effect of K, Na, and Cs on Inward Going Rectification

Potassium. The addition of K to the Na-free solution resulted in stabilization of the resting potential in the hyperpolarized state. With instantaneous CVR, the most important change occurred in the relation obtained from a low negative holding potential: the currents are shifted in the outward direction and show substantial inward rectification (Fig. 4). The difference between the CVR determined from a low and high negative level thus becomes less pronounced.

Sodium. If, instead of K, the Na concentration is increased, the membrane gradually depolarizes, and for a Na concentration of 10 to 20 mM the potential stabilizes at the low negative level. The instantaneous CVR determined from the high negative level does not show inward rectification, but instead becomes linear and very close to

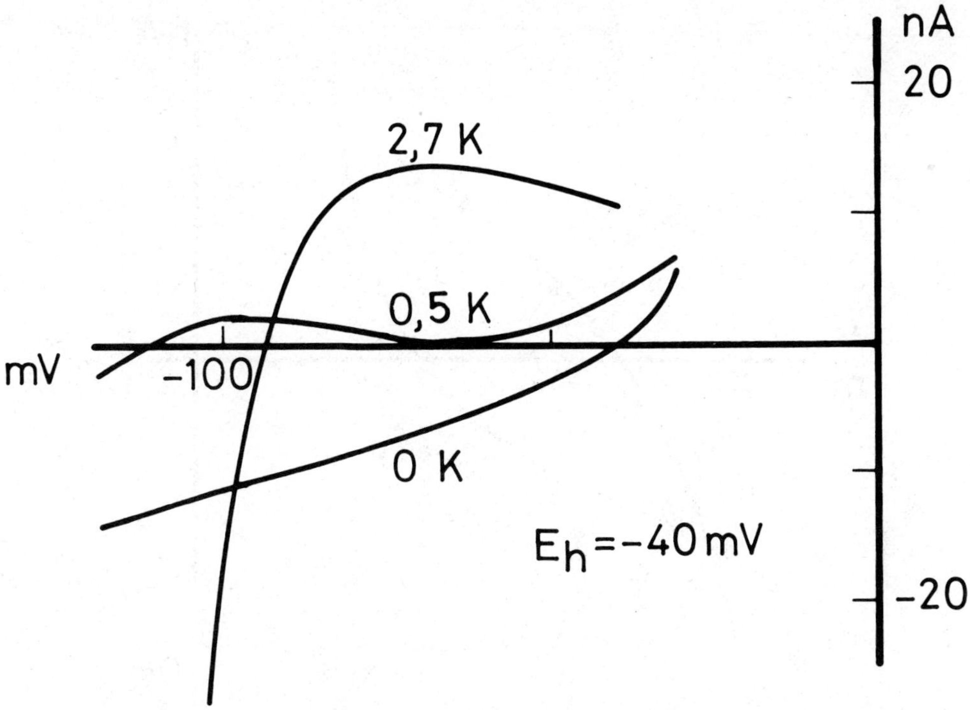

Figure 4. Effect of increasing K_o concentrations on the instantaneous current-voltage relation determined from a low level holding potential (−40 mV). Inward rectification, which is absent in K-free solution, becomes increasingly more pronounced in 0.5 and 2.7 K_o solutions.

the CVR determined from the low negative level (Fig. 5). These results suggest that Na ions, in the absence of K in the bathing solution, exert a blocking effect on the inward K rectifier.

Cesium. The effect of a variable Cs concentration on the inward rectifier properties was investigated in a Na-free solution, containing 2.7 or 5.4 mM K. As illustrated in Figure 6 the effect of Cs ions is to reduce the slope of the CVR. All CVR cross at a certain potential; this potential is dependent on K_o in a way expected for a K electrode and can be interpreted as corresponding to E_K. Positive to this potential, Cs ions shift the current in the inward direction; negative to this level, the current is more outward. Net inward, as well as net outward, K current is inhibited by Cs. The current change is greater at the higher Cs (Fig. 6).

Negative to the crossing-over potential, the slope of the CVR decreases with the extent of hyperpolarization and becomes even negative. This result strongly suggests an increase in blocking efficiency with hyperpolarization beyond E_K. From the percentage reduction in the Cs sensitive current, K_m values can be calculated. In 2.7 mM K_o, K_m varies from 0.09 mM at −140 mV to 0.43 mM at −110 mV ($N = 5$), corresponding to an e-fold change in K_m for 21 mV ($\delta = 1.28$). This sensitivity is greater than the theoretical value of 27 mV expected when the blocking particle senses the whole electric transmembrane gradient, and it suggests that probably two Cs ions are involved in the blocking mechanism. Similar results have been described for starfish egg cells (Hagiwara et al., 1976) and frog skeletal muscle (Gay and Stanfield, 1977).

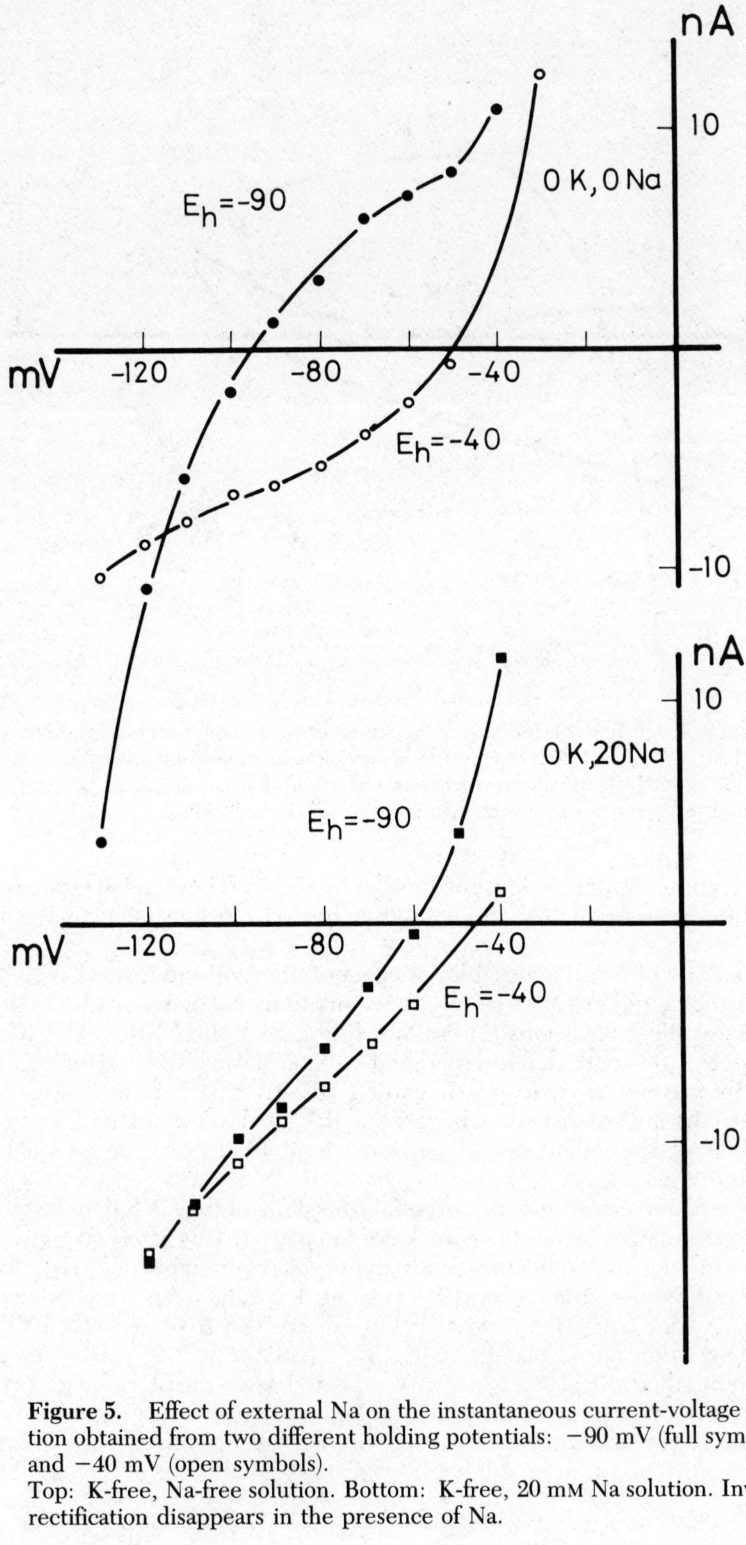

Figure 5. Effect of external Na on the instantaneous current-voltage relation obtained from two different holding potentials: −90 mV (full symbols) and −40 mV (open symbols).
Top: K-free, Na-free solution. Bottom: K-free, 20 mM Na solution. Inward rectification disappears in the presence of Na.

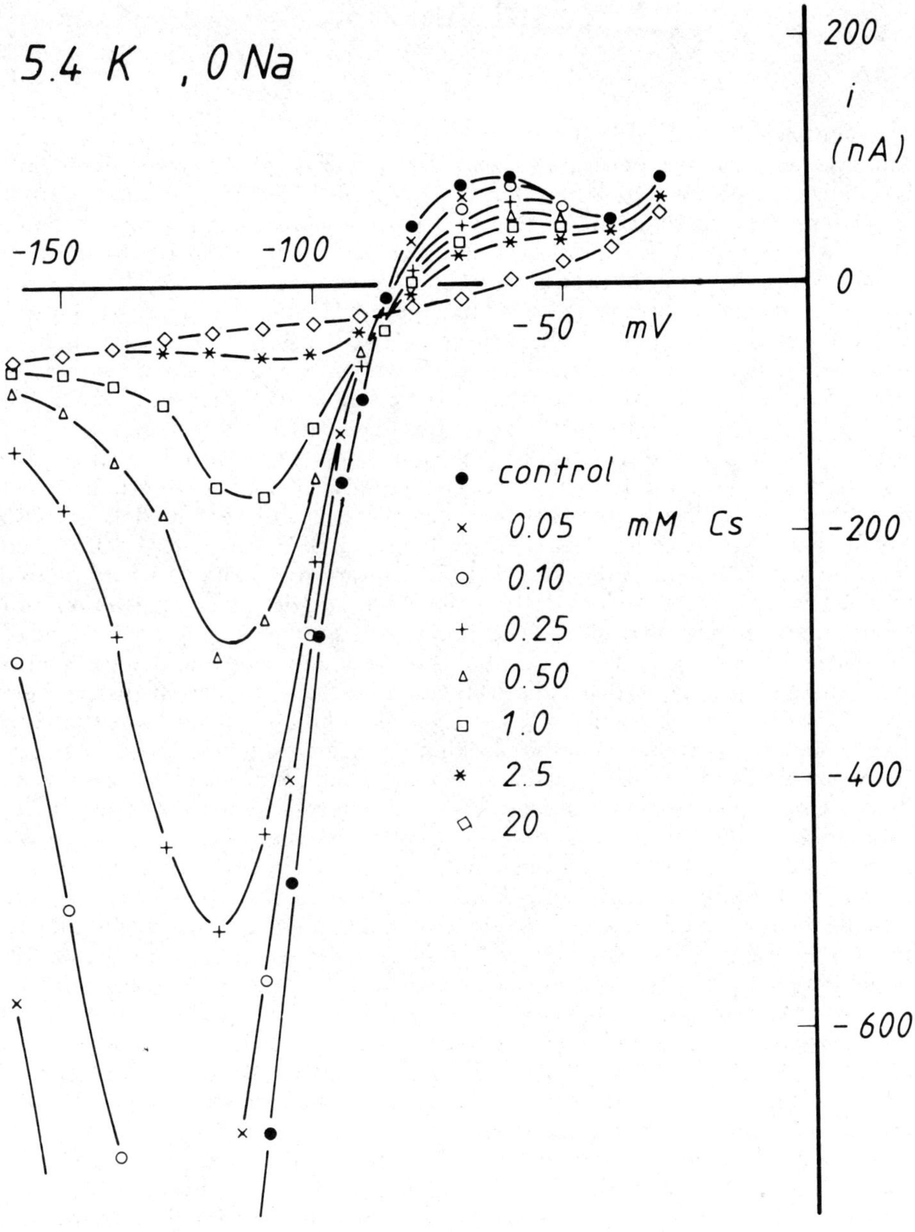

Figure 6. Current-voltage relations in Na-free, 5.4 mM K solution, containing variable concentrations of CsCl (0.05 to 20 mM). Note the negative slope of CVR at hyperpolarized levels, suggesting a potential-dependent block by Cs ions. Negative to the reversal potential, instantaneous currents were measured; positive to the reversal potential the values refer to currents measured at the end of a 5 second clamp.

DISCUSSION

The results reported in this chapter show that inward rectification is absent in a Purkinje preparation superfused with a K-free, Na-free solution when the membrane is stabilized at the low, depolarized level (for example, -50 mV). During hyperpolarizing clamps, inward rectification is induced. The induction of inward rectification is not due to a depletion of K in the intercellular clefts: a decrease in K_c should normally reduce K conductance, but the reverse phenomenon is observed. The time-dependent current changes observed during the hyperpolarizing clamps are not caused by a classical type of activation in which the state of the gate is fully determined by the potential gradient across the membrane. "Activation" occurs for potentials negative to -80 mV, whereas "deactivation" (that is, the disappearance of inward rectification) is seen in a different range of potentials (positive to -60 mV). A supplementary phenomenon that influences the orientation of the gating moiety is required. Such a phenomenon might be the binding or the access of external K ions to a certain site in the membrane. A similar assumption has been made in different models proposed to explain inward rectification (Standen and Stanfield, 1978; Ciani et al., 1978; Cleeman and Morad, 1979; Hille and Schwarz, 1978). Inward rectification, according to these models, is due to the locking-in of a blocking particle on depolarization and the unlocking on hyperpolarization. The removal of the block, however, requires the presence of K ions because the channel is opened only when an extracellular K ion replaces the blocking particle; this "activation" is thought to occur instantaneously.

To account for the results in K-free, Na-free solution, one has to assume that the change in K concentration near the blocking site is not instantaneous but that it occurs in two phases, a rapid, nearly instantaneous one and a slow one, the relative importance of both phases being dependent on K_o. During hyperpolarization in K-free solution, only the slow phase is seen; during depolarization or when K_o is increased, a rapid phase and a slow phase are observed. It is essential to note that a hyperpolarizing clamp from a holding potential of -50 mV, according to this explanation, forces K ions into the membrane but does not directly result in depletion: depletion is not possible because the rectifier channel is closed. As the rectifier becomes gradually conductive, depletion may occur. This secondary depletion will be rather ineffective in terms of current change at potentials positive to E_K due to the increase in K efflux as the rectifier opens. At potentials negative to E_K, however, the increase in K conductance and net K influx will actually deplete K from the extracellular space; this explains why the inward currents recorded during this type of clamp showed either no change or only a small time-dependent increase.

The conductance of the K inward rectifier is not only dependent on potential and K_o. Addition of 20 mM Na removed the possibility of inducing inward rectification by hyperpolarizing clamps. Addition of Cs ions equally blocked the inward rectifier channel. The block exerted by Cs was potential-dependent; that is, the block increased with hyperpolarization. It was also dependent on K_o concentration (more Cs was needed in elevated K concentrations). These results suggest an antagonistic interaction of Na or Cs ions with K ions for the same intramembranous site. The quantitative evaluation of the potential-dependent Cs block further suggests that more than one Cs ion is involved in the blocking mechanism.

REFERENCES

Baumgarten CM, Isenberg G, McDonald TF, Ten Eick RE (1977) Depletion and accumulation of potassium in the extracellular clefts of cardiac Purkinje fibers during voltage clamp hyperpolarization and depolarization. J Gen Physiol **70**:149–169

Carmeliet EE (1961) Chloride ions and the membrane potential of Purkinje fibres. J Physiol (Lond) **156**:375–388

Carmeliet E (1979a) Voltage dependent block of inward going rectification in cardiac Purkinje fibers by external Cs ions. Arch Int Pharmacodyn Ther **242**:294–295

Carmeliet E (1979b) Induction of inward going rectification in sheep cardiac Purkinje fibers. Arch Int Pharmacodyn Ther **242**:296–297

Ciani C, Krasne S, Miyazaki S, Hagiwara S (1978) A model for anomalous rectification: electrochemical-potential-dependent gating of membrane channels. J Membrane Biol **4**:103–134

Cleeman L, Morad M (1979) Potassium currents in frog ventricular muscle: Evidence from voltage clamp currents and extracellular K accumulation. J Physiol **286**:113–143

Deck KA, Trautwein W (1964) Ionic currents in cardiac excitation. Pflüg Arch **280**:63–80

Dudel J, Peper K, Rüdel R, Trautwein W (1967) The potassium component of membrane current in Purkinje fibers. Pfluegers Arch **296**:308–327

Gadsby DC, Cranefield PF (1977) Two levels of resting potential in cardiac Purkinje fibers. J Gen Physiol **70**:725–746

Gay LA, Stanfield PR (1977) Cs^+ causes a voltage-dependent block of inward K currents in resting skeletal muscle fibres. Nature **267**:169–170

Hagiwara S, Miyazaki S, Rosenthal NP (1976) Potassium current and the effect of cesium on this current during anomalous rectification of the egg cell membrane of a starfish. J Gen Physiol **67**:621–638

Hagiwara S, Takahashi K (1974) The anomalous rectification and cation selectivity of the membrane of a starfish egg cell. J Membrane Biol **18**:61–80

Hille B, Schwarz W (1978) Potassium channels as multi-ion single-file pores. J Gen Physiol **72**:409–442

Katz B (1949) Les constantes électriques de la membrane du muscle. Arch Sci Physiol **3**: 285–300

McAllister RE, Noble D (1966) The time and voltage dependence of the slow outward current in cardiac Purkinje fibres. J Physiol **186**:632–662

McDonald TF, Trautwein W (1978) Membrane currents in cat myocardium: Separation of inward and outward components. J Physiol (Lond) **274**:193–216

McGuigan JAS (1974) Some limitations of the double sucrose gap, and its use in a study of the slow outward current in mammalian ventricular muscle. J Physiol (Lond) **240**:775–806

Noble SJ (1976) Potassium accumulation and depletion in frog atrial muscle. J Physiol (Lond) **258**:579–613

Standen NB, Stanfield PR (1978) Inward rectification in skeletal muscle: A blocking particle model. Pfluegers Arch **378**:173–176

Wiggins JR, Cranefield PF (1976) Two levels of resting potential in canine cardiac Purkinje fibers exposed to sodium-free solutions. Circ Res **39**:466–474

Discussion

JOHNSON: Because of the existence of narrow intercellular clefts, I am disturbed that you use a preparation in which a sizable fraction of the membrane surface is not readily accessible to the outside bathing solution. This has two serious consequences: one is that you cannot be sure of the composition of the solution within the intercellular clefts, especially when sodium-free and potassium-free solutions are used; the second is that you must include in your membrane current interpretation the possibility of a sizable contribution of electrogenic transport current. It is my feeling, until you show otherwise, that during long clamp pulses there may occur a significant alteration of composition of the intercellular clefts, therefore creating unknown disturbances of electrogenic transport current that were not taken into account. This might give a time-dependent behavior to the ionic current in your experiment.

CARMELIET: It is certainly true that depletion and accumulation phenomena complicate the interpretation of voltage-clamp currents obtained in Purkinje fibers of the sheep heart. Perhaps I did not stress the fact that depletion currents are seen in several records obtained for hyperpolarizing clamps from a holding potential of −90 or −100 mV. What I would like to emphasize, however, is that depletion phenomena cannot explain the current changes during hyperpolarizing clamps from a holding potential of −40 or −50 mV, because with increasing hyperpolarizing steps the current pattern changes from a decreasing inward to an increasing inward current. The instantaneous current-voltage relation is linear under those conditions, suggesting that the inward rectifier is closed; depletion is not present, because an open channel is required to obtain a net inward movement of potassium ions. I also have tried to perform similar experiments in rabbit Purkinje fibers, in which cleft problems seem to be negligible. There is, however, one difficulty: rabbit Purkinje fibers do not survive well in sodium-free solutions and tend to depolarize in these conditions. In one experiment, performed in 1 mM potassium however, I was able to shift the potential from one level to the other. Another point you made was related to the contribution of electrogenic pumping (I assume you were speaking of sodium electrogenic pumping). The fibers I have used have been perfused with sodium-free solution for at least half an hour before changing to the potassium-free, sodium-free solution, in which they remained for the same time. Of course, there may always be some sodium left in the preparation, but I hope that the complication due to sodium electrogenic pumping is very small.

FOZZARD: I want to be absolutely sure that you are making the experiment in sodium-free solution. If it is indeed sodium-free, then the sodium electrogenic pump is completely blocked and cannot therefore contribute in any way. This is disappointing to me in trying to understand the phenomena, because I was attracted to the idea that it was due to sodium accumulation inside the cell. I thought this increase in inside sodium would interfere with the potassium channel, as pointed out in experiments with squid nerve. This would fit very well with the experiments made by Ellis (J Physiol **273**:211−240, 1977), in which he shows that in potassium-free solutions in presence of sodium the intracellular sodium rises. We looked at the time course of this ourselves, using sodium electrodes. We found that sodium rises in the approximate time course needed to mimic the results obtained in sodium-containing solutions, in terms of how long it takes for the fiber to change to a different potential. We can also say that in these conditions the removal of extracellular sodium causes a decrease of the intracellular sodium concentration to almost nothing within 15 min. In this way, I think that your 30-min soaking in a sodium-free solution is sufficient for intracellular sodium to vanish almost completely. I would like, therefore, to ask you if you can be absolutely sure that the phenomenon exists in sodium-free conditions. That is to say, that external sodium itself does not play any role in the phenomenon as a blocking agent in the potassium channel.

CARMELIET: I really cannot exclude the possibility that outside sodium is the blocking particle in the potassium channel. But, I should say that due to the extremely low sodium concentration that must exist at the moment of the experiment, if there is blockade of potassium channels this must be an exquisitely sensitive mechanism with respect to sodium. On the other hand, the effect of addition of external sodium is similar to what has been described in other fibers. It is not so unusual to see a blocking effect of external sodium on the potassium channel. This has been shown for other potassium channels, although not so dramatically. It is present, for instance, in skeletal muscle. It is, therefore, quite probable that external sodium blocks the potassium inward rectifier. It should be kept in mind that all these effects except the time dependence can be seen in the inward rectifier of skeletal muscle and in the inward rectifier of egg cell membranes of tunicates or starfish. In all these preparations, external potassium increases the conductance of the channel, whereas external cesium and sodium exert a blocking effect.

CRANEFIELD: Dr. Wiggins certainly saw the same phenomenology when studying the two stable levels of membrane potential in canine cardiac Purkinje fibers exposed to sodium-free solutions.

CARMELIET: I am sorry to have failed to mention the experiments by Wiggins and yourself, of which I am very much aware. In this respect, in one of the other papers you have published on sodium-free and chloride-free solutions you proposed an explanation in terms of a current-voltage relationship that had three intercepts with the voltage axis.

CRANEFIELD: Dr. Gadsby actually measured such a current-voltage relationship.

CARMELIET: Yes. This explanation, however, cannot apply to the experimental results in potassium-free, sodium-free solution. In the other paper with Wiggins, you mention that you need pulses of long duration to go from one state to the other, and this suggests that time-dependent changes in the potassium inward rectifier may play a role. These experiments were conducted in the presence of TEA, which is known to block the inward rectifier in skeletal muscle.

CRANEFIELD: Yes, but Wiggins's results were obtained well before Dr. Gadsby introduced the fast-flow system that allows for much quicker changes in external solutions.

C. COHEN: I would like to know if the voltage dependence of block by external sodium is similar to that for block by external cesium. Assuming that this voltage-dependence can be described by a Boltzmann distribution of cation binding, what fraction of the voltage across the membrane must the cations cross to reach their binding site?

CARMELIET: I did not see a potential-dependent block for the case of sodium. The results we presented were for 20 mM sodium in potassium-free media. In this situation, we observed an almost complete block of the potassium channel, and this was independent of voltage. On the other hand, the block by cesium ions is clearly potential-dependent at negative potentials. In the case of the cesium block, we found that the correction factor is about 1.27, which is similar to the values found for skeletal muscle. The cesium, therefore, is seeing more than the electrical field at the binding site.

RAMÓN: In the squid axon, this kind of effect can be obtained with high sodium inside and also with high calcium, or even with lanthanum. It would therefore seem that many cations can do it. Since your pulses were very long, can you rule out changes in the intracellular concentrations of other cations, for instance, calcium?

CARMELIET: No, I do not know what happens with intracellular calcium. I have tried to modify intracellular calcium by changing the extracellular calcium. I could not see, directly or indirectly, that the induction of inward rectifying properties was related to changes in calcium.

REUTER: I am a bit worried about the fact that you have a sodium-free solution, and therefore the sodium pump is largely blocked. I wonder what is happening to the intracellular potassium concentration. It cannot be in a steady state.

CARMELIET: The potassium concentration inside decreases with time in sheep Purkinje fibers exposed to sodium-free, potassium-free media. As far as I remember from older experiments, the half time was about 200 min.

Chapter 13

Effects of Electrogenic Sodium Extrusion on the Membrane Potential of Cardiac Purkinje Fibers

David C. Gadsby and Paul F. Cranefield

The electrical impulses that initiate each heart beat are associated with passive net fluxes of ions down their electrochemical potential gradients, sodium and calcium ions flowing into, and potassium ions out of, the cells. If the cellular content of these ions is to be kept constant, and their concentration gradients maintained, then the dissipative fluxes accompanying electrical activity must be countered by equivalent, restorative fluxes via active transport. For sodium and potassium ions, these active movements are largely accomplished by the sodium-potassium (Na^+/K^+) exchange pump and, since the human heart beats at least once a second throughout life, the electrochemical work performed by the Na^+/K^+ pump is considerable. In addition to this long-term, restorative function, however, there are two other important reasons for investigating activity of the Na^+/K^+ pump in heart cells: the first is that, by controlling the intracellular sodium ion concentration ($[Na]_i$), the sodium pump might indirectly affect the intracellular calcium ion concentration ($[Ca]_i$) (for example, via some kind of sodium-calcium exchange mechanism; see Baker et al., 1969; Glitsch et al., 1970; Mullins, 1979; Chapman, 1979), and so might modulate the strength of contraction and the size of any calcium-activated membrane conductances (for examples, see Isenberg, 1977; Marban and Tsien, 1979; Siegelbaum and Tsien, 1980). Second, Na^+/K^+ exchange is electrogenic; that is, the pump moves more sodium outwards than it does potassium inwards across the cell membrane, and so it directly generates a hyperpolarizing component of membrane current (for review, see Glitsch, 1979). Relatively small changes in pump rate can thus produce significant changes in the resting (or diastolic) potential, in the amplitude and duration of the action potential plateau, and in the rate of automaticity of cardiac cells. These pump-induced changes in the electrical activity of heart cells form the subject of this chapter.

Supported by USPHS grant #HL-14899.

METHODS

The experiments to be described were carried out on small unbranched bundles of Purkinje fibers, usually $\leqslant$ 2 mm in length and $\leqslant$ 200 μm in overall diameter, dissected from only the right ventricles of dog hearts. Visual inspection indicates that the sheath of connective tissue surrounding the bundles is usually thinner in the right than in the left ventricle, so that insertion of microelectrodes is correspondingly easier. Apart from their small size, a further advantage of these preparations for the present study (see Discussion) is that, as revealed by preliminary morphologic investigation, despite considerable variability in the size, number, and distribution of the Purkinje cells in the fiber core, the cells appear to be much more loosely packed than the cells in sheep and calf Purkinje fibers (cf. Sommer and Johnson, 1968; Eisenberg and Cohen, 1981; T.D. Pham and D.C. Gadsby, unpublished). As the diagram in Figure 1 indicates, the fibers were suspended between two fine (100 μm diameter) insect pins in the narrow channel of a modified Hodgkin-Horowicz (1959) fast-flow system. The pins were pushed into the Sylgard (#184, Dow Corning Corp., Midland, Michigan) floor of the channel. The preparations were positioned in midstream, near the tops of the pins, so that they were exposed to moving fluid on all sides, except where they rested lightly on a 100-μm wide support to facilitate microelectrode impalement (see Fig. 1). Preheated superfusion solutions continuously entered the chamber through a complex system of valves, flowed along the channel past the preparation, and were removed by suction. One output of a two-position valve (#86410, Hamilton Co., Reno, Nevada) was attached to the channel inlet by a few millimeters of silicone rubber tubing, and the other output was connected to a drain. The two inputs to that valve were supplied by the outputs from two, four-position, distribution valves (#86414, Hamilton) fitted with spring-loaded stops to permit rapid selection of a test solution for switching to the experimental chamber. At the flow rate normally used, 5 ml/min, solution changes at the middle of the channel occurred with a half-time of about 0.5 sec, as determined from the time course of establishment of the liquid junction potential on switching between Cl^--containing and Cl^--free fluids. Conventional glass microelectrodes filled with 3 M KCl were used to record membrane potentials and to inject current. One operational amplifier was used to clamp the membrane potential to the chosen level, and a second one monitored the applied current; currents were filtered (time constant, 100 msec) before they were displayed on oscilloscopes and chart-recorder.

The Cl^--containing Tyrode's solution used during dissection and throughout some experiments contained 137 mM NaCl, 4 mM KCl, 12 mM $NaHCO_3$, 1.8 mM NaH_2PO_4, 0.5 mM $MgCl_2$, 2.7 mM $CaCl_2$, and 5.5 mM dextrose. This solution was bubbled with 95% O_2 and 5% CO_2 mixture while it was being preheated. The low-Cl^- solution used in some experiments contained 146 mM Na isethionate, 4 mM K methylsulphate, 5 mM Hepes (*N*-2-hydroxyethylpiperazine-*N*′-2-ethanesulfonic acid; pH, 7.3) 0.5 mM $MgCl_2$, 2.7 mM Ca methanesulfonate, and 5.5 mM dextrose, this solution was bubbled with oxygen during preheating. In both normal and low-Cl^- solutions, K^+ concentration was varied by substitution with Na^+. All solutions were filtered before use; experiments were carried out at 36.5 ± 1° C (monitored with the small thermistor bead shown in Fig. 2). The cardiac steroid, 3-acetylstrophanthidin, was a gift from Eli Lilly & Co. (Indianapolis, Indiana) and was kept for several weeks as a refrigerated stock solution of 5 mM in ethanol.

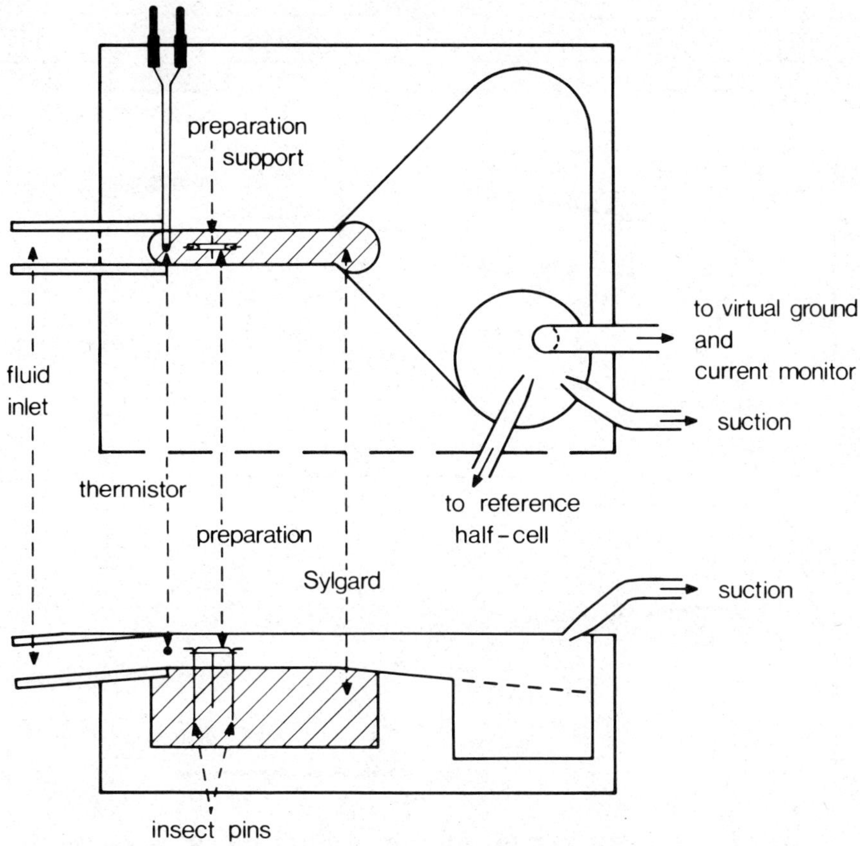

Figure 1. Schematic diagram of modified Hodgkin-Horowicz type fast-flow chamber. Superfusion fluid continuously enters the chamber via the inlet at the left, flows along the narrow channel (3-mm square cross-section), and is removed by suction at the right. The fluid inlet is set at an angle, and the upper surface is polished so that a cover slip can be used to enclose the channel when necessary. Shaped insect pins, pushed through "flaps" of the connective tissue sheath of the fiber and into the Sylgard floor of the channel, hold the fiber in midstream. A third insect pin, bent to form a rectangular hoop, gives some support during microelectrode impalements. Downstream, near the suction tube, a 3 M KCl-agar bridge connects the chamber, via an Ag/AgCl electrode, to an operational amplifier which holds the bath at ground potential and monitors applied currents; nearby, a flowing 3 M KCl bridge connects the chamber to the reference half-cell which incorporates a sintered Ag/AgCl/Pt-black pellet.

RESULTS

Some typical changes in membrane potential associated with small changes in pump rate are presented in Figure 2, which shows three different responses to brief periods of exposure to K^+-free solution, recorded in three different Purkinje fibers. In 4 mM K, low-Cl^- fluid, the N-shaped steady-state current-voltage relationship of

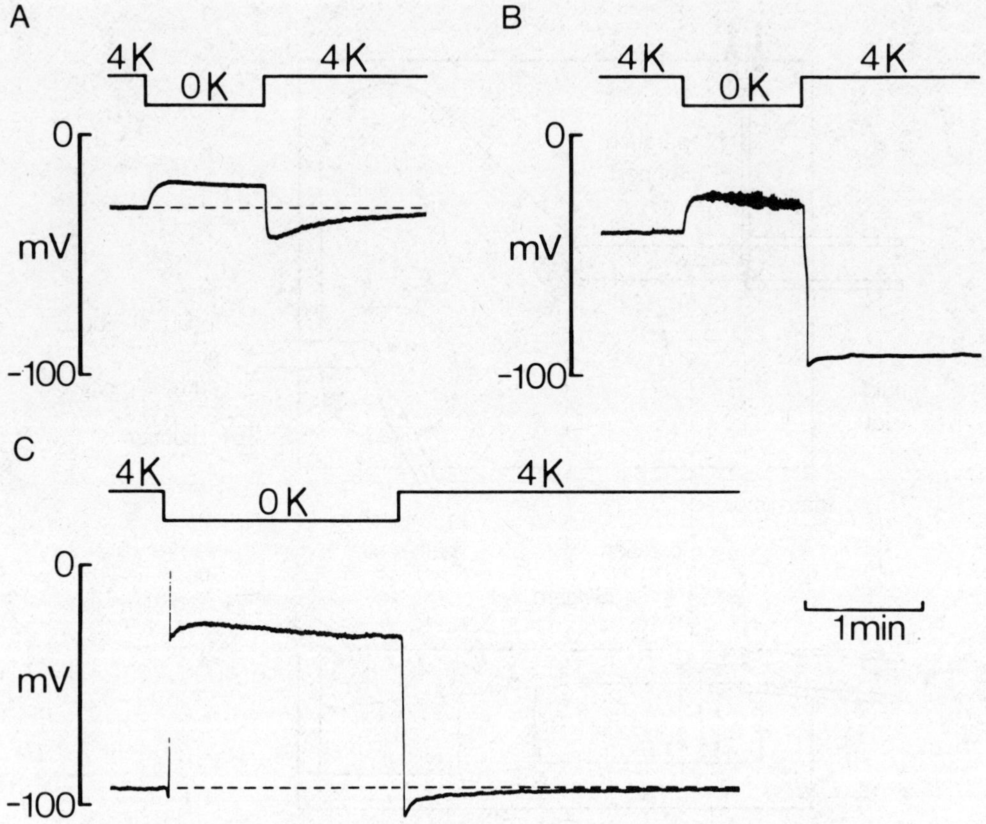

Figure 2. Membrane potential changes recorded in small canine Purkinje fibers in response to brief exposures to K^+-free solution, as indicated by the line above each record. In panels A and B, the resting potential was initially at the "lower" level, and in panel C it was initially at the "higher" level (see Gadsby and Cranefield, 1977). In all three cases, there was a maintained depolarization to about −30 mV in K^+-free solution, and there was a transient hyperpolarization on returning to 4 mM K^+ solution: the small transient hyperpolarization, lasting 5 to 10 sec, seen in B and C reflects the time course of change of K^+ concentration just outside the cell (see text), whereas the more slowly decaying hyperpolarization evident in panels A and C (the dashed lines indicate steady-state levels of resting potential) reflects temporarily enhanced electrogenic Na^+ extrusion. Low-Cl^- solutions throughout.

canine cardiac Purkinje fibers often makes three intersections with the voltage axis so that there are two possible levels of resting potential, a "lower" level near −40 mV and a "higher" level near −90 mV (Gadsby and Cranefield, 1977). In Figure 2A, the resting potential of the fiber was at the lower level in 4 mM $[K]_o$, and on switching into K^+-free solution, the membrane depolarized in spite of the fact that the K equilibrium potential, E_K, is made more negative. On returning to 4 mM $[K]_o$ after 1 min exposure to zero $[K]_o$, a transient hyperpolarization occurred, which reached a peak within a few seconds and then decayed slowly over the next minute or two. We explain this transient hyperpolarization in the following way: in 4 mM $[K]_o$, in the steady state, if the cells are neither gaining nor losing Na^+, then passive Na^+ influx into the cells must be balanced by active Na^+ extrusion. Because Na^+/K^+ exchange requires extracellular K^+, on switching into K^+-free fluid, Na extrusion is diminished while Na influx remains unchanged, with the result that $[Na]_i$ begins to rise and continues to do so as long as exposure to zero $[K]_o$ is continued, at least for several minutes (cf. Ellis, 1977; Deitmer and Ellis, 1978; Eisner et al., 1980). Because Na^+/K^+ exchange is stimulated by a rise in $[Na]_i$, on restoring extracellular K^+ the pump rate is temporarily enhanced, and hence pump current is temporarily increased, until the increment in $[Na]_i$ has been eliminated and $[Na]_i$ returned to its steady-state level. The transient hyperpolarization, then, reflects that temporary increase in the rate of electrogenic Na^+ extrusion.

In the experiment of Figure 2B, the fiber initially showed a steady resting potential at the lower level, but the transient increment in pump current resulting from the 1-min exposure to K^+-free fluid was large enough to "switch" the membrane potential permanently to the higher resting level. A similar switch can be effected by injecting a brief, weak current pulse from an external source through a second intracellular microelectrode (see Gadsby and Cranefield, 1977).

In Figure 2C, the membrane potential was initially at the high resting level and, as usual in that case, the depolarization on switching to K^+-free fluid was preceded by a brief hyperpolarization. On returning to 4 mM $[K]_o$, a similar, rapidly decaying hyperpolarization is seen to precede the small, slowly decaying, transient hyperpolarization caused by temporarily enhanced pump activity. These rapid potential changes reflect the phenomenon of "crossing over" of the steady-state, membrane K^+ current-voltage curves for different levels of $[K]_o$ (Adrian, 1965; Noble, 1965); in other words, on switching from 4 mM $[K]_o$ to zero $[K]_o$ for example, outward membrane K^+ current near the high level of resting potential is first increased, but is then reduced, as the K^+ concentration just outside the cell membrane gradually falls. In contrast to this, the monotonic depolarization seen on switching from 4 mM to zero $[K]_o$ at the lower level of resting potential (Fig. 2, A and B) indicates that in that voltage-range outward membrane K^+ current declines monotonically as $[K]_o$ falls. This difference in behavior allowed us to immediately rule out an alternative explanation for the pump-induced, transient hyperpolarization seen at the *low* resting potential following exposure to K^+-free fluid, namely, that it reflects extracellular K^+ depletion caused by the enhanced Na^+/K^+ exchange. Thus, Figure 2A shows clearly that a fall in extracellular K^+ concentration at the lower level of resting potential causes the membrane to depolarize, not hyperpolarize.

Use of a simple two-microelectrode voltage-clamp system permits the changes in net membrane current underlying the pump-induced transient hyperpolarization to be measured directly in these small Purkinje fibers, as is illustrated in Figure 3. The membrane potential changes associated with a 1-min exposure to K^+-free fluid, in a fiber already impaled with two microelectrodes but with the voltage-clamp amplifier switched off, are shown in panel Figure 3A. Because the fiber was at the lower level of resting potential, the switch to zero $[K]_o$ caused a monotonic depolarization, and on returning to 4 mM $[K]_o$ the usual transient hyperpolarization was seen. When the changes in K^+ concentration were repeated after switching on the clamp amplifier in order to hold the membrane potential at its steady resting (zero-current) level in 4 mM $[K]_o$, a maintained net inward current was recorded on switching into K^+-free fluid, and a transient net outward current, reflecting the increment in pump current, arose on returning to 4 mM $[K]_o$ (Fig. 3B). Like the transient hyperpolarization, the increment in pump current reached a peak within a few seconds and then decayed slowly over the next minute or so. On the basis of our working explanation, given above, the sharp rise in pump current indicates the time taken for diffusion equilibration of K^+ in the extracellular spaces, whereas its slow decay indicates the gradual

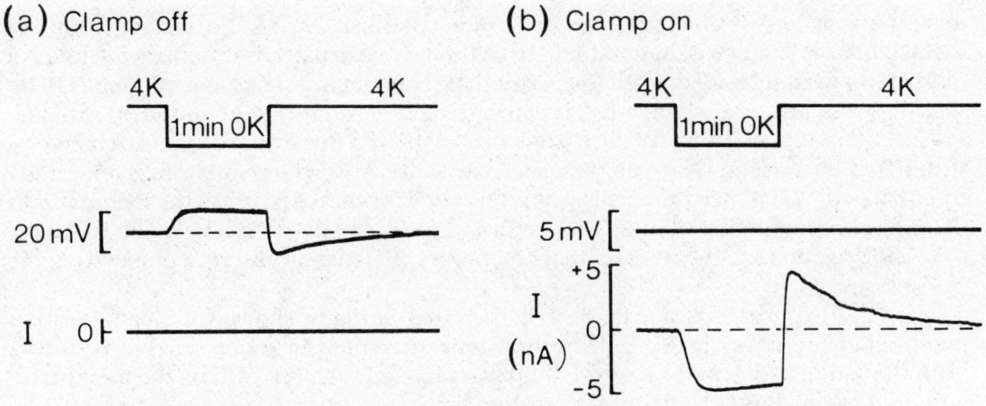

Figure 3. Changes in membrane potential (a) and in net current (b) recorded consecutively, in the same Purkinje fiber, in response to 1-min exposures to K^+-free fluid. The dashed line in (a) indicates the steady resting potential in 4 mM $[K]_o$, which was at the "lower level" of −33 mV; this was also the holding potential for (b) so that, in the steady state, the holding current was zero (dashed line). Note the different voltage calibrations in (a) and (b). Current flowing outwards across the cell membrane is defined as positive. Low-Cl^- solutions. From Gadsby and Cranefield, 1979a.

elimination of the increment in $[Na]_i$ responsible for the temporarily enhanced rate of Na^+ extrusion.

That the transient hyperpolarization and transient outward current underlying it reflect a temporary increase in the rate of Na^+/K^+ exchange is simply demonstrated by their abolition following application of a maximal concentration (2 μM) of acetylstrophanthidin, a fast-acting cardiac steroid and specific inhibitor of the Na^+/K^+ exchange pump. In Figure 4A, the top line indicates the timing of the $[K]_o$ changes, the upper record shows the transient hyperpolarization following a 1-min exposure to K^+-free fluid, and the middle record shows that the transient hyperpolarization was abolished in the presence of acetylstrophanthidin, the membrane potential on re-exposure to 4 mM $[K]_o$ returning only to the level recorded just before the period in zero $[K]_o$. The lower record shows, once again, the presence of the pump-induced hyperpolarization some 10 min after the cardiac steroid was washed out. Figure 4B shows the corresponding changes in net membrane current recorded in a voltage-clamped Purkinje fiber in a different experiment, but during an analogous series of solution changes. The upper record shows the slowly decaying, outward current transient (that is, the increment in pump current), and the middle record shows that it was absent during superfusion with acetylstrophanthidin, the membrane current level in 4 mM K^+ solution containing acetylstrophanthidin being the same before and after the exposure to K^+-free solution. The lower record confirms that the pump current transient was restored after washing out the acetylstrophanthidin.

In addition to demonstrating that micromolar concentrations of acetylstrophanthidin abolish the transient increment in pump current that follows brief periods of exposure to K^+-free fluid, Figure 4 shows that such concentrations also cause a significant depolarization of the resting membrane (Fig. 4A), or inward shift of the holding current under voltage-clamp (Fig. 4B), presumably by abolishing a steady-state component of pump current. A depolarization as large as that in Figure 4A can be explained *neither* by extracellular K^+ accumulation secondary to pump inhibition, because a rise in $[K]_o$ at the low level of resting potential causes hyperpolarization

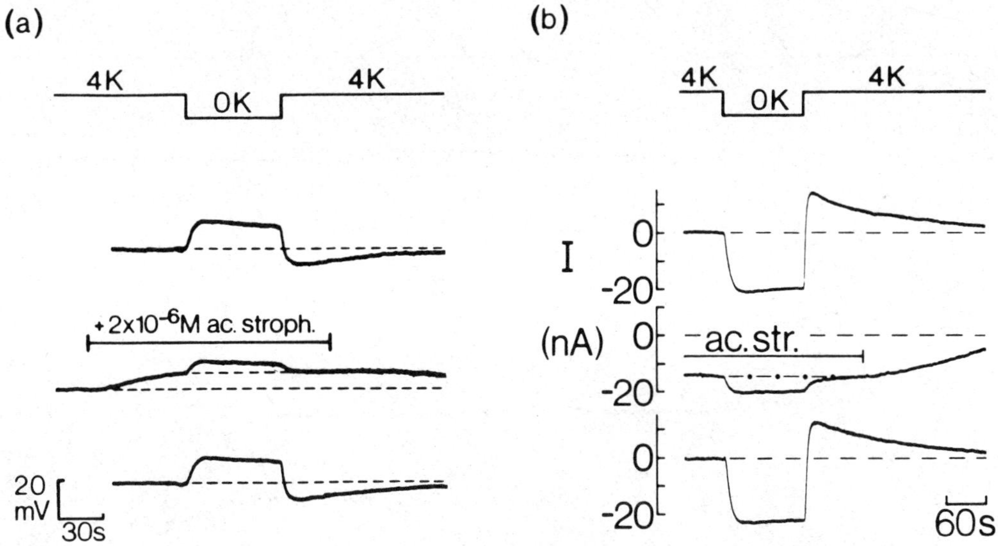

Figure 4. Abolition, by micromolar concentrations of the cardiac steroid acetylstrophanthidin, of (a) the transient hyperpolarization, and (b) the transient outward current increase under voltage clamp, following brief exposures to K^+-free fluid. In both panels, the top and bottom records show the transient changes, reflecting temporarily enhanced electrogenic Na^+ extrusion, before application of, and after recovery from acetylstrophanthidin, respectively. The middle records show, in panel (a) the steady depolarization, and in panel (b) the net inward current shift, in the presence of acetylstrophanthidin due to abolition of the steady-state, or background, component of outward pump current. (a), Resting potential, −47 mV; low-Cl^- solutions: from Gadsby and Cranefield, 1979b, with permission of the *Journal of General Physiology*. (b), Resting and holding potential, −40 mV; low-Cl^- solutions; 2 μM acetylstrophanthidin: from Gadsby and Cranefield, 1979a.

(Gadsby and Cranefield, 1977), *nor* by a fall in $[K]_i$ because, at best, that would require the cells to lose about one-third of their total K^+ content in less than a minute (see Gadsby and Cranefield, 1979b). For sake of completeness, however, it should be mentioned that although *micromolar* concentrations of acetylstrophanthidin cause an *inward* shift of holding current in voltage-clamped fibers, consistent with a reduction in steady pump current, *nanomolar* concentrations sometimes cause a small *outward* shift of holding current (Fig. 5). This is consistent with an increase in steady pump current (although alternative explanations cannot be ruled out at present) and so would seem to support other indirect evidence that low (nanomolar) concentrations of certain cardiac steroids may stimulate, rather than inhibit, the Na^+/K^+ exchange pump (see examples in DeWeer, 1970; Ghysel-Burton and Godfraind, 1975; Cohen et al., 1976; Blood, 1978).

As already mentioned, the increments in $[Na]_i$ gained during brief periods of superfusion with K^+-free fluid are expected to be increased when the durations of those periods are prolonged, so that the subsequent increments in pump current on reactivating the pump with external K^+ are likewise expected to be greater. Figure 6A shows superimposed records of current changes obtained, in the same fiber, in response to six different exposures to K^+-free fluid lasting from 15 to 180 sec, and it demonstrates that the peak amplitude of the increment in pump current increases

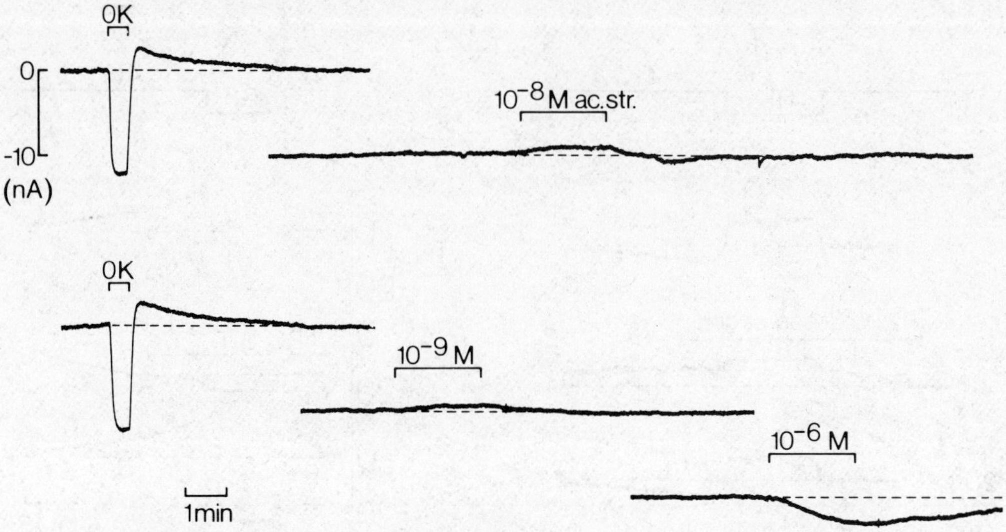

Figure 5. Net outward current shift caused by nanomolar concentrations of acetylstrophanthidin in a Purkinje fiber held at the resting potential of −33 mV in 4 mM K^+, low Cl^- solution. As usual, the two 30-sec exposures to K^+-free fluid were followed by transient increments in pump current, while the application of 1 μM acetylstrophanthidin (bottom right) caused a net inward current shift due to reduction of background pump current. One of several possible explanations for the small outward current shifts is that nanomolar concentrations of acetylstrophanthidin may stimulate, rather than inhibit, the Na^+/K^+ exchange pump.

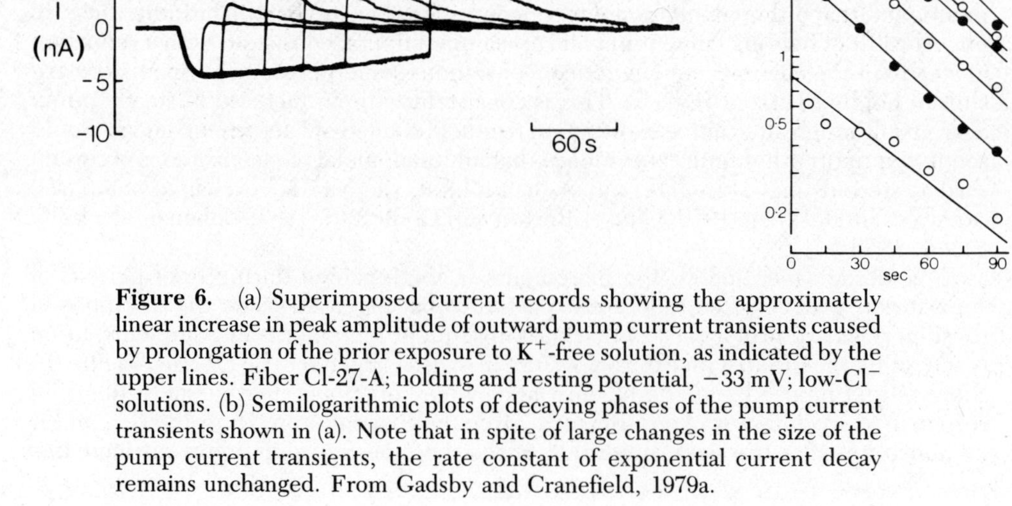

Figure 6. (a) Superimposed current records showing the approximately linear increase in peak amplitude of outward pump current transients caused by prolongation of the prior exposure to K^+-free solution, as indicated by the upper lines. Fiber Cl-27-A; holding and resting potential, −33 mV; low-Cl^- solutions. (b) Semilogarithmic plots of decaying phases of the pump current transients shown in (a). Note that in spite of large changes in the size of the pump current transients, the rate constant of exponential current decay remains unchanged. From Gadsby and Cranefield, 1979a.

approximately linearly with the duration of the exposure to zero $[K]_o$. The semilogarithmic plots of the declining phases of the outward current transients in Figure 6B reveal that the pump current increments decay with exponential time courses, and that the time constant of decay remains approximately constant, in spite of large changes in the size of the pump-current increment and, hence, of the increment in $[Na]_i$. In contrast to that independence of the time constant from the level of intracellular Na^+, however, the time constant for pump current decay changes markedly when extracellular K^+ concentration is altered: it is diminished slightly as $[K]_o$ is raised above 4 mM, and is greatly increased as $[K]_o$ is lowered below 4 mM. The $[K]_o$-dependence of the reciprocal of the time constant, that is, the rate constant for pump current decay, is illustrated in Figure 7. It appears that in canine cardiac Purkinje cells the pump rate constant is activated by external K^+ according to simple, Michaelis-Menten kinetics, with half-maximal activation occurring at 1 mM $[K]_o$.

Having demonstrated that moderate changes in the rate of Na^+/K^+ exchange can readily be induced in small Purkinje fibers, and that such changes cause measurable alterations in net membrane current and membrane potential of quiescent preparations, it was of considerable interest to investigate the effects of changes in pump rate on the electrical activity of beating fibers. Vassalle (1970) had already shown that spontaneous action potentials were temporarily abolished in cardiac Purkinje fibers following brief periods of "overdrive" (drive at rates higher than the prevailing spontaneous rate) due to the temporary stimulation of the Na^+/K^+ pump resulting from the extra Na^+ influx during the rapid drive. Figure 8, A and B, similarly, show that spontaneous action potentials arising from either the high level of resting potential (Fig. 8A), or the low level of resting potential (slow response action potentials, Fig. 8B), are temporarily abolished on returning to K^+-containing solution following brief periods of exposure to K^+-free fluid. In either case, when spontaneous action potentials reappear they do so at a rate which is initially reduced, but which gradually returns to the steady control rate. Figure 8C shows that under appropriate conditions, the increment in pump current may be large enough to cause a permanent shift of the membrane potential, from the region where spontaneous slow response action potentials are generated to a level at which the fiber remains quiescent (compare with Fig. 2B).

However, the effects of electrogenic Na^+ extrusion on the *shape* of the cardiac action potential are most easily studied in regularly stimulated fibers, because the changes in rate induced in spontaneously active fibers may themselves be expected to have some influence on action potential shape (e.g. Vick, 1971; Hauswirth et al., 1972; Boyett and Jewell, 1980). Figure 9 shows that in a Purkinje fiber driven at a rate of 1.2 Hz, a 6-min exposure to K^+-free fluid caused, on returning to K^+-containing solution, a transient reduction in action potential duration, accompanied by a temporary increase in diastolic potential. The action potentials shown below the graph were photographed at different times before and after the Na^+-loading period. Their durations, normalized with respect to the steady control duration before exposure to zero $[K]_o$, are indicated in the graph by hollow symbols: at the bottom left, the control action potential before Na^+-loading is shown superimposed on the one recorded 60 sec after returning to 4 mM $[K]_o$, and at the right, that action potential recorded after 60 sec is superimposed on those obtained after 90, 140, and 350 sec of recovery at 4 mM $[K]_o$. The points of present interest are that a brief period of exposure to K^+-free fluid is followed, on return to K^+-containing solution, by a temporary hyperpolarization during diastole, a slight reduction in plateau amplitude, and a marked reduction in plateau duration, all presumably caused by a temporary increase in sodium pump current. Moreover, the diastolic potential and action potentials gradually recover their control characteristics over a similar period of time, presumably the time required for elimination of the increment in $[Na]_i$.

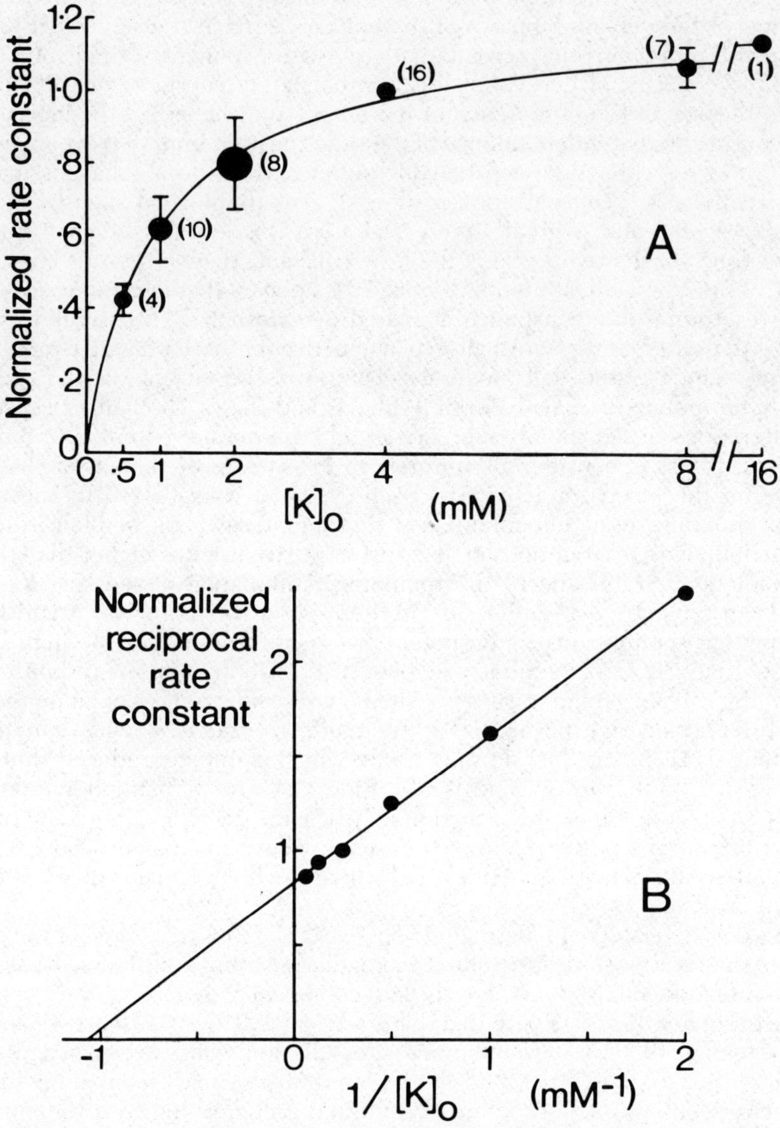

Figure 7. $[K]_o$-dependence of the rate constant for decay of the increments in pump current induced by brief exposures to K^+-free fluid of varying duration. A, Mean normalized rate constants (normalized to the average value at 4 mM $[K]_o$) are shown by circles whose diameters are equal to 2 × SEM; the vertical bars indicate ± SD, and the numbers in parentheses give the number of experiments contributing to each mean. The smooth curve is a hyperbolic function, saturating at a normalized rate constant of 1.20 and half-maximal at $[K]_o$ = 0.94 mM. B, Double-reciprocal, Lineweaver-Burk plot of mean data in A, fitted by a least-squares regression line (coefficient of determination, 0.999), from which the parameters used to construct the curve in A were determined. From Gadsby, 1980.

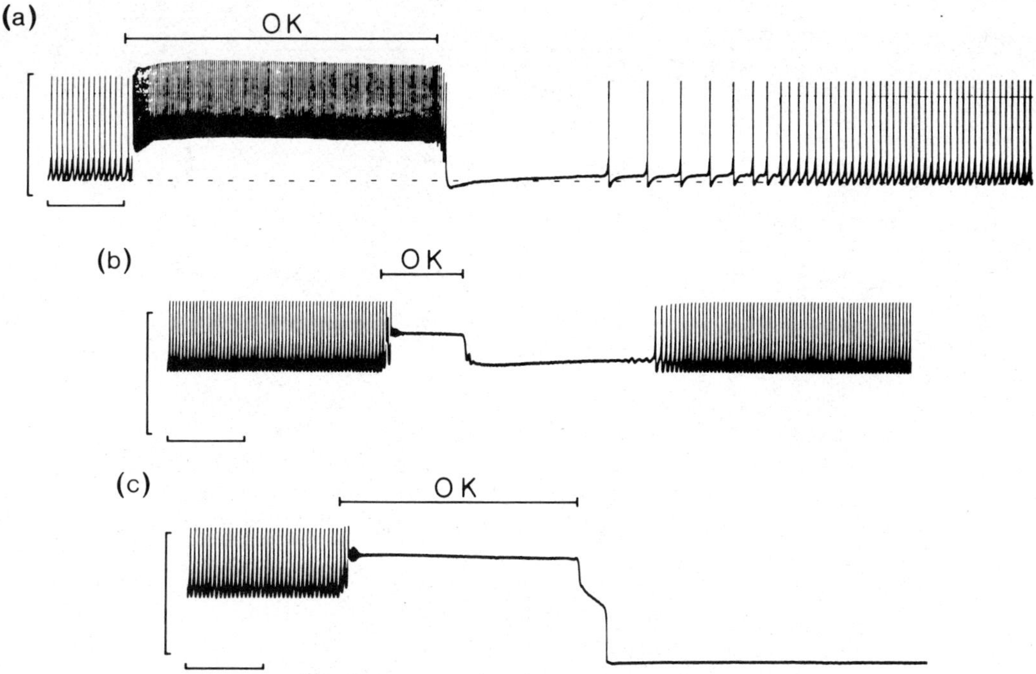

Figure 8. Effects of a temporary increase in pump rate, following brief exposures to K^+-free fluid, on action potentials arising from either the higher (a) or the lower (b and c) level of membrane potential, in spontaneously beating Purkinje fibers. The horizontal bars above the chart recordings mark the exposures to K^+-free solution; the vertical calibration bars represent 100 mV, and their upper ends indicate the zero reference potential; the horizontal calibrations are 30 sec. (a) Effects on "normal" automaticity in 4 mM K^+, Cl^--containing Tyrode's solution. The dashed line indicates the steady, control level of maximum diastolic potential, −87 mV. (b) and (c) Effects on spontaneous, slow response, action potentials in a different fiber exposed to low-Cl^- solutions; $[K]_o$ was 2 mM in (b) and 2.5 mM in (c). From Gadsby and Cranefield, 1979b, with permission of the *Journal of General Physiology*.

To establish that the transient increment in pump current is of sufficient magnitude to account for the observed, marked shortening of the action potential, however, it is necessary to measure, in the same fiber, both action potential shortening and increment in pump current caused by a given exposure to K^+-free fluid. Some results from an experiment of this kind are presented in Figures 10 and 11. The upper line in Figure 10 indicates the timing of the changes in K^+ concentration, which in this instance were between zero and 6 mM. The chart recording shows the changes in membrane potential of a small Purkinje fiber already impaled by two microelectrodes and driven at a rate of 1 Hz via external stimulating electrodes. During the 2-min exposure to K^+-free fluid, the fiber depolarized and was not excited by the extracellular stimuli. But on switching back to 6 mM $[K]_o$, the diastolic potential was temporarily increased, and the action potential duration was temporarily reduced. The storage oscilloscope photograph at the lower left shows a shortened action potential arising from an increased diastolic potential, obtained about 15 sec after switching back to 6

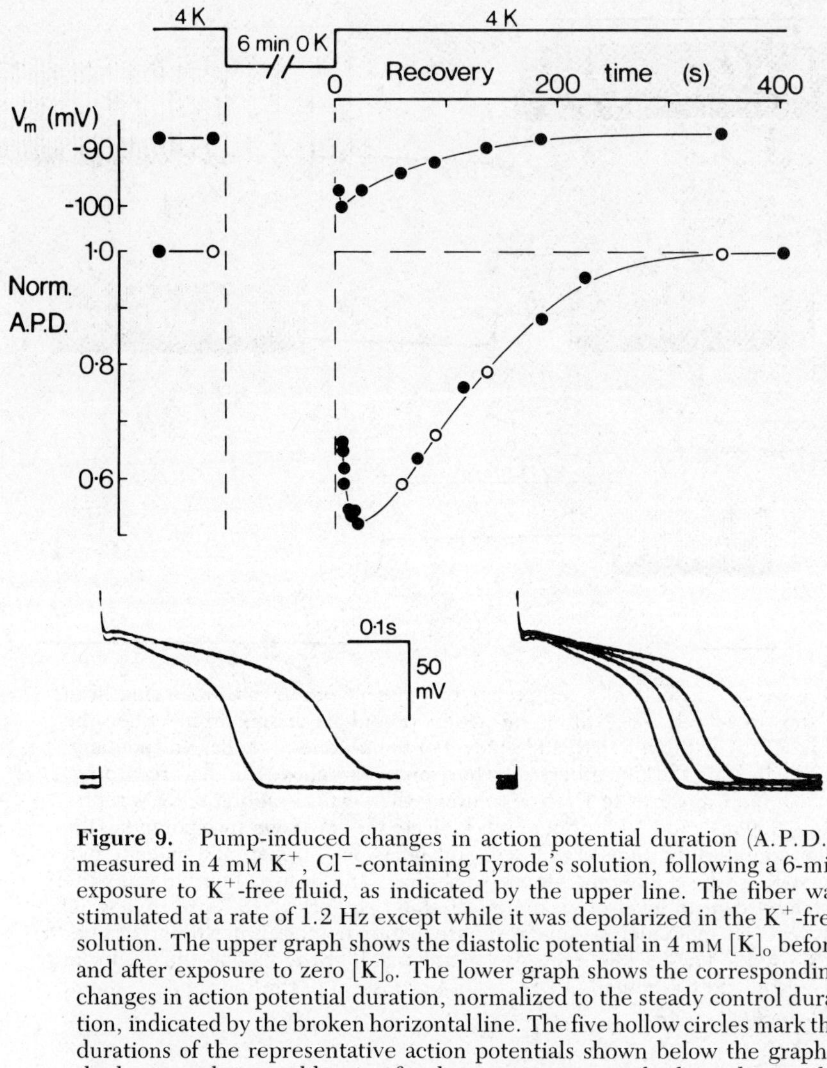

Figure 9. Pump-induced changes in action potential duration (A.P.D.), measured in 4 mM K^+, Cl^--containing Tyrode's solution, following a 6-min exposure to K^+-free fluid, as indicated by the upper line. The fiber was stimulated at a rate of 1.2 Hz except while it was depolarized in the K^+-free solution. The upper graph shows the diastolic potential in 4 mM $[K]_o$ before and after exposure to zero $[K]_o$. The lower graph shows the corresponding changes in action potential duration, normalized to the steady control duration, indicated by the broken horizontal line. The five hollow circles mark the durations of the representative action potentials shown below the graphs; the horizontal time calibration for these action potentials also indicates the zero reference potential. The shortening of the action potential caused by enhanced pump activity is associated with significant hyperpolarization of the resting membrane. Fiber Bl-20-A. From Gadsby and Cranefield, 1979b, with permission of the *Journal of General Physiology*.

mM K^+ solution, and superimposed on it is a longer control action potential recorded 10 min after the switch to 6 mM $[K]_o$, when the diastolic potential had returned to its steady control level. A few minutes later, the action potentials at the lower right were photographed, still in the presence of 6 mM $[K]_o$: the longer action potential is another control action potential, identical to the one in the left-hand photograph, and it is superimposed on an action potential shortened by injection of a steady, 12-nA hyperpolarizing current through the second intracellular microelectrode. It is apparent that injecting that time- and voltage-independent current caused both an increase in the diastolic potential and a shortening of the action potential closely similar in

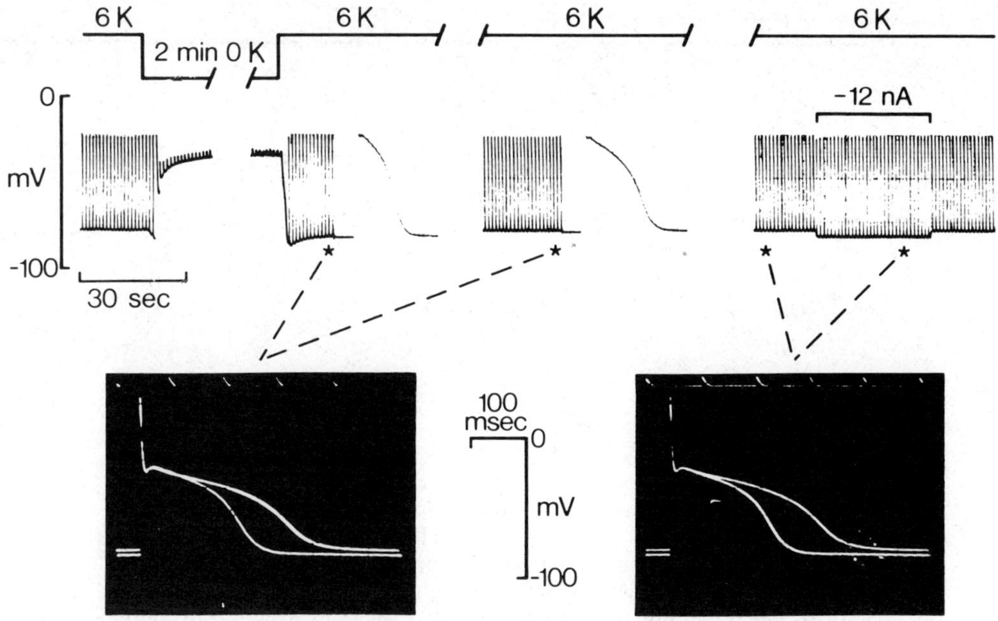

Figure 10. Action potential shortening and membrane hyperpolarization caused either by enhanced pump activity or by current injection in a Purkinje fiber impaled by two microelectrodes, exposed to 6 mM K^+, Cl^--containing solution, and driven at a rate of 1 Hz. The upper line indicates the timing of the 2-min exposure to K^+-free fluid, and also marks the three points of omission of sections of record of duration 90 sec, 10 min, and 3 min, respectively. Because of the poor frequency response of the pen, the action potential upstrokes are not seen in the chart recording, but the two high-speed chart records (for which the time calibration bar represents 500 msec) clearly show the temporary reduction in action potential duration following exposure to zero $[K]_o$. The asterisks under the chart record indicate the action potentials superimposed in the two storage oscilloscope photographs below. Note that both the action potential shortening and hyperpolarization caused by enhanced pump activity are closely approximated by injection of a steady (i.e. time- and voltage-independent), 12 nA hyperpolarizing current (indicated by bar over chart record). Fiber D7-12-D.

magnitude to those caused by the enhanced pump activity after 2 min of Na^+ loading. The current record in Figure 11 (middle trace) obtained later in the same fiber, shows that when the voltage-clamp amplifier was switched on a few seconds after raising $[K]_o$ to 6 mM, following a 2-min period of exposure to K^+-free fluid, a typical, exponentially decaying, increment in pump current was observed. More important, the amplitude of the decaying current was about 10 nA, in other words quite appropriate to account for the pump-induced changes in the action potential and diastolic potential illustrated in Figure 10.

In the experiments described so far, the technique for raising $[Na]_i$, in order to temporarily stimulate the Na^+/K^+ pump, was to *reduce* pumped *Na^+ efflux* by slowing the pump by removal of external K^+. An alternative method for raising $[Na]_i$ is to *increase Na^+ influx*, and this is readily accomplished in driven preparations simply by increasing the drive rate. As already mentioned, this technique was used by Vas-

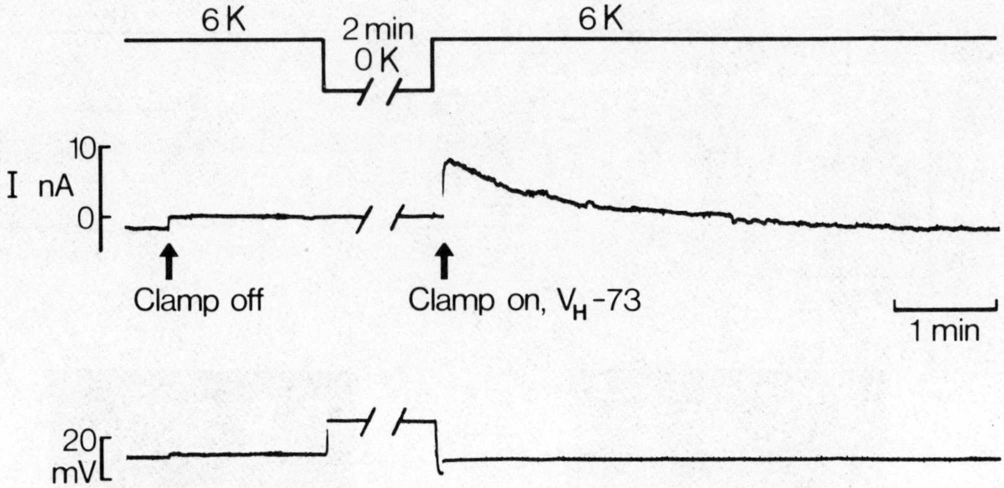

Figure 11. Direct measurement of increment in pump current on reactivation of the Na^+/K^+ pump with 6 mM K^+ solution following a 2-min exposure to K^+-free fluid, in the experiment of Fig. 10. The records in this figure were obtained from the same fiber, but 150 min later than those in Fig. 10. The upper line indicates the timing of the $[K]_o$ changes, the middle trace shows applied current, and the bottom trace shows membrane potential. At the first arrow the clamp was switched off to allow the fiber to depolarize in K+-free fluid as in Fig. 10 (in this case, the depolarization was off-scale, see bottom trace). The clamp was switched on again shortly after returning to 6 mM $[K]_o$ (second arrow) to record the slowly decaying increment in pump current, about 10 nA in total amplitude. Cl^--containing solutions throughout.

salle (1970) to demonstrate the effects of a temporary increase in the rate of electrogenic Na^+ extrusion on spontaneous action potentials in Purkinje fibers. The aftereffects of a brief period of rapid drive (labeled "overdrive" for convenience) on the shape of action potentials elicited at a relatively low basal drive rate are shown in Figure 12. The continuous chart recording in Figure 12A indicates the experimental protocol and shows the membrane potential changes (action potential upstrokes are truncated due to the inadequate frequency response of the pen) before, during, and after a 1-min period of rapid drive (2 Hz) in a fiber driven at a basal rate of 0.67 Hz. Immediately following the "overdrive," the action potential recorded after the first, longer, stimulus interval (1.5 sec) had a duration that was 80% of the control, steady-state duration at that rate (not shown). The graph in Figure 12B illustrates the time course for recovery of the duration of the action-potential at a drive rate of 0.67 Hz, in a different fiber, following a 2-min period of rapid drive at 2 Hz. The action potential duration, normalized to the control value before the "overdrive," was initially shortened to almost 70% of the control duration, and then recovered along an approximately exponential time course with a half-time of about 70 sec. The inset shows the shortened action potential, recorded 25 sec after termination of the "overdrive," superimposed on that recorded some 9 min later when the control duration had been regained; the shortening of the action potential is seen to be accompanied by a small increase in the diastolic potential, and both effects are presumably attributable to a temporary increase in pump current.

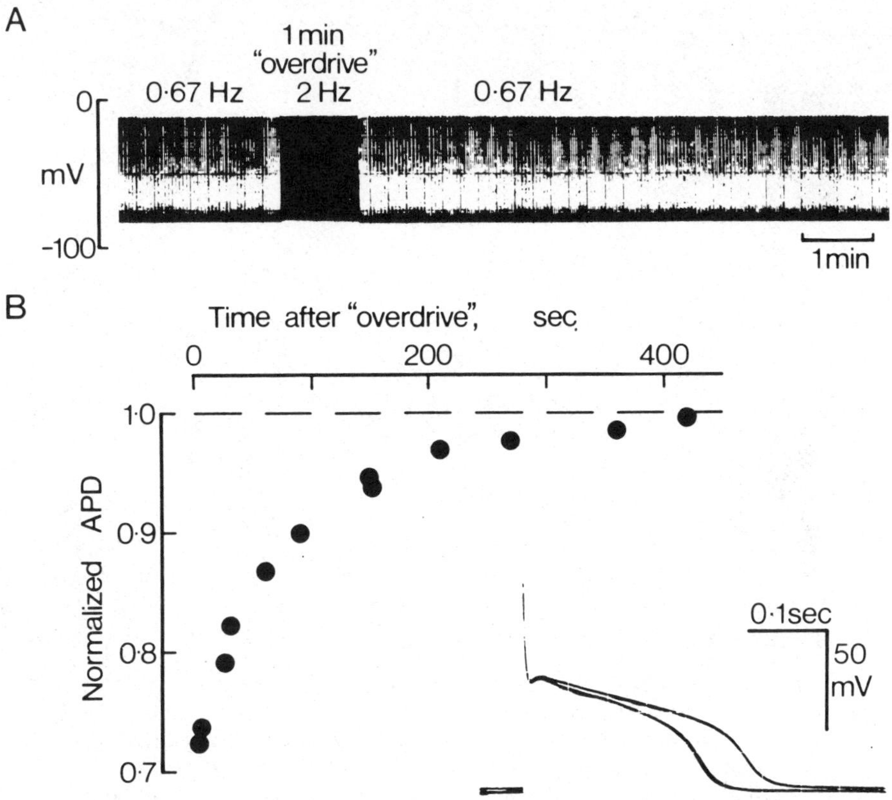

Figure 12. After-effects of brief periods of rapid drive (labeled "overdrive") on Purkinje fiber action potentials elicited at a relatively low rate in 6 mM K^+, Cl^--containing solution. A, Continuous chart recording of action potentials before, during, and after a 1-min period of overdrive. Fiber D6-25-B. B, Time course of recovery of action potential duration (normalized to the steady, control duration), in another Purkinje fiber, after a 2-min period of rapid drive: as in A, the basal drive rate was 0.67 Hz and the "overdrive" rate was 2 Hz. The inset shows two action potentials from this experiment, superimposed: the longer action potential illustrates the control shape and was photographed 9 min after the rapid drive, while the shorter action potential arising from the more negative diastolic potential was recorded just 25 sec after termination of the "overdrive." The upper end of the voltage calibration marks the zero reference potential. Fiber D6-21-C.

The small, slowly decaying, hyperpolarization that follows termination of a period of rapid drive is shown in the high-gain recording of Figure 13B, and the semilogarithmic plot of that potential change in the graph at the right (Fig. 13C) reveals that the membrane potential declined exponentially with a half-time of about 90 sec. Later during the same experiment, the voltage-clamp amplifier was switched on after termination of a 2-min period of rapid drive, in order to record the current changes responsible for the kind of transient hyperpolarization shown in Figure 13B. The current record in Figure 13A shows that cessation of the drive was followed by a slowly decaying net outward current (measured at a voltage close to the steady-state resting potential). Furthermore, as seen in the upper semilogarithmic plot in Figure

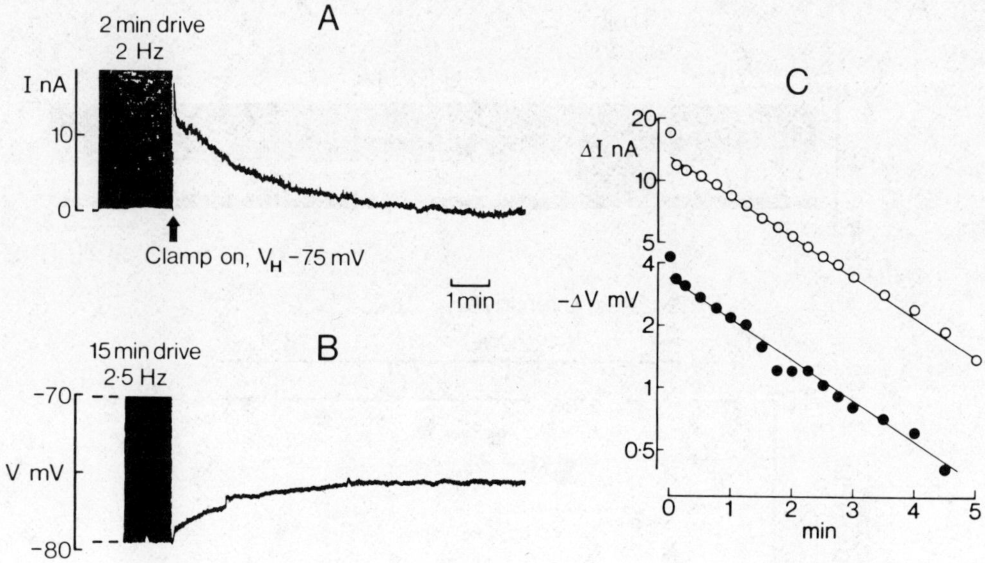

Figure 13. The post-drive hyperpolarization, and net outward current measured under voltage clamp, both decay with similar exponential time course. Panel B shows a high gain record of the decline in membrane potential, following termination of a 15-min period of stimulation at 2.5 Hz, in a small Purkinje fiber already impaled with two microelectrodes (at such gain most of the action potential is off-scale): a small rapid depolarization within the first 5–10 sec is followed by a larger, slower depolarization. The current changes in panel A were recorded in the same fiber, about 45 min later; when the voltage clamp was switched on after 2 min of stimulation at 2 Hz, a rapid decline in net outward current was followed by a much slower decline. The semilogarithmic plots in C show that membrane current (from A) and membrane potential (from B) both decline with similar exponential time courses (half-times of 94 sec, and 93 sec, respectively). Fiber D6-12-D; 6 mM K^+, Cl^--containing solution throughout; the time calibration is common to panels A and B.

13C, that outward current decayed with the same exponential time course as did the temporary hyperpolarization illustrated in Figure 13B. These results strongly suggest that the temporary reduction in action potential duration, and temporary hyperpolarization, following termination of a period of rapid drive are both caused by an exponentially decaying increment in Na^+/K^+ pump current, which itself reflects the elimination of the increment in $[Na]_i$ accumulated during the drive. This conclusion is further supported by the results of the experiment shown in Figure 14. Figure 14A shows the increment in pump current recorded in a voltage-clamped Purkinje fiber after a brief period of exposure to K^+-free fluid, and Figure 14B shows the slowly decaying outward current recorded, in the same fiber, following a period of rapid drive. Both of these decaying outward currents are shown in the semilogarithmic plots of Figure 14C, which demonstrate clearly that not only do both current increments decay exponentially, but that they do so with the same half-time, in this instance 82 sec.

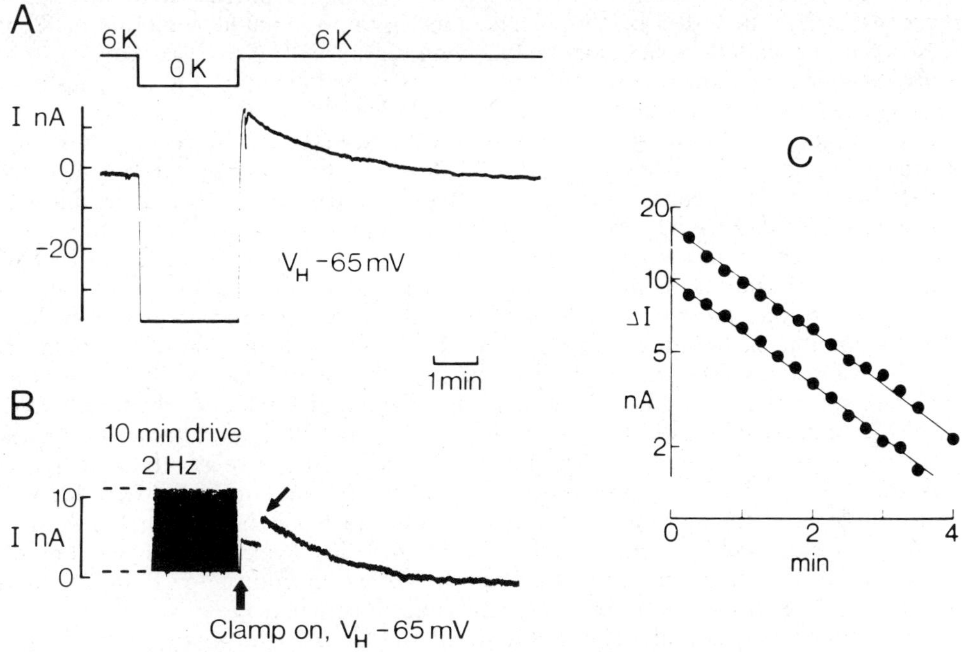

Figure 14. The slowly decaying net outward currents which follow a period of rapid drive or a brief exposure to K^+-free fluid decline with the same exponential time course. At the vertical arrow in panel B, the voltage clamp was switched on after 10 min of stimulation at 2 Hz; the diagonal arrow marks where the gain was doubled to correspond to the scale at the left. The current record in panel A begins 2 min after the end of the record in B and shows the usual, slowly decaying, increment in pump current following a 135-sec exposure to zero $[K]_o$ (the peak inward current in K^+-free fluid was off-scale). The parallel straight lines in panel C were fitted by eye to the semilogarithmic plots of the declining outward currents shown in panels A and B. Fiber D6-25-A; Cl^--containing solutions throughout; the time calibration applies to both A and B.

DISCUSSION

The results presented in this article demonstrate that, using suitably small cardiac preparations in combination with a fast-flow system, one can readily induce changes in sodium pump activity and follow the resulting changes in the resting potentials of quiescent preparations, or in the action potentials of spontaneously active or electrically stimulated preparations. Moreover, by using a two-microelectrode voltage clamp, the underlying changes in sodium pump current can be measured directly, and systematic analysis of pump current transients recorded under various conditions has allowed the Na^+/K^+ exchange pump in Purkinje cells to be characterized in some detail: thus, it appears that both the Na^+:K^+ coupling ratio of the pump and the rate constant for Na^+ extrusion remain constant, in spite of estimated increases in $[Na]_i$ of up to four- or five-fold. The coupling ratio is also unaffected by changes in $[K]_o$, whereas the rate constant for Na^+ extrusion is a saturable function of $[K]_o$ and is half-maximal at 1 mM $[K]_o$ (Gadsby and Cranefield, 1979a; Gadsby, 1980; cf. Eisner and Lederer, 1980). It seems unlikely that the pump current transients presented here are grossly distorted by the effects of any pump-mediated depletion of K^+ in restricted extracellular spaces for the following reasons: *(1)* Care was taken to study only the smaller preparations, containing few cells (indicated by the low amplitude of recorded current changes), so that extracellular diffusion distances were minimized. *(2)* The fast-flow system permitted investigation of the effects of rather small changes in pump rate, for example, those following only 1 or 2 min of Na^+-loading, so that any resulting concentration differences set up across extracellular diffusion barriers should also have been small. *(3)* If these finding were to be limited by extracellular K^+ depletion, then 1 mM would necessarily be an overestimate for the half-maximally-activating concentration of external K^+ and, because the "true" value of that concentration must be greater than zero, 1 mM also represents an upper limit for the amount of depletion accompanying half-maximal activation of the pump in these experiments (Deitmer and Ellis, 1978; Eisner and Lederer, 1980). *(4)* Preliminary morphologic studies (Eisenberg and Cohen, 1981; T.D. Pham and D.C. Gadsby, unpublished) indicate that in the small canine Purkinje fibers used for the experiments reported here, a large fraction of the cells face relatively wide spaces (on the order of 1 μm) as previously reported for rabbit Purkinje fibers (Johnson and Sommer, 1967) in which K^+ depletion currents during voltage-clamp hyperpolarizations are known to be small (Colatsky and Tsien, 1979). Preliminary measurements suggest that K^+ depletion currents are similarly small in thin canine Purkinje fibers (Cohen, Falk & Kline, 1979; D.C. Gadsby, unpublished).

The demonstration of a significant "background" or steady-state component of pump current, even in resting fibers, has important consequences for interpretation of net current changes in some voltage-clamp experiments on cardiac cells. Thus, although no marked voltage dependence of the pump current has been found (Isenberg and Trautwein, 1974), the amplitude of the steady pump current *is* expected to be a virtually instantaneous function of $[Na]_i$ and of $[K]_o$. Therefore, if changes in either of those concentrations result from voltage-clamp interventions, then allowance must be made for the concomitant modifications of pump current before any further analysis of the net changes in membrane current can be made.

Isenberg and Trautwein (1974) have shown that the steady-state pump current makes an important contribution to repolarization of the normal Purkinje fiber action potential, and this is confirmed by the experiments presented here. Those authors found that the initial effect of application of a fast-acting cardiac steroid was an inward shift of the holding current in voltage-clamped fibers (cf. Fig. 4B, above) and an increase in action potential duration in regularly stimulated fibers (Isenberg and Trautwein, 1974), both reflecting a reduction in steady-state pump current. We have shown here that a temporary increase in pump current causes a transient reduction in action potential duration, and that the time course and amplitude of the changes in pump current are appropriate to account for the observed alterations in action potential shape (see Figs. 9 to 14). It seems likely that some other well-known changes in action potential duration, for example, those resulting from modifications in the stimulation rate or in external K^+ concentration, might also be due, at least in part, to changes in the size of the pump current. Thus, an increase in drive rate is associated with a maintained reduction in action potential duration (for review, see Carmeliet, 1977) to which an increase in pump current, caused by a rise in $[Na]_i$, probably contributes. On the other hand, experimental reduction of $[K]_o$ is associated with prolongation of the Purkinje fiber action potential (e.g. Vassalle, 1965; Noble, 1965), which may be partly attributable to diminution of pump current due to reduction of the rate constant for Na^+ extrusion, based on the results illustrated in Figure 7. That observed $[K]_o$-dependence of Na^+ extrusion means that the pump rate constant is essentially maximal at a normal serum K^+ concentration of 4 to 5 mM, so that in the normal in situ heart the rate of electrogenic Na^+ extrusion is regulated almost entirely by variations in $[Na]_i$ (cf. Glitsch et al., 1976; Gadsby, 1980).

Since the component of net membrane current generated directly by the Na^+/K^+ exchange pump can clearly have a major influence on the resting or diastolic potential, on the amplitude and duration of the action potential plateau, on the rate of automaticity of cardiac Purkinje fibers, and on abnormal forms of rhythmic activity, it will be of considerable interest now to investigate the effects of, for example, various cardioactive drugs, ischemia, or anoxia, on pump function in order to aid our understanding of their effects on the electrical activity of the heart.

REFERENCES

Adrian RH (1965) Discussion, in: Symposium on physical and mathematical approaches to the study of the electrical behavior of excitable membranes. J Cell Comp Physiol **66** (suppl 2): 133–135

Baker PF, Blaustein MP, Hodgkin AL, Steinhardt RA (1969) The influence of calcium on sodium efflux in squid axons. J Physiol (Lond) **200**:431–458

Blood BE (1978) Glycoside induced stimulation of membrane Na-K ATPase—fact or artifact? *In* Biophysical Aspects of Cardiac Muscle, M. Morad (editor). New York, Academic Press, pp 379–389

Boyett MR, Jewell BR (1980) Analysis of the effects of changes in rate and rhythm upon electrical activity in the heart. Prog Biophys Molec Biol **36**:1–52

Carmeliet EE (1977) Repolarization and frequency in cardiac cells. J Physiol (Paris) **73**:903–923

Chapman RA (1979) Excitation-contraction coupling in cardiac muscle. Prog Biophys Molec Biol **35**:1–52

Cohen I, Daut J, Noble D (1976) An analysis of the actions of low concentrations of ouabain on membrane currents in Purkinje fibers. J Physiol (Lond) **260**:75–103

Cohen I, Falk R, Kline RP (1979) Voltage-clamp studies on the canine Purkinje fibre. J Physiol (Lond) **296**:72P

Colatsky TJ, Tsien RW (1979) Electrical properties associated with wide intercellular clefts in rabbit Purkinje fibres. J Physiol (Lond) **290**:227–252

Deitmer JW, Ellis D (1978) The intracellular sodium activity of cardiac Purkinje fibres during inhibition and re-activation of the Na-K pump. J Physiol (Lond) **284**:241–259

DeWeer P (1970) Effects of intracellular adenosine-5′-diphosphate and orthophosphate on the sensitivity of sodium efflux from squid axon to external sodium and potassium. J Gen Physiol **56**:583–620

Eisenberg BR, Cohen IS (1981) Morphometric analysis of dog Purkinje strands. Biophys J **33**:35a

Eisner DA, Lederer WJ (1980) Characterization of the electrogenic sodium pump in cardiac Purkinje fibres. J Physiol (Lond) **303**:441–474

Eisner DA, Lederer WJ, Vaughan-Jones RD (1980) Electrogenic Na pumping in cardiac muscle: simultaneous measurement of intracellular Na activity, membrane current and tension. J Physiol (Lond) **300**:42P

Ellis D (1977) The effects of external cations and ouabain on the intracellular sodium activity of sheep heart Purkinje fibers. J Physiol (Lond) **273**:211–240

Gadsby DC (1980) Activation of electrogenic Na^+/K^+ exchange by extracellular K^+ in canine cardiac Purkinje fibers. Proc Natl Acad Sci USA **77**:4035–4039

Gadsby DC, Cranefield PF (1977) Two levels of resting potential in cardiac Purkinje fibers. J Gen Physiol **70**:725–746

Gadsby DC, Cranefield PF (1979a) Direct measurement of changes in sodium pump current in canine cardiac Purkinje fibers. Proc Natl Acad Sci USA **76**:1783–1787

Gadsby DC, Cranefield PF (1979b) Electrogenic sodium extrusion in cardiac Purkinje fibers. J Gen Physiol **73**:819–837

Ghysel-Burton J, Godfraind T (1975) Stimulation and inhibition by ouabain of the sodium pump in guinea-pig atria. Br J Pharmac **55**:249

Glitsch HG (1979) Characteristics of active Na transport in intact cardiac cells. Am J Physiol **236**:H189–H199

Glitsch HG, Pusch H, Venetz K (1976) Effects of Na and K ions on the active Na transport in guinea-pig auricles. Pflüg Arch **365**:29–36

Glitsch HG, Reuter H, Scholz H (1970) The effect of the internal sodium concentration on calcium fluxes in isolated guinea-pig auricles. J Physiol (Lond) **209**:25–43

Hauswirth O, Noble D, Tsien RW (1972) The dependence of plateau currents in cardiac Purkinje fibres on the interval between action potentials. J Physiol (Lond) **222**:27–49

Hodgkin AL, Horowicz P (1959) The influence of potassium and chloride ions on the membrane potential of single muscle fibres. J Physiol (Lond) **148**:127–160

Isenberg G (1977) Cardiac Purkinje fibres. $[Ca^{2+}]_i$ controls steady state potassium conductance. Pflüg Arch **371**:71–76

Isenberg G, Trautwein W (1974) The effect of dihydro-ouabain and lithium-ions on the outward current in cardiac Purkinje fibers; evidence for electrogenicity of active transport. Pflüg Arch **35**:41–54

Johnson EA, Sommer JR (1967) A strand of cardiac muscle: its ultrastructure and the electrophysiological implications of its geometry. J Cell Biol **33**:103–129

Marban E, Tsien RW (1979) Ouabain increases the slow inward calcium current in ventricular muscle of the ferret. J Physiol (Lond) **292**:72P–73P

Mullins LJ (1979) The generation of electric currents in cardiac fibers by Na/Ca exchange. Am J Physiol **236**:C103–C110

Noble D (1965) Electrical properties of cardiac muscle attributable to inward-going (anomalous) rectification. J Cell Comp Physiol **66** (suppl 2):127–135

Siegelbaum SA, Tsien RW (1980) Calcium-activated transient outward current in calf cardiac Purkinje fibres. J Physiol (Lond) **299**:485–506

Sommer JR, Johnson EA (1968) Cardiac muscle: a comparative study of Purkinje fibers and ventricular fibers. J Cell Biol **36**:497–526

Vassalle M (1965) Cardiac pacemaker potentials at different extra- and intracellular K concentrations. Am J Physiol **208**:770–775

Vassalle M (1970) Electrogenic suppression of automaticity in sheep and dog Purkinje fibers. Circ Res **27**:361–377

Vick RL (1971) Action potential duration in canine Purkinje tissue: effects of preceding excitation. J Electrocardiol **4**:105–115

Discussion

HOFFMAN: I wonder if the single exponential at very short times after rapid pacing provides evidence that clefts in your preparation are well stirred, with the result that potassium accumulation does not appreciably disturb the beginning of your curve?

GADSBY: Richard Kline and Ira Cohen (Nature **286**:68, 1980) have measured the extracellular potassium changes upon rapid pacing. They show that potassium concentration in the clefts initially rises but subsequently declines to a steady-state level close to the bath concentration. This occurs as long as the sodium pump is able to cope with the increased sodium load associated with the rapid drive, so that at the end of the drive, the sodium and potassium fluxes are again in balance, and the potassium concentration in the clefts is the same as before the drive. On the other hand, on stopping the drive it is possible to see temporary depletion of cleft potassium in larger fibers due to enhanced potassium uptake by the sodium pump. In that case, because the rate constant of exponential decay of the pump current is very sensitive to external potassium concentration at values below 4 mM one would expect an initial flattening of the decay of pump current, which would then approach the correct slope as the net potassium influx declines toward zero. For this reason, I have more confidence in the final portion than I do in the initial portion of the exponential, although as you point out the fit is reasonable even at relatively short times.

FOZZARD: We tried to reproduce your experiments on action potential durations after exposure of dog Purkinje fibers to potassium-free solutions, and initially we obtained simply the opposite results. Of course, we ascribed that to the initial potassium depletion in the clefts after restoring potassium. Then we selected very small fibers of the sort you described and could reproduce your data. Therefore, if one wants to reproduce David Gadsby's experiments, one must find these small fibers. Larger Purkinje fibers in the dog will probably have cleft compartments that are not thoroughly mixed, and therefore will not reproduce the results that have been narrated here. Now, if one admits that one has the pure pump current in the measurements, it should be possible to integrate over the time and find out what is the change in the sodium concentration inside, making simple assumptions as to the volume of your tissue. So we should be able to estimate how much the sodium inside has changed under the low potassium or rapid drive conditions that you used. Have you done that?

GADSBY: We can certainly integrate under the current records. But, I am not at all comfortable about making estimates of either intracellular or extracellular volumes in these small Purkinje fibers. I think we must extract more morphologic information before attempting this. On the other hand, we have made a very simple analysis of the pump-current changes induced in resting preparations by taking away and then restoring extracellular potassium. It appears that the intracellular sodium concentration is determined only by the pump rate and the passive sodium influx. One can then predict that if the pump is switched off entirely, the time taken for the internal sodium concentration to double is equal to the time constant of the sodium pump, which in our experiments is on the order of 1.5 min.

C. COHEN: This is a followup to the question that Harry Fozzard asked. Using the data that you have presented today and the model that you have published (Proc Natl Acad Sci **77**:4035, 1980), what is the predicted increase in intracellular sodium resulting from repetitive stimulation? I am concerned about the size of the predicted increase because your model predicted a larger increase in intracellular sodium due to potassium-free solutions than has been found by Ellis (J Physiol **273**:211, 1977) or by Eisner et al (J Physiol **300**:42P, 1980).

GADSBY: With stimulation experiments I was measuring currents of about 10 nA amplitude and these do not necessarily require large increases in intracellular sodium concentration. In fact, if one makes the calculation you suggest for the Purkinje fiber of Fig. 14, by comparing the current change following the period of drive with that following the exposure to K-free solution, it appears that at the end of the 10-min period of repetitive stimulation at 2 Hz the intracellular sodium concentration was increased over its steady resting level by about 70%. Now with regard to the effects of K-free solution, the apparently divergent data of Ellis and of Eisner et al., were obtained in sheep Purkinje fibers which have very narrow extracellular clefts. It is quite clear that in these preparations a change of external solution to potassium-free does not reduce cleft potassium concentration to zero, so that the Na pump may not be switched off entirely. In other words, the results obtained with sheep Purkinje fibers during exposure to K-free solution are not necessarily comparable to ours.

I. COHEN: I would like to add that we also see these pump currents when we load the fiber with sodium using clamp pulses instead of action potentials. You can load the fiber somewhat more rapidly with this technique. When we get to very large pump currents, we can see the flattening of the initial decay that you would expect to be due to potassium depletion in the clefts, as mentioned by David Gadsby. One question I would like to ask is, in recent experiments on the TTX window current, a diffusion barrier was postulated to account for the results. Did you go back to these experiments and try to calculate what the expected accumulation of potassium should be, using the estimate for the barrier that you have? I have a feeling that the exponential decay of pump current is not actually a very sensitive measurement in the potassium range that most of us are using in these experiments.

GADSBY: On the contrary. Our analysis of the exponential decay of the sodium pump current elicited by brief exposures to potassium-free solution shows that the rate constant is an extremely sensitive function of potassium concentration below 4 mM, and is simply fitted by Michaelis-Menten kinetics with half-maximal activation occurring at 1 mM. But I should like to emphasize again that, throughout, I have tried to stick to a so-called "small signal" analysis to avoid large changes that would have to take into account a more complicated geometrical situation.

LIEBERMAN: Similar potassium-free experiments with strands of embryonic chick heart cells (20 to 30 μm, effective diameter) in the presence of chloride produces a hyperpolarization immediately after changing to potassium-free medium. Because it takes a few minutes for the preparation to depolarize in the absence of potassium, I am interested in knowing whether you have done experiments in the presence as well as in the absence of chloride.

GADSBY: All the action potential experiments I showed here were done in the presence of chloride, although the experiments shown in the initial part were done in chloride-free solutions. A brief temporary hyperpolarization lasting a few seconds was also seen in our experiments when we switched to potassium-free media, but only when the resting potential was initially at the "high level." We believe that this is because in potassium-free solution the potassium concentration in the immediate neighborhood of the membrane declines gradually over several seconds. During this change, E_K shifts in the negative direction before the decrease in potassium permeability causes the membrane to depolarize.

FOZZARD: I would like to point out that our experiments were also made in chloride-containing solutions.

REUTER: The dog Purkinje fibers, as far as I know, have another advantage over sheep Purkinje fibers: they contract a lot better. Have you tried to correlate pump stimulation or pump inhibition with the inotropic effect of acetylstrophanthidin?

GADSBY: No, we have not attempted those experiments although it would be nice to do so. It is difficult enough to work with two microelectrodes in these very small canine Purkinje fibers. For that reason, the experiments recently performed by Eisner et al., (J Physiol **300**:42P, 1980), in which they simultaneously measured membrane current, tension, and intracellular sodium in sheep Purkinje fibers, were a tremendous experimental feat.

CARMELIET: About the effects of the very small concentrations of acetylstrophanthidin you used, can you exclude effects on other membrane currents, for instance on I_{K_2}? If not, I would suggest the use of 1 mM Cs^+ or 5 mM Ba^{2+} to block the resting g_K.

GADSBY: I am not aware that a cardiac steroid like acetylstrophanthidin should affect I_{K_2}. I believe the effects observed, for example, by Cohen et al., (J Physiol *260*:75, 1976) were explained by changes in potassium concentration in the clefts of the sheep Purkinje fibers studied. Moreover, the current I_{K_2} itself is being critically reviewed at present. Also, Cs^+ most likely has more than one action, and I would wish to have a clear idea of what it does before trying those experiments.

CARMELIET: If the current that you see is due to electrogenic sodium pumping, it should be sensitive to the level at which membrane potential is set. Did you try to observe this current at different potential levels?

GADSBY: That is a very interesting question. The data produced by Isenberg and Trautwein (Pfluegers Arch **350**:41, 1974) some years ago show that within 30 sec of application of dihydro-ouabain there is a shift of the instantaneous current-voltage relationship, which is equivalent to the abolition of a voltage-independent current over the voltage range of −90 to −20 mV. Now the similarity that I showed you today of the changes in action potential shape caused by injected current or by an increment in pump current is also consistent with only a very small voltage dependence of the pump current, because the current injected from the external source was both voltage- and time-independent.

BROWN: Is there any evidence that calcium is changing inside these cells as all this is happening?

GADSBY: I would be inclined to think that intracellular calcium must be changing. But because the current increments we measure fall out so nicely according to simple prediction, it would appear that whatever calcium change occurs is too small to affect the data we obtain. Under certain conditions, however, I am able to alter the external sodium concentration in such a way as to induce current changes that are almost certainly caused by alteration of internal calcium and not simply to changes of sodium pump current.

BROWN: What I am getting at is that calcium may be acting not only on the calcium-activated potassium channel, but it may also be acting on other channels from within the membrane. For these channels, voltage profiles may be changed so the potential is not at all what you may think it is.

GADSBY: This is certainly possible. All I can say is that the current increments we study are strophanthidin-sensitive, and the data seem to fit our simple model satisfactorily.

FOZZARD: We (Sheu and Fozzard, unpublished) have made measurements of internal calcium, with a calcium electrode, in one sheep Purkinje fiber in potassium-free media. We can say that in this one experiment intracellular calcium concentration certainly changed a lot over a period of time of 2 to 3 min.

Chapter 14

The Origin of Slow Currents in Cardiac Muscle

Edward A. Johnson

Despite the controversy over the number of ionic currents that contribute to the generation of the cardiac action potential, every electrophysiologist must agree that once the crest of the action potential is reached, the net membrane current (I_m) becomes outward, so that whatever inward ionic current components exist at that time, their sum total is more than balanced by outward currents. An expectation in voltage-clamp experiments, therefore, is that after the first few milliseconds of stepping to potentials in the vicinity of the crest of the action potential I_m should be outward. In other words, if there are slow inward currents at such time, they must have inactivated or have been counterbalanced by an activated outward current, or both, such that I_m becomes outward within a few milliseconds. Whatever the composition of this net outward current, its magnitude at the potentials and times associated with repolarization of an action potential must be small, $< 1\ \mu A/cm^2$. Because the rate of change of membrane potential during repolarization is never very large, the action potential can be considered (as a first approximation) a membrane action potential, the membrane current then being equal and opposite in sign to the product of the rate of change of membrane potential and the specific membrane capacitance (see Fig. 1). This tiny outward current associated with repolarization could be the net result of relatively large inward and outward currents, the latter exceeding the former by a small amount, or it could be the result of small inward and outward currents differing by a relatively large, but same, small amount. Parenthetically, if the potassium conductance were to rectify anomalously, as is generally believed, then the magnitude of the inward component of membrane current would be reduced in proportion to the magnitude of the rectification.

The constituents of the membrane current responsible for repolarization of the cardiac action potential have been the subject of much investigation over the last 10 to 20 years, with a good deal of controversy as to the meaning and interpretation of the results. Nonetheless, it appears to be now generally (but not universally) accepted that the membrane current is composed of six or more voltage-, time-dependent ionic currents—in striking contrast to the two (Na^+ and K^+) in nerve. Putting aside for the moment the question of whether the results justify such extraordinary complexity, there is one additional component of membrane current that must be present, namely, the current generated by electrogenic active transport.

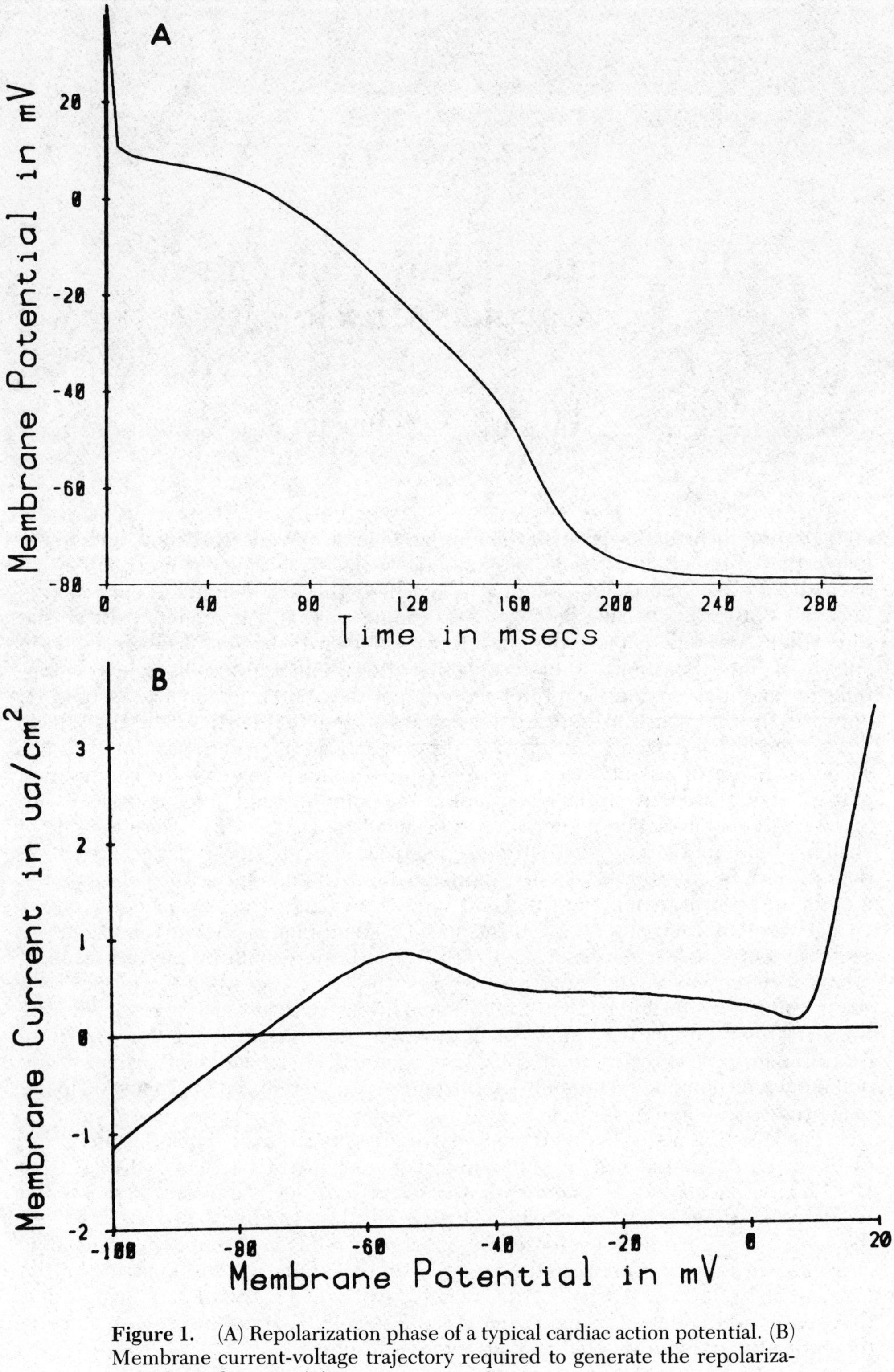

Figure 1. (A) Repolarization phase of a typical cardiac action potential. (B) Membrane current-voltage trajectory required to generate the repolarization phase shown in (A).

In a tissue that generates action potentials at a regular rate, a stationary state must eventually be reached in which the integrated passive flux of any given ion species throughout any given cardiac cycle must be exactly balanced by the integrated actively transported flux of that species during that cardiac cycle. That is to say, the ionic debt incurred in generating a cardiac action potential, however large or small, must be completely repaid by active transport within the cardiac cycle associated with that action potential (Chapman et al., 1979).

There is considerable evidence that active Na and K transport in cardiac muscle, as in many other tissues, is electrogenic. That is to say, there is a transport reaction, driven by the free energy available from adenosine triphosphate, such that:

$$x[Na^+]_i + y[K^+]_o + ATP \rightleftharpoons x[Na^+]_o + y[K^+]_i + ADP + P_i \qquad (1)$$

where $x \neq y$, $[Na^+]_i$, $[Na^+]_o$, $[K^+]_i$, $[K^+]_o$ are the intracellular and extracellular concentrations of sodium and potassium ions, and ATP, ADP, and P_i are the concentrations of adenosine triphosphate, adenosine diphosphate, and inorganic phosphate. Without exception, the experimental evidence indicates that in cardiac muscle, as well as in other tissues, $x > y$ (Thomas, 1972; Glynn and Karlish, 1975). The net active transport of Na^+ out and K^+ into the cell therefore generates an outward membrane current, which must add to the other passive components of membrane current. From the above stationary-state argument, it can be said that in any given cardiac cycle, the amount of charge carried by such active transport, relative to that carried by the passive flux of Na^+ and K^+, is equal to the difference between x and y. And it follows that the contribution of electrogenic pump current to I_m can be neglected only if this difference is negligibly small. The vast majority of evidence, however, suggests that this is not the case, the stoichiometric ratio of Na^+ to K^+ transport, $x{:}y$, being 3:2 (Thomas, 1972). Recalling again the stationary-state argument, the inescapable consequence of this fact is that the passive flux of Na^+ and K^+ must be in the same ratio—3:2. That is to say, in a given cardiac cycle in the stationary state, the charge transported by active transport (ϕ_p) relative to that carried by the passive flux of Na^+ (ϕ_{Na}) and K^+(ϕ_K), must be in the ratio $\phi_{Na}{:}\phi_K{:}\phi_p = 3{:}2{:}1$. A charge equal in magnitude to one half that carried by potassium or one third that of sodium cannot be judged insignificant. Moreover, because the duration of a cardiac action potential is comparable to that of an entire cardiac cycle, the instantaneous flux carried by the pump (the pump current J_p) must be comparable in magnitude to the passive ionic currents, I_{Na} and I_K.

Thus, if J_p is significant in comparison to the passive currents I_{Na} and I_K, can J_p be constant, independent of transmembrane potential and time? The answer is no, for J_p must depend on the transmembrane potential, V. For Reaction 1 to proceed to the right, that is, for the forward rate of the reaction, r_f, to exceed the backward rate, r_b (with the consequent net extrusion of Na^+ and uptake of K^+), the free energy available from the splitting of ATP ($\hat{Ç}$) must exceed the sum of that conserved in the electrochemical work performed in moving three Na^+ ions up their respective electrochemical gradient

$$3\,R\,T \ln \frac{[Na^+]_i}{[Na^+]_o} + 3\,F\,V \qquad (2)$$

plus the work performed in moving two K^+ ions up their respective electrochemical gradient

$$2\,R\,T \ln \frac{[K^+]_o}{[K^+]_i} - 2\,F\,V \qquad (3)$$

(V measured inside with respect to outside of the cell). Associated with this net forward transport will be a current, $J_p = F(r_f - r_b)$.

The electrochemical work conserved in Reaction 1 can be increased (or decreased) by increasing (decreasing) not only the chemical concentration gradients but also the electrical gradient. Imagine the resting potential of a quiescent cell in stationary state (r_f exceeding r_b by an amount that exactly balances the passive ion fluxes) to be slowly increased in the negative direction, as in a voltage-clamp experiment. A potential V_r would eventually be reached where the electrochemical work conserved by Reaction 1 would exactly balance the energy available from ATP ($\hat{Ç}$), and the reaction would come to thermodynamic equilibrium ($r_f = r_b$), the pump current declining to zero in the process:

$$\hat{Ç} = 3\,R\,T \ln \frac{[Na^+]_i}{[Na^+]_o} + 2\,R\,T \ln \frac{[K^+]_o}{[K^+]_i} + F\,V_r \tag{4}$$

which on rearranging gives

$$V_r = -\frac{R\,T}{F}\left[3 \ln \frac{[Na^+]_i}{[Na^+]_o} + 2 \ln \frac{[K^+]_o}{[K^+]_i} - \frac{\hat{Ç}}{Rt}\right] \tag{5}$$

Were the potential increased beyond this point, then the electrochemical work would exceed the energy available from ATP and $r_f < r_b$; net overall transport would then run in a backward direction to the left in reaction 1, with the generation of an *inward* pump current (and ATP). From this argument, the transport reaction must have a current-voltage relationship, one which passes through a reversal potential V_r given by Eq. 4 (Chapman and Johnson, 1978). Although the form of this current-voltage relationship is not known with certainty, it can be shown, again thermodynamically, that the forward and backward rate coefficients of Reaction 1, k_f and k_b, must be functions of membrane potential, such that

$$\frac{k_f\,(V)}{k_b\,(V)} = \exp\left(\frac{F\,V}{R\,T}\right) \tag{6}$$

Of the possible forms permitted within the boundaries of this constraint (Chapman and Johnson, 1978; Chapman et al., 1979), the one most consistent with experimental observation is one that describes a pump current that is largely independent of potential in the physiologic range of potentials, the potential dependence of reaction 1 being confined to the backward reaction with the forward rate coefficient independent of potential. Given this form for the current-voltage relationship (see Fig. 2), the exact relationship for any particular cell is, as I shall show, completely defined. For any given energy available from ATP, the reversal potential is determined by the internal and external concentrations of sodium ($[Na^+]_i$, $[NA^+]_o$) and potassium ions ($[K^+]_i$, $[K^+]_o$), respectively, through Eq. 4. In addition, the ordinate scale for the pump current for any given circumstance, for example, the resting state, is determined by the resting passive Na^+ and K^+ fluxes, because these in turn determine the active transport (and hence pump current) necessary to counterbalance them at the resting potential.

I can best demonstrate that there are no arbitrarily adjustable parameters in the definition of the pump I-V relationship by describing how the pump mechanism is combined with a system of passive permeabilities (of the minimum degree of complexity) to produce a resting membrane slope resistance and a resting transmembrane potential and action potential typical of cardiac muscle.

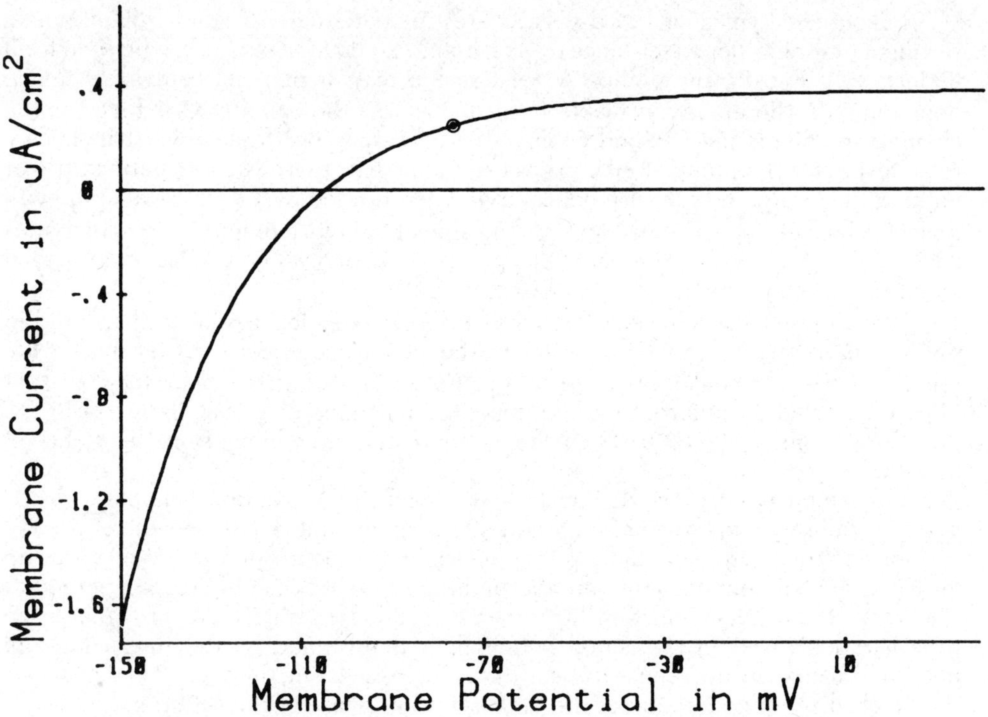

Figure 2. Form of the pump I-V relationship that was chosen as the most consistent with experimental observation: the pump acts as a constant current source over most of the physiological range of membrane potentials. The relationship plotted here is that for the quiescent cell in stationary state in Figure 3A. Circled point on the curve is the pump current for this cell at the resting potential.

I shall assume for the purpose of this demonstration that only two ionic currents are involved in the generation of the action potential, namely, sodium (I_{Na}) and potassium (I_K), these currents being governed by their respective membrane permeabilities, P_{Na} and P_K, with their respective I-V relationships obeying the constant-field equations (Goldman, 1943):

$$I_K = \frac{P_K F^2 V}{RT}\left[\frac{[K^+]_o - [K^+]_i \exp\left[\frac{FV}{RT}\right]}{\exp\left[\frac{FV}{RT}\right] - 1}\right] \tag{7}$$

and

$$I_{Na} = \frac{-P_{Na} F^2 V}{RT}\left[\frac{[Na^+]_o - [Na^+]_i \exp\left[\frac{FV}{RT}\right]}{\exp\left[\frac{FV}{RT}\right] - 1}\right] \tag{8}$$

I shall further assume, for the sake of simplicity, that P_K is a constant, independent of voltage and time, and that P_{Na} is an instantaneous function of potential only.

I choose, as typical of a cardiac cell, a resting potential of around −80 mV and a resting membrane slope resistance (r_m) of around 20,000 $\Omega \cdot cm^2$. As can be seen from its form (see Fig. 2), the pump I-V relationship may or may not contribute to r_m, depending on the energy available from ATP, $\hat{Ç}$. If the value of $\hat{Ç}$ is high, or the chemical gradients low, or both, then V_r (Eq. 4) may be so negative that the I-V relationship for the pump at −80 mV is essentially flat, thereby contributing little or nothing to r_m—r_m in such case being largely determined by P_K. For example, with typical values of ion concentrations and a value of −44 kJ/mol for $\hat{Ç}$, P_K contributes 25.2, P_{Na} contributes 132.4, and the pump contributes 277.1 $k\Omega \cdot cm^2$ to a total membrane slope resistance of 19.7 $k\Omega cm^2$.

Were I to choose a lower value for $\hat{Ç}$ or larger chemical gradients than I did in my first example, V_r would be closer to the resting potential, and the pump I-V relationship would contribute more to r_m. For example, with a value for $\hat{Ç}$ of −41 kJ/mol (and slightly different internal ion concentrations), P_K contributes 41.9; the pump, 84.9; and P_{Na}, 237.0 $k\Omega \cdot cm^2$ to a total resting membrane slope resistance of 25.1 $k\Omega \cdot cm^2$.

For the purposes of the demonstration, I shall choose the first example with a $\hat{Ç}$ of −44 kJ/mol. As can be seen from Figure 3, the quiescent cell defines the entire I-V relationship for J_p and I_K, whereas it defines only two points on the I-V relationship for Na^+: the Na^+ equilibrium potential and the value of I_{Na} at the resting potential. The rest of the I_{Na}-V relationship, or rather the I_{Na} trajectory throughout the repolarization phase of the action potential, is determined by the time course of potential change during repolarization. But before discussing this, I shall first consider the mechanism of generation of the depolarization phase of the action potential.

There is general agreement, I think, among cardiac electrophysiologists that this phase is generated by the rapid activation and subsequent inactivation of an inward sodium current, similar to that found in the squid and other large axons, as well as the frog node of Ranvier. Recent studies of this current in cardiac muscle confirm this (Colatsky and Tsien, 1979; Lee et al., 1979; Ebihara et al., 1980). Voltage-clamp analysis of this fast current in tissue-cultured embryonic chick heart cells shows that the kinetics of the current are similar, if not identical, to those of the squid axon, lending support to the idea that chick heart cells, at least, and the squid giant axon share the same kind of sodium-carrying mechanism (Ebihara et al., 1980; Ebihara and Johnson, 1980).

For various reasons, which I have no time to go into here, there is no equivalent quantitative description of the membrane current underlying the repolarization phase of the action potential. Even the separation of the membrane current into its active and passive components has not been accomplished, nor does it seem feasible at the present time. Although the magnitude and time course of the passive and active components of membrane current during the repolarization phase of the action potential are not known, we do know the I_m-V trajectory for any given action potential (as described earlier; see Fig. 1). Because I am assuming, for the sake of simplicity, that both P_{Na} and P_K are independent of time, the I_{Na}-V relationship that I require is simply the difference between the overall I_m-V relationship given by this trajectory and the sum of the J_p and I_K curves that I derived earlier from other considerations. A simple voltage dependency for P_{Na} that will generate I_{Na}-V relationships of this form is an exponential increase on depolarization to some maximum value. That is to say,

$$P_{Na} = \bar{P}_{Na} \cdot f(V) \tag{9}$$

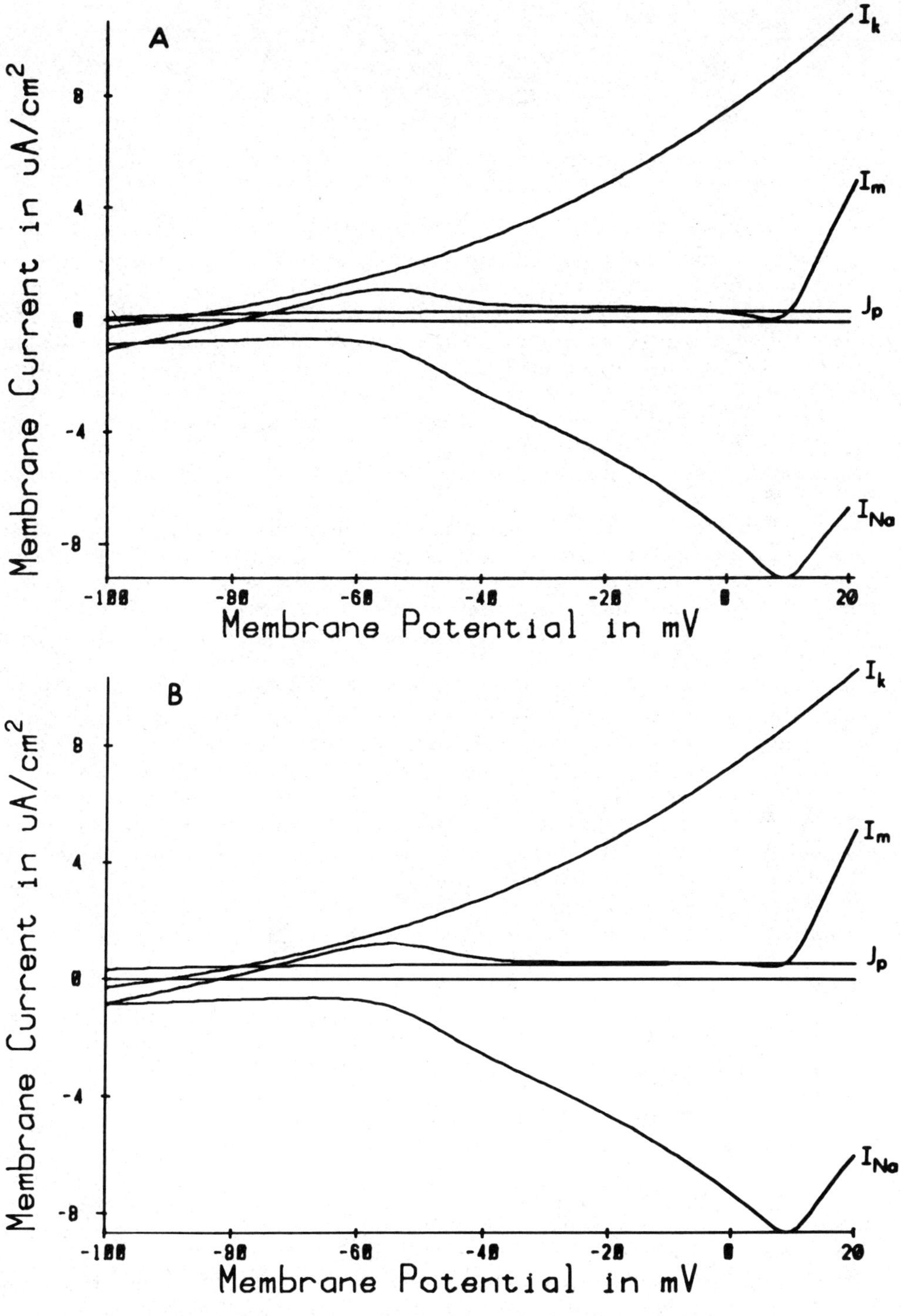

Figure 3. I_{Na}, I_K, J_p, and net I_m versus potential relationships for the quiescent cell in steady-state (A) and the cell stimulated at 1 Hz in stationary state (B).

where $\bar{P}_{Na}$ is a constant and

$$f(V) = \frac{\exp\left[3\,\dfrac{V-\alpha}{60}\right]}{\exp\left[\dfrac{-V-50}{5}\right]+1} + \beta - \frac{\exp\left[3\,\dfrac{V-10}{60}\right] - \gamma}{\exp\left[\dfrac{-V+10}{2}\right]+1} \tag{10}$$

where α, β, and γ are adjustable parameters to give a desired I_{Na}-V relationship.

The set of ionic and pump current vs. V curves that combine to give the I_m-V curve that generated the action potential first shown in Figure 1b is shown in Figure 3a. These I-V curves are for a quiescent cell, however. That is to say, they are consistent with a stationary state only at the resting potential, because only at this potential are the passive ionic and active fluxes in the required ratio of 3:2:1, as shown in Figure 4a.

Imagine now that I "excite" the cell with the I-V relationships of Figure 3, simulating the depolarization phase (for reasons of economy in computation time) by simply displacing the membrane potential to some chosen crest potential and, at the same time, adding an increment in Na^+_i equal to the corresponding charge displacement. The membrane potential/membrane current thereafter follows that I_m-V relationship shown in Figure 3. It is immediately obvious from this figure that once the membrane potential is away from the rest potential, the cell is no longer in stationary state: the ratio I_{Na}:I_K:J_p throughout the entire action potential is never in the required ratio of 3:2:1. As a consequence, the cell incurs a finite loss of K^+ and gain of Na^+ in each cycle, which, although small, eventually accumulate to cause sufficient stimulation of pump activity to counterbalance the increase in passive fluxes. In addition, the I-V relationships themselves must also change so that the pump current and ionic currents *integrated* over any given cardiac cycle are in the required ratio.

How these compensatory changes come about requires a quantitative description of the way that active Na and K transport (that is, J_p) adapts to meet the changing loads imposed by changes in electrical activity. In studies of active transport in many different kinds of cells, the rate is governed by the activities of the transported ions themselves on either side of the membrane. How r_f depends on K^+_o, K^+_i, Na^+_o, and Na^+_i (as measured, for example, by the rate of efflux of ^{24}Na) is sufficiently well known (albeit approximately in some instances) to permit explicit equations to be written for r_f and r_b of Reaction 1 purely on the basis of thermodynamic arguments. These equations that incorporate such experimentally determined dependencies explicitly describe how J_p varies as a function of potential and chemical composition ($[Na^+]_o$ . . . [ATP], [ADP], $[P_i]$). These equations are listed below; their derivation is described in Chapman et al. (1979).

$$J_p = k\left[[Na^+]_i^3[K^+]_o^2 - [Na^+]_o^3[K^+]_i^2 \exp\frac{\hat{Ç} - FV}{RT}\right] \tag{11}$$

Were the pump reaction (Eq. 1) to obey mass action kinetics, the specific reactivity k in this equation would be constant. Not surprisingly, experimental observation has shown that the reaction exhibits non-mass-action kinetics: the forward rate has a first-order kinetic dependence on internal sodium concentration in the physiologic range and an exponential dependence on $[K^+]_o$ with a concentration constant of 2.5 mM (Aiton et al., personal communication). I have assumed that the reverse rate is saturated by internal potassium and has a first-order dependence on external sodium.

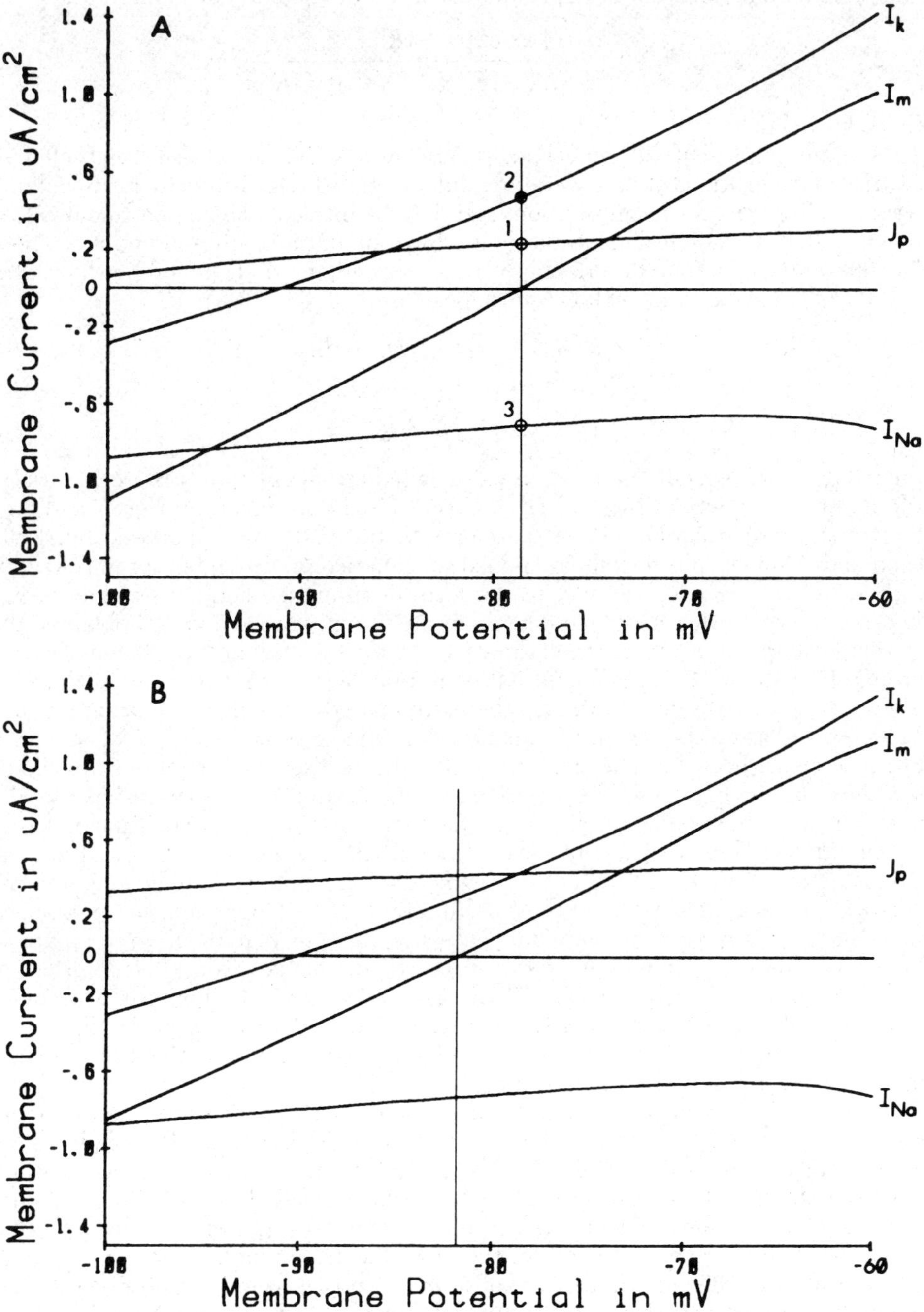

Figure 4. Expanded form of the current voltage relationships shown in Figure 3 for potentials in the neighborhood of the resting potential: (A) quiescent cell, (B) cell stimulated at 1 Hz.

Thus, a functional form for the specific reactivity for the 3:2 stoichiometry is

$$k = \bar{k} \frac{(1 - \exp(-[K^+]_o/2.5))}{[Na^+]_0^2 \cdot [K^+]_o^2 \cdot [Na^+]_1^2 \cdot [K^+]_i^3} \qquad (12)$$

where $\bar{k}$ is a constant.

For the simplest of cell geometries—an isolated, small, smooth-surfaced cell, free of surface invaginations or narrow intercellular clefts—I can assume that extracellular space is of fixed chemical composition, and that the intracellular compartment is well stirred so that its chemical composition is a function of time only and not of position. The differential equations describing the time-dependency of the membrane potential V_m, $[Na^+]_i$, and $[K^+]_i$ in such circumstances are

$$-C_m\dot{V} = I_{Na} + I_K + J_p \qquad (13)$$

$$[\dot{Na}^+]_i = (-I_{Na} - \tfrac{3}{2}J_p)\tfrac{\sigma}{F} \qquad (14)$$

$$[\dot{K}^+]_i = (-I_K + 2J_p)\tfrac{\sigma}{F} \qquad (15)$$

where C_m is the specific membrane capacitance (1 $\mu F/cm^2$), σ is the cell surface: volume ratio, and where I_{Na} and I_K in Eqs. 13 to 15 are given by Eqs. 7 and 8.

Given these equations, I can therefore compute how my hypothetical cell will respond to changes in intracellular and extracellular composition, either imposed, or as the result of electrical activity in the form of simulated action potentials. After choosing values for the model parameters in the way described above, I obtained the I-V relationships for a quiescent cell shown in Figure 3a by solving the system of Eqs. 7 through 15 (with no "excitation") until the internal ion concentrations reached steady values. Using these as initial values, I then "stimulated" the cell at a constant rate of 1 Hz and solved again the system of equations until the ion concentrations at any given time in a cardiac cycle became constant, giving the new set of I-V relationships shown in Figure 3b. In Figure 4, the I_{Na}-V, I_K-V, J_p-V, and I_m-V relationships for the quiescent (4A) and stimulated cell (4B) in stationary state are plotted in expanded form for potentials in the vicinity of the resting potential. As seen from Figure 4B for the stimulated cell, I_{Na}, I_K, and J_p at the resting (diastolic) potential are no longer in the ratio 3:2:1; indeed, at no time are they in this ratio. On the other hand, computation of the *integrated* currents over a cardiac cycle shows them to be in the required ratio. At the resting (diastolic) potential, the ratio $I_{Na}:I_K:J_p$ changes from 3.00:2.00:1 (Fig. 4A) for the quiescent cell to 1.72:0.72:1.00 for the cell at 1 Hz (Fig. 4b). Moreover, during stimulation of the previously quiescent cell at 1 Hz, the integrated flux ratios $\phi_{Na}:\phi_K:\phi_p$ changed slowly over a period of 2 to 3 min from 6.64:5.64:1.00 for the first action potential to 3.00:2.00:1.00.

The time scale over which such changes in pump activity and hence pump current occur is determined by factors such as the surface to volume ratio of the cell and the energy available from ATP. The half time for equilibration of internal concentrations for cells of the size of mammalian ventricular cardiac cells is of the order of 1 to 2 min, and as Figures 5 through 7 show, the resulting changes in J_p produced by such concentration changes readily account for the slow changes in shape of the action potential that follow the changes in the rate of stimulation that have been observed experimentally. Indeed, the closeness with which changes in J_p alone mimic the experimental observations suggests that time-dependent changes in I_m on the time-scale of 10's of seconds result from changes in J_p alone and not from changes in membrane permeability.

The behavior of the smooth-surfaced cell (Johnson et al., 1980) also mimics other well-known electrophysiologic observations, such as the diastolic hyperpolarization

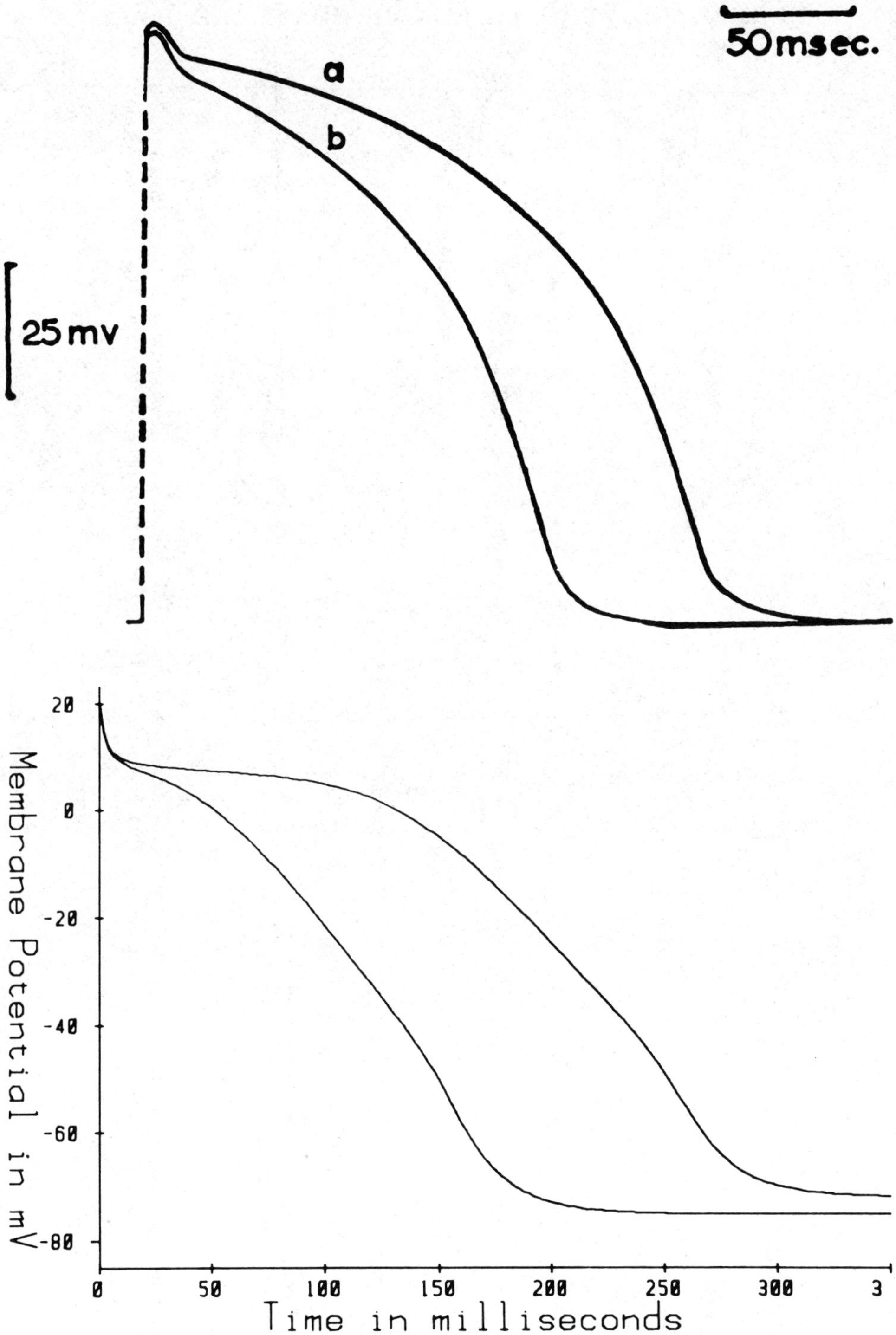

Figure 5. (A) (top panel) Action potential recorded from rabbit ventricular muscle (38°C). Action potential labeled (a) was recorded shortly after stimulation at 1.5 Hz following a 3 min period of rest. Action potential labeled (b), steady-state action potential at 1.5 Hz. [Redrawn from Gibbs, Johnson and Tille (1963).] (B) (bottom panel) Model Cell: Initial (a) and final action potentials (b) at 1 Hz after 3 min rest. [Reproduced from Johnson (1979).]

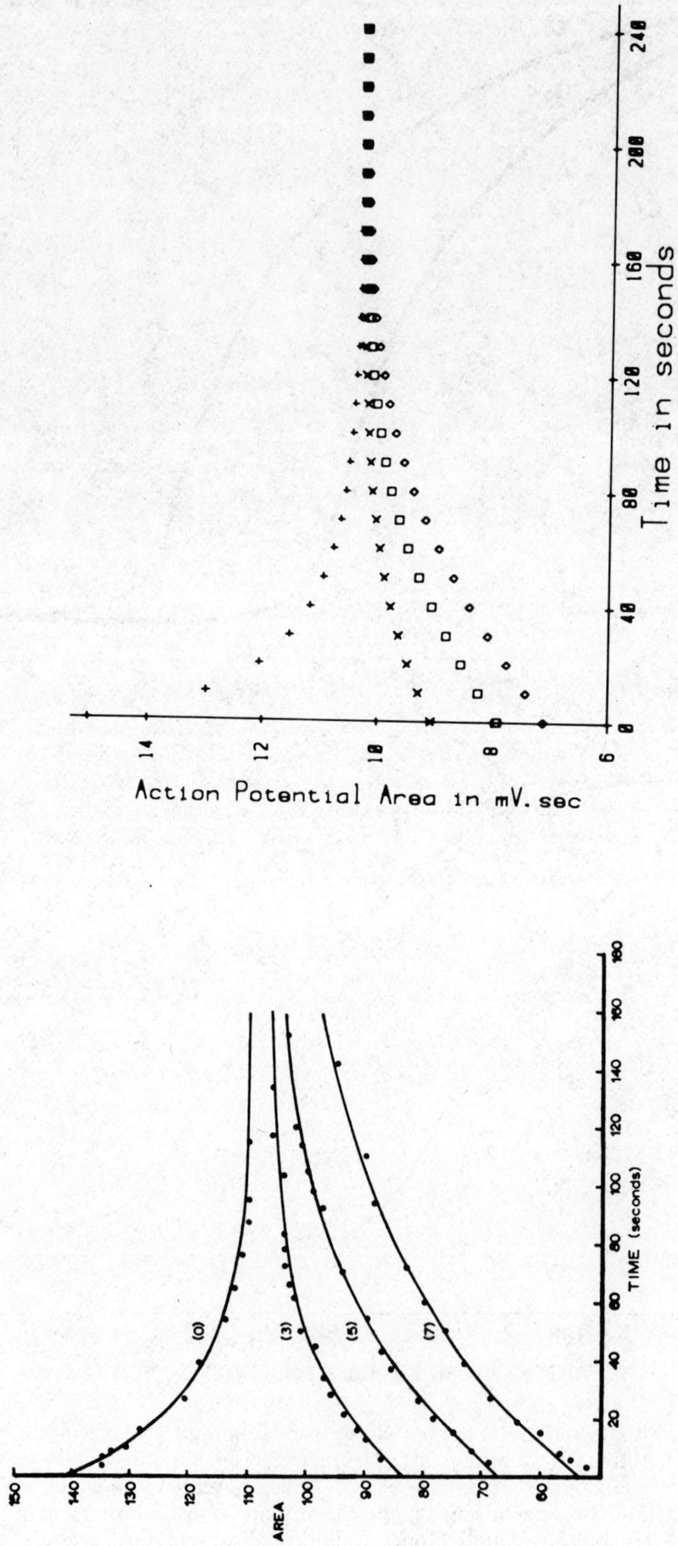

Figure 6. (A) (left panel) Area of action potentials recorded at 1.5 Hz as a function of time after 2–3 minutes of stimulation at a variety of conditioning rates given in the figure. Redrawn from Gibbs, Johnson and Tille (1963). Rabbit ventricular muscle (38°C). (B) (right panel) Model Cell: Similar experimental protocol to that of (A). +, 0 Hz; ×, 2 Hz; □, 4 Hz; ◇, 7 Hz. Cell surface/volume ratio 1/1μ. Ĉ = −41 kJ/mol. [Reproduced from Johnson (1979).]

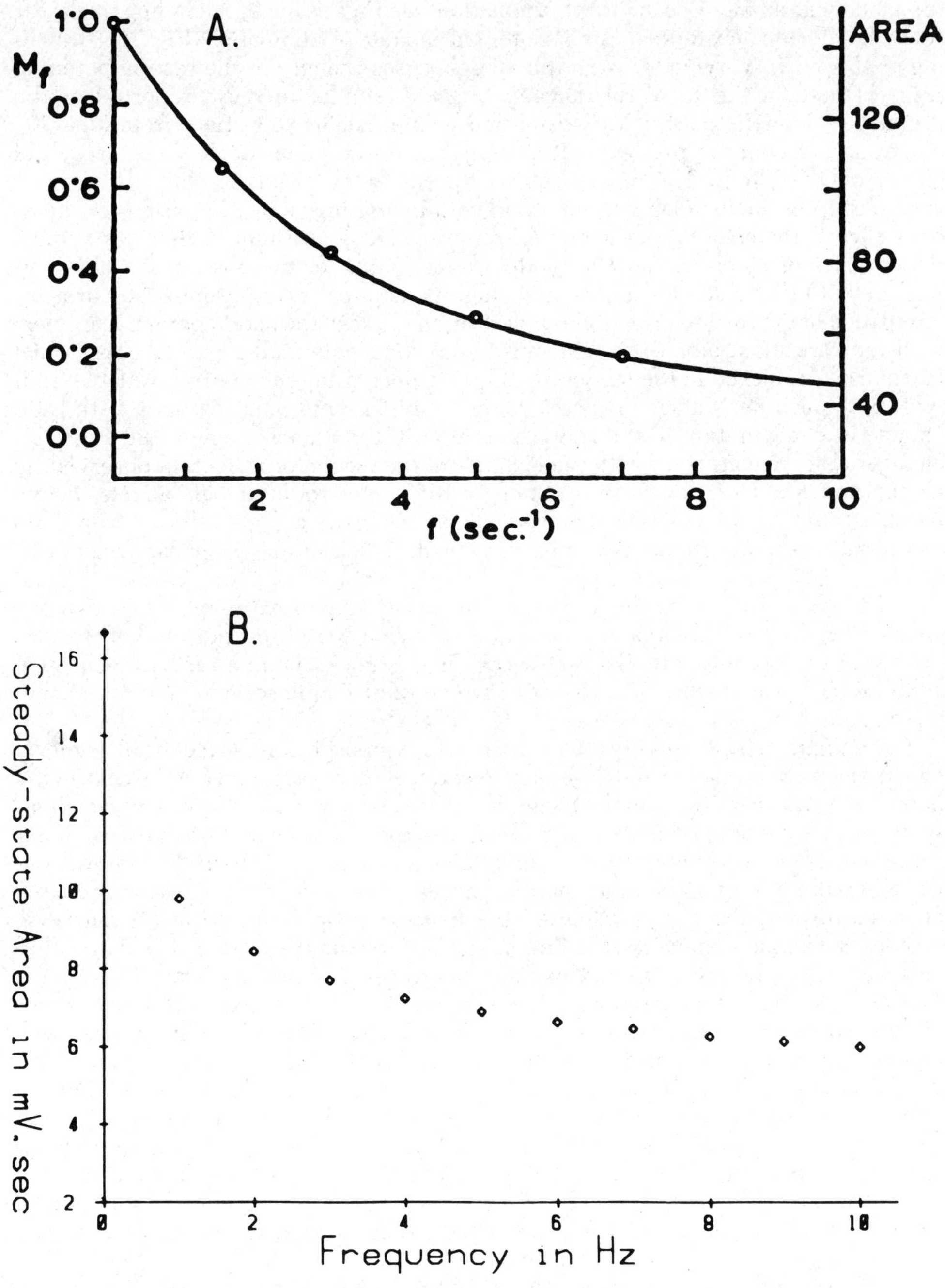

Figure 7. (A) Steady-state area (right-hand ordinate) of action as a function of the rate of stimulation. Redrawn from Gibbs, Johnson and Tille (1963). Rabbit ventricular muscle (38°C). (B) Model Cell: Steady-state area of action potential as a function of rate of stimulation. Cell surface/volume ratio 1/0.3μ. Ç = −42.5 kJ/mol. [Reproduced from Johnson (1979).]

seen following an increase in rate of stimulation (see Figs. 8 and 9), including the linear relation between maximum diastolic potential and rate of stimulation (Fig. 10) (Browning et al., 1979). Varying $[K^+]_o$ in the model causes changes in the resting potential (Fig. 11) and in the I_m-V relationship (Fig. 12) similar to those reported in the literature (Carmeliet, 1961; McAllister and Noble, 1966). Deviations from ideal K^+ electrode behavior are predicted at both high and low values of $[K^+]_o$ as a result of effects on the pump. The model not only predicts the observed shift of the I_m-V relationship in the depolarizing direction with increasing $[K^+]_o$, but also the "cross-over effect," the crossing of the curve for normal $[K^+]_o$, without having to assume a dependency of P_k on $[K^+]_o$. The model also accounts for the observation of Weidmann (1956) that a sudden injection of high-potassium perfusate into the coronary circulation of the turtle during the repolarization phase of the action potential accelerated repolarization, albeit to a less negative resting potential (Fig. 14). Myocardial ischemia is mimicked in the model by suddenly decreasing the energy available from ATP by a small percentage. This results in an initial rapid depolarization with little change in configuration of the action potential in the plateau region (see Fig. 13), changes that are consistent with the changes in the magnetocardiogram observed by Cohen and Kaufman, 1975. In addition to these electrophysiologic effects, active transport and its association with passive ion transport are also shown to greatly complicate the interpretation of isotopic ion flux measurements (Chapman et al., 1979).

But what of the slow currents seen in voltage-clamp experiments, which are on the time-scale of a fraction of a second rather than 10's of seconds, and of changes in shape of the action potential that occur on the time-scale of a cardiac cycle such as those shown in Figure 15? How can we account for these more rapidly changing currents?

As remarked by Eisenberg (1980) in a recent symposium on the electrophysiologic effects of ion accumulation and depletion in extracellular space, none of the cells in the body, except perhaps those in the blood, have free access to a well-stirred extracellular space. A sizeable fraction of the plasmalemma of most cells faces a small extracellular space, either in the form of narrow intercellular clefts, as in tightly-packed multicellular tissues (for example, the brain, cardiac muscle, the lens of the eye, to name a few), or as narrow tubular invaginations of the plasmalemma in the form of transverse tubules, such as in skeletal muscle fibers. The surface:volume ratio of such extracellular spaces is two to three orders of magnitude greater than that of extracellular space. Therefore, with all other conditions the same, the time-scale of concentration changes in these spaces, compared with those I have just described for intracellular space, will be two to three orders of magnitude faster. Recently, Dr. Mailen Kootsey and I have investigated the electrophysiologic consequences of such changes by modifying our original model of a smooth-surfaced cell to include the effects of ion accumulation and depletion and electrodiffusion in a narrow cleft (Kootsey et al., 1980). Figure 16 gives the diagrammatic representation of this model cell in which a single compartment represents intracellular space, a distributed compartment represents the cleft, and a space in which the ion concentrations are parameters represents extracellular space. Ions in the cleft were assumed to move under the influence of diffusion *and* electrical forces, that is, ion movements were described by an electrodiffusion equation for each of the important ions in question: Na^+, K^+, and Cl^-. The parameters for our preliminary exploration of the behavior of this new model were those appropriate for the ungulate Purkinje fiber (see Table 1) and the diffusion coefficients for K^+, Na^+, and Cl^- were assumed to be equal to the values measured in bulk solution at the same activity: 2.04×10^{-8}, 1.39×10^{-8}, and 2.11×10^{-8} cm^2/msec, respectively.

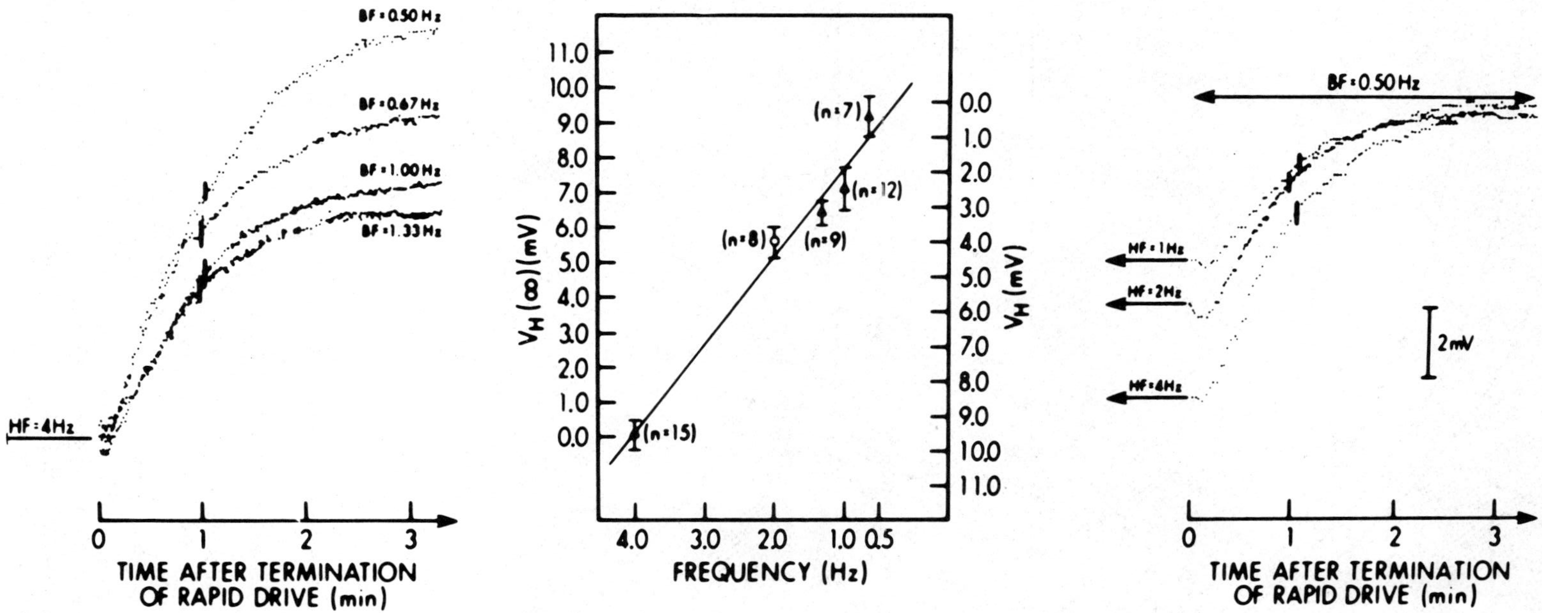

Figure 8. Rate dependent changes in maximum diastolic potential in cat Purkinje fibers. Left-hand panel: maximum diastolic potential as a function of time after switching from stimulation at 4 Hz to a variety of different lower stimulation rates as indicated in figure. Right-hand panel: Maximum diastolic potential as a function of time after stimulation at a variety of stimulation rates as indicated in figure to the one rate of 0.5 Hz. Center panel: Steady-state maximum diastolic potential as a function of stimulation frequency. (Reproduced from Browning et al., 1979.)

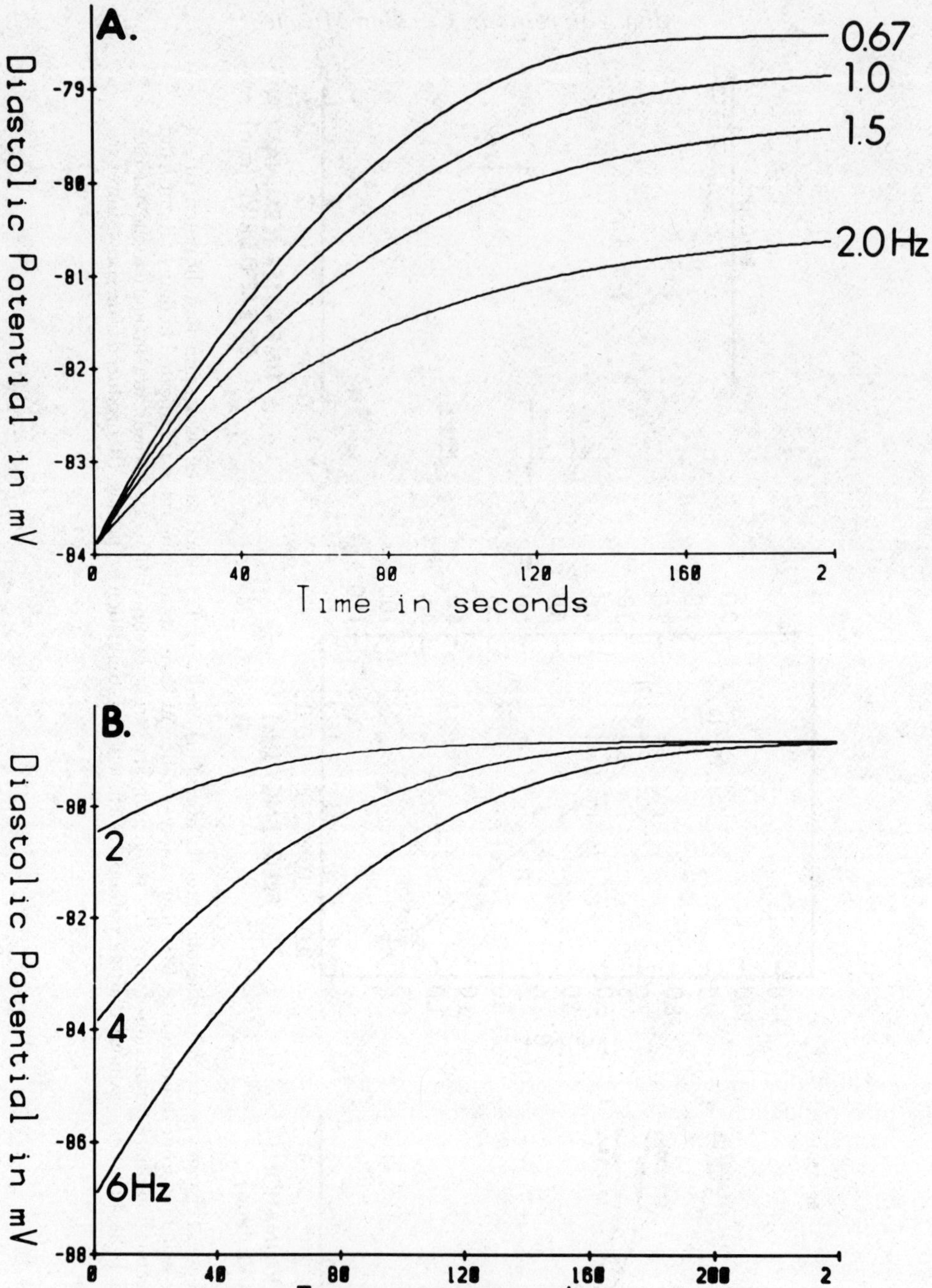

Figure 9. Model Cell: Maximum diastolic potential and the rate of stimulation. Simulation of the experimental results from cat Purkinje fibers of Figure 9. (A) Maximum diastolic potential as a function of time after switching from stimulation at 4 Hz to a variety of different lower stimulation rates as indicated in figure. (B) Maximum diastolic potential as a function of time after stimulation at a variety of stimulation rates as indicated in figure to the one rate of 1 Hz. Cell surface/volume ratio 1/0.3μ. Ç̂ = −42.5 kJ/mol. [Reproduced from Johnson (1979).]

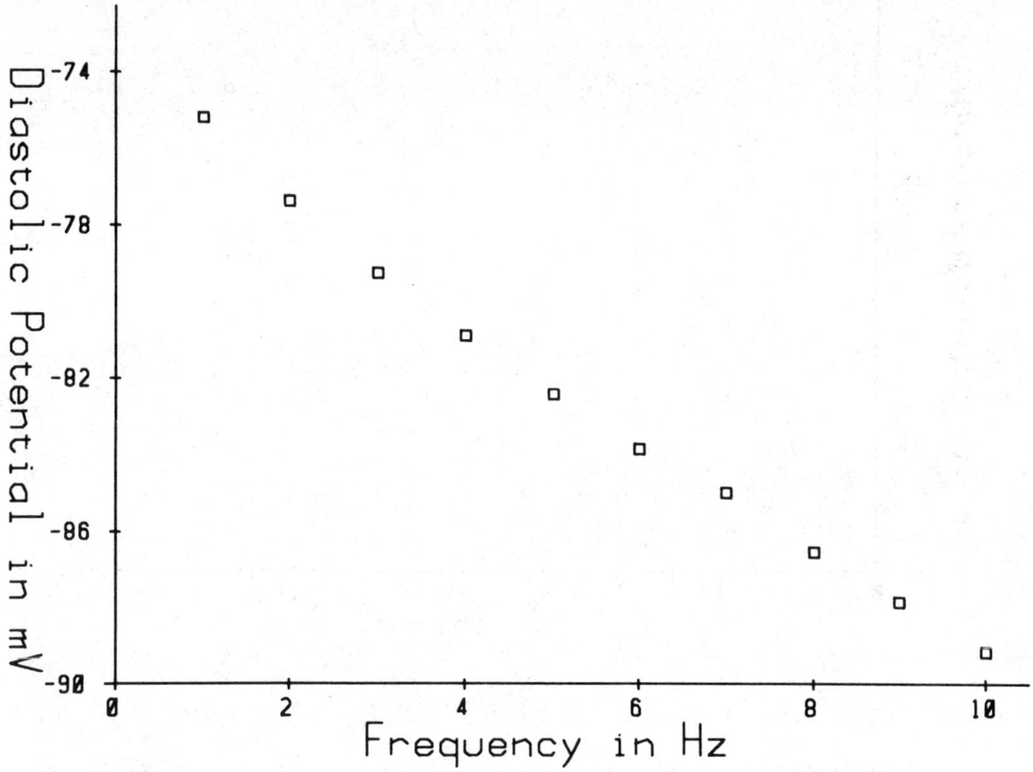

Figure 10. Model Cell: Steady-state maximum diastolic potential as a function of stimulation frequency. c.f. center panel of Figure 9. Cell surface/volume ratio 1/0.3μ. Ç = −42.5 kJ/mol. [Reproduced from Johnson (1979).]

Figure 17 shows one well-known electrophysiologic effect predicted by the cleft model. The first action potential shown in the upper panel of the figure is that produced by a single stimulus after a long pause. The action potential generated by a second stimulus applied 500 msec later is considerably shorter in duration. Clearly, the time-dependency of the I_m-V relationship that is responsible for this change in configuration of the action potential cannot have arisen from time-dependent changes in membrane permeabilities because the model specifically made these independent of time. The time dependency must have arisen from changes in active transport brought about by changes in chemical composition of the cleft. Figure 18 shows the K^+ concentration at the bottom of the cleft as a function of time after the moment of initiation of the action potential. As shown in the figure, the K^+ concentration in the cleft (for example, at the bottom) rises steadily throughout the action potential to reach a maximum value some three times that in the bulk extracellular space. During the fast phase of repolarization, $[K^+]$ in the cleft begins to fall and continues to do so in diastole to approach its initial value at 1000 msec. The changes in $[K^+]$ with distance down the cleft are shown in Figure 19 for various times after the upstroke of the first action potential shown in Figure 17. Note that, at depths greater than 40 to 50 μm, the chemical composition of the cleft is essentially independent of that of bulk extracellular space, the deeper part of the cleft acting essentially as a closed compartment.

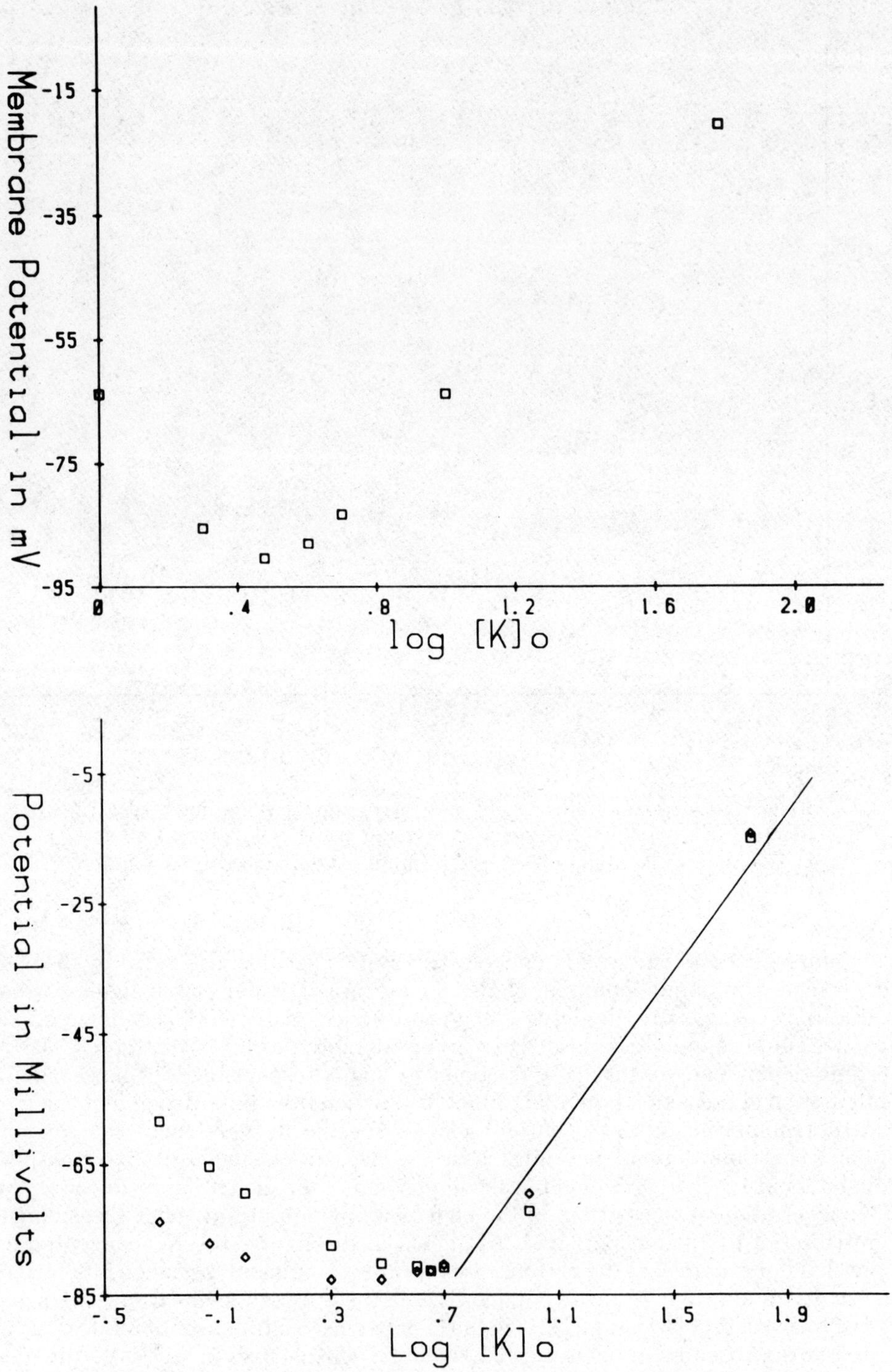

Figure 11. (A) (top panel) Membrane potential as a function of outside potassium ion concentration, $[K^+]_o$. (dog Purkinje fiber) (courtesy A. Stagg). (B) (bottom panel) Model Cell: Membrane potential as a function of outside potassium ion concentration, $[K^+]_o$. [□, initial value and ◇, final value of membrane potential. [Reproduced from Johnson (1979).]

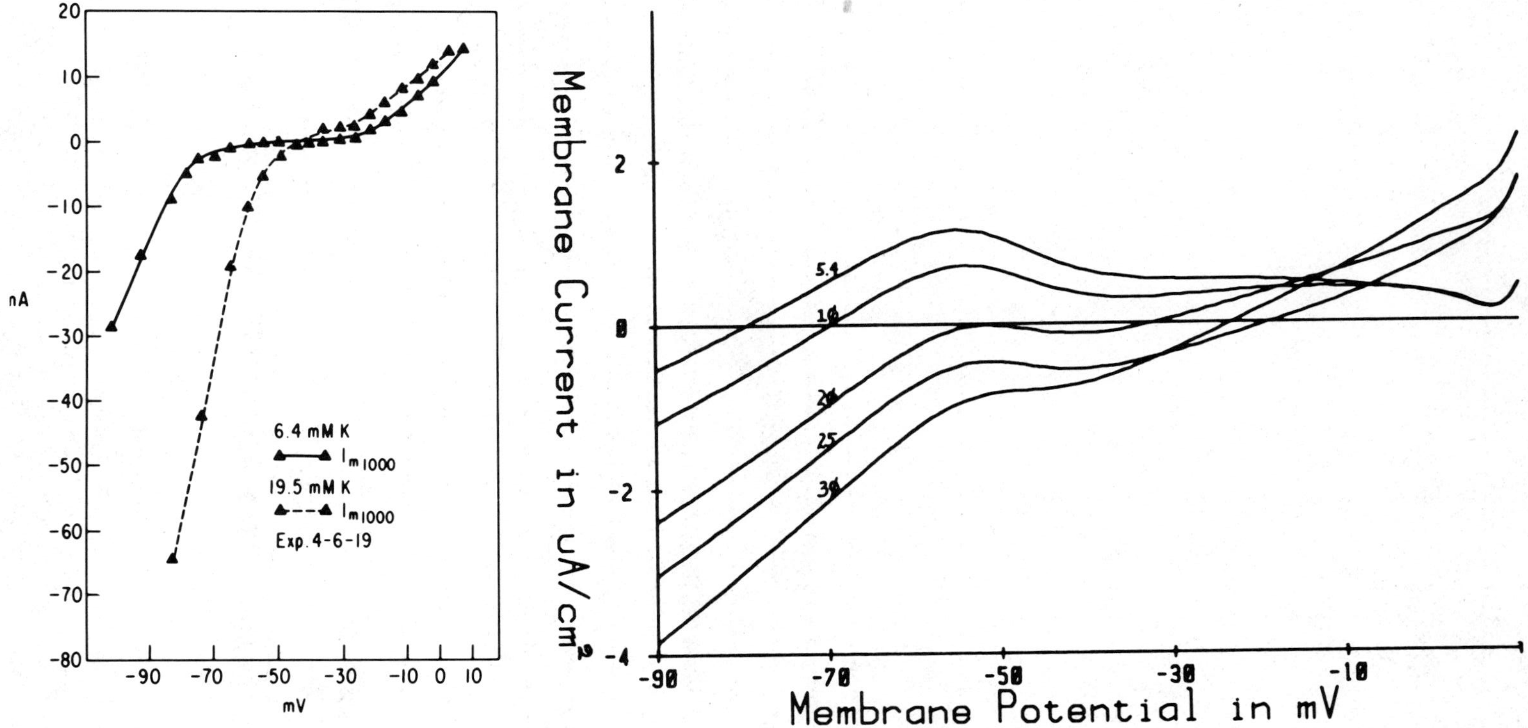

Figure 12. (A) (left panel) Quasi steady-state current voltage relationships for a tissue-cultured "synthetic strand" of cardiac muscle. Effects of an increase in extracellular potassium ion concentration. (Shigeto, Lieberman and Johnson, unpublished) (B) (right panel) Model Cell: Effects of changes in extracellular potassium ions concentration. Simulation of the experimental results of (A); numbers above curves give $[K^+]_o$ in mM. [Reproduced from Johnson (1979).]

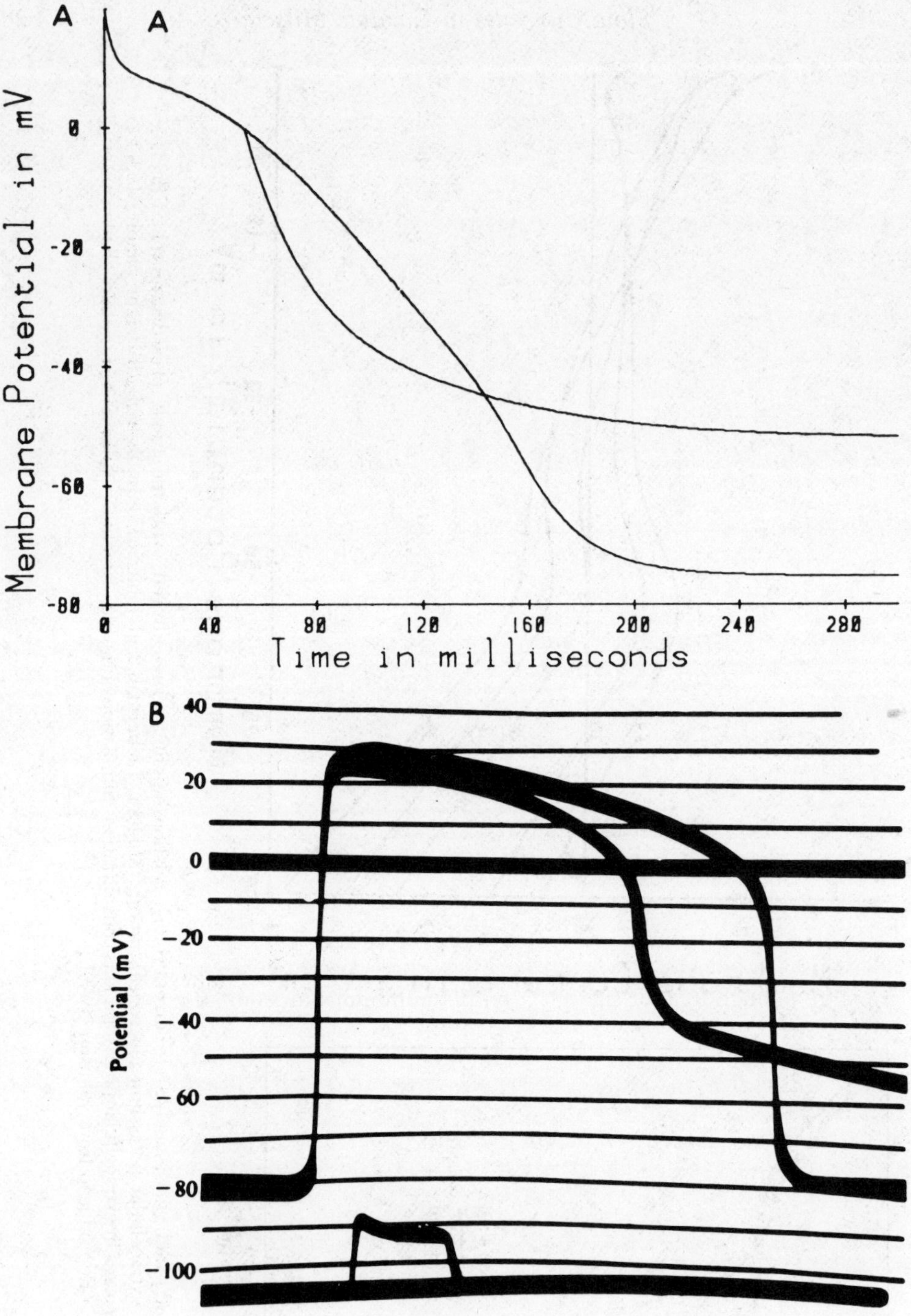

Figure 14. A: Response of model action potential to a sudden increase in $[K^+]_o$ (5.4 to 30 mM) together with an equivalent reduction in $[Na^+]_o$. [Reproduced from Johnson, Chapman and Kootsey, 1980).] B: Response of turtle ventricular action potential to a sudden injection of a high concentration of K^+ into the coronary circulation. (Reproduced from Weidmann, 1958).

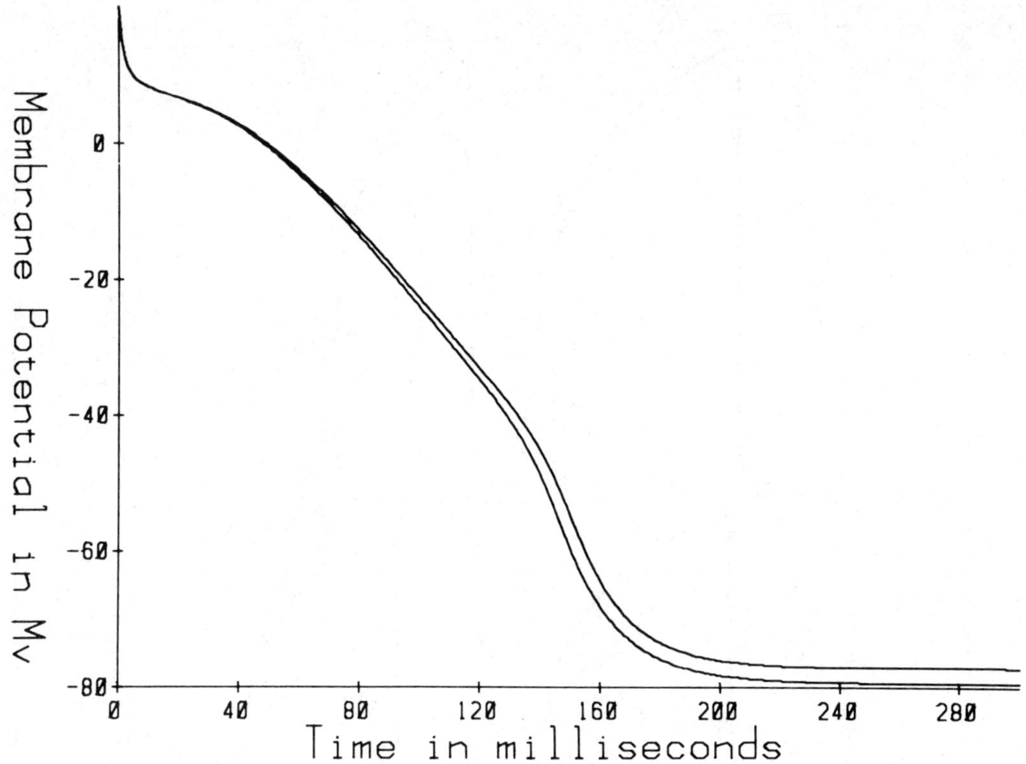

Figure 13. Model Cell: Simulation of the effects of anoxia. Immediate effect (depolarization) of a 6.6% reduction in the energy available from ATP. [Reproduced from Johnson (1979).]

This change in [K^+] and the corresponding change in cleft sodium concentration are large enough to alter significantly the membrane current-voltage relationship. A current-voltage relationship that generated an action potential of normal duration in the smooth-surfaced cell model was so distorted that the duration was abnormally short. To generate an action potential of reasonable duration, the quiescent membrane current-voltage relationship had to be made to cross the voltage axis (see lower panel of Fig. 17, quiescent cell curve). During the course of the action potential, the change in chemical composition caused the current-voltage relationship to shift upwards in the plateau region, eliminating the region of inward current (see lower panel of Fig. 17, t = 300 msec curve) and initiating fast repolarization. The necessity for the quiescent current-voltage relationship to cross the axis implies that if the capacity of the pump were decreased (for example by cooling), the cell might have a second stable state at a less negative potential because the chemical stimulation of the pump may be insufficient to raise the current-voltage relationship above the voltage axis.

The reason for the shortening of the second action potential is now clear. This action potential is initiated before the current-voltage relationship has returned to its quiescent form. In the plateau region, the current-voltage curve does not dip as far below the axis and, thus, requires less time to drift up to the axis. The duration of the plateau is a measure of the time taken for the curve to be lifted just beyond the voltage axis.

The changes in sodium and potassium ion concentrations in a cleft can therefore be substantial and clearly could be responsible for currents on the time scale of tens to

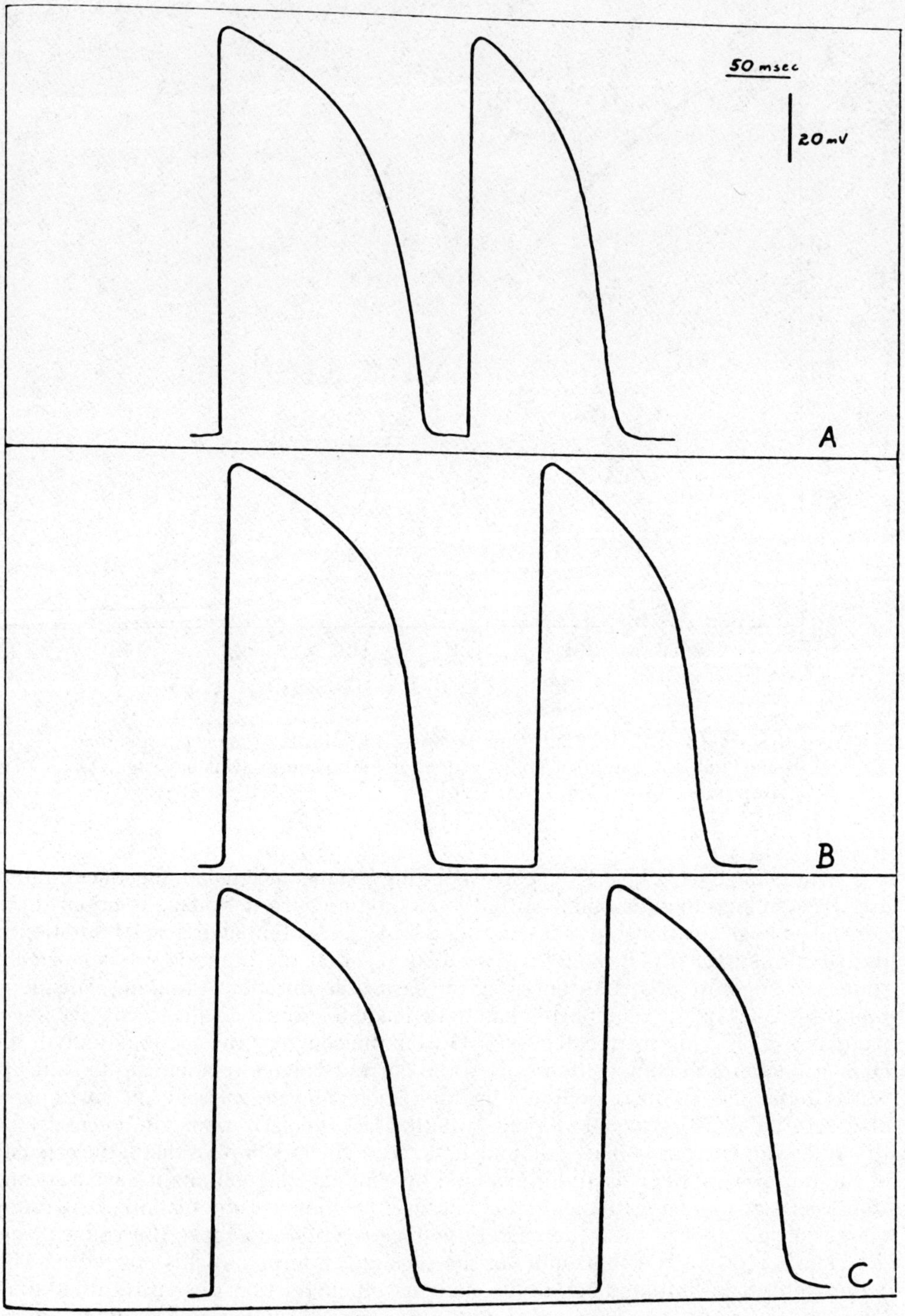

Figure 15. Response of frog ventricular muscle to an extra stimulus applied at varying intervals after an extra action potential evoked at a low (0.33 Hz) constant rate (T.W. Anderson and E.A. Johnson, unpublished results).

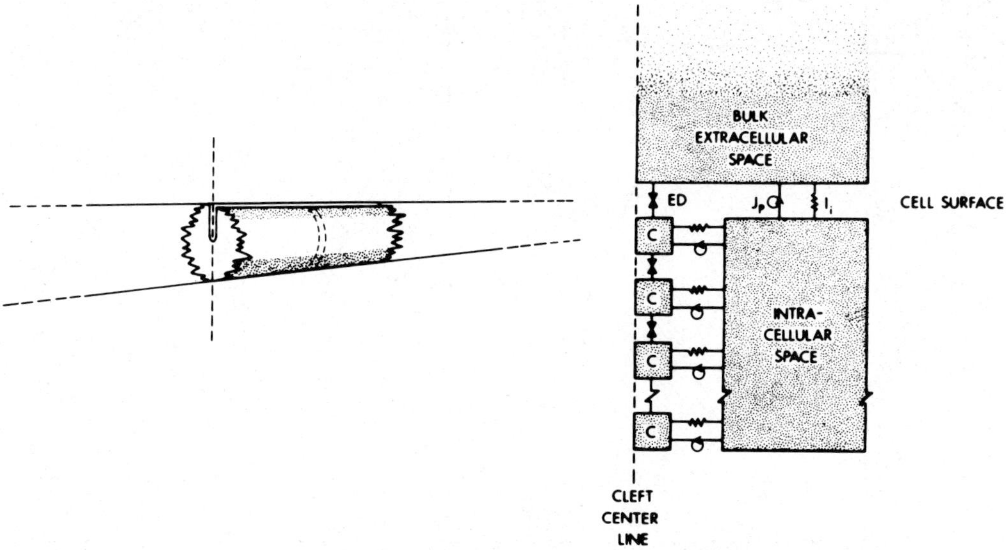

Figure 16. A (left panel): Idealized cylindrical cell with groove-like cleft forming an extracellular compartment. B (right panel): Block diagram of model. C = cleft segment; ED = coupling by electrodiffusion; J_p = pump current; I_i = passive current. [Reproduced from Kootsey, Johnson and Chapman (1980).]

Table 1
Parameter Values and Initial Conditions

$[Na^+]_i$	= 9.6 mM	D_K	= 2.04×10^{-8} cm²/msec
$[Na^+]_o$	= 140 mM	D_{Na}	= 1.39×10^{-8} cm²/msec
$[K^+]_i$	= 130 mM	D_{Cl}	= 2.11×10^{-8} cm²/msec
$[K^+]_o$	= 4.0 mM	V_{rest}	= −90 mV
$[Cl^-]_i$	= 139.6 mM	Δx	= 10 μm
$[Cl^-]_o$	= 144 mM	Δt	= 0.1 msec
surf/vol (IC comp.)	= $10^6 m^{-1}$		
cleft width	= 30 nm		
cleft length	= 100 μm		
cleft/total (membrane area)	= 0.8		

hundreds of milliseconds, namely, the shortening of an extra action potential. These results are only the beginning of our study of the contribution that clefts make to the electrophysiology of cardiac muscle. We are curious to see how much of the electrophysiology on this time scale can be accounted for by this model, including voltage-clamp currents. Indeed, we believe that the major obstacles to be overcome, before the generation of the cardiac action potential is understood, have moved from concern with *voltage inhomogeneity* to concern with *chemical inhomogeneity* and its resultant effects on *active* as well as *passive* transport.

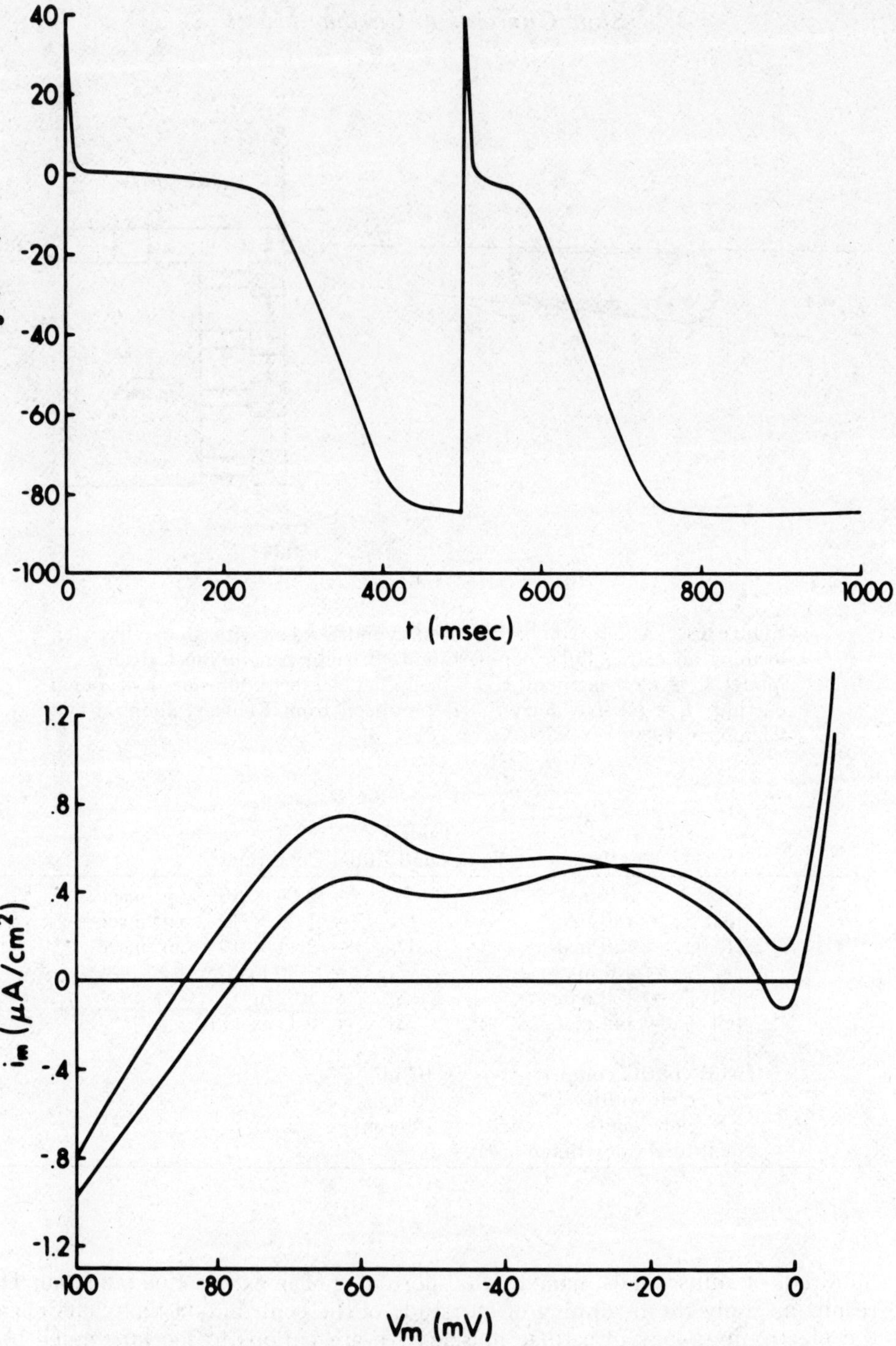

Figure 17. (A) Response of model to two stimuli after long quiescent period. The surface transmembrane potential is shown as a function of time. (B) Current-voltage relationship for membrane at the bottom of the cleft at two instants during the simulated experiment shown in upper panel. I-V relationship for quiescent cell: upper curve to left, lower curve to right of the crossover. Remaining curve is I-V relationship 300 msec after first stimulus (see upper panel). [Reproduced from Kootsey, Johnson and Chapman (1980).]

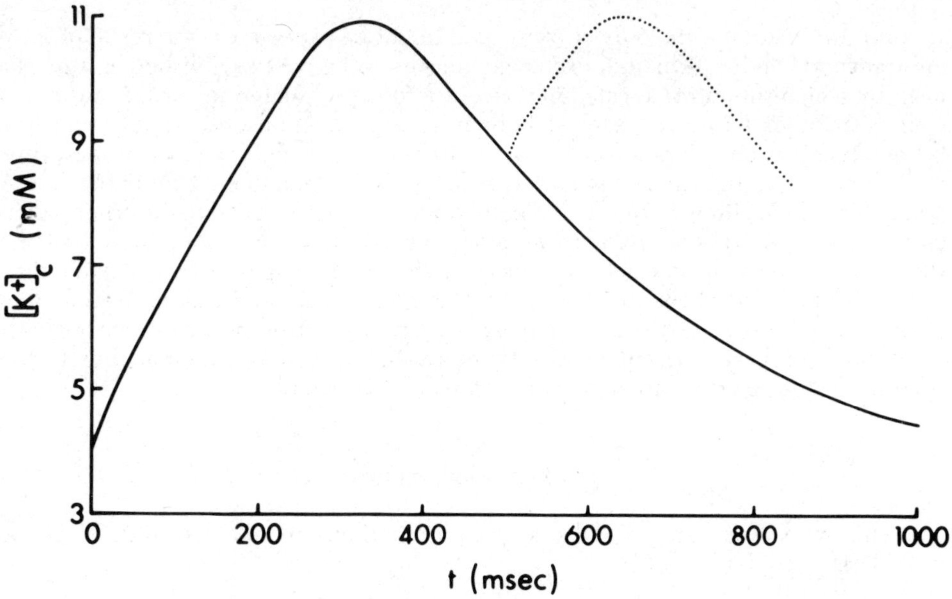

Figure 18. Potassium concentration at the bottom of a 100 μm deep cleft as a function of time after a single stimulus (solid line) and an extra stimulus (dotted line), i.e., during the first (solid line) and extra action potential (dotted line) in the upper panel of Figure 17.

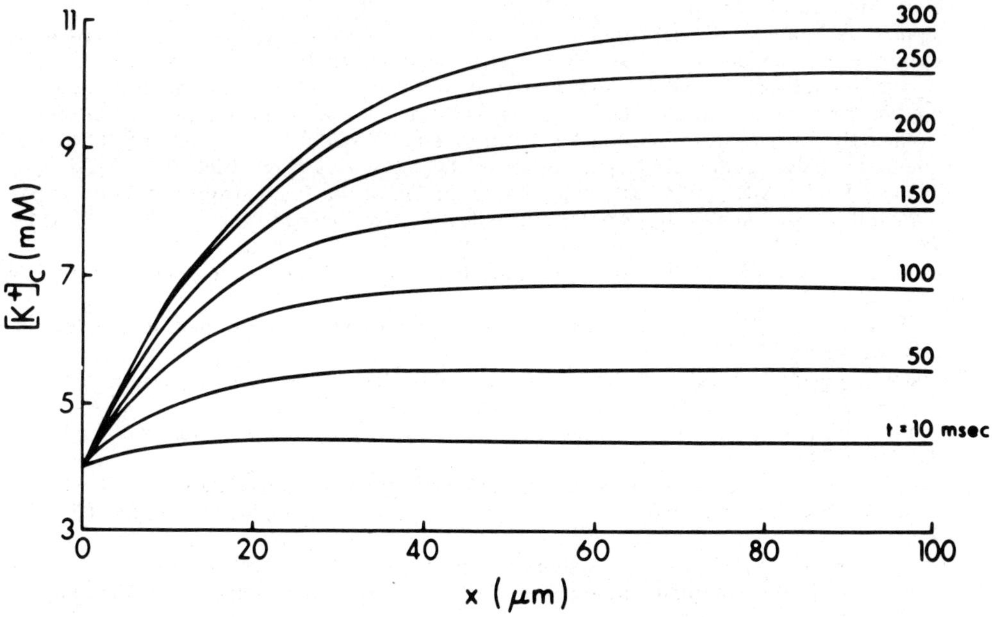

Figure 19. Potassium concentration along the cleft at several times after the first stimulus (0 time) of the simulation shown in upper panel of Figure 17. The distance x is measured from the mouth of the cleft. [Reproduced from Kootsey, Johnson and Chapman (1980).]

But these are not the only currents that might be expected as the result of active ion transport. Sodium-calcium exchange appears to be well established as a mechanism by which the internal calcium concentration is regulated in cardiac muscle, as well as in other tissues. It seems, both from experimental observations and from thermodynamic considerations, that such an exchange is electrogenic: at least three Na^+ ions moving into the cell in exchange for one Ca^{++} ion moved out of the cell. As pointed out by Mullins (1979), such electrogenic current must add to the other passive currents, contributing an *outward* membrane current during the action potential as the exchange mechanism runs in reverse (a Ca^{++} ion moving *into* the cell while three Na^+ ions move *out* of the fiber), whereas later, for example, in diastole, contributing an *inward* current as the mechanism runs forward, extruding Ca^{++} ions out of the fiber. Such diphasic current on the time scale of an action potential thus further complicates the picture, to an as yet undetermined extent.

Acknowledgment

This work was supported by a grant from the National Institutes of Health (2-POI-HL 12157).

REFERENCES

Browning DJ, Tiedemann JS, Stagg AL, Benditt DG, Scheinmann MM, Strauss HC (1979) Aspects of rate-related hyperpolarization in feline Purkinje fibers. Circ Res **44**:612–624

Carmeliet E (1961) Chloride and Potassium Permeability in Cardiac Purkinje Fibres. Bruxelles, Press Acad. Europ.

Chapman JB, Johnson EA (1976) Current-voltage relationships for theoretical electrogenic sodium pump models. Proc Aust Physiol Pharmacol Soc **7**:69P

Chapman JB, Johnson EA (1978) The reversal potential for an electrogenic sodium pump: A method for determining the free energy of ATP breakdown? J Gen Physiol **72**:403–408

Chapman JB, Kootsey JM, Johnson EA (1979) A kinetic model for determining the consequences of electrogenic active transport in cardiac muscle. J Theor Biol **80**:405–424

Cohen D, Kaufman LA (1975) Magnetic determination of the relationship between the S-T segment shift and the injury current produced by coronary artery occlusion. Cir Res **36**:414–424

Colatsky TJ, Tsien RW (1979) Sodium channels in rabbit cardiac Purkinje fibers. Nature **278**: 265–268

Ebihara L, Johnson EA (1980) Fast sodium current of cardiac muscle. A quantitative description. Biophys J **32**:779–790

Ebihara L, Shigeto N, Lieberman M, Johnson EA (1980) The initial inward current in spherical clusters of chick embryonic heart cells. J Gen Physiol **75**:437–456

Eisenberg RS (1980) Structural complexity, circuit models and ion accumulation. Fed Proc **39**:1540–1543

Gibbs CL, Johnson EA, Tille J (1963) A quantitative description of the relationship between the area of rabbit ventricular action potentials and the pattern of stimulation. Biophys J **3**:443–458

Glynn IM, Karlish SJD (1975) The sodium pump. Ann Rev Physiol **37**:13–55

Goldman DE (1943) Potential, impedance, and rectification in membranes. J Gen Physiol **27**:37–60

Johnson EA (1979) The genesis of the cardiac action potential: Chemical and electrical considerations. Proc Aust Physiol Pharmacol Soc **10**:59–72

Johnson EA, Chapman JB, Kootsey JM (1980) Some electrophysiological consequences of electrogenic Na, K transport in cardiac muscle: A theoretical study. J Theor Biol **87**:737–756

Kootsey JM, Johnson EA, Chapman JB (1980) Electrochemical inhomogeneity in ungulate Purkinje fibers: Model of electrogenic transport and electrodiffusion in clefts. Proc. Int. Cong. Physiol. Sci., Budapest. *In* Adv Physiol Sci, Vol. 8, Cardiovascular Physiology: Heart, Peripheral Circulation and Methodology, edited by A.G.B. Kovach, E. Menos, G. Rubanyi. pp 83–92

Lee KS, Weeks TA, Kao RL, Akaike N, Brown AM (1979) Sodium current in single heart muscle cells. Nature **278**:269–271

McAllister RE, Noble D (1966) The time and voltage dependence of the slow outward current in cardiac Purkinje fibers. J Physiol (Lond) **186**:632–662

Mullins LJ (1979) The generation of electric currents in cardiac fibers by Na/Ca exchange. Am J Physiol **236**:C103–C110

Thomas RC (1972) Electrogenic sodium pump in nerve and muscle cells. Physiol Rev **52**: 563–594

Vassalle M (1970) Electrogenic suppression of automaticity in sheep and dog Purkinje fibers. Circ Res **27**:361–377

Weidmann S (1956) Resting and action potentials of cardiac muscle. Ann NY Acad Sci **65**: 663–678

Discussion

FOZZARD: Could you give us an idea of the behavior of your model during intracellular sodium under any controlled conditions, such as going from the resting state up to a frequency of 1 Hz?

JOHNSON: The change in internal sodium could be immeasurably small to rather large. It all depends on how far away from equilibrium the pump is working at a given moment. Take for example the situation in which the forward pump rate for extrusion is 1 and the backward pump rate is close to 0. This means a very large departure from thermodynamic equilibrium for the pump. In this case, if we want to double the pump current, that is, to make it 2, we would have to double the forward pump rate, and this would probably require a very sizable increase in internal sodium. On the other hand, if the forward pump rate is 1000 and the backward pump rate is 999, the net outward pumping is also 1. In this situation however, you may need only a small or even undetectable increase in internal sodium to double the pump current; that is, to make the pump current go from a net value of 1 to a value of 2 by making, e.g., the forward rate go from 1000 to 1001. In other words, depending on how close to equilibrium you are, you may or may not require a large change of internal sodium concentration to get a doubling of the pump rate.

CARMELIET: I see two problems with your model. The first one is that you should expect a Goldman type of current-voltage relationship when you are in a sodium-free medium. The second is that, at least in sheep or dog Purkinje fibers, when you turn the extracellular potassium to zero the efflux of radioactive potassium also decreases.

JOHNSON: I can answer both these points. First, I have no particular objection to the potassium channel showing anomalous rectification. Indeed, we could have chosen to make g_K an instantaneous function of V rather than g_{Na} in which case g_K would have exhibited anomalous rectification. Our choice of g_{Na} (V) was to emphasize that, in the absence of anomalous rectification, behavior generally thought to require it still occurred. It is possible that in a sodium-free medium sodium would be maintained in narrow extracellular clefts to such a degree that much of the nonlinearity imparted by sodium to the I-V relationship would be retained. In answer to your second question, there are two ways for a radioactive potassium ion to leave the cell. One is via the passive potassium channel, the other is via the transport mechanism. This transport mechanism is a reversible reaction, net transport being the difference between unidirectional forward and reverse reaction rates. Even at equilibrium, when no net transport of Na or K occurs, the unidirectional rates are not 0 but have finite values. Indeed the unidirectional reverse rate would be measured by the rate of efflux of radioactive potassium via the mechanism. When the fiber is placed in K-free medium, which is known to inhibit Na,K transport, it is not unlikely that the observed drop in radioactive K efflux is not due to a decrease in efflux via a passive channel (anomalous rectification) but to a decrease in the unidirectional reverse rate of the pump caused by the drop in outside potassium.

Chapter 15

The Slow Inward Current and Its Modulation by Neurotransmitters

Harald Reuter

About 15 years ago, three independent studies (Reuter, 1966; Niedergerke and Orkand, 1966; Hagiwara and Nakajima, 1966) suggested that calcium (Ca) influx could contribute considerably to the total membrane current flowing during the cardiac action potential. But, the main evidence for a Ca-dependent slow inward current, as distinguished from the fast excitatory Na current, was obtained from voltage-clamp studies (Reuter, 1967; Reuter and Beeler, 1969; Rougier et al., 1969). To date, the slow inward current (i_{si}) has been observed in all vertebrate cardiac tissues investigated (for recent reviews see Reuter, 1979; Carmeliet and Vereecke, 1979), including single cardiac cells (Isenberg and Klöckner, 1980) and cardiac cells in tissue culture (Ebihara et al., 1980). As I have pointed out, details of the kinetic properties and ion selectivities of the slow inward current may not be identical in various cardiac tissues, but the basic features of this current component (Ca dependence, TTX insensitivity, sensitivity to drugs and ions that suppress Ca currents in other excitable tissues, voltage ranges of activation and inactivation of i_{si}, and so on) are very similar (Reuter, 1979). I shall briefly summarize, in this review, some of the basic properties of i_{si}, including its sensitivity to β-adrenergic and muscarinic cholinergic neurotransmitters and drugs.

THE SLOW INWARD CURRENT (i_{si})

Figure 1, (recording from a cow ventricular trabecula), demonstrates that i_{si} is the main inward current during the plateau phase of the action potential. Moreover, Kass et al. (1979) have shown a correlation between i_{si} and the upstroke velocity ($\dot{V}_{max}$) of a "slow response," that is, an action potential after complete inactivation of i_{Na}. Also, the role played by i_{si} in oscillatory phenomena in ventricular cardiac muscle (Reuter and Scholz, 1968; Katzung, 1975) has been simulated by a computer model on the basis of the kinetic properties of i_{si} (Beeler and Reuter, 1977). The importance of i_{si} for

Supported by the Swiss National Science Foundation.

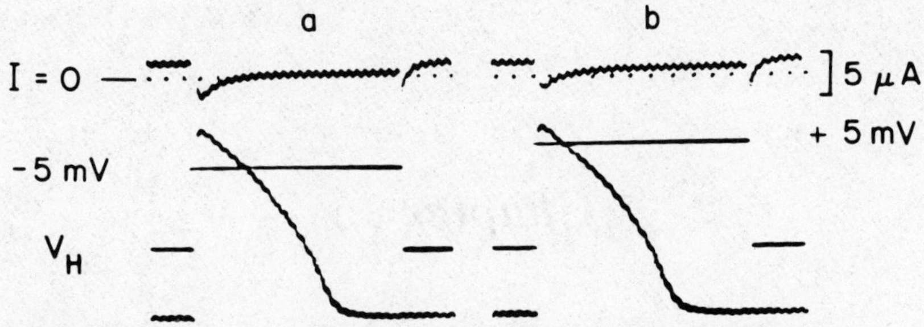

Figure 1. Relation between i_{si} (upper traces) and action potentials (lower traces). Voltage-clamp steps (500 msec duration) from a holding potential (V_H = −45 mV) to −5 mV (a) and +5 mV (b) produce inward currents which partially inactivate. Cow ventricular trabecula, single sucrose-gap voltage-clamp method (see Reuter and Scholz 1977a).

natural pacemaker action potentials in the sinus node and atrioventricular node has recently been demonstrated (Noma et al., 1980a; 1980b). These results establish the major role of i_{si} in generating cardiac action potentials under normal and abnormal conditions.

What are the charge carriers of i_{si}? The high sensitivity of i_{si} to variation of the external Ca ion concentration ($[Ca]_o$) and its relative insensitivity to the external Na ion concentration ($[Na]_o$) has already been established in early experiments (for review, see Reuter, 1973). Relative permeabilities for Ca, Na, and K ions have been estimated from reversal potential (V_o) measurements of i_{si} (Reuter and Scholz, 1977a) on the basis of experiments similar to that shown in Figure 2. Instantaneous current-voltage relationships yielded apparent reversal potentials in normal Tyrode's solution around +40 mV (+44 mV in Figure 2). Similar or slightly more positive val-

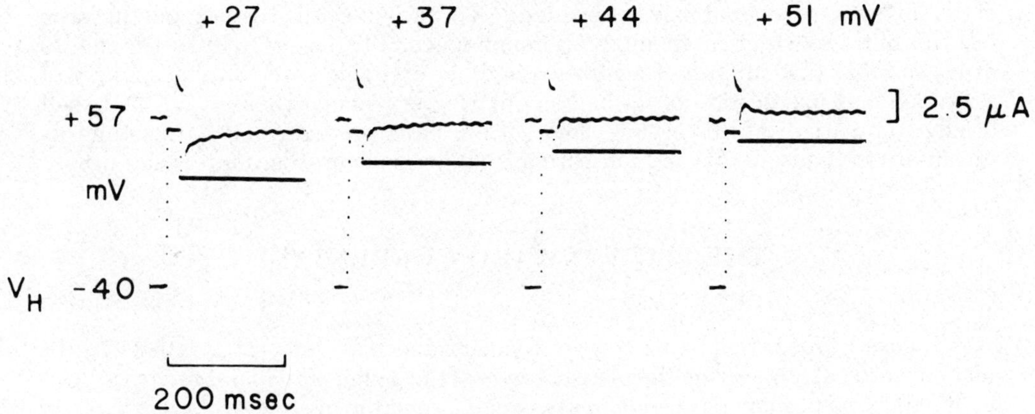

Figure 2. Membrane current (upper traces) flowing upon two step displacement of membrane potential from a holding potential (V_H) of −40 mV; first step always to +57 mV, second steps to voltages indicated above current records. Note reversal of tail currents at second voltage step; reversal potential +44 mV. Sheep ventricular trabecula, single sucrose-gap voltage-clamp method.

ues have been obtained for other preparations by various investigators (Ochi, 1970; Trautwein, 1975; Noma et al., 1980a). Reuter and Scholz (1977a) showed that V_o could be shifted by changing $[Ca]_o$ and $[Na]_o$. Application of the constant-field theory (an error in Eq. 2 in Reuter and Scholz [1977a] has been corrected in J Physiol **268**:574, 1977) led to the relative permeability sequence: $P_{Ca} : P_{Na} : P_K \approx 1 : 0.01 : 0.01$; in other words, the ion channels responsible for i_{si} are highly selective for Ca ions. The Ca selectivity must be considered as a lower limit, because it is not completely clear whether experiments like those in Figure 2 determine the true V_o of i_{si}, or whether an overlapping K outward current, which depends on $[Ca]_i$ (Siegelbaum and Tsien, 1980), is responsible for the apparent reversal of i_{si}. In both cases, changes in $[Ca]_o$ would shift the apparent V_o along the voltage axis. Sr and Ba ions, but not Mg ions, effectively replace Ca ions as charge carriers of i_{si}.

Typical current-voltage relationships and steady-state activation and inactivation variables (d_∞ and f_∞) of i_{si} are shown in Figure 3. There is a large region of overlap between d_∞ and f_∞, which is responsible for the hump in the instantaneous current-voltage relation (open circles) and for part of the negative slope of the steady-state current-voltage relation (closed circles). But these latter phenomena vary considerably between different cardiac preparations (see Trautwein and McDonald, 1978a; Reuter and Scholz 1977a). In addition to the overlap between d_∞ and f_∞, i_{si} may not inactivate completely as was first suggested for calf Purkinje fibers by Kass et al. (1976). Similarly, this explanation can be extended to the results obtained from cow ventricular trabeculae (Fig. 4). Compared with a 30-msec voltage-clamp pulse, the tail current at the end of the voltage step is reduced by only about 50% after a 280-msec pulse, and pulse prolongation caused only a slight reduction in the size of the tail current. In cat papillary muscles, inactivation of i_{si} seems to be more complete (Trautwein and McDonald, 1978b). Rate constants of activation and inactivation of i_{si} and those of recovery from inactivation seem to vary considerably from preparation to preparation and particularly among different animal species.

NEUROTRANSMITTER ACTIONS ON i_{si}

β-Adrenergic catecholamines greatly increase i_{si}, whereas muscarinic cholinergic substances have an opposite effect (reviewed by Reuter, 1980). A detailed analysis of the action of catecholamines on i_{si} in mammalian ventricular muscle (Reuter, 1974; Reuter and Scholz, 1977b) showed that the increase in i_{si} by β-adrenergic drugs is not accompanied by changes in the kinetic properties of this current. Figure 5 shows that adrenaline (0.2 μM) increases the peak inward current without changing the time course of inactivation (time constants indicated by arrows). As judged by the size of the tail currents at the end of the clamp pulses, adrenaline seems to increase the conductance, $\bar{g}_{si}$. The similar time course of relaxation of the tail currents indicates identical rates of closing of the i_{si} channels in the absence and presence of the neurotransmitter. A more complete analysis of these results is shown in Figure 6 where tail currents have been measured with two different pulse protocols. Figure 6A shows the results obtained with short (20 msec) activating clamp steps. The tail currents were always measured at the holding potential, V_H. The resulting activation curves indicate that adrenaline causes an increase in the limiting conductance, $\bar{g}_{si}$, without any shift of the voltage range of activation. The notion of an increase in $\bar{g}_{si}$ is supported by Figure 6B, where the slopes of instantaneous current-voltage relations show an increase in $\bar{g}_{si}$ as identical to that in Figure 6A without a change in the reversal

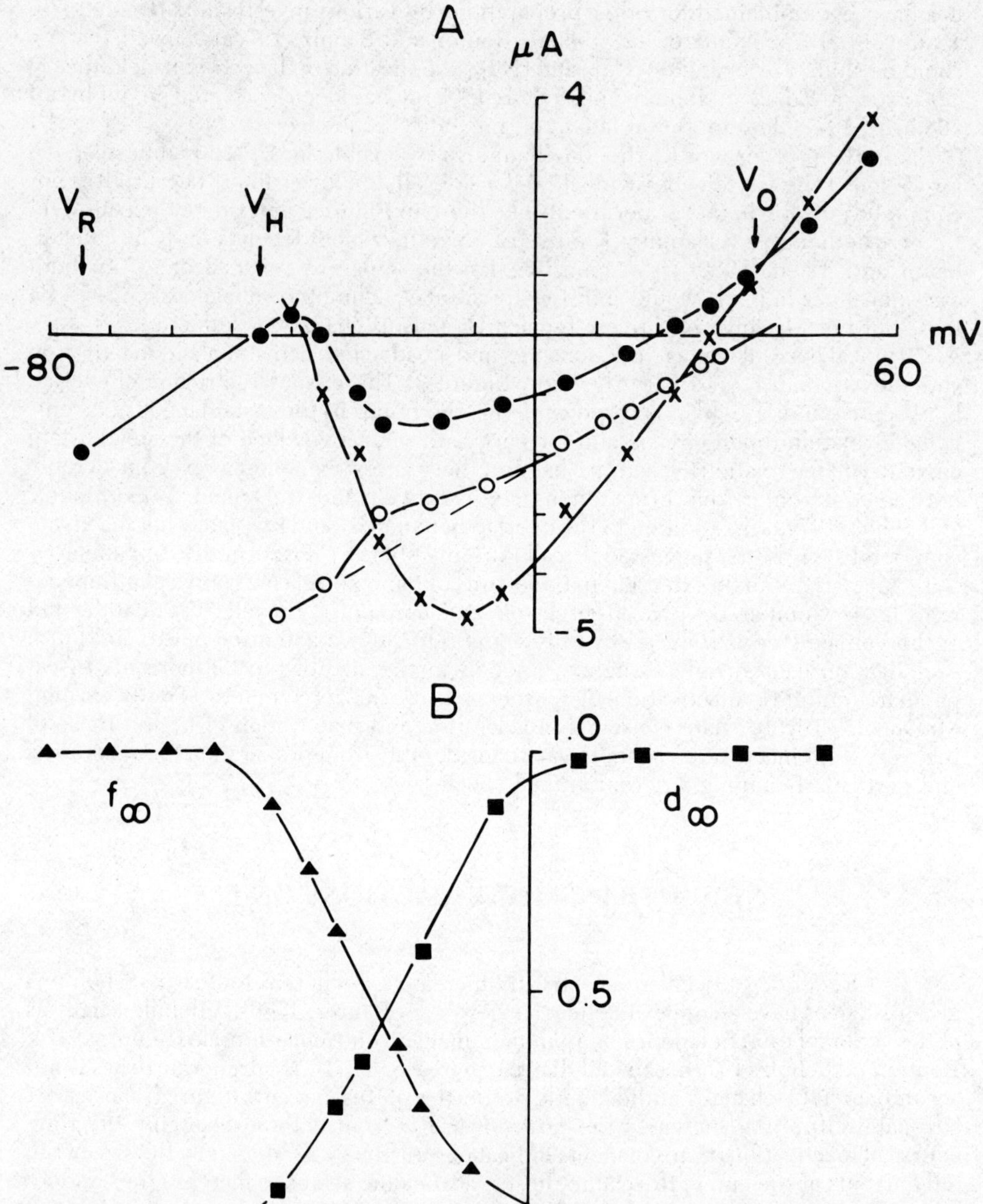

Figure 3. (A) Current-voltage relations of peak i_{si} (x) and of current at the end of a 500-msec clamp step (●) cross over at +37 mV; an identical reversal potential (V_o) was obtained from the instantaneous current voltage relation of i_{si} (○). Resting potential (V_R) −75 mV, holding potential (V_H) −45 mV. (B) Voltage ranges of steady-state activation (d_∞) and inactivation (f_∞) measured in the same experiment as (A). Experimental results obtained from the same cow trabecula as in Fig. 1.

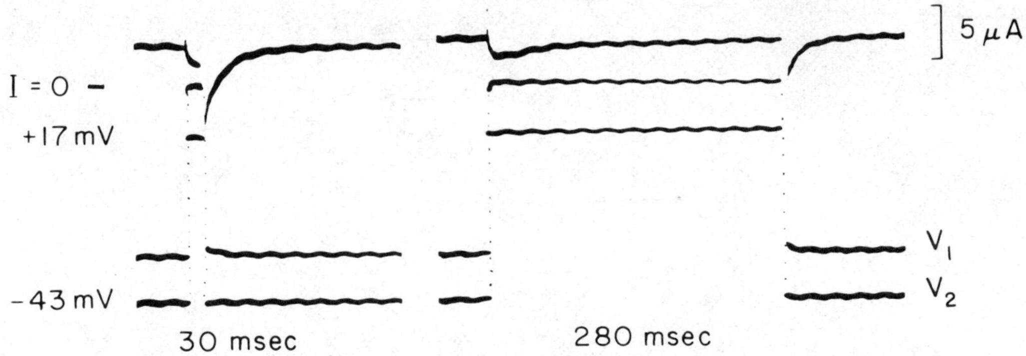

Figure 4. Membrane currents (upper traces) measured during short (30 msec) and long (280 msec) voltage-clamp steps from a holding potential of −43 mV to +17 mV. Note tail currents at the end of the clamp steps. Cow ventricular trabecula; single sucrose-gap voltage-clamp method with two intracellular microelectrodes (V_1 and V_2). Voltage was controlled at V_2 and longitudinal uniformity of voltage distribution was checked by V_1.

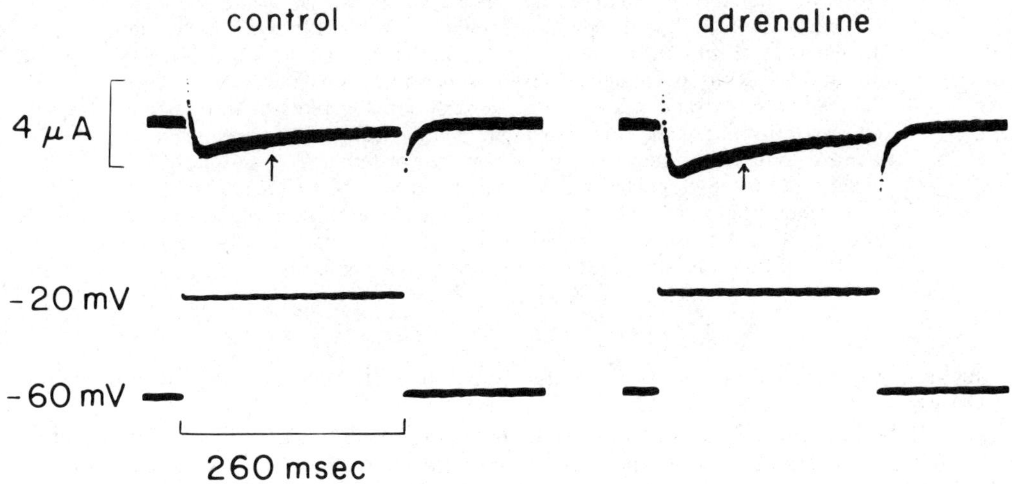

Figure 5. Voltage-clamp steps (lower traces) and corresponding membrane currents (upper traces) under control conditions and in the presence of adrenaline (0.2 μM); cow trabeculae, single sucrose-gap voltage-clamp method. Note that the rates of inactivation (time constants indicated by arrows) of the slow inward current are *unchanged* by adrenaline.

potential. These results have been interpreted by Reuter and Scholz (1977b) to indicate that the availability of functional Ca channels is regulated by β-adrenergic agonists. Similar results have recently been reported by Noma et al. (1980a) for the rabbit sinus node.

The cholinergic agonists, acetylcholine and carbachol, reduce i_{si} in frog atria (Giles and Noble, 1976), mammalian atria (Ten Eick et al., 1976) and ventricle (Ochi and Hino, 1978). Although a detailed kinetic analysis of this cholinergic effect is still

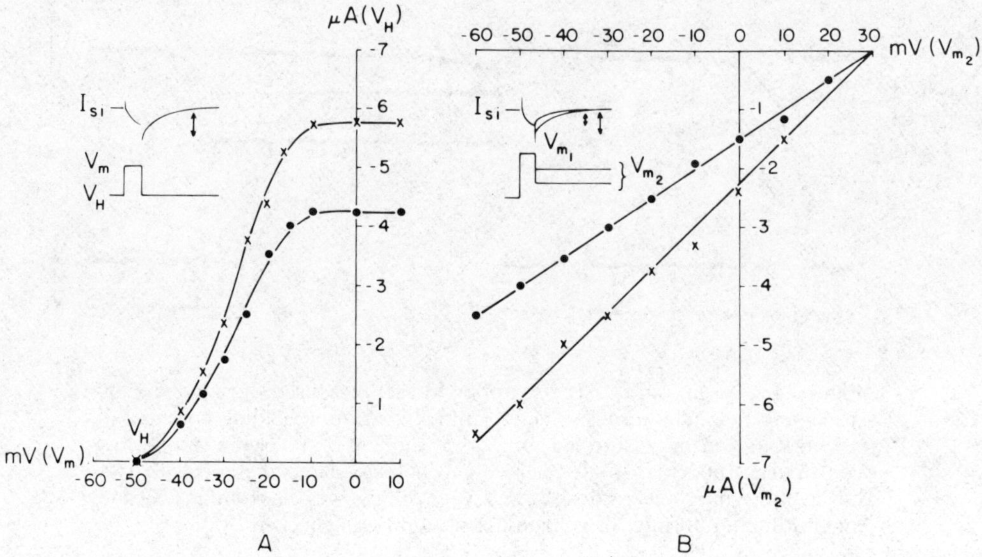

Figure 6. (A) Activation curves of i_{si} measured in absence (•) and presence (x) of adrenaline (10^{-6} M) in a cow ventricular trabecula. Plotted are maximal tail currents *(ordinate)* recorded at V_H and activated at V_m *(abscissa)* during short (20 msec) voltage clamp steps *(inset)*; maximal tail currents were obtained from extrapolation to time zero of semilog plots of the current traces. (B) Instantaneous current-voltage relation from the same experiment as in (A); plotted are maximal tail currents recorded at V_{m_2} and activated by short (20 msec) depolarizing clamp steps to V_{m_1} = +10 mV (*inset*); *abscissa*: membrane potential V_{m_2}, where tail currents were measured in absence (•) and presence (x) of adrenaline (10^{-6}M). Note that clamp step V_{m_1} to +10 mV was sufficient to fully activate i_{si} (see [A]).

lacking, the published results are consistent with a reduction of $\bar{g}_{si}$ by muscarinic drugs.

If the interpretation is correct that changes in $\bar{g}_{si}$ reflect variations in the availability of functional ion channels, the regulation of these ion channels by β-adrenergic and muscarinic cholinergic neurotransmitters is probably not a direct consequence of the transmitter-receptor reactions.

Figure 7 illustrates possible mechanisms for the regulation of membrane permeabilities by neurotransmitters. Although ion channels in end-plates are the classical example for a direct reaction between acetylcholine-receptor binding and channel opening, in the heart, the probability of voltage-dependent Ca channels to open during depolarization may be regulated by metabolic intermediates. An increase in cyclic AMP, as a result of β-adrenoceptor stimulation, may somehow (for example, via phosphorylation reactions) increase the probability of Ca channels to open in cardiac cell membranes, and thereby enhance the conductance g_{si}. Cyclic AMP analogues have indeed been shown to have an effect on i_{si} similar to that of β-adrenergic catecholamines. A reduction in cyclic AMP, or an increase of cyclic GMP, or both, produced by muscarinic cholinergic receptor stimulation in the heart, may have an opposite effect on the probability of functional Ca channels to enter an open state in cardiac cell membranes.

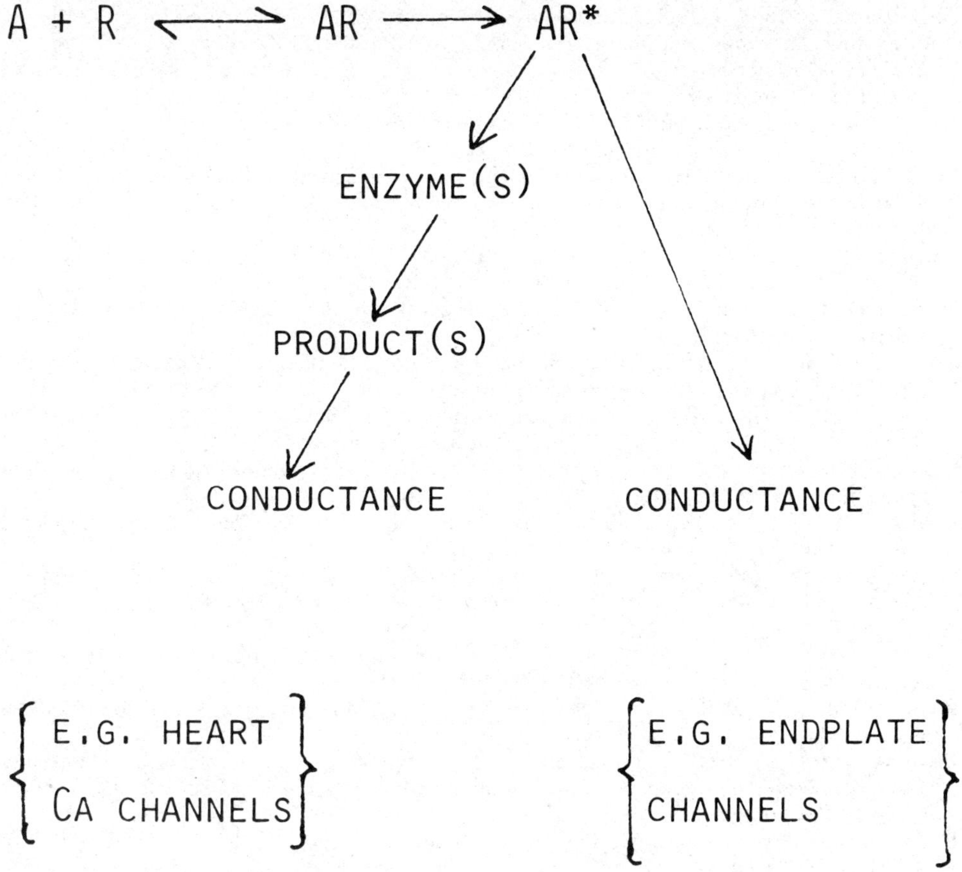

Figure 7. Schematic diagram of possible regulation of membrane ion channels by neurotransmitters. A = agonist, R = receptor, AR* = activated agonist-receptor complex.

From a functional point of view, the changes of i_{si} observed in the working myocardium and in pacemaker tissues contribute greatly to the inotropic and chronotropic effects of adrenergic and cholinergic neurotransmitters and drugs.

REFERENCES

Beeler GW, Reuter H (1977) Reconstruction of the action potential of ventricular myocardial fibres. J Physiol **268**:177–210

Carmeliet E, Vereecke J (1979) Electrogenesis of the action potential and automaticity. In Handbook of Physiology—The Cardiovascular System I. 1979, pp 269–334

Ebihara L, Shigeto N, Lieberman M, Johnson EA (1980) The initial inward current in spherical clusters of chick embryonic heart cells. J Gen Physiol **75**:437–456

Giles W, Noble SJ (1976) Changes in membrane currents in bullfrog atrium produced by acetylcholine. J Physiol **261**:103–123

Hagiwara S, Nakajima S (1966) Differences in Na and Ca spikes as examined by application of tetrodotoxin, procaine, and manganese ions. J Gen Physiol **49**:793–806
Isenberg G, Klöckner V (1980) Glycocalyx is not required for slow inward calcium current in isolated rat heart myocytes. Nature **284**:358–360
Kass RS, Siegelbaum S, Tsien RW (1976) Incomplete inactivation of the slow inward current in cardiac Purkinje fibres. J Physiol **263**:127–128P
Kass RS, Siegelbaum SA, Tsien RW (1979) Three-micro-electrode voltage clamp experiments in calf cardiac Purkinje fibres: is slow inward current adequately measured? J Physiol **290**: 201–225
Katzung BG (1975) Effects of extracellular calcium and sodium on depolarization-induced automaticity in guinea pig papillary muscle. Circ Res **37**:118–127
Niedergerke R, Orkand RK (1966) The dual effect of calcium on the action potential of the frog's heart. J Physiol **184**:291–311
Noma A, Kotake H, Irisawa H (1980a) Slow inward current and its role mediating the chronotropic effect of epinephrine in the rabbit sinoatrial node. Pflüg Arch **388**:1–9
Noma A, Irisawa H, Kokobun S, Kotake H, Nishimura M, Watanabe Y (1980b) Slow current systems in A-V node of the rabbit heart. Nature **285**:228–229
Ochi R (1970) The slow inward current and the action of manganese ions in guinea pig's myocardium. Pflüg Arch **316**:81–94
Ochi R, Hino N (1978) Depression of slow inward current by acetylcholine in mammalian ventricular muscle. Proc Japan Acad **54** (B):474–477
Reuter H (1966) Strom-Spannungsbeziehungen von Purkinje-Fasern bei verschiedenen extrazellulären Calcium-Konzentrationen und unter Adrenalineinwirkung. Pflüg Arch **287**: 357–367
Reuter H (1967) The dependence of slow inward current in Purkinje fibres on the extracellular calcium-concentration. J Physiol **192**:479–492
Reuter H (1973) Divalent cations as charge carriers in excitable membranes. Prog Biophys Mol Biol **26**:1–43
Reuter H (1974) Localization of *beta* adrenergic receptors and effects of noradrenaline and cyclic nucleotides on action potentials, ionic currents and tension in mammalian cardiac muscle. J Physiol **242**:429–451
Reuter H (1979) Properties of two inward membrane currents in the heart. Ann Rev Physiol **41**:413–424
Reuter H (1980) Effects of neurotransmitters on the slow inward current. In The Slow Inward Current and Cardiac Arrhythmias, edited by DP Zipes, JC Bailey, V Elharrar. The Hague, Martinus Nijhoff Publishers
Reuter H, Beeler GW (1969) Calcium current and activation of contraction in ventricular myocardial fibers. Science **163**:399–401
Reuter H, Scholz H (1968) Ueber den Einfluss der extracellulären Ca-Konzentration auf Membranpotential und Kontraktion isolierter Herzpräparate bei graduierter Depolarisation. Pflüg Arch **300**:87–107
Reuter H, Scholz H (1977a) A study of the ion selectivity and the kinetic properties of the calcium-dependent slow inward current in mammalian cardiac muscle. J Physiol **264**:17–47
Reuter H, Scholz H (1977b) The regulation of the calcium conductance of cardiac muscle by adrenaline. J Physiol **264**:49–62
Rougier O, Vassort G, Garnier D, Gargouil YM, Coraboeuf E (1969) Existence and role of a slow inward current during the frog atrial action potential. Pflüg Arch **308**:91–110
Siegelbaum SA, Tsien RW (1980) Calcium-activated transient outward current in calf cardiac Purkinje fibres. J Physiol **299**:485–506
Ten Eick R, Nawrath H, McDonald TF, Trautwein W (1976) On the mechanism of the negative inotropic effect of acetylcholine. Pflüg Arch **361**:207–213
Trautwein W (1975) The slow inward current in mammalian myocardium. Eur J Cardiol **1**: 169–175
Trautwein W, McDonald TF (1978a) Current-voltage relations in ventricular muscle preparations from different species. Pflüg Arch **374**:79–89
Trautwein, W, McDonald TF (1978b) Membrane conductance measurements in cat ventricular muscle. J Mol Cel Cardiol **10**:387–394

Discussion

JOHNSON: We have in our model a small sodium current that inactivates rapidly, not as fast as the usual fast sodium channel activation, which is of the order of milliseconds, but perhaps ten times slower than that, in the order of tens of milliseconds. As far as I can see, this sodium current that we point out could well account for many of the effects that you show. This current also has a reversal potential right about the reversal potential of your slow inward current. I wonder why you bring in the notion of a calcium current when you could just say it was a sodium current, or even add to it a little bit of potassium permeability to make the reversal potential a little negative in relation to the sodium equilibrium potential. Can you be absolutely sure that your current reverses at the potential beyond, that is more positive than the sodium equilibrium potential? If that is the case I agree you need another current.

REUTER: No, I am not sure that the reversal potential of the slow inward current is beyond the sodium equilibrium potential. But, I should point out that the slow inward current can also be observed in the absence of external sodium in which case its reversal potential is certainly beyond that of the sodium equilibrium potential. That this current is very sensitive to external calcium and little sensitive to external sodium is the very same argument that has been applied to implicate calcium channels in other excitable tissues. Also, the blockers that are being used to define calcium channels like methoxyverapamil (D-600), cobalt, and others eliminate this slow inward current. This is an indication that this current is at least different from the usual sodium current. That these currents can generate slow response action potentials in the presence of high tetrodotoxin concentrations is also evidence for this difference. This last result, associated with the slow inward current increasing, and its reversal potential shifting with increasing external calcium, is a fairly good indication of the calcium nature of this current. It could not be explained readily by surface-charge effects, as such effects would not explain why the current is maintained in the presence of a high tetrodotoxin concentration and abolished with lanthanum or high magnesium.

LIEBERMAN: A recent paper from the laboratory of Galper and Catterall (Dev Biol **65**:216–227, 1978) shows that D-600 blocks sodium influx in embryonic heart cells. Would you care to comment on this finding?

REUTER: This is actually not a new finding. It has also been shown by Bayer et al. (Naunyn-Schmiedeberg's Arch Pharmacol **290**:81, 1975) that D-600 in high concentration decreases the sodium influx. You need a much higher concentration of D-600 to block sodium channels, however, than you need to block the slow inward current. Unfortunately, there is no drug that is as specific for the calcium channel as tetrodotoxin is for the fast sodium channel. Now, if the slow inward current is a sodium current, then the channels through which it is carried must have completely different properties than the usual fast sodium channels, because they are entirely insensitive to tetrodotoxin.

FOZZARD: Most of the protocols used to look at the slow inward current use holding potentials to −45 mV or so to get rid of the fast sodium spike. Although this is an eminently reasonable approach, I have often been concerned with it. A recent report by Adams and Gage (J Physiol **289**:143–161, 1979) using neurons shows what you call the f_∞ curve to be biphasic. It peaked at about −40 or so, but was much more inactivated in the region of the normal resting potentials. Do you feel that the evidence in neuron is valid, and do you think that there is any evidence for that in heart muscle?

REUTER: This was analyzed about ten years ago by Neher (J Gen Physiol **58**:36, 1971) and was shown to be due to a fast potassium current that is activated at negative potentials. This potassium current messes up the inactivation curve at very negative potentials. This outward current was called the *A* current, and it is not present in the heart.

BROWN: The *A* current is a potassium current that has activation kinetics as fast as that of the sodium system, is inactivated at about −40 mV, and is activated as you go more negative to this voltage. This potassium channel can be blocked by 4-AP. The biphasic effect mentioned by Fozzard for the inactivation curve of the calcium channel is a possibility, but this effect may be excluded in the case of heart muscle, as Reuter has just mentioned. I would also like to state that I am a firm believer in the existence of calcium channels. You can dialyze neurons both inside and outside with solutions that are entirely free of sodium and potassium and do it for 5 hours, so that there is no sodium and no potassium left either inside the cells or in clefts. In these conditions, the sodium-potassium pump and the calcium-sodium pump are not working. After this time you still see an inward current that is insensitive to tetrodotoxin and is sensitive to calcium. This current is, in fact, dependent on the amount of extracellular calcium present.

REUTER: You can also see this type of behavior in single cardiac cells.

BROWN: I have two other questions. First, are you sure that what you call the reversal potential is indeed related to a contribution of an outward current carried by potassium or cesium through the calcium channel? Or is there possibly another set of channels that is carrying outward current? In this respect it would be interesting to examine the tail current during the slow inward current and see if you can spot an inward tail followed by an outward tail.

REUTER: There might be a transient outward current that could contribute to the appearance of a reversal potential in that region. This outward current would have to depend on the internal calcium concentration and could be a potassium current activated by calcium. In this case it would be difficult to differentiate between these two possibilities, that is, a current carried through the calcium channel or an outward current that is activated by calcium. But, there is one strong argument against this, and that is the epinephrine effect. It has been shown that epinephrine increases appreciably the inward calcium current, and yet its reversal potential stays constant. This should not be expected if the reversal potential were determined by a summation of two currents, a calcium current potentiated by epinephrine and an unchanged outward potassium current. But, I cannot answer completely your question because I am not sure whether there is an outward-going potassium current sensitive to calcium.

I. COHEN: I am confused with the argument concerning adrenaline, because if the outward current is sensitive to internal calcium, the increase in inward calcium movement through the slow channel due to adrenaline would also enhance the outward-going potassium current, and the reversal potential might not be changed.

REUTER: If the sensitivity of both systems to calcium is exactly the same then you might be right, but this would, I think, be a fortuitous situation. I cannot, however, give a more definite answer to the question.

Chapter 16

Pacemaker Activity in Cardiac Purkinje Fibers: A Voltage Clamp Analysis

Ira S. Cohen, Robin T. Falk, and Richard P. Kline

The development of the voltage clamp by Marmont (1949) and its subsequent application by Hodgkin and Huxley (1952) to the study of excitability in the squid giant axon have provided the necessary technical and theoretical framework for much of the recent research on cardiac pacemaker activity. As in many applications of an ideal theoretical or experimental concept designed for a simpler experimental system, however, the use of the voltage clamp to study cardiac membrane conductances and the application of the Hodgkin-Huxley theory have met with only limited success.

In the following pages, we will discuss the application of the voltage clamp to the study of pacemaker activity in cardiac Purkinje fibers. The anatomy of the Purkinje fiber (where much of the membrane surface area faces narrow intercellular clefts) creates special problems in the interpretation of many voltage-clamp measurements. These narrow clefts can result in time-dependent extracellular [K^+] changes in response to changes in membrane potential.

In the first part of this article, we discuss the purpose of each of five voltage-clamp measures used in the analysis of Purkinje fiber pacemaker activity. We then reconsider each measure in the light of experimental evidence of [K^+] fluctuations during voltage steps (see Fig. 3). In the second section we examine the development of our present understanding of the pacemaker mechanism.

PART I - VOLTAGE CLAMP ANALYSIS

(A) Analysis of a Current in the Absence of Extracellular Ionic Concentration Changes

One aim of applying the voltage clamp to the cardiac Purkinje fiber is to characterize the time and the voltage dependence of the membrane currents that underlie pacemaker activity. There are five measures of a novel time-dependent current that are used frequently, and each provides some information on the nature of the conductance change. We will consider each in turn.

(i) The Rate of Change of the Slope Conductance

Figure 1 demonstrates schematically the experimental protocol designed to examine this property. Small short voltage clamp steps are superimposed on a larger step that induces the time-dependent current. On the assumption that the superimposed steps are small enough and short enough not to perturb the time course of the current during the voltage clamp step, this measurement should provide information as to whether the membrane resistance is increasing or decreasing as a function of time and consequently whether channels are opening or closing during the voltage clamp step.

To understand this measure more fully, consider a membrane with a conductance that is time-dependent (gated) and voltage-dependent, $g_1(v,t)$, and a background conductance that is voltage- but not time-dependent, $g_2(v)$.

At any voltage v,

$$I(v,t) = g_1(v,t)(v - V_1) + g_2(v)(v - V_2) \quad (1)$$

where V_1 and V_2 are the reversal potentials (see next section) for g_1 and g_2.

Then the slope conductance is obtained by differentiating the membrane current with respect to voltage:

$$\frac{dI}{dv} = \frac{dg_1}{dv}(v,t)(v - V_1) + g_1(v,t) + \frac{dg_2}{dv}(v)(v - V_2) + g_2(v) \quad (2)$$

Equation 2 can be reexpressed: the conductance, g_1, can be written as the product of a fully activated conductance and the fraction of open channels,

$$g_1(v,t) = N_1(t)\bar{g}_1(v) \quad (3)$$

where N_1 (t) is the fraction of open channels that is assumed to be time dependent, but not instantaneously voltage dependent, and $\bar{g}_1(v)$ is the fully activated conductance (all channels open). Substituting into Eq. 2

$$\frac{dI}{dv} = N_1(t)\frac{d\bar{g}_1}{dv}(v)(v - V_1) + N_1(t)\bar{g}_1(v) + \frac{dg_2}{dv}(v)(v - V_2) + g_2(v) \quad (4)$$

Considering now the rate of change of the slope conductance with time, we differentiate Eq. 4 by

$$\frac{d}{dt}\left[\frac{dI}{dv}\right] = \frac{dN_1(t)}{dt}\left[\frac{d\bar{g}_1(v)}{dv}(v - V_1) + \bar{g}_1(v)\right] \quad (5)$$

Thus, the rate of change of the slope conductance is proportional to the rate of change of the fraction of open channels. But because $d\bar{g}_1(V) \div dV$ can be positive or negative, there is no guarantee that the sign of the slope conductance change and that of the rate of change of the fraction of open channels will be the same. Thus, to interpret this measure accurately, we need to know the voltage dependence of the fully activated conductance and the driving force. In the special case of a voltage-independent, fully activated conductance (that is, a linear relation between a fully activated current and voltage), $d\bar{g}_1/dv = 0$; and thus

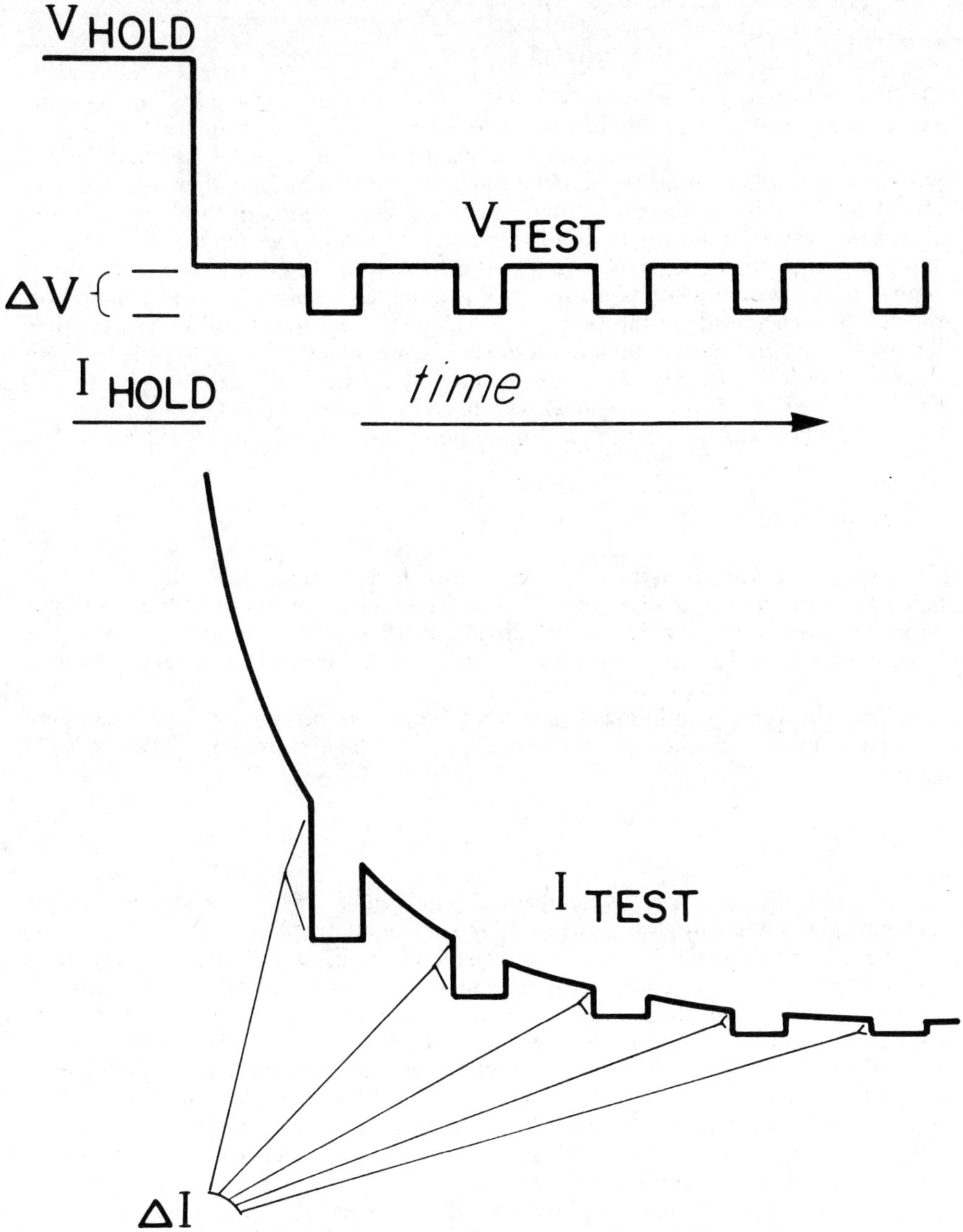

Figure 1. A schematic representation of the method of measuring the slope conductance during hyperpolarizing voltage-clamp pulses. During a hyperpolarizing test pulse from V_{hold} to V_{test}, small hyperpolarizing voltage clamp pulses of magnitude ΔV are superimposed. On the assumption that the small pulses are short enough not to perturb the gating variable, the slope conductance can be assessed. The magnitude of the slope conductance at each point in time is the magnitude of the current jump in response to each small voltage pulse, ΔI, divided by the magnitude of the pulse, ΔV.

$$\frac{d}{dt}\left[\frac{dI}{dv}\right] = \frac{dN_1(t)}{dt}\bar{g}_1(v) \tag{6}$$

The fully activated conductance then is the constant of proportionality between the rate of change of the slope conductance and the rate of change of the fraction of open channels. Under these special conditions, channel opening will be associated with a positive d/dt[dI/dV], and the channel closing will be associated with a negative one.

It is important to recognize that a negative slope region of the fully activated current-voltage relation (where $d\bar{g}_1/dV$ would be negative) does not necessarily guarantee a disagreement in sign between the measured d/dt[dI/dv] and the rate of change of the fraction of open channels. For example, even if $d\bar{g}_1(v)/dV$ is negative, the absolute magnitude of the term, $dg_1(v)/dV \cdot (V - V_1)$ must still be greater than that of $\bar{g}_1(v)$ for the sign of the measured slope conductance change to disagree with the actual sign of $dN_1(t)/dt$. Conversely, if a fully activated I-V exhibits inward rectification, $d\bar{g}_1(v)/dV$ will be negative even in a positive slope region, and, therefore, the sign of the measured d/dt[dI/dV] need not reflect the sign of $dN_1(t)/dt$.

(ii) The Reversal Potential

The potential at which the unidirectional ion fluxes through the ionic channel are balanced to provide zero net current flow is called the reversal potential for an ionic current. Besides allowing for the calculation of driving force on ionic current flow through the channel at any potential, the position of the reversal potential gives useful clues to the ion selectivity of the channel.

With the same assumptions concerning the time-dependent and time-independent membrane conductances that led to Eqs. 1–3, the first time derivative of Eq. 1 gives

$$\frac{dI}{dt} = \frac{dN_1(t)}{dt}\bar{g}_1(v)(v - V_1) \tag{7}$$

The reversal potential is defined as the potential at which ionic current through the channel is identically zero at all times. The current flow approaches zero, only if (*a*) the clamp test potential is equal to the reversal potential, (*b*) the gating variable does not change at the test potential, or (*c*) the single channel conductance is near zero. To be certain that neither alternative b nor c have reduced the time-dependent current to near zero, we have to give a larger test pulse to make the time-dependent current change sign. This would not be expected for the gating or single channel conductance alternatives. A schematic illustration of a reversal-potential measurement is shown in Figure 2. Voltage clamp test pulses VT5, VT6, and VT7, respectively, are increasing inward, remaining constant, and increasing outward. The absence of time-dependent current at VT6, along with the difference in direction of time-dependent current at smaller and larger test pulse amplitudes, defines the reversal potential.

A comparison of VT6 with V_K, V_{Na}, V_{Cl}, or V_{Ca} should indicate which ion or combination of ions might pass through the channel. Changing extracellular ion concentrations and observing changes in the reversal potential can define the channel selectivity.

(iii) The Activation Curve

To assess the voltage dependence of the gating reaction controlling an ionic channel, we construct the activation curve. At any given potential, the activation curve

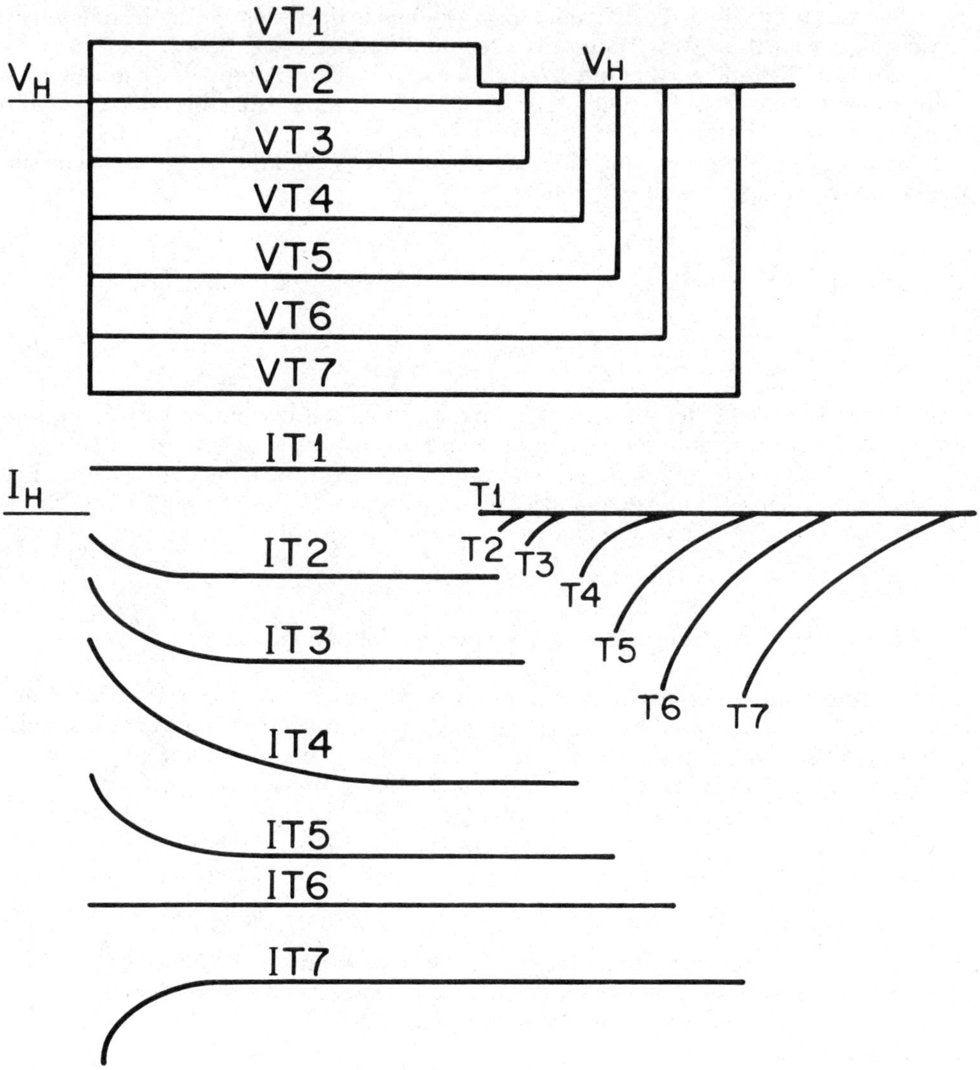

Figure 2. A schematic view of the voltage-clamp pulses required for a complete analysis of an unknown time-dependent conductance. These pulses along with the accompanying current tails should allow construction of the activation curve, the time constant versus voltage curve, and the rectifier ratio. The reversal potential of the channel can also be estimated. For details, see sections A(ii) to A(v).

gives the fraction of gating particles that are in the open position. On the assumption that only one gate controls each channel, the activation curve will give the fraction of channels open in the steady state at each potential.

Figure 2 shows schematically how data for an activation curve might be obtained from tail currents in response to voltage clamp steps throughout the activation range.

The amplitude of any tail current at V_H (which we denote by T_x) following a voltage clamp test pulse (VT_x) is given by

$$T_x = \bar{g}_1(v)(v_H - V_1)\,(N_{VT_{x_\infty}} - N_{v_{H_\infty}}) \tag{8}$$

thus, the magnitude of the tail current is proportional to the difference in the fraction of channels open in the steady state at the test and holding potential.

To obtain the total current due to all the channels at any potential, we must apply voltage clamp steps from the holding potential in the depolarizing direction to obtain the largest tail current, and then in the hyperpolarizing direction to obtain the largest tail current. T_{Total}, representing the current flow at the holding potential when all the channels are open, is then given by

$$T_{total} = T_{Dep} - T_{Hyp} = \pm \bar{g}_1(v_H)\,(v_H - V_1) \qquad (9)$$

Then, the fraction of channels opened or closed by any test pulse is just

$$\frac{T_x}{T_{total}} = N_{VT_{x_\infty}} - N_{v_{H_\infty}} \qquad (10)$$

Then, if we know whether channels are opened or closed by hyperpolarization (see Section A (i)) the activation curve can be constructed.

Sample test pulses generating the maximum tail currents in the depolarizing (T1) and hyperpolarizing (T6) direction are given in Figure 2. Tail currents T2 to T5 in Figure 2 are needed to characterize the slope of the activation curve.

(iv) The Gating Time Constant as a Function of Voltage

The membrane current due to a gated conductance has a characteristic time course. For a channel gated by a single first-order kinetic process, the current should be exponential. The characteristic time constant, for a given potential, is the time necessary for 63% of the ensemble of gating reactions to occur.

Figure 2 schematically shows the data necessary to construct the time constant against voltage curve. For each voltage step, the time-dependent current at the test potential is given by

$$I(t) = [N_\infty + (N_0 - N_\infty)e^{-t/\tau}]\bar{g}_1(v)(v - V_1) \qquad (11)$$

where N_o is the fraction of channels open in the steady state at the holding potential, N_∞ is the fraction of channels open in the steady state at the test potential, τ is the characteristic time constant at the test potential, and $\bar{g}_1(v)$ is the conductance if all the gated channels are open.

Factoring and reorganizing, we get

$$I(t) = \bar{g}_1(v)(v - V_1)(N_0 - N_\infty)e^{-t/\tau} + N_\infty \bar{g}_1(v)(v - V_1) \qquad (12)$$

and because the steady-state current through the gated channel at the test potential is given by

$$I(t = \infty) = N_\infty \bar{g}_1(v)(v - V_1) \qquad (13)$$

then,

$$I(t) - I(t = \infty) = \bar{g}_1(v)(v - V_1)(N_0 - N_\infty)e^{-t/\tau} \qquad (14)$$

and a plot of log $(I(t) - I_\infty)$ versus time has a slope of $-1/\tau$. Thus, at any voltage, the time constant is obtainable from the time course of the membrane current.

A τ versus a v-curve can be constructed from Figure 2 by analyzing test-pulse currents IT2 to IT6 in the manner described above.

(v) The Rectifier Ratio

In the first section, interpreting slope conductance relied on a knowledge of the voltage dependence of the fully activated conductance. The rectifier function is constructed to provide that information.

For any voltage step from a holding potential V_A to test potential V_B, the time-dependent current at the test potential is given by

$$[I(t=0) - I(t=\infty)]_{v=V_B} = (N_{A_\infty} - N_{B_\infty})\bar{g}_1(V_B)(V_B - V_1) \qquad (15)$$

and the tail current at the holding potential is

$$[I(t=0) - I(t=\infty)]_{v=V_A} = (N_{B\infty} - N_{A\infty})\bar{g}_1(V_A)(V_A - V_1) \qquad (16)$$

the ratio of these currents ($R_{B/A}$) is given by

$$R_{B/A} = \frac{[N_{A\infty} - N_{B\infty}]}{[N_{B\infty} - N_{A\infty}]} \frac{\bar{g}_1(V_B)(V_B - V_1)}{\bar{g}_1(V_A)(V_A - V_1)} = -\frac{\bar{I}_B}{\bar{I}_A} \qquad (17)$$

where $\bar{I}_B$ is the current obtained at voltage B if all the gated channels are open, and $\bar{I}_A$ is the current obtained at voltage A if all the gated channels are open.

If the reversal potential and activation curve for the conductance are known, then the voltage dependence and magnitude of the fully activated conductance is obtainable. A knowledge of the rectification properties of the channel can be useful in analyzing the energetics of the ion permeation mechanism.

(B) Potassium Concentration Changes and the Interpretation of Voltage-Clamp Measures

In the introduction, we mentioned that narrow intercellular spaces in Purkinje fibers can cause accumulation or depletion of ions. Figure 3 shows measurements of changes in the extracellular K^+ concentration during voltage-clamp pulses in a canine Purkinje fiber of small radius. The two-microelectrode voltage-clamp technique was used along with an extracellular double-barreled K^+-selective microelectrode. On depolarizing from −50 to −32 mV, there is an increase in cleft $[K^+]$ greater than 0.7 mM. On hyperpolarization to −66, −80, and −95 mV, the $[K^+]$ decreases by 0.5, 0.9, and 1.3 mM, respectively.

Results with these K^+-selective microelectrodes are in contrast to previous indications, obtained by indirect measurements, of only minimal K^+ accumulation and depletion in the canine Purkinje fiber (Cohen and Falk, 1980). Indirect electrophysiologic evidence favoring the preparation was obtained from (1) estimates of the extracellular series resistance, by measuring the final time course of the decay of the capacity transient in normal and low ionic strength solution during a voltage-clamp step (Fozzard, 1966; Cohen and Falk, 1980), and (2) measurements of the ratio of the magnitude of the proposed depletion current to the magnitude of the instantaneous jump in current during a hyperpolarizing membrane potential (Baumgarten et al., 1977; Cohen and Falk, 1980). Also, morphometric analysis of the canine Purkinje fiber performed on voltage-clamped preparations indicates that only 33% of the membrane surface area faces <0.1-μ clefts, and about 20% of the total fiber volume is extracellular (B. Eisenberg, personal communication). These three methods of estimating the possible significance of extracellular K^+ accumulation and depletion in the sheep Purkinje fiber have indicated the expectation of substantially larger K^+ fluctuations.

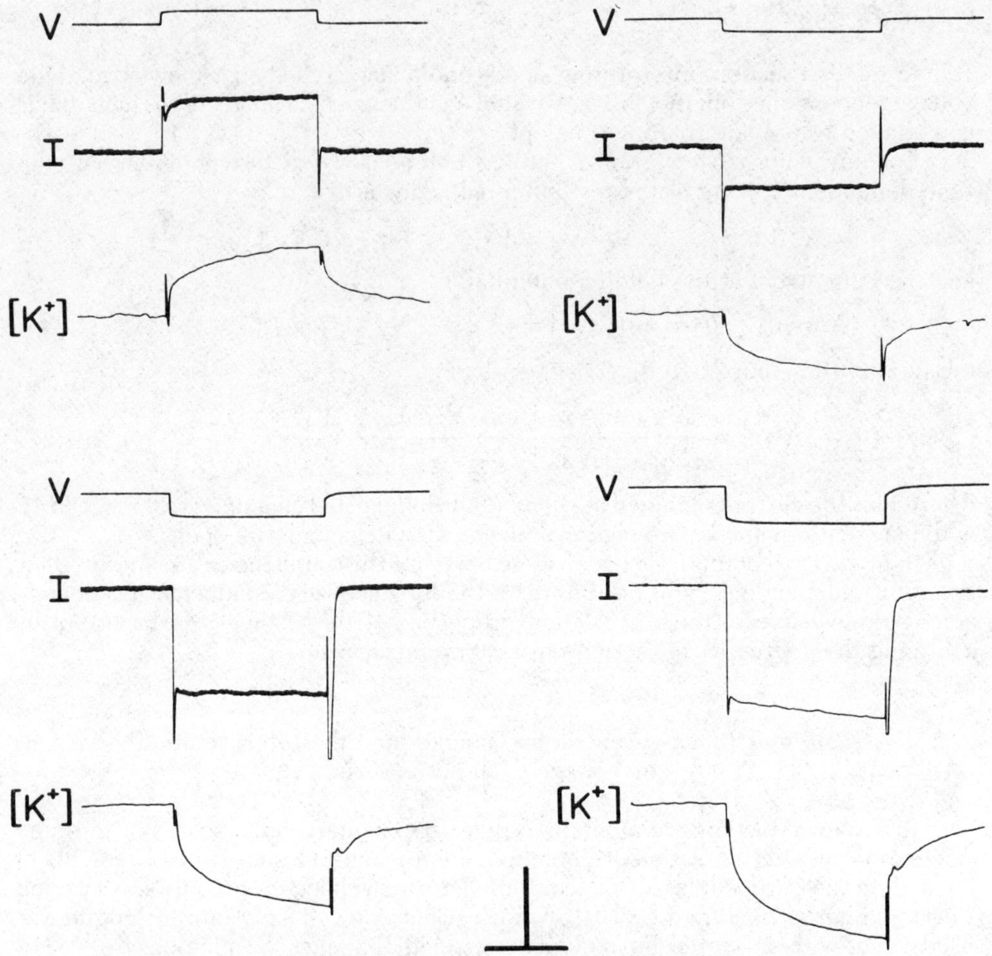

Figure 3. Results from an experiment in which membrane currents were recorded from a Purkinje fiber in the presence of an extracellular K^+-selective microelectrode. The vertical bar represents 50 mV on the voltage scale, 0.7 mM on the K^+ scale (this is approximate as the scale is nonlinear), and 50 nA on the current scale for all but the lower right figure where it represents 100 nA. The horizontal bar is 4 seconds. The holding potential was −50 mV, and the test pulses were to −32, −66, −80, and −95 mV. Note that the membrane current is constant at −66 and −80 mV, but the extracellular $[K^+]$ is changing. A discussion of the interpretation of these measurements is included in the text. The bulk $[K^+]$ was 4 mM, the temperature was 27° C. Kline et al. (unpublished observation).

Difficulties in the interpretation of extracellular K^+ selective electrode measurements do exist, however. The magnitude of the K^+ fluctuation can depend on the position of the microelectrode within the extracellular space. If the tip is pressing on the membrane or blocking a narrow cleft, an artifactually large $[K^+]$ change could be recorded. Therefore, it is worth noting that the K^+ fluctuations in response to voltage-clamp pulses in two additional canine Purkinje fibers were of similar magnitude and time course. Also slight movements of the electrode once it was positioned beneath the connective tissue sheath did not appreciably affect the magnitude or time course of the K fluctuation. Nevertheless, additional tests are necessary to evaluate the spatial variation in the magnitude and time course of K^+ concentration changes before quantitative use of the available data can be made.

The fluctuation in extracellular $[K^+]$ illustrated in Figure 3 has several consequences. First, the background current becomes time dependent because of a time-dependent driving force, and possibly a time-dependent conductance (if $g_2 = f(K)$). Second, the gated current, if it is K^+ selective, has a time-dependent driving force, and also possibly a time-dependent conductance (if $\bar{g}_1 = f(K)$). These additional time-dependent currents complicate the interpretation of the five voltage-clamp measures discussed in section A. These complications are discussed below.

(i) The Slope Conductance

In the previous section, we showed that the rate of change with time of the slope conductance was proportional to the rate of change of the fraction of open channels. Thus, this measure can be useful in assessing whether a conductance is activating (channels opening) or deactivating (channels closing) over a given voltage range.

Consider now a slightly more complete description of the conductances of Section A. The background conductance g_2 is voltage dependent, at least it is, in part, K^+ selective, and like many cardiac conductances, it also depends on the external $[K^+]$. The gating conductance $\bar{g}_1$, has similar ion transfer properties to the background conductance (K^+ selective, with a conductance that depends on the external $[K^+]$).

Under these assumptions,

$$I = N_1(t)\bar{g}_1(v,K)(v - V_1(K)) + g_2(v,K)(v - V_2(K)) \tag{18}$$

and

$$\frac{dI}{dv} = N_1(t)\bar{g}_1(v,K) + N_1(t)(v - V_1(K))\frac{\partial \bar{g}_1}{\partial v}(v,K) + g_2(v,K) + \frac{\partial g_2}{\partial v}(v,K)(v - V_2(K)) \tag{19}$$

Taking the first derivative of the slope conductance,

$$\begin{aligned}\frac{d}{dt}\left[\frac{dI}{dv}\right] = {} & \frac{dN_1(t)}{dt}\left[\bar{g}_1(v,K) + (v - V_1(K))\left[\frac{\partial \bar{g}_1(v,K)}{\partial v}\right]\right] \\ & + \frac{dK}{dt}\left[N_1(t)\frac{\partial \bar{g}_1(v,K)}{\partial K} + N_1(t)(v - V_1(K))\frac{\partial}{\partial K}\left[\frac{\partial \bar{g}_1(v,K)}{\partial v}\right]\right. \\ & -N_1(t)\frac{\partial \bar{g}_1}{\partial v}(v,K)\frac{dV_1(K)}{dK} + \frac{\partial g_2(v,K)}{\partial K} + (v - V_2(K)) \\ & \left.\frac{\partial}{\partial K}\left[\frac{\partial g_2(v,K)}{\partial v}\right] - \frac{dV_2(K)}{dK}\frac{\partial g_2}{\partial v}(v,K)\right]\end{aligned} \tag{20}$$

Equation 20 illustrates the difficulty in interpreting the rate of change of the slope conductance when the extracellular $[K^+]$ is varying during the flow of time-dependent current. The first term on the right hand side of the equation is the same as it is in Eq. 5, and so it is necessary to know the voltage dependence of the fully activated conductance. The second term depends on the rate of change of [K^+], dK/dt, and is not proportional to the rate of change of the fraction of open channels. Thus, no simple proportionality exists between the rate of change of the slope conductance and the rate of change of the fraction of open channels.

Is the second term significant? No conclusive statement can be made on the importance of the time-dependent conductance changes induced by changes in cleft [K^+] during voltage-clamp pulses (see Appendix for some limiting cases). But, the large depletion currents in Na^+-free solution observed in sheep Purkinje fibers (Baumgarten et al., 1978) suggest that significant effects would not be surprising. The new model proposed by DiFrancesco and Noble (1980) for pacemaker activity (Part II) requires that depletion currents on hyperpolarizing voltage-clamp steps be large, and it postulates that these currents can result in an apparent reversal of an inward pacemaker current at negative potentials. Recent attempts (Cohen and Falk, unpublished observations) to measure the change in slope conductance with time in the pacemaker range of potentials of the canine Purkinje fiber have given equivocal results. Representative examples of this data are shown in Figure 4. These results should be compared with those of DiFrancesco (1980a), in which a clear increase in slope conductance during hyperpolarization was reported, and with those of Vassalle (1966), in which a decrease in slope conductance during hyperpolarization was reported (see Part II). These latter two studies consist of data obtained from the ungulate Purkinje fiber.

(ii) The Reversal Potential

As mentioned previously, at the reversal potential, the time-dependent current is zero at all times, thus dI/dt is 0. Now, consider estimates of the reversal potential in the presence of K^+ accumulation. Taking the derivative of Eq. 18 with respect to time gives

$$\frac{dI}{dt} = \frac{dN_1(t)}{dt}\,\bar{g}_1(v,K)(v - V_1(K)) + \frac{dK}{dt}\Big[N_1(t)(v - V_1(K))\,\frac{\partial \bar{g}_1(v,K)}{\partial K}$$

$$-N_1(t)\,\bar{g}_1(v,K)\,\frac{dV_1(K)}{dK} + (v - V_2(K))\,\frac{\partial g_2}{\partial K}\,(v,K) - g_2(v,K)\,\frac{dV_2(K)}{dK}\Big] \quad (21)$$

There is no value of V for which dI/dt should be identically zero for all time. For that matter, neither term should be identically zero for all time. The measured current reversals will be functions of the time-dependent and time-independent K^+ conductances, and the K^+ dependencies of their individual reversal potentials. The true value at rest of the reversal potential of the gated membrane conductance simply can not be obtained from the membrane current.

Under such circumstances, we might expect measured reversals for the pacemaker current to be complex. Figure 5 from Cohen et al. (1976) illustrates that such complex reversals are frequently seen.

(iii) The Activation Curve

As mentioned previously, the activation curve provides information on the voltage dependence of the gating reaction. This information is obtained from analysis of tail-current magnitudes. The magnitude of the tail current in the first section was shown to be proportional to the fraction of channels opening or closing. Now consider how a time-varying extracellular [K^+] will affect this proportionality.

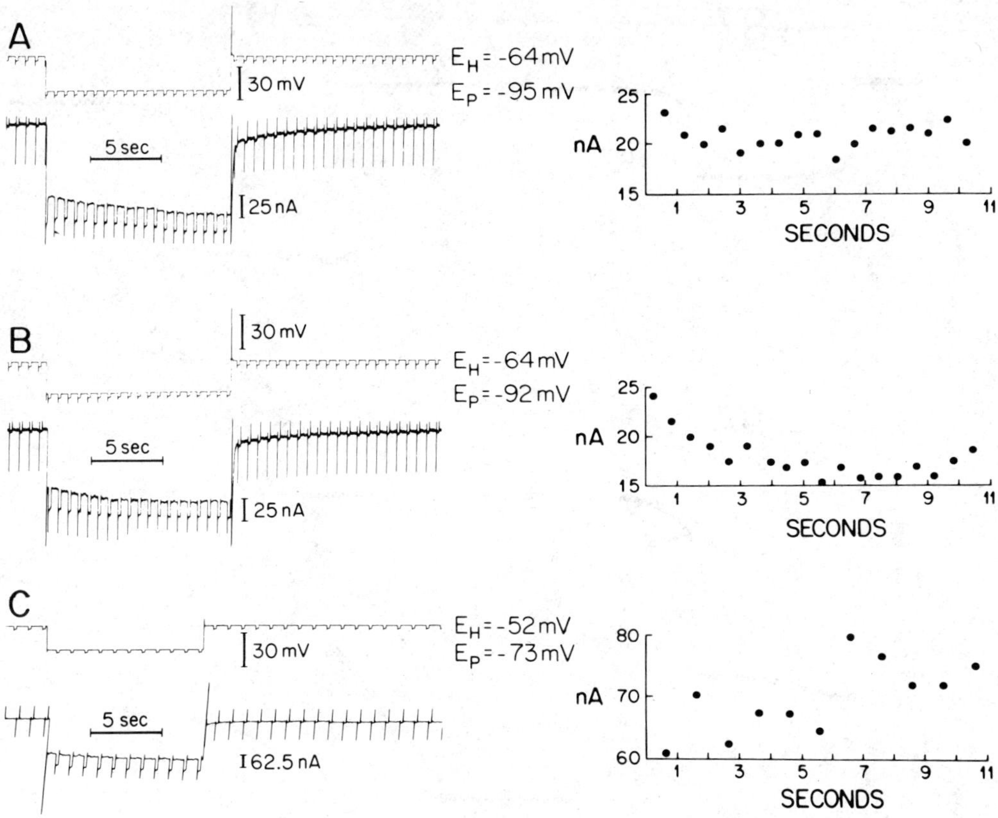

Figure 4. Examples of experiments designed to investigate the magnitude of the slope conductance in canine Purkinje fibers. Voltage-clamp pulses were applied as indicated. The magnitude of the current, ΔI, in response to the small hyperpolarizing voltage pulses is plotted on the right of each pulse. ΔI is constant during the upper pulse, decreases significantly during the middle pulse, and increases during the bottom pulse. For each pulse, the reversal potential of the pacemaker current was at least 15 mV more negative than the test pulse potential. The upper two pulses were recorded from one Purkinje fiber, and the lower pulse was recorded from a second Purkinje fiber. These results are representative of slope conductance measurements from more than 10 canine Purkinje fibers.

The membrane current is expressed by

$$I = N_1(t)\,\bar{g}_1\,(v,K)(v - V_1(K)) + g_2(v,K)(v - V_2(K)) \qquad (22)$$

When a voltage step is applied from the test potential A to the holding potential B

$$I(t = 0) = N_{A\infty}[\bar{g}1_{K_{T=0}}(v_B)][v_B - V1_{K_{T=0}}] + g2_{K_{T=0}}(v_B)[v_B - V2_{K_{T=0}}]$$

At $t = \infty$,

$$I(t = \infty) = N_{B\infty}[\bar{g}1_{K_{T=\infty}}(v_B)][v_B - V1_{K_{T=\infty}}] + g2_{K_{T=\infty}}(v_B)\,[v_B - V2_{K_{T=\infty}}]$$

where $K_{T=0}$ is the $[K^+]$ at $t = 0$, and $K_{T=\infty}$ is the $[K^+]$ at $t = \infty$.

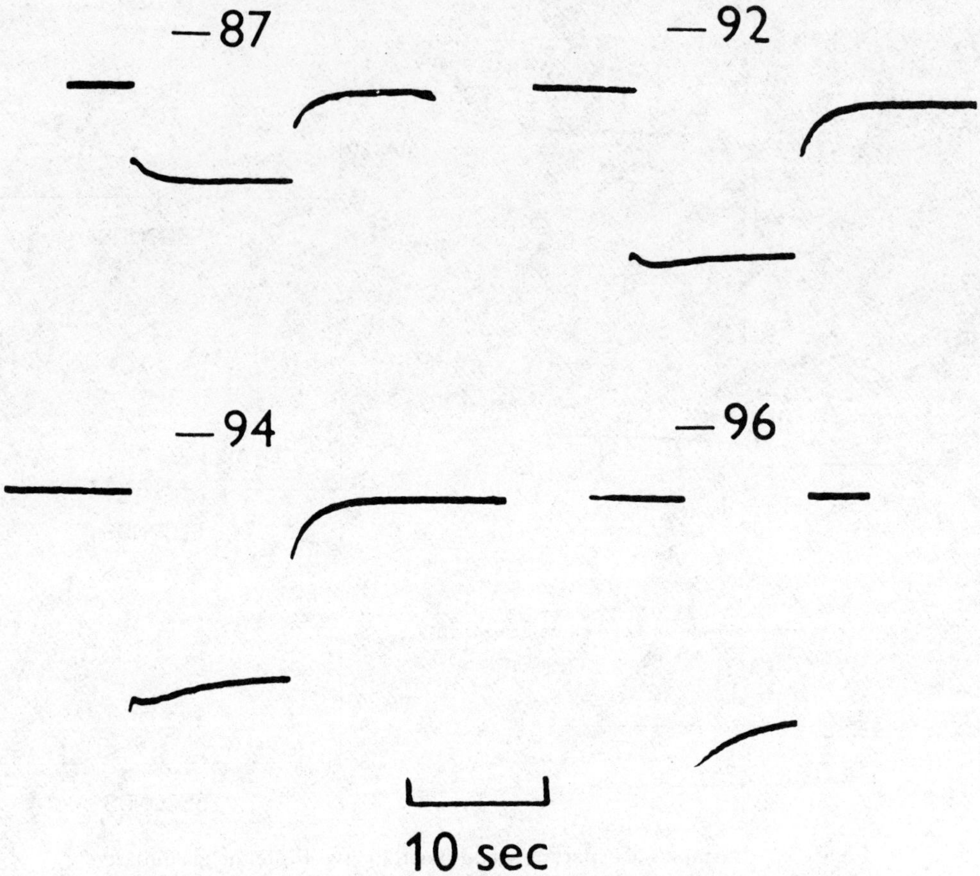

Figure 5. An example of a complex reversal of the pacemaker current in a sheep Purkinje fiber, from an experiment performed by Cohen et al. (1976). At potentials near the reversal potential, the time-dependent current is biphasic.

Therefore, the amplitude of the time-dependent current is

$$I(t=0) - I(t=\infty) = N_{A\infty}[\bar{g}1_{K_{T=0}}(v_B)][v_B - V2_{K_{T=0}}] + g2_{K_{T=0}}(v_B)[v_B - V2_{K_{T=0}}] - N_{B\infty}[\bar{g}1_{K_{T=\infty}}(v_B)][v_B - V1_{K_{T=\infty}}] + g2_{K_{T=\infty}}(v_B)[v_B - V2_{K_{T=\infty}}] \quad (23)$$

Thus, a simple proportionality does not exist between the change in the gating variable, ($N_{A\infty} - N_{B\infty}$), and the magnitude of time-dependent current ($I_{t=0} - I_{t=\infty}$). Also, there is no simple protocol for evaluating the voltage range of activation of the gated membrane current. Measurements of this property of the gating variable will be contaminated by the time-dependent current now being contributed by the partially K^+-specific background conductance.

(iv) The Time Constant versus Voltage Curve

The rate of movement of the population of gating particles is a function of the transmembrane voltage (see Section A(iv)). This dependence on transmembrane voltage produces a membrane current that is most rapid at the extremes of gating activation and slowest at the midpoint of activation (Hodgkin and Huxley, 1952). But when the [K^+] changes during the current flow, the time-dependent membrane current can no longer be characterized in these simple terms.

The membrane current is expressed by

$$I(t,v,K) = N_1(t)\bar{g}_1(v,K)(v - V_1(K)) + g_2(v,K)(v - V_2K))$$

and if the gating reaction is first order, then

$$I(t,v,K) = [N_\infty + (N_0 - N_\infty)e^{-t/\tau}]\bar{g}_1(v,K)(v - V_1(K)) + g_2(v,K)(v - V_2(K)) \quad (24)$$

By reorganizing the terms, we get

$$I(t,v,K) = [(N_0 - N_\infty)e^{-t/\tau}\, \bar{g}_1(v,K)(v - V_1(K))] + N_\infty \bar{g}_1(v,K)(v - V_1(K)) + g_2(v,K)(v - V_2(K)) \quad (25)$$

and

$$I(t = \infty) = N_\infty \bar{g}_1(v,K_{T=\infty})\,(v - V_1(K_T = \infty)) + g_2(v,K_T = \infty)\,(v - V_2(K_T = \infty))$$

Subtracting $I(t{=}\infty)$ from $I(t,v,K)$, we get

$$I(t,v,K) - I(t = \infty) = (N_0 - N_\infty)e^{-t/\tau}\bar{g}_1(v,K)(v - V_1(K(t))) + N_\infty \bar{g}_1(v,K(t))(v - V_1(K(t))) + g_2(v,K(t))(v - V_2(K(t))) - N_\infty \bar{g}_1(v,K_{T=\infty})(v - V_1(K_{T=\infty})) - g_2(v,K_{t=\infty})(v - V_2(K_{T=\infty})) \quad (26)$$

Because $\bar{g}_1$ and V_1 are a function of K^+, and the [K^+] is time dependent, a plot of $\log(I(t) - I(t{=}\infty))$ versus t will not have slope $-1/\tau$. The slope will vary with time because the [K^+] varies with time. Also, the second and third terms on the right-hand side of the equation, which were time independent in section A(iv), are now time dependent. Thus, it appears that no simple relationship exists between the time course of the gating reaction and the time course of the membrane current.

One implication of these results is that the time course of the time-dependent current might be expected to vary with the extracellular [K^+] at a given potential (see our Fig. 6 and Fig. 6 of Noble and Tsien, 1968).

(v) The Rectifier Ratio

The rectifier ratio, like the activation curve, requires the measurement of the magnitude of gated membrane currents. The underlying assumption is that the magnitude of the gated current at a given potential is linearly proportional to the fractional change in gating activation. If this assumption is valid, the voltage dependence of the conductance can be obtained. In a previous section (B(iii)), we saw that tail currents were no longer proportional to the gating change in the presence of K^+ accumulation. We now examine the rectifier properties under similar conditions.

The time-dependent current in response to a voltage-clamp step from voltage A to voltage B is given by

$$I_B = I_B(t = 0) - I_B(t = \infty) = N_{A\infty}(\bar{g}_{1_{K_{T=0}}})(V_B)\,[V_B - V_{1_{K_{T=0}}}] + g_{2_{K_{T=0}}}(V_B)(V_B - V_{2_{K_{T=0}}}) - N_{B\infty}(\bar{g}_{1_{K_{T=\infty}}}(V_B)[V_B = V_{1_{K_{T=\infty}}}] + g_{2_{K_{T=\infty}}}(V_B)(V_B - V_{2_{K_{T=\infty}}}) \quad (27)$$

And similarly, a voltage clamp step from voltage B to voltage A is given by

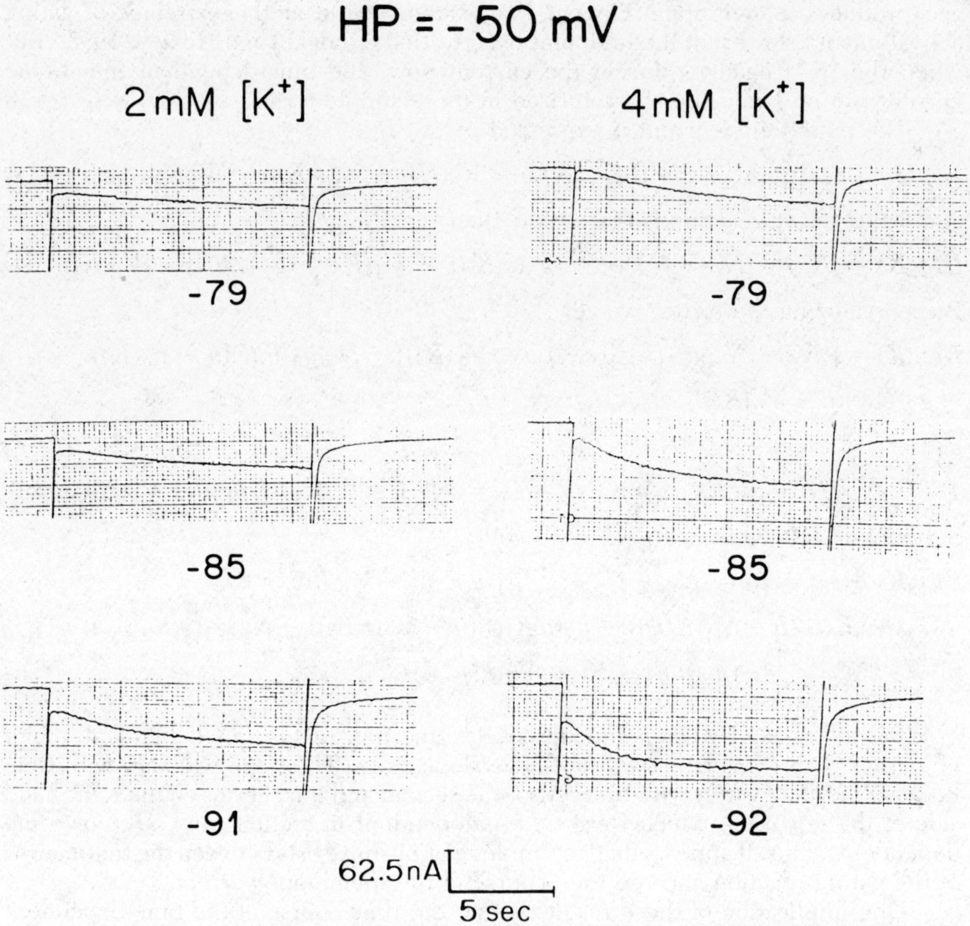

Figure 6. An example of the [K⁺] dependence of the time course of the time-dependent current at a variety of potentials. These results were recorded from a canine Purkinje fiber at 37° C.

$$I_A = I_A(t = 0) - I_A(t = \infty) = N_{B_\infty}(\bar{g}_{1_{K_{T'=0}}}(V_A)[V_A - V_{1_{K_{T'=0}}}] + g_{2_{K_{T'=0}}}(V_A)(V_A - V_{2_{K_{T'=0}}}) - N_{A_\infty}(\bar{g}_{1_{K_{T'=\infty}}}(V_A)[V_A - V_{2_{K_{T'=\infty}}}] + g_{2_{K_{T'=\infty}}}(V_A)(V_A - V_{1_{K_{T'=\infty}}})) \tag{28}$$

where the subscripts $K_{T=0}$, and $K_{T=\infty}$ refer to the [K⁺]'s immediately after stepping from voltage A to voltage B and in the steady state at voltage B, and the subscripts $K_{T'=0}$, and $K_{T'=\infty}$ refer to the [K⁺]'s immediately after stepping from voltage B to voltage A and in the steady state at voltage A.

The rectifier ratio, $R_{B/A}$, is

$$R_{B/A} \frac{I_B}{I_A} \tag{29}$$

Under these circumstances the rectifier ratio is not simply proportional to the ratio of the fully activated currents.

Conclusion - Part I

In summary, the analysis of a Hodgkin-Huxley conductance involves the construction of a number of functions by manipulating the time-dependent current observed in response to voltage-clamp steps. But, if the $[K^+]$ varies while the membrane current is flowing, these same functions will reveal little about the characteristics of the gating and ion transfer function for the channel under study. With this difficulty in mind, we will now review the available voltage-clamp data on pacemaker activity of Purkinje fibers.

PART II - VOLTAGE CLAMP ANALYSIS OF PACEMAKER ACTIVITY

A K^+ Conductance Activated by Depolarization

(a) The Basis of the Hypothesis

In 1951, Weidmann attempted to determine changes in membrane conductance during the action potential by superimposing repetitive, small, negative current pulses during action potentials that were being recorded from sheep Purkinje fibers. The magnitude of the resulting voltage deflections increased during the pacemaker potential, suggesting that the membrane conductance might be decreasing. But, even if the possibility of K^+ fluctuations (see Part I) is ignored, channel opening still could not be distinguished from channel closing because the membrane potential was changing. Vassalle (1966) used a modification of this technique for voltage-clamp conditions. Following an action potential, he clamped the membrane potential at the maximum diastolic potential and observed a current that became increasingly inward with time. Small hyperpolarizing voltage-clamp steps of short duration were superimposed during the voltage clamp to estimate the change in the slope conductance as a function of time (see part I, Figs. 1 and 4). The slope conductance decreased with time, suggesting that the activation of the pacemaker current decayed during diastole (channels were closing).

Noble and Tsien (1968) performed a classic voltage-clamp analysis, as described in part I of this review, on the pacemaker current of sheep Purkinje fibers. They found that the time-dependent current reversed direction at potentials near the expected potassium equilibrium potential and that the current exhibited a high K^+ selectivity, seemingly indicating that the major ion carrying the current was K^+. These findings were confirmed by Peper and Trautwein (1969). From analysis of the time-dependent currents, Noble and Tsien (1968) constructed an activation curve, time-constant curve, and rectifier-function curve (see part I C, D, E). The current was fully activated at -60 mV and fully deactivated by -90 mV. The tail currents were exponential, and the time constant versus voltage curve was bell shaped with its midpoint at half activation. The time constant ranged from several hundred milliseconds at -60 or -90 mV to several seconds at -75 mV. These results suggested that the gating mechanism controlling the pacemaker conductance could be described by a first-order kinetic process. In addition, the rectifier function for the pacemaker current showed a negative slope. That is, the current through the open channel decreased at positive potentials. Thus, although the pacemaker channels were assumed open at plateau potentials, they passed little current.

Noble and Tsien (1968) were able to reconstruct the pacemaker potential on the computer by using the information on the gating and ion transfer properties that they obtained from analysis of the voltage clamp records. In addition, the increase in the rate of diastolic depolarization seen in the presence of adrenalin was explained, within the framework of the analysis, as resulting from a positive shift of the gating and ion transfer properties along the voltage axis (Hauswirth et al. (1968), Tsien (1974a, 1974b).

(b) Difficulties with the Hypothesis

Initial difficulties with the hypothesis were recognized by Noble and Tsien (1968), for although the reversal of the pacemaker current occurred near V_K, it always seemed somewhat more negative. This difficulty in the measured reversal potential was illustrated further by the data of Peper and Trautwein (1969). Their reversal potential for the pacemaker current showed a 61-mV change for a tenfold change in the extracellular $[K^+]$, as predicted for a K^+ specific current. But, the extrapolated intercept on the abscissa ($[K^+]_o$ axis) was greater than 220 mM. The intercept represented the extracellular $[K^+]$ when the reversal potential was 0 mV, and thus the extracellular $[K^+]$ equaled the intracellular $[K^+]$. The 220 mM was a much greater concentration than expected for intracellular $[K^+]$. For example, values for the intracellular K^+ activity of between 110 and 130 mM, with an activity coefficient of 0.75, were recently obtained for the canine Purkinje fiber (Miura et al., 1977).

Cohen et al. (1976) reinvestigated the reversal potential of the pacemaker current. For a range of extracellular $[K^+]$'s between 2.7 and 8 mM, the reversal potential always occurred negative to the predicted value of V_K. Furthermore, in some fibers it was not possible to obtain a reversal of the pacemaker current. These investigators interpreted these measurements as indicating a steady-state K^+ depletion in the clefts of the Purkinje fiber. Baumgarten and Isenberg (1977) provided substantial evidence for K^+ depletion occurring during hyperpolarizing voltage-clamp steps, and DiFrancesco et al. (1979) showed that the reversal potential for the pacemaker current is altered by hyperpolarizing or depolarizing prepulses delivered prior to the test pulse. The overall conclusion from these studies was that the time course of the measured membrane currents and the measured reversal potential were contaminated by a concomitant depletion of K^+ from the narrow clefts of the Purkinje fiber. The importance of this finding to the interpretation of the pacemaker current is readily apparent from the first part of this article.

Actually, the first evidence of accumulation of K^+ in the sheep Purkinje fiber came from the current-clamp studies of McAllister and Noble (1966). Upon termination of prolonged depolarizing currents, the membrane remained depolarized, and only slowly hyperpolarized with time. This was surprising, for the depolarizing current increased g_K. The investigators argued that substantial K^+ accumulated in the extracellular spaces of the Purkinje fiber, which decayed slowly over tens of seconds.

Anatomical evidence for narrow extracellular spaces in the sheep Purkinje fiber that might result in a significant extracellular $[K^+]$ dependence on membrane potential comes from studies of Hellam and Studt (1972) and Mobley and Page (1971). The intercellular clefts in the sheep Purkinje fiber were found to be approximately 300 to 400 Å in diameter. Clefts of this size comprise 0.2% of the fiber volume and face 80% of the fiber membrane area. Given the long duration of cardiac membrane currents and the large surface-to-volume ratio, it is not surprising that K^+ can accumulate or deplete in these narrow spaces.

The discussion presented in Part I of this review emphasized that K^+ accumulation and depletion should distort more parameters than just the measured reversal potential. If the original records in several papers are reexamined, the following deviations from simple Hodgkin-Huxley behavior can be observed. (*1*) The time course of the membrane current often is not exponential and is frequently biphasic (Fig. 6 of Noble and Tsien, 1968; Fig. 1 of Hauswirth et al., 1968; Figs. 2–4 of Cohen et al., 1976; Figs. 2–4 of Baumgarten and Isenberg, 1977; Fig. 2 of DiFrancesco et al., (1979). (*2*) The time course of the current depends on the extracellular $[K^+]$ (Fig. 6 of Noble and Tsien; Fig. 6 of this chapter). (*3*) The time course of the current at the holding potential depends on the test-pulse potential (Fig. 1 of Cohen et al., 1976b).

These results suggested that the initial hypothesis was incomplete and required modification. More recent experiments have led investigators to suggest, however, that an altogether different ionic mechanism may underlie the pacemaker current.

An Inward Current Activated by Hyperpolarization

(a) The Basis of the Hypothesis

Noma et al. (1977) studied the rabbit sinoatrial node and presented evidence for a time-dependent, increasing inward current present at potentials negative to −50 mV. This current (I_h) did not reverse direction at potentials as negative as −80 mV in 10 mM $[K^+]$ (Yanagihara and Irisawa, 1980). But, I_h has been found to be sensitive to changes in extracellular $[K^+]$ (DiFrancesco and Ojeda, 1980). Yanagihara and Irisawa (1980) also investigated the effects of barium on I_h. Barium has been shown to reduce the current flowing through inwardly rectifying K^+ channels in both vertebrate and invertebrate skeletal muscle and to increase the current flowing through the slow inward channels (Standen and Stanfield, 1978; Shibata, 1973; Hagiwara et al., 1974). Yanagihara and Irisawa reported that although barium blocked the time-dependent K^+ current seen with depolarizing pulses (thought to be similar to I_x in the Purkinje fiber), I_h, the inward current, on hyperpolarizing it negative to −50 mV, was still present. This finding, combined with the absence of a current reversal near the expected V_K led these investigators to conclude that I_h was an inward current activated by hyperpolarization. (On reinspection, the time-dependent current flowing on hyperpolarization to −73 mV from a holding potential of −10 mV is reduced by approximately 30% from the control value in Ba^{2+}-containing solution, and the time-dependent current flowing on hyperpolarization to −81 mV is reduced by approximately 40%.) Yanagihara and Irisawa also determined the reversal potential of I_h by applying a constant test pulse to −85 mV while varying the holding potential from −2 to −63 mV, in Tyrode's solution containing D 600, 5×10^{-8} g/ml, (to reduce the slow inward current). The current tails reversed direction at approximately −25 mV, lending added support to their conclusion that I_h was generated by a Na^+- and K^+-selective channel that activated on hyperpolarization.

DiFrancesco (1980b) recognized the apparent similarity between this channel and the pacemaker channel in Purkinje fibers. He applied Ba^{2+}, thereby eliminating much of the time-independent K^+ conductance. Most importantly, the reversal of the pacemaker current was eliminated. On the basis of these measurements, and an increasing slope conductance measured on hyperpolarization (1980a) (in contrast to the earlier results of Vassalle [1966]), DiFrancesco proposed that the pacemaker current in Purkinje fibers was an inward current activated by hyperpolarization. The differences between the DiFrancesco hypothesis and the original Noble and Tsien hypothesis are illustrated in Figure 7. The reversal of the pacemaker current in normal solution near V_K was presumed to be due to depletion of K^+, creating a time-dependent balancing current through the background K^+ permeability (DiFrancesco and Noble, 1980). Ba^{2+} blocks the background K^+ current, and so eliminates the reversal near V_K. The actual reversal of the pacemaker current has been proposed to occur near −20 mV, and the current is proposed to be carried by Na^+ and K^+ (DiFrancesco, 1980b).

(b) Difficulties with the Hypothesis

Experimental manipulations basic to the development of the new hypothesis were performed in a solution containing Ba^{2+}. Ba^{2+} was presumed to block background K^+ permeability, with little or no effect on the pacemaker current. Recent experiments on the canine Purkinje fiber by Cohen and Falk (1980) suggest that Ba^{2+} reduces the time-dependent current positive to the predicted value of V_K for both 2

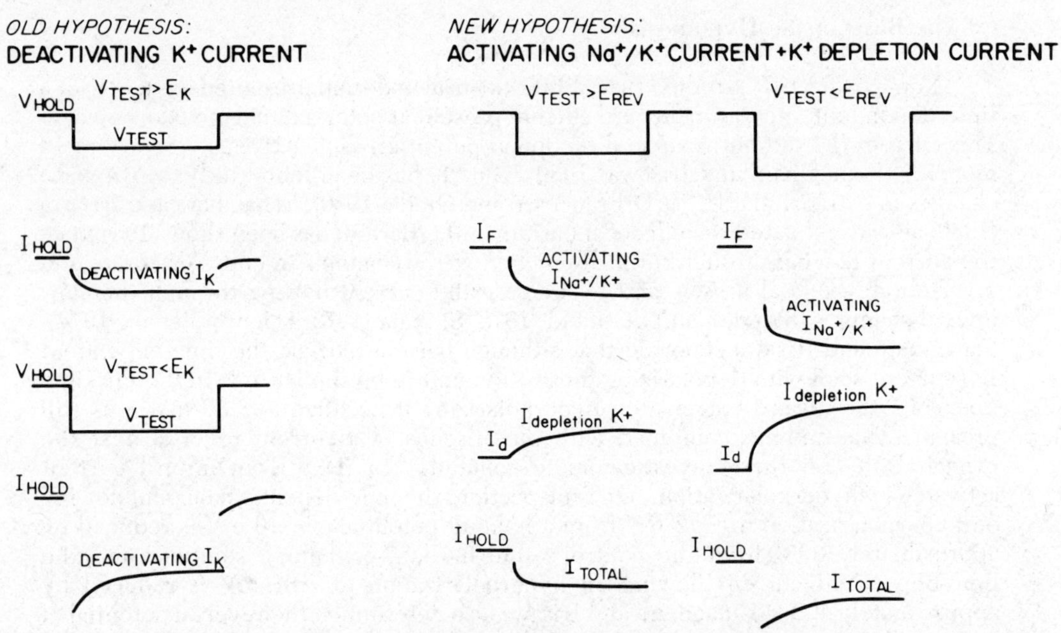

Figure 7. Schematic view of the differences between the Noble and Tsien (1968) and DiFrancesco (1980) hypotheses for the pacemaker current in Purkinje fibers. In the old hypothesis, the pacemaker current was deactivating on hyperpolarization and carried by K^+. The reversal of the current occurred near the K^+ equilibrium potential due to the K^+ specificity of the gated current. In the new hypothesis, the gated current is carried by Na^+ and K^+. The reversal of the current is assumed due to depletion of K^+ creating a time-dependent balancing current. This causes an apparent reversal of the time-dependent current near to but somewhat more negative than the potassium equilibrium potential. The instantaneous jump in current in both hypotheses is caused, in part, by the voltage dependence of gated current and, in part, by the voltage dependence of the other membrane currents.

and 4 mM extracellular [K^+]. This reduction depends on potential and can be near total at potentials positive to −70 mV. This effect of Ba^{2+} on the magnitude of the time-dependent current in canine Purkinje fibers is illustrated in Figure 8. In agreement with DiFrancesco's results from the sheep Purkinje fiber, the pacemaker current reversal, which is initially present, is removed by barium and reappears following return to the control solution.

In simulating the pacemaker current reversal in the sheep Purkinje fiber, DiFrancesco and Noble (1980) assumed a 7% extracellular space in contrast to the 0.2% extracellular space reported in the morphometric studies of Hellam and Studt (1974) and Mobley and Page (1972). Furthermore, to make the apparent reversal K^+-specific, they assumed the magnitude of the depletion to increase dramatically with hyperpolarization and extracellular [K^+]. Experiments in Na^+-free solution in sheep Purkinje fibers (Baumgarten et al., 1977) suggest this may not be the case.

Activation curves and rectifier functions have been constructed on the new hypothesis, but even in Ba^{2+} the membrane currents are often not exponential (Fig. 1 of DiFrancesco, 1980b). Because the current in the presence of Ba^{2+} is postulated to be carried in part by K^+ (DiFrancesco, 1980b), depletion of K^+ from the intercellular spaces might still distort the measured Hodgkin-Huxley parameters. This presence of [K^+] fluctuations in barium-containing solution would be particularly important in evaluating experiments on the selectivity of the pacemaker channel. The actual reversal potential of the pacemaker current has been proposed to occur at approximately −20 mV. The slow inward current and I_x are also present in the plateau range of potentials. DiFrancesco (1980b) identified the current tails near the reversal potential as the pacemaker current by applying the envelope test (Noble and Tsien, 1968). But, because the current at negative potentials does not appear to be exponential, it is difficult to evaluate the details of this test. These experiments were performed in high extracellular K^+ (up to 36 mM) where the K^+ component of the pacemaker current is expected to be large. Therefore, K^+ depletion may be significant and may be the cause of the nonexponentiality of the pacemaker current at some potentials.

Finally, because the current is assumed to be carried in part by K^+, the new hypothesis still does not provide a clear explanation for the absence of a pacemaker current in Na^+-free solution.

Despite these difficulties, the new hypothesis provides a novel and interesting explanation of confusing experimental results.

Conclusion-Part II

Initial voltage-clamp studies suggested that the pacemaker current in Purkinje fibers was activated by depolarization and was K^+ specific. But, this interpretation of the results became uncertain as further evidence indicated the presence of significant extracellular [K^+] changes in the intercellular spaces during voltage-clamp pulses.

More recently, it has been suggested that the pacemaker current is an inward current activated by hyperpolarization. Results from experiments in which Ba^{2+} was used to "unmask" the pacemaker current, by removing background K^+ permeability, constitute a substantial portion of the evidence upon which this new hypothesis is based. Ba^{2+} also apparently affects the pacemaker current and, therefore, perturbs the current it is designed to unmask. Moreover, K^+ depletion is likely to exist even in the presence of Ba^{2+}, because the remaining pacemaker current is still assumed to be carried in part by K^+. This depletion could still distort attempts to analyze gating and ion transfer properties of the pacemaker channel.

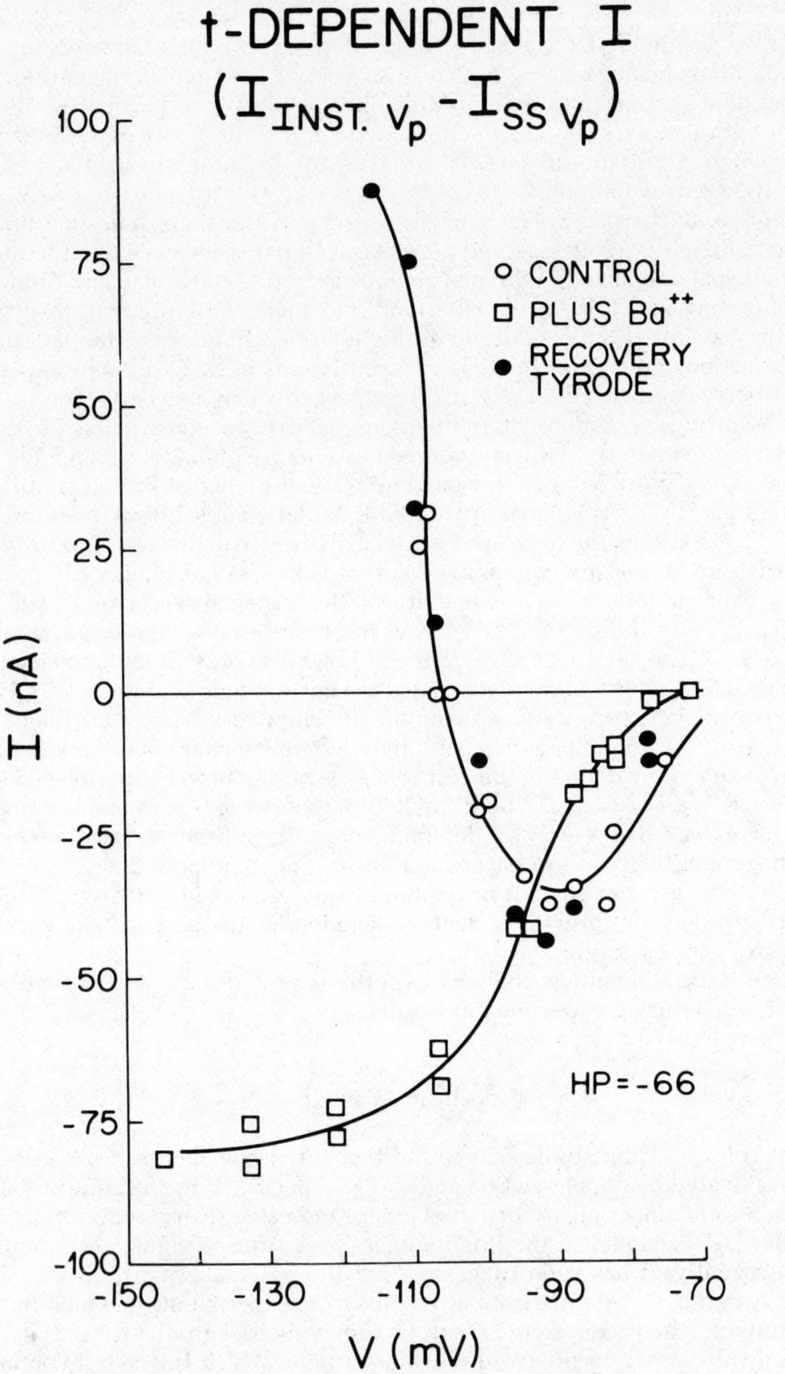

Figure 8. The results of an experiment examining the effects of Ba^{2+} on the pacemaker current in a canine Purkinje fiber. Ba^{2+} reduces the magnitude of the time-dependent current at potentials positive to the potassium equilibrium potential. This is inconsistent with a simple blockage of a K^+-depletion current. Ba^{2+} therefore appears to block the pacemaker current itself. This has serious implications for the use of Ba^{2+} as a probe of the pacemaker current. The temperature was 36° C.

An understanding of the pacemaker activity of Purkinje fibers may require a shift in focus away from the classic Hodgkin-Huxley analysis and towards the application of a variety of alternative approaches.

Because $[K^+]$ fluctuations do occur in the pacemaker range of potentials, a concentration oscillator (Attwell, Eisner and Cohen, 1979) should be considered. The $[K^+]$ oscillations might affect time-independent ionic channels or the Na^+-K^+ exchange pump. In either case, the current will have a time course similar to the K^+ oscillation (although not necessarily identical to it, unless the current is linear with changes in $[K^+]$).

Although the voltage clamp is powerful when applied to the appropriate experimental preparation, anatomical properties of the Purkinje fiber preclude simple application of the technique. The presence of $[K^+]$ fluctuations provide a challenge for the experimenter. Only when those properties of the pacemaker due to membrane conductances are separated from those properties due to $[K^+]$ oscillations will a convincing understanding of the pacemaker mechanism be obtainable.

Acknowledgements

The authors would like to thank Dr. W.G. Van der Kloot for helpful criticism of the manuscript. I.C. was supported by an RCDA from the NIH-NHLBI, and research grants from the NIH and the AHA in collaboration with its Dutchess County Affiliate. R.K. was supported by a grant from the AHA and is a recipient of a Young Investigator Award from the NIH-NHLBI.

REFERENCES

Attwell D, Eisner DA, Cohen I (1979) Voltage clamp and tracer flux data: effects of a restricted extracellular space. Quart Rev Biophys **12**:213–261

Baumgarten CM, Isenberg G (1977) Depletion and accumulation of potassium in the extracellular spaces of cardiac Purkinje fibres during voltage clamp hyperpolarization and depolarization. Pflüg Arch Ges Physiol **368**:19–31

Baumgarten CM, Isenberg G, McDonald TF, Ten Eick RE (1977) Depletion and accumulation of potassium in the extracellular clefts of cardiac Purkinje fibres during voltage clamp hyperpolarization and depolarization. Experiments in Na-free bathing media. J Gen Physiol **70**:149–169

Cohen I, Daut J, Noble D (1976) The effects of potassium and temperature on the pacemaker current i_{K2} in Purkinje fibres. J Physiol **260**:55–74

Cohen I, Falk R (1980) The pacemaker current in canine Purkinje fibres (presented at the Cambridge meeting of the Physiological Society). J Physiol (in press)

DiFrancesco D (1980a) Evidence that 'i_{K2}' in Purkinje fibres is an inward current activated on hyperpolarization. J Physiol **305**:64p–65p

DiFrancesco D (1980b) The pacemaker current i_{K2} in Purkinje fibres is carried by sodium and potassium. (presented at the Cambridge meeting of the Physiological Society). J Physiol (in press)

DiFrancesco D, Noble D (1980) Reconstruction of Purkinje fibre currents in sodium-free solution. (presented at the Cambridge meeting of the Physiological Society). J Physiol (in press)

DiFrancesco D, Ohba M, Ojeda C (1979) Measurement and significance of the reversal potential for the pacemaker current (i_{K2}) in sheep Purkinje fibres. J Physiol **297**:135–162

DiFrancesco D, Ojeda C (1980) Properties of the pacemaker current i_f in the sinoatrial node of the rabbit: a comparison with the current i_{K2} in Purkinje fibres. J Physiol (in press)

Fozzard H (1966) Membrane capacity of the cardiac Purkinje fibre. J Physiol **182**:255–267

Hagiwara S, Fukuda J, Eaton D (1974) Membrane currents carried by Ca, Sr, and Ba in barnacle muscle fibre during voltage clamp. J Gen Physiol **63**:564–578

Hauswirth O, Noble D, Tsien RW (1968) Adrenaline: A mechanism of action on the pacemaker potential in cardiac Purkinje fibres. Science **162**:916–917

Hellam DC, Studt JW (1974) A core conduction model of the cardiac Purkinje fibre based on structural analysis. J Physiol **243**:637–660

Hodgkin A, Huxley A (1952) A quantitative description of membrane current and its application to conduction and excitation in nerve. J Physiol **117**:500–544

Marmont G (1949) Studies on the axon membrane. 1. A new method. J Cell Comp Physiol **34**:351–382

McAllister E, Noble O (1966) The time and voltage dependence of the slow outward current in cardiac Purkinje fibres. J Physiol **186**:632–662

Miura DS, Hoffman B, Rosen MR (1977) The effect of extracellular potassium on the intracellular potassium ion activity and transmembrane potentials of beating canine cardiac Purkinje fibres. **69**:463–473

Mobley BA, Page E (1972) The surface area of sheep cardiac Purkinje fibres. J Physiol **220**: 547–563

Noble D, Tsien RW (1968) The kinetics and rectifier properties of the slow potassium current in cardiac Purkinje fibres. J Physiol **195**:185–214

Peper K, Trautwein W (1969) A note on the pacemaker current in Purkinje fibres. Pflüg Arch Ges Physiol **309**:356–361

Shibata J (1973) The effects of barium on the action potential and the membrane current of sheep heart Purkinje fibres. J Pharm Exp Ther **185**:418–426

Standen and Stanfield (1978) A potential and time-dependent blockade of inward rectification in frog skeletal muscle fibres by barium and strontium ions. J Physiol **280**:169–191

Tsien RW (1974a) Effects of epinephrine on the pacemaker potassium current of cardiac Purkinje fibres. J Gen Physiol **64**:293–319

Tsien RW (1974b) Mode of action of chronotropic agents in cardiac Purkinje fibres. J Gen Physiol **64**:320–342

Vassalle M (1966) Analysis of cardiac pacemaker potential using a "voltage clamp" technique. Am J Physiol **210**(6):1335–1341

Weidmann S (1951) Effect of current flow on the membrane potential of cardiac muscle. J Physiol **115**:227–236

Yanagihara K, Irisawa H (1980) Pacemaker potential generated by the slow inward current in rabbit sinoatrial node cell. Pflüg Arch (in press)

APPENDIX: THE TIME COURSE OF [K^+] CHANGES IN THE EXTRACELLULAR SPACE

In the preceding sections we have often referred to the term, dK/dt, the rate of change of the extracellular K^+ concentration following a clamp step from holding potential (V_H) to the test potential (V_T). Among the factors affecting this time course are: *(1)* the time course of diffusional equilibration between the extracellular space and the bathing solution; *(2)* the ratio of extracellular volume to membrane area; *(3)* the activity and K^+ dependence of the Na^+-K^+ pump; *(4)* the potential and K^+ dependence of the passive time-independent and time-dependent currents; and *(5)* the time constant ($1/\lambda$) of the gating process at the test potential.

The assumptions of the model discussed in this section are described in detail in Attwell et al., (1979). The model is a diffusion model with three compartments: intracellular, extracellular, and bulk (or perfusate) compartments. Movement between the first two compartments is defined by both the transmembrane passive efflux and by the active uptake of K^+. Movement between the latter two compartments is defined by diffusion with a single time constant ($1/\alpha$) (see Eqs. 1 and 2 in Attwell et al., 1979). For simplicity, we assume that the cleft volume per unit area of membrane is equal to one. All quantitative values of current are given in millimoles per second (we divide by F, the Faraday). In this section we consider only one conductance, whose fully activated rectifier is given by $\bar{g}_1$ and whose gating variable is given by N(t). The steady-state values of extracellular $[K^+]$ are K_H and K_T at the holding (V_H) and test (V_T) potentials.

The K^+ concentration of the cleft (called K_c in Attwell et al., 1979) is here referred to as K. The bulk $[K^+]$ is referred to as K_B.

Let $\Delta_1(I_K)$ be the instantaneous change in current on voltage clamping from V_H to V_T:

$$\Delta_1(I_K) = N_{V_H}(t^\infty)[\bar{g}_1(V_H)(V_H - V_K) - \bar{g}_1(V_T)(V_T - V_K)] \qquad \text{I}$$

The time-dependent change in current can be written:

$$\Delta_2(I_K) = [N_{V_H}(t^\infty) - N_{V_T}(t^\infty)][\bar{g}_1(V_T)(V_T - V_K)] \qquad \text{II}$$

We initially consider the simplified case where $\bar{g}_1(V)$ is K^+ independent and the change in $[K^+]$ induces only a small change in the driving force (ΔV_K), or

$$\left(\frac{\Delta V_K}{V - V_K}\right) \cong 0 \qquad \text{III}$$

In this first case, we consider gating effects to be minimal, that is the time-independent current jump is large compared with the time-dependent current, or

$$\Delta_1(I_K) >> \Delta_2(I_K) \qquad \text{IV}$$

At the holding potential (V_H), a steady state K_H can exist and is given by the equation

$$\frac{dK(t)}{dt} = 0 = -\alpha(K_H - K_B) + N_{V_H}(t^\infty)\bar{g}_1(V_H)(V_H - V_K) \qquad \text{V}$$

When the clamp potential is shifted from V_H to V_T, an instantaneous change in current $\Delta_1(I_K)$ is induced (see Eq. I). The new steady-state $[K^+]$ at V_T, (K_T), is given by

$$\frac{dK(t)}{dt} = 0 = -\alpha(K_T - K_B) + N_{V_T}(t^\infty)\bar{g}_1(V_T)(V_T - V_K) \qquad \text{VI}$$

The time course of the $[K^+]$ change can be shown to be given by

$$K(t) = (K_H - K_T)e^{-\alpha t} + K_T \qquad \text{VII}$$

where K_H and K_T can be solved for in equations V and VI.

If we assume a K^+ dependence of either $\bar{g}_1(V)$ or V_K, and include in our model a Na^+-K^+ pump whose rate is sensitive to changes in $[K^+]$, the behavior of $[K^+]$ following the clamp step is modified. In this treatment, only linear, first-order terms are considered, because ΔK is assumed to be small. The general equation (V, VI) now becomes

$$\frac{dK(t)}{dt} = -\alpha(K(t) - K_B) + N_{V_T}(t^\infty)\bar{g}_1(V_T)(V_T - V_K) - P(1 + (K(t) - K_H)\delta p)$$

$$+ (K(t) - K_H)\delta_I \qquad \text{VIII}$$

where the effect of the pump on the $[K^+]$ is given by $-P(1+ (K(t) - K_H)\delta p)$ and $(P\delta p)$ is the coefficient of the linear K^+-dependent term. Likewise, the linear K^+ dependence of the K^+ current is given by the product of $K(t)-K_H$ and the coefficient δ_I. This modification affects the solution for K(t) (Eq. VII) in two ways. First, the values of both K_H and K_T are altered. Second, the time constant of the exponential decay term is changed from $1/\alpha$ to $1/\alpha' = 1/(\alpha + P\delta p - \delta_I)$ (see Attwell, et al., 1979; DiFrancesco and Noble, 1980).

Both the terms $P\delta p$ and δ_I can be shown to be dependent on the bulk K^+ concentration (K_B) and the holding potential (V_H), because these parameters determine K_H. If we assume that the K^+ dependence of the pump is given by the function $(K/K+\sigma)$, where σ is the half-maximal activation value for K, then the linear dependence of the pump varies with the derivative of this term, and for any K,

$$\delta p \sim \frac{\partial}{\partial K}\left(\frac{K}{K+\sigma}\right) = \frac{\sigma}{(K+\sigma)^2}$$

Thus, in a neighborhood around K_H,

$$\delta p \sim \frac{\sigma}{(K_H+\sigma)^2} \qquad \text{IX}$$

due to the assumptions of linearity and small K changes.

The polarity of the term δ_I depends on the relation of V_T to the crossover potential of $\bar{g}_1(V)$ at the two steady-state K^+ concentrations (K_H and K_T). The magnitude of this term depends on the exact value of the difference term:

$$\bar{g}_1(V_T, K_H) - \bar{g}_1(V_T, K_T)$$

Consider now the case where the time-dependent change in K^+ current is dominant, but in which the effects of K^+ on the rectifier are neglected.

The following equation defines this case.

$$\frac{dK(t)}{dt} = -\alpha(K(t) - K_B) + \Delta_2 (I_K)e^{-\lambda t}$$

where $\Delta_2(I_K)$ is given by Eq. II and λ is the time constant of the gating at $V = V_T$.

K(t) can then be shown to be given by

$$K(t) = K_T + \left[\frac{\Delta_2(I_K)}{\alpha - \lambda}\right]\left[e^{-\lambda t} - \left(\frac{\lambda}{\alpha}\right) e^{-\alpha t}\right] \qquad \text{XI}$$

where $K_T = K_H - [\Delta_2(I_K)/\alpha]$. XII

The limiting cases for the solution in Equation XI are:
(1) for $\lambda >> \alpha$ (gating fast, compared with diffusion)

$$K(t) = K_T + \frac{\Delta_2(I_K)}{\alpha} e^{-\alpha t} \qquad \text{XIII}$$

and *(2)* for $\alpha >> \lambda$ (gating slow, compared with diffusion)

$$K(t) = K_T + \frac{\Delta_2(I_K)}{\alpha} e^{-\lambda t} \qquad \text{XIV}$$

For other cases, the $[K^+]$ decay is the difference of two exponential terms but can often be incorrectly interpreted as a single exponential with a time constant larger than both time constants $1/\alpha$ and $1/\lambda$.

If in addition to the time-dependent change $\Delta_2(I_K)$ we reintroduce the time-independent current change $\Delta_1(I_K)$ to equation X, the solution would be similar to that given by Eq. XI, but with the coefficients of the two exponential terms altered and the value of K_T different.

For the more complicated case where we also reintroduce the $[K^+]$ dependence of the Na^+-K^+ pump, the effective diffusional time constant, $1/\alpha'$, is again modified. But for a nonlinear Na^+-K^+ pump-dependence on $[K^+]$ and even a linear dependence of the rectifier on $[K^+]$, the time constants themselves will be time dependent.

Summary

(1) During hyperpolarizing voltage clamp steps, if gating has minimal effects on the net K^+ outward currents but there is a large time-independent decrease in these currents, then the $[K^+]$ decays exponentially with a time constant that is dependent on the diffusional characteristics of the extracellular space.

(2) If, in addition, there are significant effects of the $[K^+]$ changes on the time-independent current or on a K^+-modulated pump, the total change in steady state $[K^+]$ in going from V_H to V_T will change, as will the time constant. If a decreased $[K^+]$ leads to decreased net K^+ efflux, the total change in $[K^+]$ will be larger and the process slower (that is, a larger time constant). If a decreased $[K^+]$ implies more net K^+ efflux, the total change in $[K^+]$ will be smaller and the process faster (a smaller time constant).

(3) If gating occurs at the same time as the $[K^+]$ declines, then the $[K^+]$ decay will generally be slower than either the gating $(1/\lambda)$ or diffusion $(1/\alpha)$ time constants indicate. If the $[K^+]$ changes alter the pump rate or the time-independent currents in the presence of gating, the time constants defining the $[K^+]$ decay during the clamp can themselves become time-dependent, defying meaningful attempts at exponential analysis.

(4) For situations where the clefts are very small and K^+ also accumulates in the larger extracellular spaces, then a four-compartment model would be needed, because cleft $[K^+]$ and average extracellular $[K^+]$ would vary with different magnitudes and time courses. In fact, for sufficiently small clefts, one must consider whether the short-test pulses, which are used to measure changes in slope conductance and are considered too short to affect gating processes, may actually alter cleft $[K^+]$.

Discussion

CRANEFIELD: For the sake of argument, what if Ba^{2+} abolishes the normal pacemaker current *and simultaneously creates a new pacemaker current that has different properties*? What would you say to that?

I. COHEN: This is one of the suggestions we made when we reported our results to The Physiological Society. Indeed the suggestion was made that barium was abolishing something that was very much like i_{K_2}.

PAGE: For the last couple of days, I have been hearing everybody speak of the volume of the clefts. As this seems to be a very crucial issue, I would like to put the question in perspective. When I first reported a measurement of this value in the early 70s, we were interested in looking at the membrane capacity in terms of an evaluation of the true surface area of the Purkinje fiber. In this study, we made an incidental observation about the volume of the clefts, and this has been very widely cited. Subsequently, Hellam and Studt (J Physiol **243**:637–660, 661–694, 1974), in what I think is a very fine study, came up with somewhat different figures, but these are not very helpful either in terms of evaluating the volume of the clefts. So what I would like to point out is that nobody so far has measured cleft volume with the accuracy that seems to be necessary for the electrophysiologists. This measurement is possible, but has not yet been made. I would go as far as to say that no one has yet estimated the cleft volume.

REUTER: Do you have any explanation for the absence of pacemaker potential in rabbit Purkinje fibers?

I. COHEN: One very interesting experiment, which I have tried to induce Colatsky and Tsien to do, is to expose rabbit Purkinje fibers to barium. Under these conditions, one might expect to see a pacemaker current. But Tsien tells me that he only saw a pacemaker current once out of 20 experiments in normal Tyrode. This is in keeping with the fact that rabbit Purkinje fibers do not often show pacemaker potentials. Do you have any suggestions?

REUTER: No, I have no really good suggestions, except that cleft spaces and pump activity may be involved again. Maybe in the rabbit you do not have these narrow clefts, and therefore you do not see the pacemaker currents.

I. COHEN: Well, the canine Purkinje fiber has a cleft geometry that is not dissimilar to that of the rabbit. Yet, the pacemaker current *is* clearly present in the dog. To know whether the difference in cleft space in the rabbit and in the dog is actually important, we would need the morphometric results which are presently in preparation by Brenda Eisenberg and myself.

CARMELIET: I would like to state that you do see diastolic depolarization in rabbit Purkinje fibers provided the extracellular potassium is low enough. The cell hyperpolarizes and the diastolic depolarization ensues. Yet, you do not see in this voltage range a pacemaker current like that of sheep Purkinje fibers. Also, barium is able to induce a pacemaker potential in rabbit Purkinje fibers.

JOHNSON: What assumptions did Noble make in his model to get a relationship between membrane potential and outside potassium that was shifted in the voltage axis as much as 18 mV?

I. COHEN: The only necessary assumption is that the reversal potential must be negative to the cross over. This must be true to allow the depletion current and the inward current to be flowing in different directions. Then, what he needed was an extremely flat relationship up to the voltage where you get to E_K. From this voltage on, he had to make the current voltage relation very steep so that he could then produce the reversal potential at the desired potential.

Chapter 17

Developmental Aspects of Cardiac Excitation: Active Transport

Melvyn Lieberman, C. Russell Horres, James F. Aiton, Norikazu Shigeto, and David M. Wheeler

During the past decade, electrophysiologists have sought to understand the cardiac action potential by studying its development in the embryo. To understand the mechanisms responsible for the generation of transmembrane potentials, they have studied the movements of ions down their electrochemical gradients (for recent reviews, see Sperelakis [1980] and DeHaan [1980a]). During electrical activity in embryonic heart cells, as in other excitable cells, the transmembrane sodium (Na) gradient is directed inward, whereas the potassium (K) gradient is directed outward; and cardiac muscle is repetitively generating action potentials. Thus, to maintain intracellular homeostasis, a mechanism capable of extruding Na and K against their respective electrochemical gradients must exist to balance the passive Na and K fluxes. Because embryonic cardiac muscle cells are characterized by a large surface area to volume ratio and a high membrane permeability (Carmeliet et al., 1976), an active transport system must play a major role in maintaining steady-state conditions. Such a mechanism takes on an even greater fundamental significance if the active Na extrusion is not balanced by an equal uptake of K, for then an electrogenic pump current must contribute to the resting and action potentials of cardiac cells.

This chapter will highlight briefly, from an historical perspective, evidence that supports the presence of an Na-K pump in embryonic heart muscle, from both intact and tissue-cultured preparations. As in adult cardiac muscle, the morphology and cellular heterogeneity of intact embryonic heart muscle impedes the identification of the basic biological mechanisms associated with ion transport and electrical activity of the cardiac membrane (Lieberman et al., 1978; Horres et al., 1979a). Consequently, we have directed our efforts to heart cells in tissue culture because of their physiologic stability, minimal diffusion distance, and morphologically simple extracellular space. The results obtained from electrophysiologic and radiotracer studies of cultured heart cells provide new insights into the physiologic implications of active transport on cardiac cell function.

EMBRYONIC HEART MUSCLE

Transmembrane action potentials recorded from defined regions of embryonic chick hearts at the primitive tubular stage of development are remarkably similar to those obtained from older embryonic and adult heart cells (Fig. 1) (Lieberman and Paes de Carvalho, 1965). The ionic mechanism underlying the depolarization phase of the cardiac action potential at these early stages of differentiation is attributed to an inward current activated by conductance mechanisms associated with calcium (DeHaan, 1980b) and sodium (Sperelakis, 1980). With development, the density of

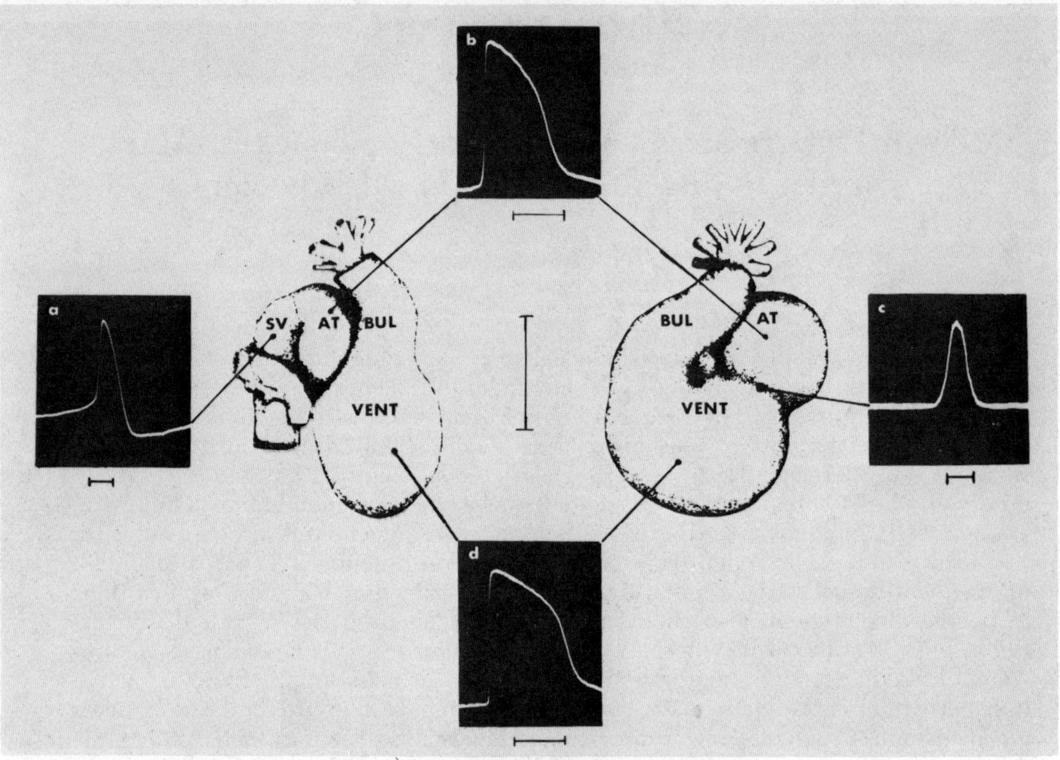

Figure 1. Transmembrane potentials from the sinus venosus (SV), atrium (AT), atrioventricular canal, and ventricle (VENT) of a 72-hour chick embryo heart. Vertical bar, 50 mV. Horizontal bars, 100 msec. Modified after Lieberman and Paes de Carvalho (1965).

sodium channels in the membrane is thought to increase, such that the inward current becomes associated with a sodium-specific conductance mechanism that is sensitive to the Na channel blocking agent, tetrodotoxin. Although there is evidence that the configuration of the embryonic action potential changes in response to an increase in extracellular potassium (Yeh and Hoffman, 1968) and that membrane permeability to potassium appeared to increase as a function of embryonic age in the study of Carmeliet et al. (1976), the ionic mechanism associated with repolarization is still in question. We still need to distinguish between the relative contributions of an outwardly activated potassium current and a slowly inactivating inward sodium current. Not to be overlooked, in this regard, is the possible contribution of an electrogenic mechanism for active transport.

In embryonic chick hearts between the ages of 2 and 18 days, the resting membrane potential is less negative than the calculated potassium equilibrium potential is, and the difference between the potentials declines with development (McDonald and DeHaan, 1973; Fozzard and Sheu, 1980). The increase in resting membrane potential during the early stages of cardiac development is caused by a progressive increase in P_K (Sperelakis and Shigenobu, 1972; Carmeliet et al., 1976) or maturation of the Na-K pump (Fozzard and Sheu, 1980). Because the electrochemical gradient for potassium in the early embryonic heart is outwardly directed, the net passive efflux of potassium must be balanced by the active transport of potassium into the cell. The presence of a membrane-bound Na-K-ATPase enzyme in early embryonic chick hearts, albeit of low specific activity, is sufficient to maintain the normal concentration gradients of sodium and potassium (Sperelakis, 1972). Additional evidence to support the presence of an active transport mechanism in the embryonic heart is that ouabain markedly inhibits Na-K ATPase activity (Sperelakis and Lee, 1971) as well as ^{24}Na efflux and ^{42}K influx (Klein and Evans, 1961). Furthermore, in the presence of ouabain (10^{-4} M), the loss of cell potassium can be reasonably well accounted for by a reciprocal exchange with sodium (McDonald and DeHaan, 1973). In the embryonic chick heart during hypoxia, several parameters of cell membrane function support the hypothesis that changes in intracellular ion contents and membrane potential are probably due to the inhibition of active Na-K transport (Vleugels et al., 1976). In older embryonic hearts, the substantial effects of hypoxia on the cardiac action potential are probably related to the high values obtained for ATPase activity (Sperelakis, 1972) and potassium permeability (Carmeliet et al., 1976) in these preparations.

The concept that an active transport process, responsible for maintaining the transmembrane sodium and potassium gradients in embryonic ventricular muscle, can be electrogenic was tested by Sano et al. (1975). Prolonged periods of cooling preparations in a low-K Tyrode's solution caused a significant decline in the resting membrane potential, which when rewarmed in a 5.4 mM-K Tyrode resulted in a hyperpolarization in excess of the mean resting membrane potential of control muscle fibers. In accord with the data cited above, the average values obtained from rewarmed older (15 day) hearts were greater than those from the 6-day embryonic chick heart. Unfortunately, the fundamental test for electrogenic transport, that is, whether the potential during the hyperpolarization exceeded the potassium equilibrium potential, could not be resolved because the intracellular K content at the time of reactivation was not measured.

TISSUE-CULTURED HEART CELLS

Our laboratory studied active transport in the embryonic heart cell membrane by using tissue-cultured preparations of heart cells designed to minimize problems created by extracellular diffusion delays. To achieve this experimental criterion, we developed a multistranded preparation of heart cells grown as thin annuli around a nylon monofilament (Horres et al., 1977). The preparation was mechanically stable, able to be stimulated electrically, and sufficiently thin (60 to 100 μm in diameter inclusive of the 20 μm nylon core) to avoid the complications of tracer reflux on radiotracer kinetics (Horres et al., 1979a), as well as to allow for the recording of transmembrane potentials during extremely rapid changes of ionic composition in the extracellular spaces of the preparation.[1] As a consequence, we were able to inhibit and stimulate active transport more quickly than the time reported for many experiments using complex naturally occurring preparations of cardiac muscle. The problems of extracellular ion accumulation or depletion which occur in diffusion-limited preparations with changing activity of the transport mechanism and/or membrane permeability were sufficiently small in the cultured heart cell preparation. Thus, we could observe the effects of stimulation of active transport on membrane potential before a change in intracellular ion content could occur.

The possibility that an active membrane transport process in cardiac muscle could be electrogenic and contribute to the steady-state resting potential has been discussed in the literature for more than 20 years (for review, see Glitsch, 1979). A question pertinent to this hypothesis is whether the experimental evidence in support of electrogenic transport satisfactorily excludes any contribution of a change in membrane permeability during the time course of the measured event. In cardiac muscle, the relationship between membrane potential and extracellular potassium concentration deviates markedly from the Nernst equation at low K_o. Although the decline in resting membrane potential in nominally K-free solutions has been attributed to a decrease in K permeability (Carmeliet, 1961), recently our laboratory has obtained evidence that challenges this interpretation (Horres et al., 1979a). Figure 2 summarizes the values obtained for membrane potentials (E_m) from a series of single impalements maintained throughout several rapid changes in extracellular K from a control value of 5.4 mM. For concentrations of K_o greater than 10 mM, the relationship between E_m and K_o was linear with a slope predicted by the Nernst equation for a K-selective membrane. When K_o was changed from 5.4 mM to a nominally K-free solution, within 2 sec the maximum resting (diastolic) potential increased (became more negative), as expected from the increased electrochemical gradient for K, and only after 5 min did it decline to a value of −42 mV (Fig. 3). The deviation of the instantaneous membrane potential from the Nernst equation between 1 and 10 mM K could be accounted for by a finite permeability of the membrane to sodium. Furthermore, in the absence of K_o, the rate of ^{42}K efflux from the preparation increased, and direct measurements of intracellular K and Na concentration revealed a 50% decrease in K_i and a 400% increase in Na_i (Fig. 4A). These data could be accounted for by the presence of a large gradient for net K efflux and the inhibition of active transport, rather than to a decrease in potassium permeability. We found support for this hypothesis when we added 10^{-4} M ouabain to perfusates containing 2.7 and 5.4 mM K (Fig. 2). In each case, within 3 min after switching to the ouabain-containing solution, the cells depolarized to approximately −50 mV, a value comparable to the depolarized potential obtained in the K-free perfusate.

The results presented thus far cannot be attributed solely to inhibition of an electrogenic active transport mechanism because of the observed decrease in the electrochemical gradient. But, as illustrated in Figure 3, the reintroduction of 5.4 mM K did not produce a further decrease in membrane potential, but rather hyperpolar-

[1]The perfusion apparatus for electrical measurements consisted of a shallow-walled, silicone rubber chamber (fluid capacity approximately 1.0 ml) that was molded to the dimensions of the U-shaped preparation support and housed in a thermostatically controlled aluminum block mounted to the stage of an inverted microscope. Fluid flow in the chamber was essentially laminar so that visual distortions were avoided at flow rates as high as 25 ml·min^{-1} when the preparation was viewed with a television microscopy system. An electrically controlled air-actuated diverter valve (Horres et al., 1979b) enabled the entire volume of the chamber to be replaced within 2 sec. Conventional microelectrode recording techniques were used to record transmembrane potentials from the cultured heart cells during rapid changes of the perfusate.

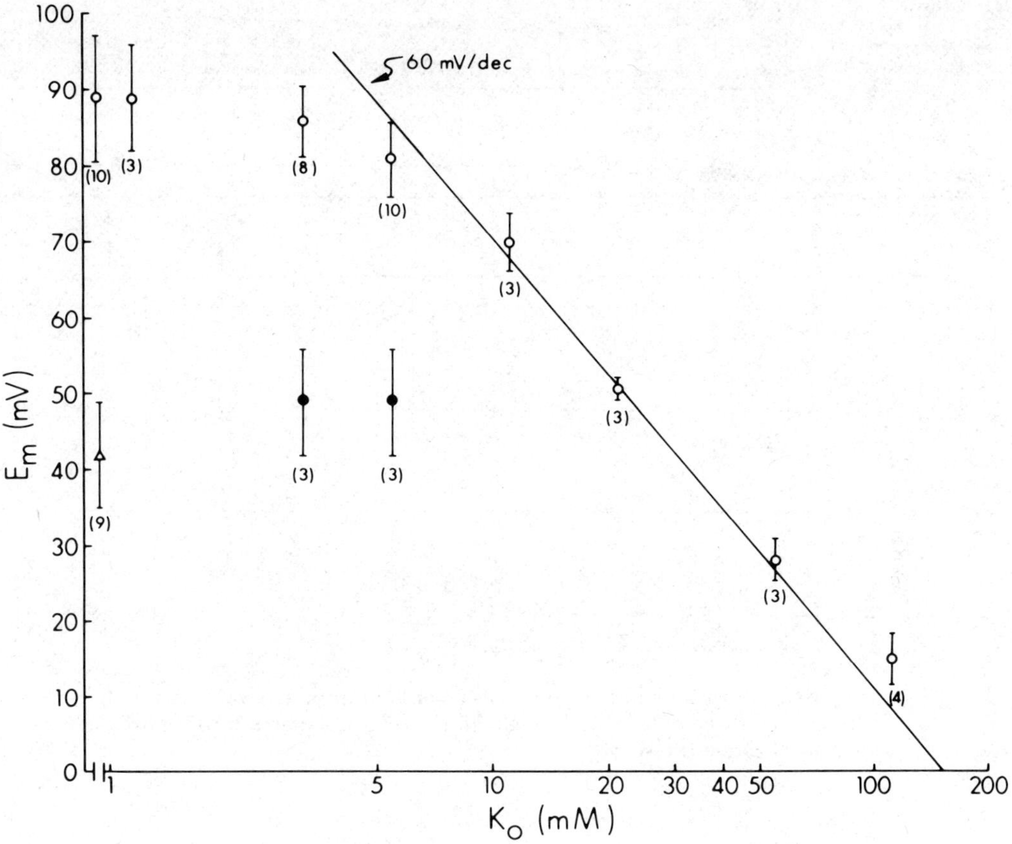

Figure 2. Resting membrane potential as a function of external potassium for growth-oriented embryonic heart cells in tissue culture. Open circles represent a continuous series of measured values obtained immediately after a rapid solution change for a single impalement. Open triangle is the potential recorded after several minutes in K-free solution. Closed circles are potentials obtained three minutes after the addition of 10^{-4} M ouabain. Parentheses enclose number of experiments; values are mean ± SD.

ized the membrane by approximately 50 mV to a value of −89 mV within 2 sec.[2] Because the hyperpolarization preceded the recovery of Na and K to their control values in 5.4 mM K (Fig. 4B), the electrochemical gradient alone could not account for the observed change in membrane potential. That the average potential observed on reexposure to 5.4 mM K exceeded the calculated K equilibrium potential by 13 mV provided the critical evidence in support of an electrogenic transport mechanism in cultured embryonic heart cells. Although the data did not address the stoichiometry of the Na-K coupled transport, the kinetics of Na loss and K gain during recovery of intracellular ionic concentration (Fig. 4B) are consistent with a coupling ratio of 3Na:2K.

[2]In spontaneously beating preparations, it was not uncommon to wait as long as 4 min for the reappearance of action potentials following active transport inhibition by K-free solutions. But, electrically stimulated preparations were observed to reinitiate the action potentials immediately after they reached the maximal level of hyperpolarization.

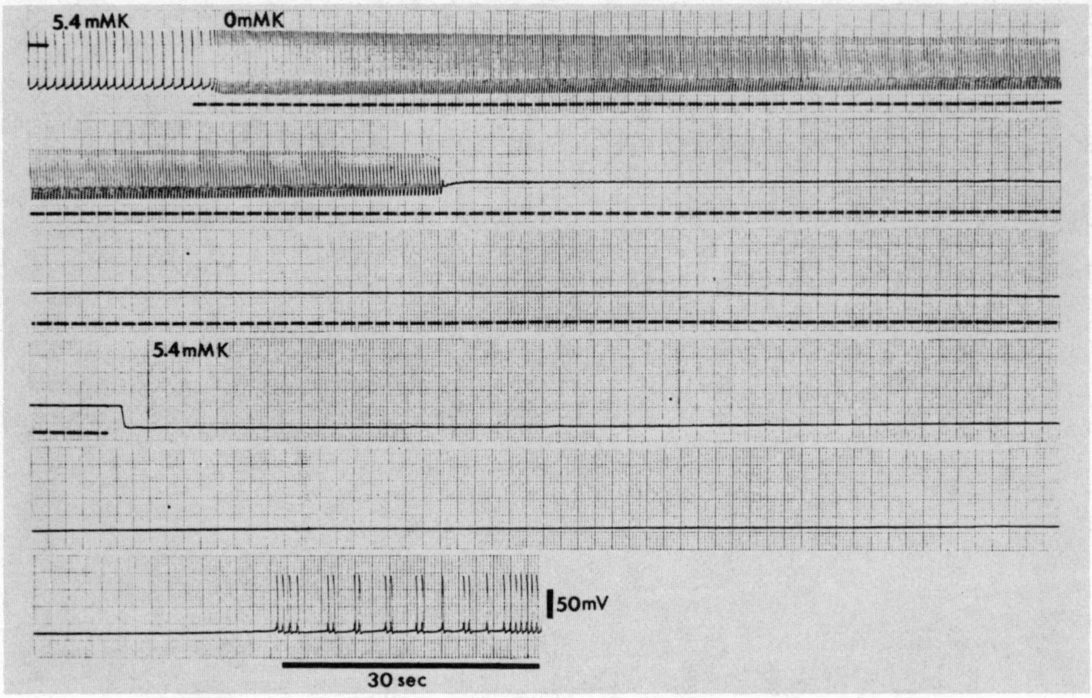

Figure 3. Transmembrane potentials recorded continuously from growth-oriented cultured heart cells during inhibition (0 mM K) and reactivation (5.4 mM K) of active transport.

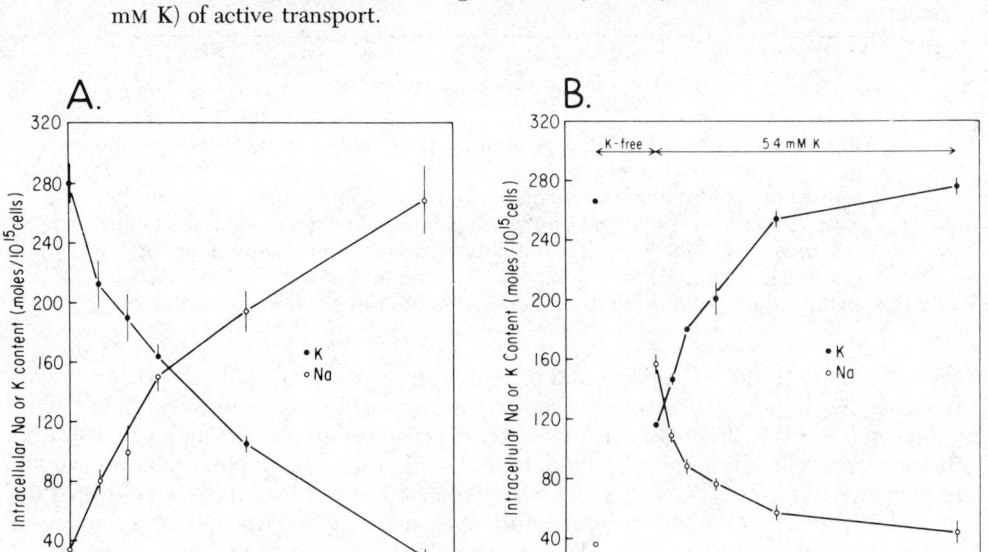

Figure 4. Panel A. Effect of K-free solution on intracellular sodium and potassium content of confluent cultures of muscle-enriched heart cells. Panel B. Recovery of sodium and potassium content following reactivation of Na-K transport. Each value represents mean ± SD of 3 to 11 preparations.

Activation of the Na-K pump in many cells, including cardiac muscle cells, is dependent on the concentration of K_o (Glitsch et al., 1976; Gadsby and Cranefield, 1979). Thus, we studied this relationship by measuring the amplitude and time course of the change in membrane potential following reactivation of active transport over the range from 0.54 to 20 mM K. Reintroduction of 1 to 20 mM K to transport-inhibited preparations markedly hyperpolarized the membrane potential by approximately 50 mV, whereas the maximal hyperpolarization attained in the presence of 0.54 mM K was approximately 33 mV (see Fig. 5). Furthermore, the values obtained for the maximal rates of hyperpolarization varied tenfold, from 4.1 ± 1.0 to 41.4 ± 8.0 $mV{\cdot}sec^{-1}$ (mean ± SD), on the reintroduction of 0.54 and 5.4 mM K, respectively. The data in Figure 5 show that, depending on the K concentration during a 10-sec interval of pump activation, reperfusion with K-free solution causes the membrane to depolarize rapidly and to initiate transiently spontaneous activity. In this circumstance, the transient appearance of spontaneous action potentials could be related to temporal changes in the current-voltage relationship produced during the brief reactivation of the electrogenic Na-K pump (Gadsby and Cranefield, 1977; Eisner and Lederer, 1980).

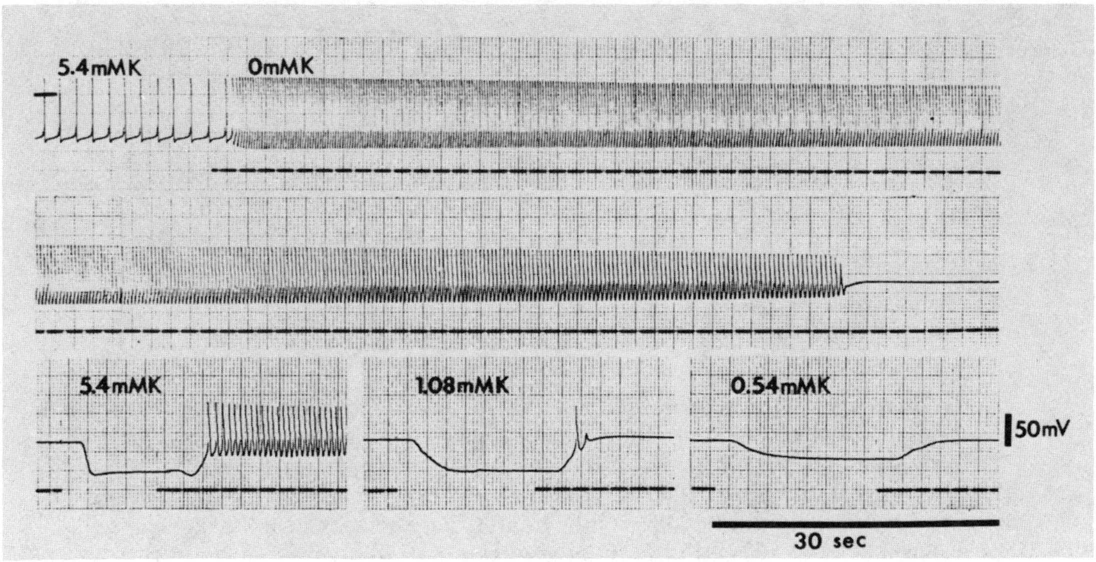

Figure 5. Recordings of transmembrane potentials during inhibition of active transport by K-free solution. Lower panels indicate the effect of a 10-sec exposure to different levels of K followed by the response upon reintroducing the K-free solution.

Rate-dependent changes in membrane potential described by the phenomenon of "overdrive suppression" of automaticity (Vassalle, 1970), presumed to be due to stimulation of electrogenic transport, have recently been demonstrated in spherical aggregates of cultured embryonic chick heart cells (Pelleg et al., 1980), as well as with growth-oriented heart cells in our laboratory (unpublished observation). To further characterize stimulation of Na-K transport, we used muscle-enriched monolayer cultures to evaluate ^{42}K influx as a function of K_o (Fig. 6). The measurements were made approximately 10 min after potassium was removed from the medium, at which time Na_i was elevated to values three times that of control. When these were compared with the ^{42}K influx of control preparations, stimulation of active transport in the Na-loaded cells also appeared to saturate at 5.4 mM K_o, with half-maximal

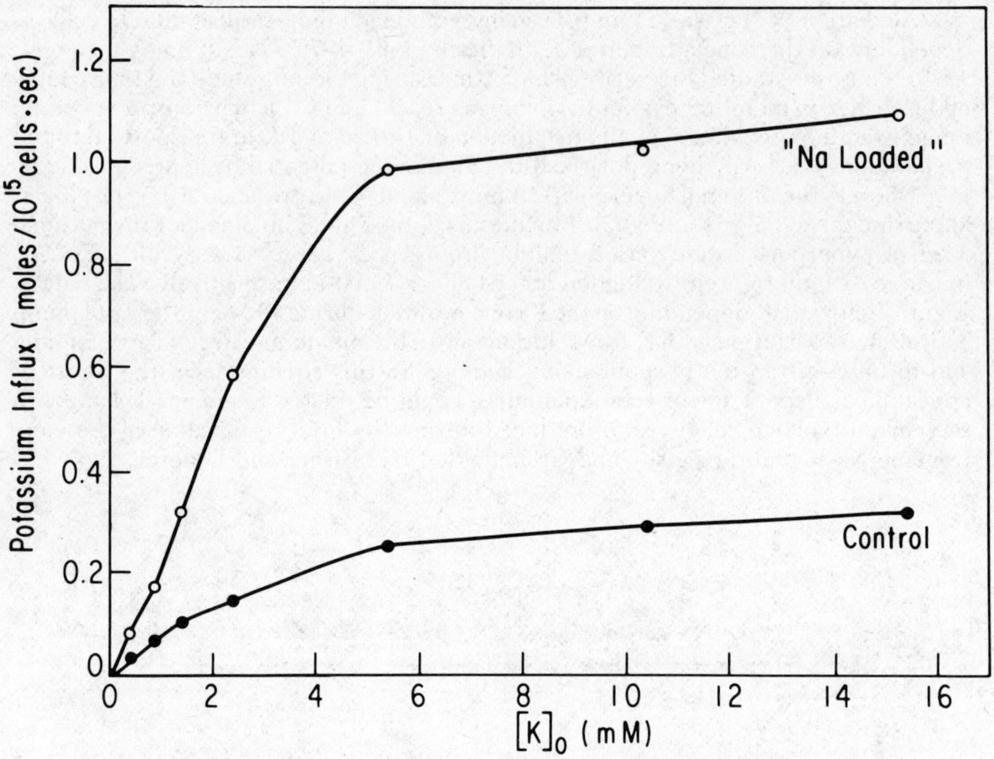

Figure 6. ^{42}K uptake as a function of external K for preparations in steady-state (control) and during recovery from K-free perfusion ("Na loaded").

stimulation at 2 mM K_o, comparable to the value reported by Glitsch et al. (1978) for activation of the electrogenic sodium pump in guinea-pig atria.

Early studies with cultured heart cells reported the specific activity of the Na-K-ATPase to be tenfold lower than it was in intact embryonic chick hearts, although ouabain (5×10^{-4} M) inhibited 96% of the total ATPase activity in cultured heart cells (Sperelakis and Lee, 1971). Subsequent studies reported a gain in sodium that was closely paralleled by a loss of potassium when cultured heart cells were exposed to 10^{-4} M ouabain (McDonald and DeHaan, 1973). In growth-oriented heart cells exposed to 10^{-4} M ouabain, ^{42}K influx was reduced by an average of 72% (Lieberman et al., 1978). Recently, we observed that after a 10-min exposure to the same concentration of ouabain the K/Na ratio declined from 8.3 to 1.6. The effectiveness of ouabain in blocking the activity of the Na-K pump was also evident in the transmembrane potentials recorded from a cultured heart cell preparation (Fig. 7). With 10^{-3} M ouabain, in the presence of 5.4 mM K, the membrane depolarized within 3 min. But, when ouabain was removed, activation of the electrogenic response proceeded more slowly than the onset of hyperpolarization did when the preparation was returned to 5.4 mM K after K-free perfusion (see Fig. 3). This experiment also demonstrated an advantage of the cultured embryonic chick heart cell preparation for studying the effects of cardiac glycosides on membrane transport, namely, the relatively rapid dissociation of ouabain, even at high concentrations, from binding sites on the cell membrane. Figure 8 illustrates the rapid release of ouabain, a result that is in marked contrast to the slow release of ^{3}H-ouabain (T½ = 11 hours) obtained with neonatal

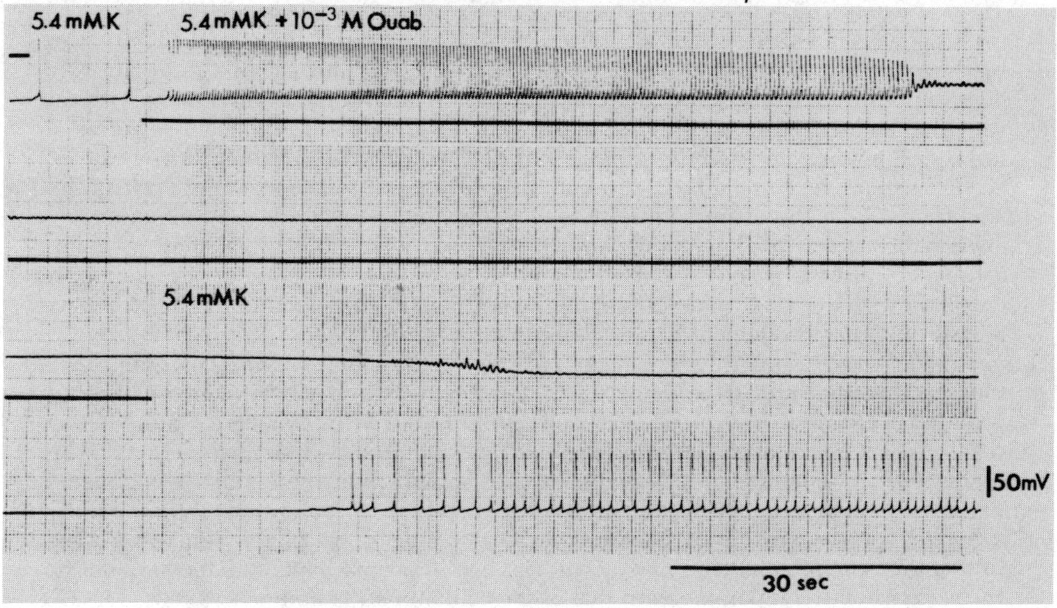

Figure 7. Transmembrane potentials recorded continuously from growth-oriented cultured heart cells during active transport inhibition by 10^{-3} M ouabain and recovery in 5.4 mM K.

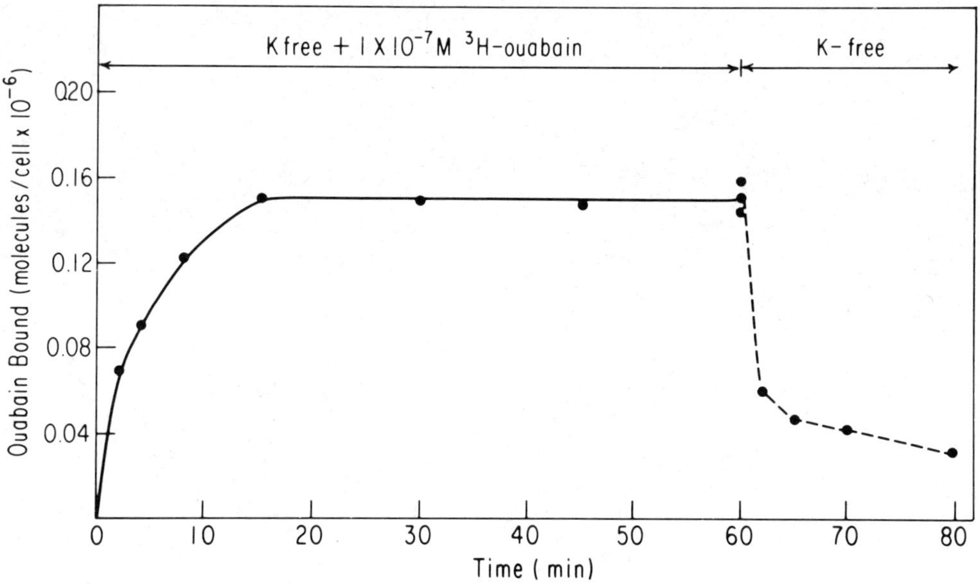

Figure 8. Time course of ^{3}H-ouabain binding and release in confluent cultures of heart cells. Each point represents a single observation. T½ for release of ouabain is approximately 2 min.

rat heart cells in culture (McCall, 1979). Preliminary data obtained from ^{3}H-ouabain binding studies indicate that muscle-enriched heart cell cultures have approximately 800 Na pump sites per square micrometer, a value in reasonable agreement with results obtained by McCall (1979). Using the values obtained for ouabain-sensitive K influx (11 pmoles·cm^{-2}·sec^{-1} [Horres, 1975]), we calculated the turnover rate of each transport site to be 40 sec^{-1}, assuming 2 K ions are transported per cycle of the Na pump. From the estimated net loss of positive ions during the 30-sec period following the return to 5.4 mM K (see Fig. 4), we were able to calculate a pump turnover rate of 210 sec^{-1}. This five-fold stimulation of the pump rate compares favorably with the magnitude of active transport stimulation obtained from ^{42}K-influx measurements for values of $K_o \geq 5.4$ mM (see Fig. 6).

To arrive at a quantitative analysis of the stoichiometry of the Na-K pump, we measured the sodium tracer kinetics under steady-state conditions in the growth-oriented preparation. Cultured heart cells equilibrated with ^{24}Na were rapidly *superfused* with a nonradioactive solution while we monitored the tissue activity. The extracellular component of ^{24}Na efflux was separated from the cellular components by initially superfusing each preparation with a cold (6° C) solution and then rapidly switching to a warm (37.5° C) solution. The cellular ^{24}Na efflux from contractile preparations (stimulated at 150 beats·min^{-1}) exhibited two exponential components, the slower being comparable with that of the contaminating nonmuscle cells (Fig. 9). The mean efflux rate constants for contractile preparations perfused with a physiologic solution containing 5 mM K were, respectively, 3.11 and 0.35 min^{-1} for the two components. Although the rate constants of these preparations agree well with those obtained by McCall (1978) in tissue-cultured rat heart cells, we differ in the interpretation of the cellular identification of the slowest component, which he attributes to the muscle cells. The average intracellular sodium concentration, as determined by

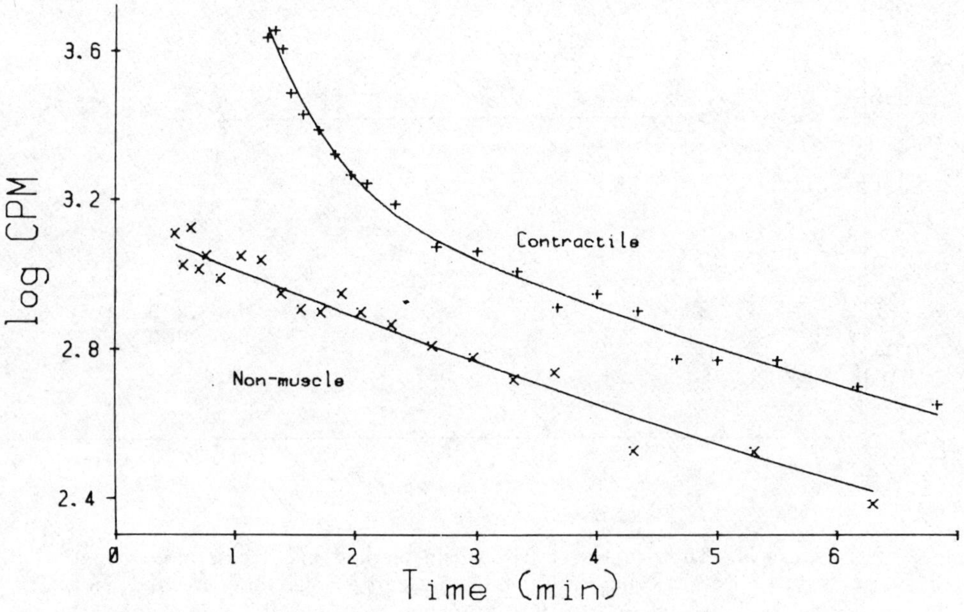

Figure 9. Comparison of the ^{24}Na efflux curves of a nonmuscle and contractile preparation in 5 mM K.

isotopic uptake and flame photometry, was 17 mM in contractile preparations and 18 mM in nonmuscle preparations. The steady-state, transmembrane sodium fluxes computed from these data were 98 $\text{pmoles}\cdot\text{cm}^{-2}\cdot\text{sec}^{-1}$ for muscle cells and 5.4 $\text{pmoles}\cdot\text{cm}^{-2}\cdot\text{sec}^{-1}$ for nonmuscle cells.

In the presence of 10^{-4} M ouabain, sodium efflux kinetics of the muscle cells was reduced by approximately 16%, and thus only a relatively small fraction of the total Na efflux can be attributed to the activity of the Na-K pump. Biedert et al. (1979) similarly reported that 10^{-6} M ouabain reduced the rate constant for ^{24}Na efflux by 34% in monolayers of chick embryo heart cells. Although the values of sodium efflux obtained by Biedert et al. (1979) were somewhat different from those obtained in our preparations, they do compare reasonably well with the slow component (nonmuscle) of contractile preparations. Table 1 summarizes the data obtained for ^{24}Na kinetics and transmembrane flux in the growth-oriented preparation of embryonic chick heart cells. The large value of 98 $\text{pmoles}\cdot\text{cm}^{-2}\cdot\text{sec}^{-1}$ for the ouabain-insensitive, unidirectional sodium efflux in the cardiac muscle cell was an unexpected finding because the result obtained from previous measurements of potassium influx in similar preparations was 15 $\text{pmoles}\cdot\text{cm}^{-2}\cdot\text{sec}^{-1}$ (Horres, 1975).

The rapid sodium flux indicates that in most, if not all, diffusion-limited preparations of embryonic and adult cardiac muscle, ^{24}Na tracer techniques cannot be used to study transmembrane sodium exchange. In growth-oriented cultured heart cells, the large ouabain-insensitive fraction and the greater magnitude of sodium over potassium fluxes demonstrate that mechanisms other than the Na-K pump contribute significantly to sodium exchange across embryonic cardiac muscle cells.[3] It is clear, however, from net content changes during pump inhibition, that Na-K ATPase is a major determinant of cellular homeostasis. Although the ouabain-sensitive sodium efflux is only a small fraction of the total Na efflux and represents a small difference between two large numbers, it is tempting to compare the calculated value of 16 $\text{pmoles}\cdot\text{cm}^{-2}\cdot\text{sec}^{-1}$ for ouabain-sensitive sodium efflux with the value of 11 $\text{pmoles}\cdot\text{cm}^{-2}\cdot\text{sec}^{-1}$ for ouabain-sensitive potassium influx and arrive at a pump stoichiometry of 3Na:2K.

Table 1
Average Values of Transmembrane Sodium Efflux from Tissue-Cultured Chick Heart Cells

	Muscle	Nonmuscle
Na efflux rate constant (min^{-1})		
5 mM K	3.11[a]	0.42
	0.35[b]	
0 K + 10^{-4} M Ouabain	2.85[a]	0.17
	0.17[b]	
Intracellular Na concentration (mM)	17	18
Sodium efflux ($\text{pmoles}\cdot\text{cm}^{-2}\cdot\text{sec}^{-1}$)	98	5.4

[a]Fast compartment
[b]Slow compartment

[3]In a previous report, Na-K pump inhibition of cultured embryonic chick heart cells promoted the appearance of electron-dense deposits, possibly $CaPO_4$, in the mitochondria of muscle cells (Aiton et al., 1978; see also Friedman et al., 1980). Measurements of total cell calcium by atomic absorption spectroscopy and ^{45}Ca exchange showed that incubation of preparations in K-free medium resulted in a threefold increase in total calcium content (Murphy et al., 1981).

CONCLUSION

Tissue-cultured preparations of embryonic heart cells have proven to be capable of providing an important model system for the study of rapid radiotracer flux and electrophysiologic measurements. As we expand our knowledge of the cellular physiology of adult and embryonic hearts, it is becoming apparent that passive processes alone cannot account for all of the electrophysiologic and ion transport phenomena associated with the resting and active states of cardiac muscle. Because an electrogenic potential also seems to affect automaticity and may also contribute to the membrane potential under conditions that tend to depolarize heart muscle, for example, hypoxia, it is particularly important to design experiments capable of providing accurate information about the electrogenic capabilities of active transport. Indeed, a thorough understanding of the electrogenically active transport processes, as well as those that are electroneutral, is essential if we are to fully and quantitatively comprehend the mechanisms underlying the generation of the embryonic and adult cardiac action potential.

Acknowledgments

This work was supported in part by grants from the National Institutes of Health (HL-12157, HL-17670, HL-07101), North Carolina Heart Association and the Insurance Medical Scientist Scholarship Fund (DMW). We wish to thank Dr. Elizabeth Murphy for critically reviewing the manuscript, Owen Oakeley for technical advice, and Carol Clyman for secretarial assistance.

REFERENCES

Aiton JF, Stubbs FB, Lorenz JJ, Lieberman M (1978) Heart cells in tissue culture: a model for myocardial ischemia. Fed Proc **37**:229 (Abstract)

Biedert S, Barry WH, Smith TW (1979) Inotropic effects and changes in sodium and calcium contents associated with inhibition of monovalent cation active transport by ouabain in cultured myocardial cells. J Gen Physiol **74**:479–494

Carmeliet EE (1961) Chloride and Potassium Permeability in Cardiac Purkinje Fibers. Bruxelles, Editions Arscia, SA

Carmeliet EE, Horres CR, Lieberman M, Vereecke JS (1976) Developmental aspects of potassium flux and permeability of the embryonic chick heart. J Physiol (Lond) **254**:673–692

DeHaan RL (1980a) Differentiation of excitable membranes. Curr Topics Develop Biol **16**: 117–164

DeHaan RL (1980b) Development of rhythmic activity in cardiac cells. *In* Physiology of Atrial Pacemaker and Conductive Tissues, edited by RC Little, Mt. Kisco, New York, Futura Publ Co, pp 21–53

Eisner DA, Lederer WJ (1980) Characterization of the electrogenic sodium pump in cardiac Purkinje fibers. J Physiol (Lond) **303**:441–474

Fozzard H, Sheu SS (1980) Intracellular potassium and sodium activities of chick ventricular muscle during embryonic development. J Physiol (Lond) **306**:579–586

Friedman I, Schwalb H, Hallaq H, Pinson A, Heller M (1980) Interactions of cardiac glycosides with cultured cardiac cells: II. Biochemical and electronmicroscopic studies on the effects of ouabain on muscle and non-muscle cells. Biochim Biophys Acta **598**:272–284

Gadsby DC, Cranefield PF (1977) Two levels of resting potential in cardiac Purkinje fibers. J Gen Physiol **70**:725–746

Gadsby DC, Cranefield PF (1979) Electrogenic sodium extrusion in cardiac Purkinje fibers. J Gen Physiol **73**:819–837

Glitsch HG (1979) Characteristics of active Na transport in intact cardiac cells. Am J Physiol **236**:H189–H199

Glitsch HG, Pusch H, Venetz K (1976) Effects of Na and K ions on active Na transport in guinea-pig auricles. Pflüg Arch **365**:29–36

Glitsch HG, Grabowski W, Thielen J (1978) Activation of the electrogenic sodium pump in guinea-pig atria by external potassium ions. J Physiol (Lond) **276**:515–524

Horres CR (1975) Potassium Tracer Kinetics of Growth Oriented Heart Cells in Tissue Culture. Ph.D. Dissertation, Duke University Medical Center

Horres CR, Lieberman M (1977) Compartmental analysis of potassium efflux from growth-oriented heart cells. J Membr Biol **34**:331–350

Horres CR, Lieberman M, Purdy JE (1977) Growth orientation of heart-cells on nylon monofilament: Determination of the volume-to-surface area ratio and intracellular potassium concentration. J Membr Biol **34**:313–329

Horres CR, Aiton JF, Lieberman M (1979a) Potassium permeability of embryonic avian heart cells in tissue culture. Am J Physiol **236**:C163–C170

Horres CR, Aiton JF, Lieberman M, Johnson EA (1979b) Electrogenic transport in tissue cultured heart cells. J Mol Cell Cardiol **11**:1201–1205

Klein RL, Evans ML (1961) Effects of ouabain, hypothermia and anoxia on cation fluxes in embryonic chick heart. Am J Physiol **200**:735–740

Lieberman M, Paes de Carvalho A (1965) The electrophysiological organization of the embryonic chick heart. J Gen Physiol **49**:351–363

Lieberman M, Horres CR, Purdy JE, Halperin LR (1978) Development of electrical activity in embryonic myocardial cells. *In* Fetal and Newborn Cardiovascular Physiology, edited by LD Longo, DD Reneau, New York, Garland Press, vol 1, pp 237–255

McCall D (1979) Cation exchange and glycoside binding in cultured rat heart cells. Am J Physiol **236**:C87–C95

McDonald TF, DeHaan RL (1973) Ion levels and membrane potential in chick heart tissue and cultured cells. J Gen Physiol **61**:89–109

Murphy E, Aiton JF, Horres CR, Lieberman M (1981) Na-K pump inhibition and calcium accumulation in cultured heart cells. Fed Proc **40**:617 (abstract)

Pelleg A, Vogel S, Belardinelli L, Sperelakis N (1980) Overdrive suppression of automaticity in cultured chick myocardial cells. Am J Physiol **238**:H24–H30

Sano T, Hiraoka M, Sawanobori T (1975) Electrogenic contribution to resting potential in different cardiac tissues. *In* Developmental and Physiological Correlates of Cardiac Muscle, edited by M Lieberman, T Sano. New York, Raven Press, pp 299–310

Sperelakis N (1972) (Na^+, K^+)-ATPase activity of embryonic chick heart and skeletal muscles as a function of age. Biochim Biophys Acta **266**:230–237

Sperelakis N (1980) Origin of the cardiac resting potential. *In* Handbook of Physiology—The Cardiovascular System I, edited by RM Berne, N Sperelakis. Baltimore, Williams and Wilkins Company, pp 187–267

Sperelakis N, Lee EC (1971) Characterization of (Na^+, K^+)-ATPase isolated from embryonic chick hearts and cultured chicks heart cells. Biochim Biophys Acta **233**:562–579

Sperelakis N, Shigenobu K (1972) Changes in membrane properties of chick embryonic hearts during development. J Gen Physiol **60**:430–453

Vassalle M (1970) Electrogenic suppression of automaticity in sheep and dog Purkinje fibers. Circ Res **27**:361–377

Vleugels A, Carmeliet E, Bosteels S, Zaman M (1976) Differential effects of hypoxia with age on the chick embryonic heart: Changes in membrane potential, intracellular K and Na, K efflux and glycogen. Pflüg Arch **365**:159–166

Yeh BK, Hoffman BF (1968) The ionic basis of electrical activity in embryonic cardiac muscle. J Gen Physiol **52**:666–681

Discussion

FOZZARD: One of your slides showed the data of McDonald and DeHaan (J Gen Physiol **61**:89–109, 1973) for the hyperpolarization with maturation of embryonic chick heart cells. In the same slide, you had calculated the potassium equilibrium potential from their measurements of intracellular potassium, showing that the potassium equilibrium potential becomes less negative with age. It made no sense to us that the cells would have more potassium in the immature stage and lose potassium as they mature, especially if the sodium potassium pump is becoming more and more effective with age. I am also concerned about the high level of intracellular sodium that is shown in your preparation, and I wonder if these results may be contaminated by methodologic error. Sheu and I (J Physiol **306**:579–586, 1980) measured sodium and potassium activity with ion-sensitive electrodes and found that the sodium inside was indeed high or higher for the very young and immature cells and went down to about 7 mM by 18 days. On the other hand, potassium was lower in the very young cells and went up as the cells matured. This is what we would expect if the sodium pump became more effective with maturation. I wonder then if you could comment on possible inaccuracies of the chemical methods for measuring intracellular ionic concentrations as opposed to what I modestly propose as an accurate and sensitive method using ion selective electrodes.

LIEBERMAN: What I can offer in support of the data that I showed is that values obtained by atomic absorption spectroscopy and those obtained with tracer methods were virtually identical. To be sure, there could be some problems associated with the analysis of these data because of the need to obtain accurate measurements of dry tissue mass from preparations on the order of 0.3 mg. Another possible source of error could be the value used for cellular water that we have taken from previous measurements of the preparation (Horres et al., J Mem Biol **34**:313, 1977).

Whether values of physiologic significance should be obtained from concentration or activity measurements is a question that continues to pose a problem. Ion-selective electrodes should provide more reliable information for calculations of electrochemical potentials but will be of limited value for measurements of ion fluxes that require a knowledge of the exchangeable component. To be sure, other problems are associated with ion-selective electrodes, for example, the electrodes are calibrated in solutions that differ in composition from the cytoplasm, and impalement of cells may alter their ion content. I should say, however, that I have no personal data that would lead me to challenge the values that you have obtained with the ion selective electrode.

GADSBY: I have a bit of a problem with your evidence for 3:2 stoichiometry of the Na/K pump. I think you determined the uptake of potassium and the loss of sodium with a flame photometer, and under those conditions you cannot distinguish between net active movements and net passive movements. I think you also said that in similar experiments the membrane hyperpolarized negative to E_K. At that point, there should be net passive influx of potassium so that, as far as I can see, the uptake rate of potassium and the extrusion rate of sodium have to be the same when measured chemically. This is because any discrepancy between the active, pumped sodium and potassium fluxes must be balanced by the net passive flux. In other words, the hyperpolarizing current of sodium ions generated by the pump is usually exactly balanced by the passive inward potassium current (plus any chloride current) that flows in response to the hyperpolarization. The only way you can get a 3:2 stoichiometry for Na and K movements determined chemically is by having an infinitely large membrane chloride conductance, which would prevent the membrane from hyperpolarizing beyond the potassium equilibrium potential.

LIEBERMAN: For reasons that you have stated, calculation of the active potassium influx could actually be overestimated. But, the stimulated active transport is capable of producing fluxes that can transiently exceed passive movements by several fold. We are also aware that chloride may play a role in shunting the magnitude of the electrogenic response in this preparation.

HOFFMAN: You showed a rapid loss of ouabain when you shifted from potassium-free media with ouabain to 5.4 mM potassium in ouabain-free media. You have attributed the fast loss of ouabain to a wash-out response. I am wondering if changing two things at the same time, that is, removing ouabain and increasing potassium, could not create two phases in your washout curve. At the beginning, there would be a faster phase induced by the increase in extracellular potassium, and the second phase would then be a slower phase of true loss of ouabain from the tissue. I feel that doing the two changes at the same time may render the data difficult to interpret.

LIEBERMAN: The point of the data was to show that ouabain can be removed very rapidly from the cultured heart cell preparations.

Chapter 18

Mechanisms for Muscarinic Inhibition of Calcium-Dependent Action Potentials and Contractions in Developing Ventricular Muscle: The Role of Cyclic AMP

Achilles J. Pappano and Rebecca L. Biegon*

The parasympathetic and sympathetic divisions of the autonomic nervous system help to maintain homeostasis by their contrasting or antagonistic effects. Levy (1971) has reviewed the nature of this antagonism in cardiac function, using appropriately the term "accentuated antagonism" to describe the enhanced inhibitory effects of vagal stimulation that are experimentally induced by stimulating, simultaneously, sympathetic fibers. These inhibitory effects of vagal stimulation, also called "muscarinic inhibition," have a presynaptic and a postsynaptic component. The presynaptic component depends on neurally released acetylcholine (ACh) to inhibit the release of norepinephrine (NE) from adrenergic nerve endings (Löffelholz and Muscholl, 1970). The postsynaptic component of muscarinic inhibition depends largely on a sympathetic adrenergic transmitter to reduce the accumulation of adenosine 3′,5′-cyclic monophosphate (cyclic AMP) (reviewed by Levy, 1971).

Investigators are greatly interested in both components. Cyclic AMP is viewed as the metabolic control point by which the sympathetic transmitter augments the secondary inward current (i_{si}) and contractions in cardiac muscle (reviewed in Niedergerke and Page, 1977; Reuter and Scholz, 1977; Tsien, 1977). Also, the antagonistic effects of ACh and NE on i_{si} display Hodgkin-Huxley kinetics; that is, i_{si} is a voltage- and time-dependent current susceptible to control in various ways (reviewed in Reuter, 1979 and in these proceedings).

This chapter describes experiments we performed to study the mechanisms of muscarinic inhibition in ventricular muscle. We have given considerable attention to the intracellular reactions that may explain muscarinic inhibition of i_{si} and contractions. These mechanisms may differ, however, from those in atrial muscle (for discus-

---

The research was supported by a grant from USPHS (HL-13339).
*Recipient of a fellowship from the American Heart Association of Greater Hartford, Inc.

sion see Biegon and Pappano, 1980). For our experiments, we have chosen avian ventricular muscle because an unfolding of the reaction pathways seems to occur during ontogenetic development in that tissue.

METHODS

The procedures used to inactivate the fast Na^+ current and thereby permit study of Ca^{2+}-dependent action potentials have been described (Pappano, 1970). By this method, a 25 mM K^+ solution was used to inactivate the fast Na^+ current by depolarization; K^+ was substituted isotonically for Na^+. The electrophysiologic methods used to record Ca^{2+}-dependent action potentials and the maximum rate of rise ($\dot{V}_{max}$) of these potentials in cells from the right ventricle of embryonic and hatched chick hearts are given elsewhere (Biegon and Pappano, 1980). The force of contraction from isolated right ventricular tissue was obtained by the techniques described in a previous report from this laboratory (Higgins and Pappano, 1981). A radioimmunoassay method (New England Nuclear) was used to estimate cyclic AMP content. Cyclic AMP phosphodiesterase activity of homogenates of ventricular muscle was assayed by a two-step radioisotope procedure adapted from that described by Thompson et al. (1979) and applied to the avian heart (Biegon et al., 1980). Adenylate cyclase activity was determined according to the method given by Salomon (1979). Chick right ventricular tissue was excised, rinsed in Tyrode's solution, and homogenized at 50 mg wet wt/ml in 10 mM Tris-HCl (pH, 7.8), 1 mM dithiothreitol (DTT), and 0.2 mM $MgCl_2$ in a Duall homogenizer. Reaction mixtures (0.1 ml) contained 25 mM Tris-HCl (pH, 7.8), 3 mM $MgCl_2$, 1 mM DTT, 1 mM cyclic AMP, 0.3 mM ATP, 1 to 3 × 10^{-6} cpm of α^{32}P-ATP, and 1 mg of ventricular tissue. The reaction was initiated by adding tissue homogenate and incubating it for 10 min at 30° C (the reaction was linear for more than 20 min). Approximately 0.05 to 0.1% of the substrate (α-^{32}P-ATP) was converted to cyclic AMP; the substrate and product were separated by a sequential chromatographic method with Dowex and alumina.

RESULTS

Properties of the β-Adrenergic Mechanism in Avian Ventricular Muscle

It has been previously shown that the embryonic chick heart displays a positive chronotropic effect to catecholamines on the 2nd day after fertilization, soon after spontaneous contractions begin (Markowitz, 1931). McCarty et al. (1960) were the first to report that a β-adrenergic receptor is activated by catecholamines to elicit the positive inotropic and positive chronotropic effect. The positive inotropic effect of catecholamines in avian ventricular muscle can be detected as early as the 3rd (Frieswick et al., 1979) and 4th (Higgins and Pappano, 1980) incubation days. But, before the 3rd day, inotropic effects of catecholamines are technically difficult to detect in the avian ventricle. Electrophysiologic experiments (Pappano, 1981) reveal that isoproterenol (ISO) increases the amplitude and duration of Ca^{2+}-dependent action potentials in ventricular cells from the 3rd incubation day (53 to 65 hours after fertilization). The Ca^{2+}-dependent action potentials are also obtained in a 25 mM K^+

solution, which depolarizes the membrane and inactivates the fast Na^+ current (Iijima and Pappano, 1979).

In addition to their effects on contractility and Ca^{2+}-dependent action potentials, catecholamines also increase the accumulation of cyclic AMP in the embryonic avian heart. In the earliest measurements, done on the 4th incubation day, norepinephrine (NE) and ISO caused a marked increase of cyclic AMP (Polson, et al., 1977; Renaud et al., 1978). The accumulation of cyclic AMP preceded the positive inotropic effect, and both actions were blocked by propranolol (Polson et al., 1977). These results are consistent with the hypothesis that the positive inotropic effect and the increased membrane permeability to Ca^{2+} by catecholamines in the embryonic avian heart (reviewed by Pappano, 1981), as in the adult heart (reviewed by Tsien, 1977), are the result of increased accumulation of cyclic AMP.

Our results supported the hypothesis that cyclic AMP mediates these effects (see Fig. 1). Experiments were done with right ventricles from 18-day embryonic chicks (3 days before hatching). After a 30-min equilibration period, the tissues were exposed to ISO for 2 min, and the change in force of contraction was recorded with a force-displacement transducer. At the end of the 2-min exposure, the tissue was quickly removed from the bath and homogenized in ice-cold 5% trichloroacetic acid solution and prepared for assay of cyclic AMP. The data in Figure 1 were obtained from the average increase in tension and cyclic AMP at each concentration of ISO ($N \geq 4$ measurements). The concentration-effect relationships for the accumulation of cyclic AMP and for the increase in twitch tension by ISO were essentially the same. The ED_{50} (concentration to evoke 50% of maximum effect) for ISO was 5×10^{-8} M for

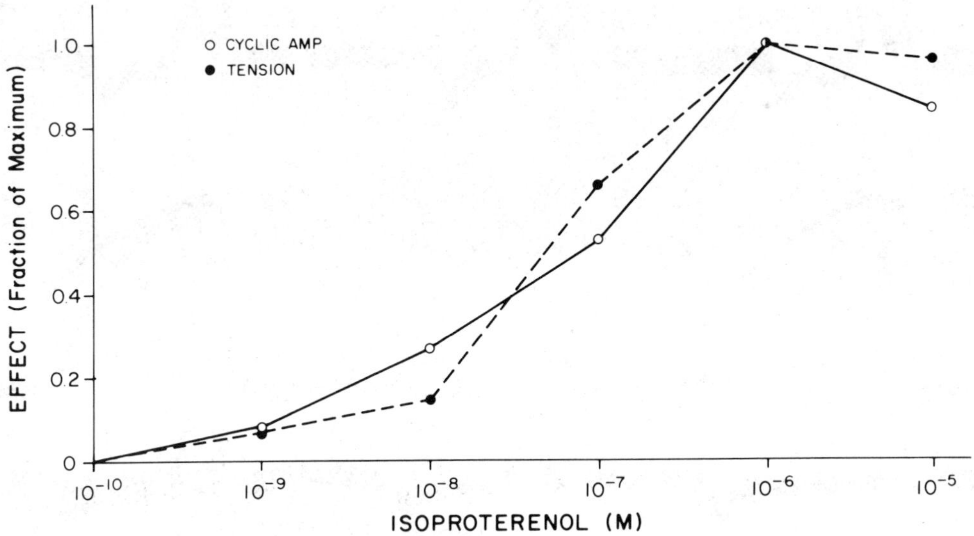

Figure 1. Stimulation of cyclic AMP accumulation (○) and twitch tension (●) by ISO in right ventricles from 18-day embryonic chicks. Ordinate: increase of cyclic AMP and twitch tension as a fraction of maximum effect; abscissa: concentration of ISO. Each point is the mean of at least 4 measurements in different preparations. The tissues were stimulated at 3 Hz with supramaximal rectangular pulses. The basal value of cyclic AMP was 0.68 ± 0.07 pmole/mg wet wt and cyclic AMP attained a maximal value of 1.30 ± 0.24 pmole/mg wet wt in the presence of 10^{-6} M ISO. Twitch tension increased to $283 \pm 45\%$ above control levels in the presence of 10^{-6} M ISO.

twitch tension and 7.5×10^{-8} M for cyclic AMP accumulation. Taken together, these results provide considerable support for the role of cyclic AMP as an intracellular mediator of the effect of β-receptor agonists on g_{Ca} (membrane Ca^{2+} conductance underlying Ca-dependent action potentials) and on contractility in ventricular muscle of the embryonic chick heart.

Muscarinic Inhibition—Blockade of Cyclic AMP Production Before Hatching

Acetylcholine (ACh), itself, had a negligible effect on the Ca^{2+}-dependent action potential and contractions in ventricles from embryonic chicks. However, ACh inhibited the ventricular function augmented by ISO. This inhibitory effect of ACh, which has been termed "indirect" (Biegon and Pappano, 1980), is illustrated in Figure 2. Acetylcholine did not inhibit the "basal" Ca^{2+}-dependent action potential (Fig. 2B), whereas it inhibited that portion of the Ca^{2+}-dependent action potential augmented by ISO (Fig. 2E).

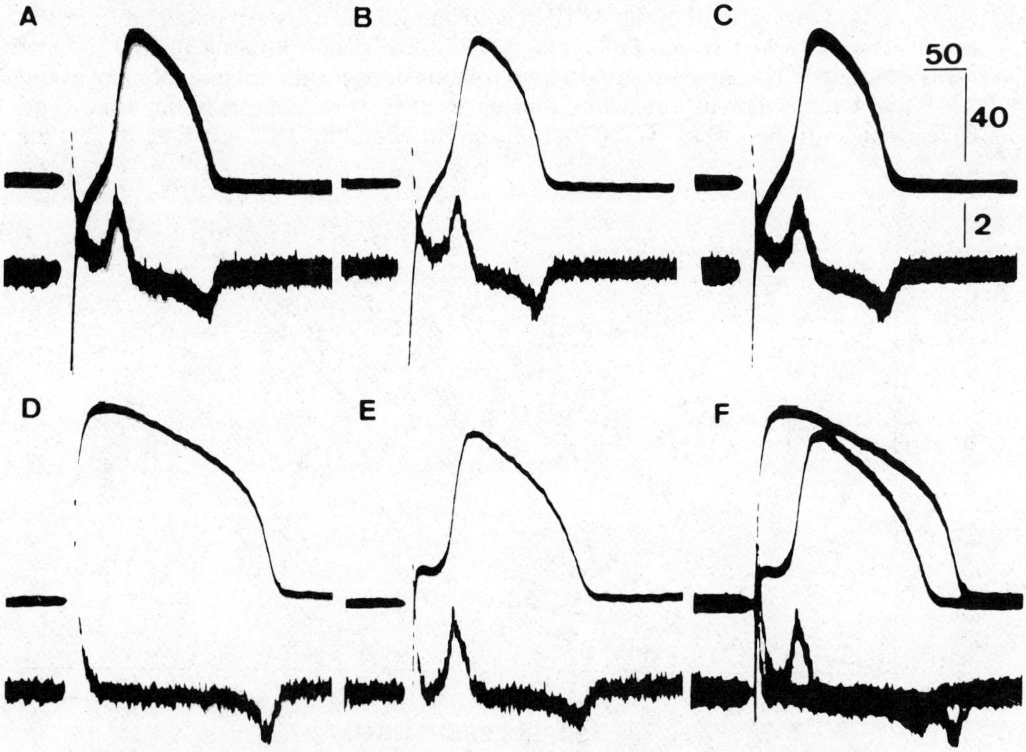

Figure 2. Inhibition by ACh of the stimulatory effect of ISO on Ca^{2+}-dependent action potential in cell of the right ventricle from the 18th incubation day. Horizontal calibration for time (50 msec) and vertical calibrations for voltage (40 mV) and $\dot{V}_{max}$ (2 V/sec) in C apply to all records. A: control in 25 mM $[K^+]_o$. B: After 4 min in 10^{-5} M ACh. C: A and B superimposed. D: After removal of ACh and addition of 10^{-6} M ISO. E: ACh (10^{-5} M) added in the presence of ISO. F: D and E superimposed (from Biegon and Pappano, 1980; reproduced with permission from the American Heart Association).

This inhibitory effect of ACh was observed as early as the 7th incubation day, was mimicked by the addition of carbamylcholine, and was reversibly antagonized by atropine. Therefore, the "indirect" inhibitory effect of ACh was mediated by a muscarinic cholinergic receptor. Muscarinic inhibition did not occur when the Ca^{2+}-dependent action potential was augmented by elevation of external Ca^{2+} or when the Ca^{2+}-dependent action potential was initiated from a more negative resting potential in the presence of tetrodotoxin. Inhibition by ACh also does not occur when external Ca^{2+} is used to increase the Ca^{2+}-dependent action potential in mammalian ventricle (Inui and Imamura, 1977).

That cyclic AMP reduction may be the mechanism of "indirect" muscarinic inhibition has been indicated by the results of experiments on ventricles from the 18th incubation day, in which ACh (10^{-6} M) had no effect on the basal concentration of cyclic AMP but reduced the accumulation of this cyclic nucleotide caused by ISO (10^{-6} M) (Biegon and Pappano, 1980). We corroborated these results by directly examining the rate of cyclic AMP synthesis by adenylate cyclase in broken cell preparations from the 18th embryonic day (Fig. 3). In embryos of this age, isoproterenol (10^{-6} M) significantly increased the rate of cyclic AMP synthesis, whereas ACh (10^{-6} M) alone had no significant effect. In the presence of ISO, however, ACh reduced the rate of cyclic AMP synthesis by as much as 0.22 pmole/mg wet wt/min, an 85% reduction of the change in cyclic AMP synthesis caused by ISO. The inhibitory effect of ACh was competitively antagonized by atropine. At 10^{-4} M, ACh had no effect on Ca^{2+}-dependent action potentials, and it produced a small but statistically

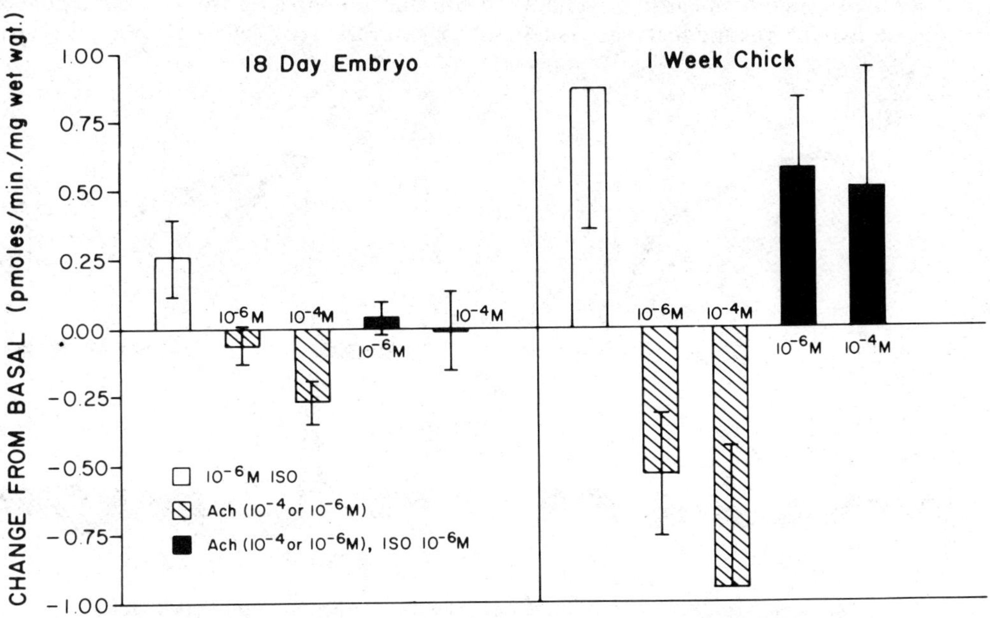

Figure 3. Changes in the activity of adenylate cyclase caused by ACh and ISO, alone and in combination, in ventricular homogenates from the 18th incubation day and one week after hatching. Ordinate: change in adenylate cyclase from basal levels. The basal level of adenylate cyclase was 1.65 ± 0.24 pmole cyclic AMP/min/mg wet wt in 18-day embryos and 3.56 ± 0.83 pmole cyclic AMP/min/mg wet wt in 1-week hatched chicks. The legend applies to both ages. For additional details, see Results.

insignificant reduction of cyclic AMP content in the 18-day embryonic ventricle (Biegon et al., 1980). But, when we examined the rate of cyclic AMP synthesis, we found that 10^{-4} M ACh had reduced cyclic AMP synthesis by 0.27 ± 0.079 pmole/mg wet wt/min in homogenates from the ventricle of 18-day embryos. This result is even more striking because a positive inotropic effect can be observed in the 18-day embryonic ventricle exposed to ACh at concentrations $\leq 10^{-5}$ M. Apparently the positive inotropic effect of high concentrations of ACh is not mediated by increased synthesis of cyclic AMP (Biegon et al., 1980).

After Hatching

By 1 week after hatching, ACh consistently inhibited Ca^{2+}-dependent action potentials and contractions in the absence of added catecholamines. The inhibition also occurred in preparations from chicks treated 24 hours prior to the experiment with 6-hydroxydopamine to deplete transmitter from adrenergic nerves and from preparations superfused with propranolol (Biegon and Pappano, 1980). An example of this form of muscarinic inhibition, termed "direct," is given in Figure 4. In the presence of 3×10^{-7} M propranolol, increasing concentrations of ACh decreased the duration, amplitude, and $\dot{V}_{max}$ of Ca^{2+}-dependent action potentials (Fig. 4B). At higher concentrations (10^{-5} and 10^{-4} M), the rate of repolarization increased in the presence of ACh. Interestingly, the "indirect" inhibitory effect of muscarinic agonists continued after hatching. "Direct" and "indirect" muscarinic inhibition after hatching occurred over the same concentration range (10^{-7} to 10^{-4} M) of ACh.

Measurements of cardiac cyclic AMP content in ventricles from hatched chicks showed two interesting features. The basal concentration of cyclic AMP increased by

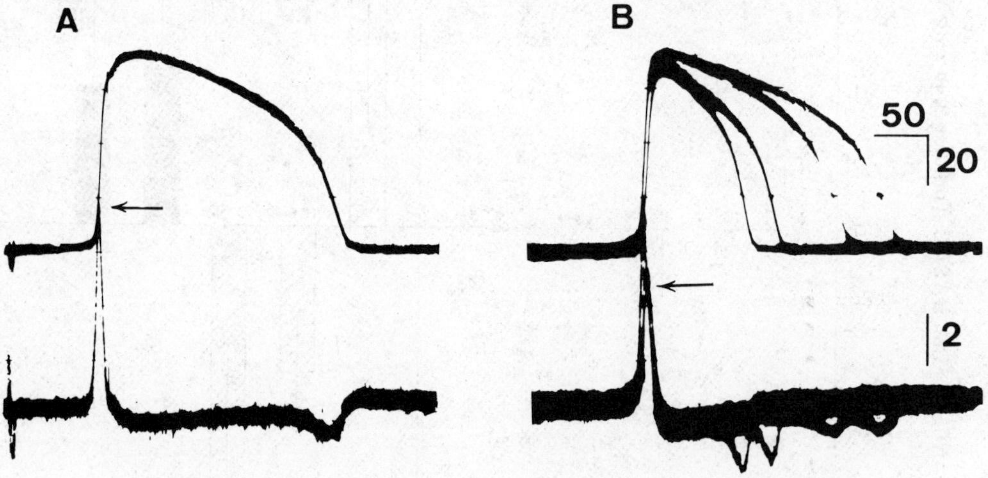

Figure 4. Inhibition by ACh of Ca^{2+}-dependent action potentials in ventricular cell from chick, 9 days after hatching. Calibration format as in Figure 2. Propranolol (3×10^{-7} M) present in all solutions. A: control in 25 mM $[K^+]_o$. B: Superimposed action potentials at 5 minutes after 10^{-7}, 10^{-6}, 10^{-5}, and 10^{-4} M ACh; the briefest action potential is in 10^{-4} M ACh. The smallest $\dot{V}_{max}$ signal in B is indicated by the arrow (from Biegon and Pappano, 1980; reproduced with permission of the American Heart Association).

50% when compared with that on the 18th incubation day, and it significantly decreased when ACh (10^{-6} M) was added (Biegon and Pappano, 1980). These changes in cyclic AMP content were associated with similar alterations in the rate of synthesis of cyclic AMP by homogenates of right ventricle from chicks 7 days after hatching (Fig. 3). The basal rate of cyclic AMP synthesis increased over twofold between the 18th embryonic day and 7 days after hatching. Moreover, ACh (10^{-6} M) significantly reduced the rate of cyclic AMP synthesis by 0.53 pmole/mg wet wt/min when tested in the absence of added catecholamine. Finally, the increase in the rate of cyclic AMP synthesis by ISO was reduced by 33% in the presence of ACh (10^{-6} M). At 10^{-4} M, ACh reduced the basal rate of cyclic AMP synthesis by 0.95 ± 0.514 pmole/mg wet wt/min.

The relationship of "indirect" and "direct" muscarinic inhibition to cyclic AMP synthesis and accumulation is shown in Figure 5, which summarizes the results of experiments that measured the effects of ACh and ISO, alone and in combination, on cyclic AMP content and contractions. Twitch tension was assigned a value of 100% at the basal level of cyclic AMP on the 18th incubation day (open circles denote cyclic AMP, 0.43 pmole/mg wet wt). Whereas 10^{-6} M ACh had a negligible effect on cyclic AMP content and twitch tension at the 18th incubation day (a), ACh reduced both significantly at 7 days after hatching (a′). The positive inotropic effect and the accumulation of cyclic AMP caused by ISO were greater after hatching (b′) than they were in the embryo (b). (The reduced sensitivity to ISO at the 18th incubation day might be related to the "subsensitivity" of the β-adrenergic mechanism at this age, as reported previously by our laboratory [Löffelholz and Pappano, 1974; Higgins and Pappano, 1981].) Interestingly, in the presence of ACh and ISO, there was a proportionately greater reduction of contractility than there was of cyclic AMP content both before (c) and after (c′) hatching. This phenomenon could be due to *(1)* a nonlinear relationship between cyclic AMP production and contractility or *(2)* an inhibitory effect of ACh unrelated to the synthesis of cyclic AMP. The experiments with isobutylmethylxanthine (IBMX) were done to test the latter possibility.

Muscarinic Inhibition—Blockade of the Effects of Accumulated Cyclic AMP

According to the cyclic AMP hypothesis, substances that interfere with the degradation of cyclic AMP by phosphodiesterase (PDE) should mimic the effects produced by activation of adenylate cyclase (reviewed in Tsien, 1977). The PDE inhibitor, IBMX, like ISO, reduces the time to peak tension, increases peak force, and accelerates the rate of relaxation of ventricular muscle (Korth, 1978). A similarity in the actions of ISO and IBMX is also observed in the embryonic avian heart (Biegon et al., 1980).

In our experiment, IBMX increased the force of contraction and the amplitude, duration, and $\dot{V}_{max}$ of Ca^{2+}-dependent action potentials. An example of the actions of IBMX on the Ca^{2+}-dependent action potential is given in Figure 6. Unlike the effects of ISO, those of IBMX were not inhibited by propranolol.

The stimulatory effects of IBMX on Ca^{2+}-dependent action potentials and contractions were inhibited by ACh, as shown in Figure 7 for the action potentials in a ventricular cell from the 7th incubation day. Again ACh had no effect on the Ca^{2+}-dependent action potential in the absence of IBMX (Fig. 7B), whereas it opposed the increase in amplitude, $\dot{V}_{max}$, and duration produced by IBMX (Fig. 7E).

Cyclic AMP accumulation and twitch tension increased in ventricular muscle exposed to IBMX (Table 1). A low concentration of ACh (10^{-6} M) did not significantly change the basal level of cyclic AMP or the accumulation of cyclic AMP caused by

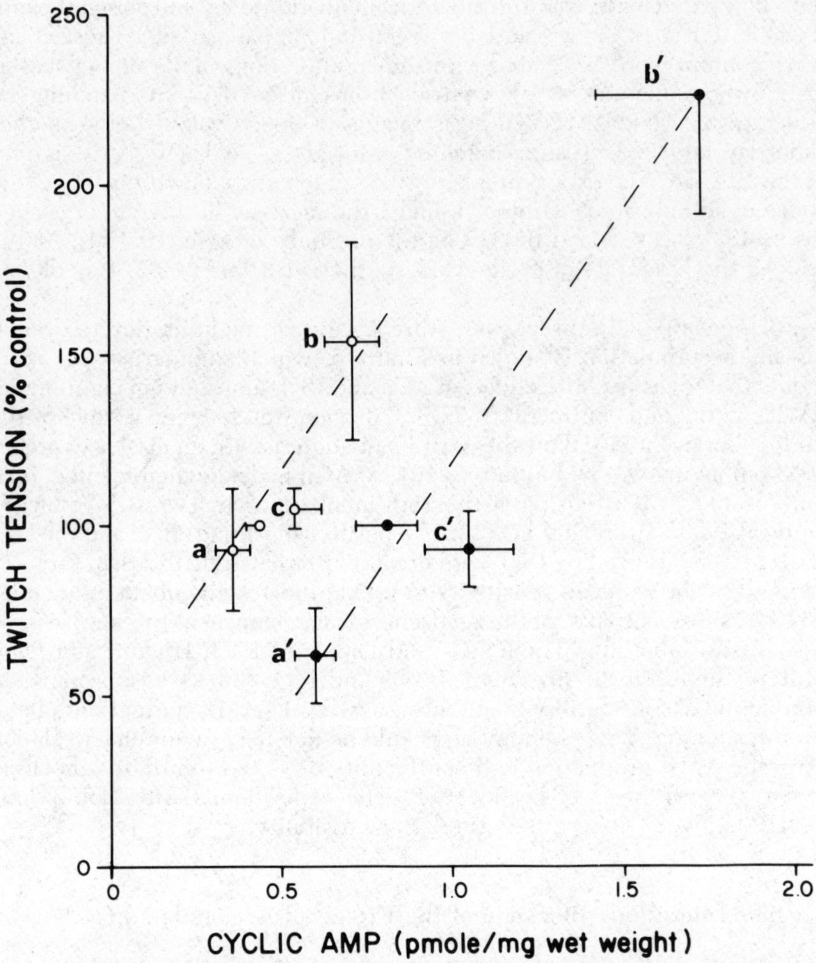

Figure 5. Changes in twitch tension and cyclic AMP content caused by ACh and ISO, alone and in combination, in ventricles from the 18th incubation day (non-filled circles) and from one week after hatching (filled circles). Twitch tension set at 100% in the absence of drug additions. a,a′:10^{-6} M ACh; b,b′:10^{-6} M ISO; c,c′:10^{-6} M ACh plus 10^{-6} M ISO in 18 day embryos and one week after hatching chicks, respectively. For additional details, see Results.

IBMX. The positive inotropic effect of IBMX was, however, completely blocked by ACh (10^{-6} M). These results indicate that a low concentration of ACh can inhibit the positive inotropic effect of accumulated cyclic AMP without changing the accumulation of the nucleotide caused by IBMX. On the other hand, the effects of a high concentration (10^{-4} M) of ACh include a reduction of the accumulation of cyclic AMP and of the positive inotropic effect of IBMX (Table 1). The actions of 10^{-4} M ACh seem even more complex because the drug has a small but statistically insignificant effect on basal cyclic AMP, but it increases the force of contraction.

Isobutylmethylxanthine inhibited PDE in homogenates of ventricular muscle prepared from 18-day embryos. The concentration of IBMX required to inhibit PDE activity by 50% was 3×10^{-6} M (Biegon et al., 1980). At 3×10^{-4} M, IBMX maximally inhibited PDE activity in vitro. Acetylcholine (10^{-4} M) had no effect on PDE activity in the absence or presence of IBMX (Biegon et al., 1980).

As noted above, the stimulatory effect of IBMX on Ca^{2+}-dependent action potentials and contractions occurs in the presence of propranolol. The positive inotropic effects of IBMX and of theophylline are competitively antagonized by adenosine. The apparent dissociation constant for adenosine with the receptor mediating the positive inotropic effect of the methylxanthines is about 1.5×10^{-5} M, as determined by an analysis of Schild plots (LaMothe and Pappano, unpublished observation).

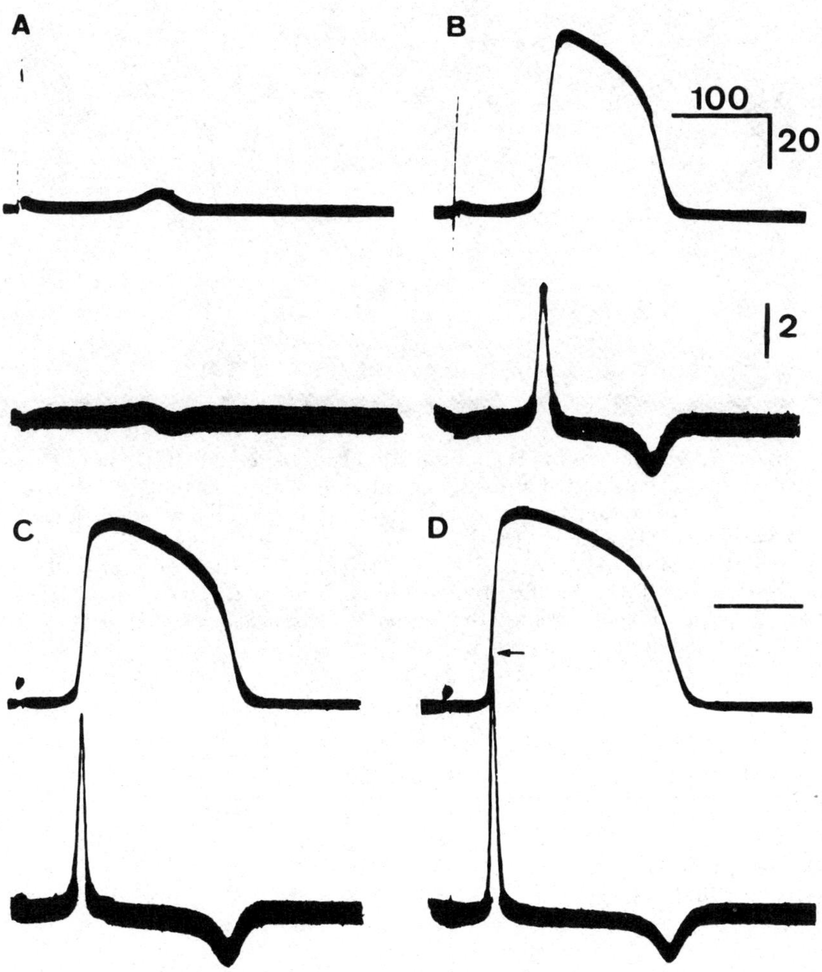

Figure 6. Stimulation of Ca^{2+}-dependent action potential by IBMX (3×10^{-4} M) in a ventricular cell from the 18th incubation day. Calibration format as in Figure 2. A: control (electrotonic potential) in 25 mM $[K^+]_o$. B, C and D: at 1, 2 and 3 min, respectively, after addition of IBMX. Arrow indicates top of $\dot{V}_{max}$ signal in D (from Biegon et al., 1980; reproduced with permission of the *Journal of Pharmacology and Experimental Therapeutics*).

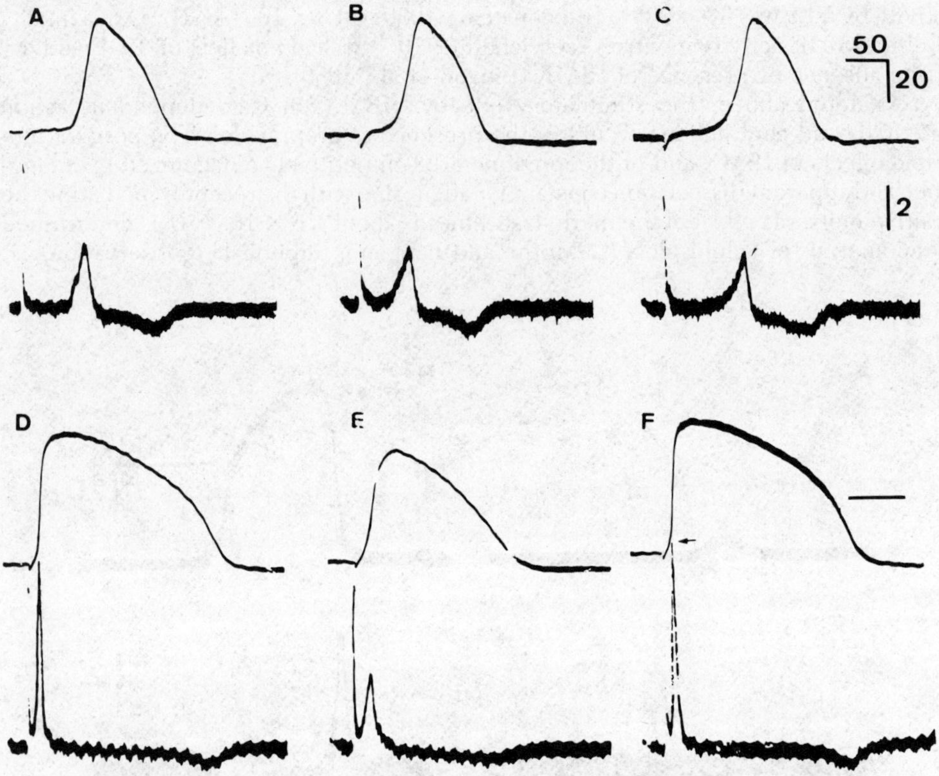

Figure 7. Inhibition by ACh of the stimulatory effect of IBMX on Ca^{2+}-dependent action potential in right ventricular cell from the 7th incubation day. Calibration format as in Figure 2. A: control Ca^{2+}-dependent action potential in 25 mM $[K^+]_o$. B: 5 min after 10^{-5} M ACh. C: 10 min after removal of ACh. D: in 3×10^{-4} M IBMX. E: 10^{-5} M ACh in the presence of IBMX. F: after removal of ACh (from Biegon et al., 1980; reproduced with permission of the *Journal of Pharmacology and Experimental Therapeutics*).

Table 1
Effects of ACh and IBMX on Cyclic AMP and Twitch Tension[a]

Condition	Cyclic AMP (pmole/mg wet wt)	Tension (%)
Basal	0.71 ± 0.03 (11)	100
ACh (10^{-6}M)	0.65 ± 0.04[b] (8)	99 ± 3 (7)
IBMX (3×10^{-4}M)	1.05 ± 0.10[c] (8)	232 ± 18 (7)
ACh (10^{-6}M), IBMX (3×10^{-4}M)	0.99 ± 0.14[d] (7)	91 ± 9 (5)
Basal	0.67 ± 0.04 (21)	100
ACh (10^{-4}M)	0.57 ± 0.03[b] (9)	147 ± 10 (8)
IBMX (3×10^{-4}M)	1.01 ± 0.05[c] (7)	195 ± 17 (5)
ACh (10^{-4}M), IBMX (3×10^{-4}M)	0.70 ± 0.06[b,e] (7)	96 ± 7 (5)

[a]This table is taken from Biegon et al. (1980). Ventricles from 18-day embryos were exposed to ACh for 6 min, to IBMX alone for 3 min, or to IBMX for the last 3 min of a 6-min exposure to ACh. Tension was recorded simultaneously in most experiments.
[b]Not significantly different from basal.
[c]Significantly different from basal ($P<0.05$).
[d]Not significantly different from IBMX alone.
[e]Significantly different from IBMX alone ($P<0.01$).

Muscarinic Inhibition—Blockade of the Effects of Cholera Toxin

Cholera toxin, which can activate irreversibly adenylate cyclase by virtue of its ability to promote ADP-ribosylation of a GTP-dependent binding protein and thereby inhibit GTPase activity (Cassel and Pfeuffer, 1978), has a positive inotropic effect in the 4-day embryonic chick heart (Hedtke et al., 1976). The positive inotropic effect is associated with an accumulation of cyclic AMP. The accumulation of cyclic AMP can be considered the result of persistent and irreversible activation of adenylate cyclase by cholera toxin.

In preliminary experiments, cholera toxin (5 μg/ml) had a positive inotropic effect in a ventricle isolated from chicks on the 12th to 18th incubation day. The results of one of these experiments is shown in Figure 8. Before the introduction of cholera toxin, ACh (10^{-6} M) had a negligible effect on contractility (the slight reduction in

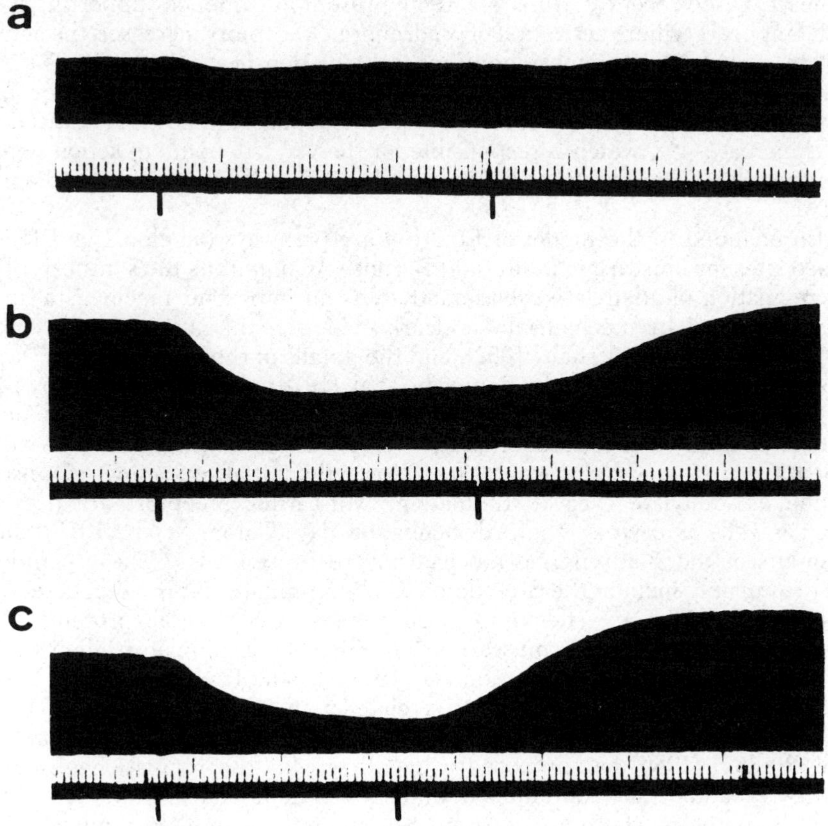

Figure 8. Inhibition by ACh of the positive inotropic effect of cholera toxin in right ventricle from the 12th incubation day. The muscle was stimulated at 3 Hz with supramaximal rectangular pulses throughout the experiment. Upper trace in each pair is twitch tension and lower trace is time (interval between largest upward deflections is one minute). A: control in Tyrode's solution (twitch tension was 300 mg). B: At 3 min after the end of a 3-hour exposure to cholera toxin (5×10^{-6} g/ml). C: At 60 min after removal of cholera toxin. The first downward deflection signal in A, B and C indicates introduction of 10^{-6} M ACh. The second downward deflection signal in A and B indicates removal of ACh whereas in C, this signal indicates addition of 3×10^{-7} M atropine to the ACh-containing solution.

tension was associated with fluid change). After 3 hours in cholera toxin, the tissue exhibited an increased twitch tension of 30%. After the tissue was washed in Tyrode's solution, lacking cholera toxin, for 3 min and then ACh (10^{-6} M) was reintroduced, a prompt and sustained inhibition (50%) of contraction force occurred (Fig. 8B). The inhibitory effect of ACh was demonstrated again at 1 hour after cholera toxin was removed. (Fig. 8C). The inhibition by ACh was muscarinic, for it was antagonized by atropine (Fig. 8C).

DISCUSSION

There is considerable support for the cyclic AMP hypothesis in the embryonic avian heart. Quite recently, Au et al. (1980) presented evidence supporting it in the neonatal rat heart, where activation of β-adrenergic receptors increased the activity of adenylate cyclase and brought about an accumulation of cyclic AMP. The results obtained in other laboratories and our own (see Results section for summary) are also consistent with the hypothesis that the accumulation of cyclic AMP caused by β-agonists increases g_{si}, which is responsible for the Ca^{2+}-dependent action potential, and contractility. The features of this hypothesis are illustrated in the diagram of Figure 9.

Also included in the model of Figure 9 are pathways (labeled I and II) of the proposed sites for muscarinic inhibition. Because ACh inhibits the synthesis of cyclic AMP, regulation of adenylate cyclase activity is an important mechanism for muscarinic inhibition. This mechanism was clearly evident in the earliest studies of cardiac adenylate cyclase (Murad et al., 1962), and the details of the mechanism in the heart have been described elegantly by Watanabe et al. (1978) and more recently by Birdsall et al. (1980). If we assume that muscarinic inhibition in the avian heart includes inhibition of adenylate cyclase activation, there are two questions that we must consider. The first is, what is the limiting factor in the initial appearance of muscarinic inhibition of adenylate cyclase stimulation? Muscarinic receptors are present on ventricular cells as early as the 3rd incubation day (Galper et al., 1977), and the components of the β-adrenergic mechanism are present also. These components would presumably include the β-receptor, GTP-binding proteins, adenylate cyclase, protein kinase, and Ca^{2+}-effectors (g_{si} channels and contractile proteins). In the presence of all these elements, muscarinic inhibition of the stimulatory effects of ISO is not evident until the 7th incubation day (Biegon and Pappano, 1980). We have considered the hypothesis that the delay is related to the synthesis and incorporation of a GTP-binding protein specifically needed to mediate muscarinic inhibition. In this regard, Rodbell (1980) has proposed a hypothesis for the regulation of adenylate cyclase by excitatory and inhibitory hormones and neurotransmitters. According to Rodbell's hypothesis, there are separate RN_s (receptor-stimulatory nucleotide regulatory component) and RN_i (receptor-inhibitory nucleotide regulatory component) complexes in the cell membrane coupled to adenylate cyclase. If this model were applied to the embryonic heart, it could be that the synthesis and incorporation of the N_i component is the limiting feature in the initial appearance of muscarinic inhibition via pathway I in the embryonic avian ventricle. Alternatively, the avian heart may have only one kind of nucleotide regulatory component, which displays a recognition site for muscarinic receptor several days after it displays a recognition site for β-adrenergic receptor. Whatever the mechanism, it seems reasonable that a GTP-dependent process is essential for muscarinic inhibition. Evidence from adult vertebrate hearts

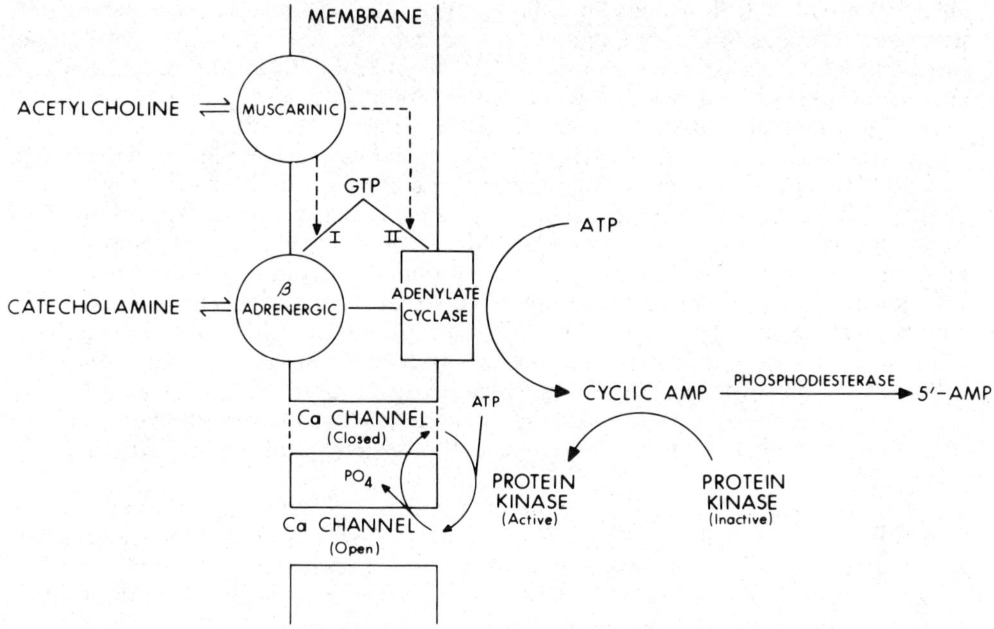

Figure 9. Model for muscarinic inhibition of Ca^{2+}-dependent action potentials. The muscarinic and β-adrenergic receptors, GTP-binding protein, and adenylate cyclase are components of the plasma membrane (Ross et al., 1977; Watanabe et al., 1978). Cyclic AMP activates a protein kinase that phosphorylates a membrane site and increases the number of g_{Ca} sites activated at a given voltage; dephosphorylation of the membrane site decreases g_{Ca} (Sperelakis and Schneider, 1976; Niedergerke and Page, 1977; Reuter and Scholz, 1977; Pappano and Carmeliet, 1979). Muscarinic drugs affect activation of adenylate cyclase by "indirect" (I) and "direct" (II) pathways with mechanism I present before hatching and mechanisms I and II present after hatching (from Biegon and Pappano, 1980; reproduced with permission of the American Heart Association).

indicates that the coupling of β-receptor to adenylate cyclase is impaired by muscarinic drugs because these drugs act on a GTP-dependent regulatory component that links the two (Watanabe et al., 1978; Birdsall et al., 1980; J.H. Brown, 1980).

The second question implicit in assuming that muscarinic inhibition includes inhibition of adenylate cyclase is, what is the nature of the transition that permits "direct" inhibition of adenylate cyclase after hatching? After hatching, the basal activity of adenylate cyclase and basal concentration of cyclic AMP are greater than they are on the 18th embryonic day, when "direct" inhibition is lacking. It may be speculated that "direct" inhibition of adenylate cyclase after hatching results from an increase of cyclic AMP in a compartment sensitive to ACh. This increase may arise from enhanced stimulation of basal adenylate cyclase by endogenous GTP. Watanabe et al. (1978) noted that muscarinic inhibition of adenylate cyclase in canine ventricle required GTP and could be observed in the absence as well as the presence of catecholamine. Interestingly, although muscarinic inhibition of basal adenylate cyclase can be demonstrated in tissue homogenates, ACh does not change the contractility of mammalian ventricular muscle). Alternatively, the appearance of "direct" muscarinic inhibition may require only a quantitative change in the basal level of adenylate cyclase (that is, a change unrelated to a change in GTP regulation). Basal cyclase may be higher, however, in younger embryos than it is in older embryos. Up to this point, we have not discussed why high concentrations (10^{-4} M) of ACh inhibit significantly adenylate cyclase on the 18th embryonic day yet do not inhibit Ca^{2+}-dependent action potentials or contractions. Indeed, contractility increases in the presence of high ACh concentration (Biegon et al., 1980). Perhaps a qualitative change in the activation of cyclic AMP-dependent protein kinases is essential for the inhibitory effects of ACh on cardiac cell function after hatching. Activation of adenylate cyclase by two different hormones need not be associated with similar changes in cell function (Hayes et al., 1980; or for a similar view in connection with hormonal activation of guanylate cyclase, Lincoln and Keely, 1980). In the study by Hayes et al., both epinephrine and PGE_1 simulated the accumulation of cyclic AMP and activated protein kinase in the isolated perfused rat heart, yet only epinephrine was associated with an increase of phosphorylase activity and of contractility. These results are consistent with the hypothesis that there are compartments of cyclic AMP-dependent protein kinase with unequal access to the enzymes that regulate glycogen metabolism and contractility (Hayes et al., 1980).

Summarily, the "indirect" and "direct" inhibitory effects of muscarinic drugs are referable, in part, to the development of pathways (I and II) between muscarinic receptor and the site of GTP-dependent regulation of adenylate cyclase. But, there is reason to suspect that muscarinic inhibition can also occur by mechanism(s) in addition to adenylate cyclase inactivation.

Experiments with the PDE inhibitor IBMX lend additional support to the cyclic AMP hypothesis in the embryonic heart. These experiments also indicate that muscarinic inhibition can occur through a mechanism that requires the accumulation of cyclic AMP and yet does not inactivate adenylate cyclase or interfere with the accumulation of cyclic AMP. It is reasonable to conclude that muscarinic inhibition, observed with low concentrations of ACh in embryonic ventricles treated with IBMX, occurs at some site in the reaction beyond cyclic AMP, perhaps the activation of protein kinases or membrane protein phosphorylation at the Ca^{2+} channel (Biegon et al., 1980). Muscarinic inhibition of contractility in embryonic hearts treated with cholera toxin could also occur without a reduction in cyclic AMP. For example, J.H. Brown (1980) reported that carbamylcholine (Carb) did not inhibit the accumulation of cyclic AMP caused by cholera toxin, yet it inhibited the accumulation of cyclic AMP caused by ISO in mouse atria treated with cholera toxin. In the embryonic chick ventricle, interestingly, muscarinic inhibition of g_{si} and of contractility can occur only after accumulated cyclic AMP has activated these processes and regardless of whether ISO, IBMX, or cholera toxin is used to bring about cyclic AMP accumulation.

By contrast, the ability of high concentrations of ACh to inhibit the effects of IBMX includes a reduction of cyclic AMP accumulation, as well as blockade beyond cyclic AMP (Biegon et al., 1980). In the canine ventricle, carbamylcholine reduces the accumulation of cyclic AMP and opposes the positive inotropic effect of theophylline, an inhibitor of PDE (Endoh, 1980). Although inhibition of adenylate cyclase by carbamylcholine may be considered a mechanism for reduced accumulation of cyclic AMP in canine ventricle, the choline ester may stimulate PDE activity (Endoh, 1980). In our experiments, the effect of ACh on cyclic AMP accumulation in the chick ventricle is not explained by an action on PDE or on the inhibition of PDE by IBMX. It is speculated that IBMX may activate adenylate cyclase indirectly by virtue of its ability to block an inhibitory effect of endogenous adenosine on this enzyme (Biegon et al., 1980). Adenosine inhibits the accumulation of cyclic AMP caused by ISO in the mammalian ventricle (Dobson, 1978; Schrader et al., 1979), and this inhibitory effect of adenosine is, in turn, opposed by methylxanthines (Schrader et al., 1979). Preliminary experiments indicate that adenosine competitively interacts with a membrane site also responsive to IBMX and theophylline; the apparent K_D for adenosine is about 15 μM. If methylxanthines, but not other inhibitors of PDE, interact with the adenosine receptor in the embryonic heart, as is the case in the adult amphibian heart (Hartzell, 1979), and if this interaction is relevant to the positive inotropic effect of IBMX, then perhaps this interaction is a site of ACh action. This speculation about the mechanism of muscarinic inhibition of cyclic AMP content in embryonic hearts can be tested initially by investigating the interactions among ACh, adenosine, and various classes of PDE inhibitors on twitch tension.

Muscarinic cholinergic receptors have a reaction latency of ≥ 100 msec as compared with the much briefer latency (< 1 msec) at nicotinic cholinergic receptors (Purves, 1978). Therefore, the effects of muscarinic substances are perhaps mediated by the production of an intracellular messenger, like cyclic GMP. Linden and Brooker (1979), in a critical analysis of the role of cyclic GMP as a mediator of muscarinic inhibition in the adult heart, reported that the time course and the concentration-dependence for the synthesis of this cyclic nucleotide are insufficient to explain muscarinic inhibition (see also B.S. Brown et al., 1980; and for additional criticism, J.H. Brown, 1980). In the embryonic chick ventricle, the negative chronotropic effect of muscarinic agonists is associated with significant increases of cyclic GMP because both effects of muscarinic agonist appear at the same time during development, that is, after the 6th incubation day (Renaud et al., 1980). It was concluded that accumulation of cyclic GMP is not essential for the negative chronotropic effect of muscarinic agonists because these agents have a negative chronotropic effect unaccompanied by accumulation of cyclic GMP in heart cell reaggregates. There are, however, many conflicting views in this area. Watanabe and Besch (1975) showed that muscarinic inhibition in the guinea pig ventricle is related to the synthesis of cyclic GMP and that accumulation of this nucleotide is associated with inhibition only after cyclic AMP levels are increased by ISO. More recently, Lincoln and Keely (1980) suggested that there may be several intracellular compartments of cyclic GMP in adult rat heart and that only some of these are coupled to the activation of protein kinases. In view of these considerations, it would be instructive to determine if muscarinic inhibition is associated with increased synthesis of cyclic GMP in the embryonic avian heart. Such experiments may suggest a possible intracellular mechanism by which muscarinic substances inhibit functions dependent on cyclic AMP-dependent protein kinases without changing the synthesis of cyclic AMP itself.

Finally, attention to the role of changes in cyclic nucleotide metabolism should not obscure consideration of other mechanisms for muscarinic inhibition. The inhibition of adenylate cyclase by carbamylcholine (Carb) in WI-38 fibroblasts may be related to the production of phosphatidic acid in the membranes of these cells (Clark et al., 1980). Phosphatidic acid, which mimics the inhibitory effect of Carb on intact cells, accumulates in the plasma membrane of Carb-treated cells. The alteration of membrane phospholipid composition produced under these conditions can regulate adenylate cyclase activity (Clark et al., 1980). However, regulation of adenylate cyclase may be an epiphenomenon of muscarinic inhibition. For example, the effects of β-agonist on calcium permeability in reticulocytes have been attributed to reduced membrane viscosity (Hirata et al., 1979). Occupation of β-receptors by agonist relieves inhibition of methyltransferases in the membrane, and the resulting increase in phosphatidylcholine production diminishes membrane viscosity and increases Ca^{2+} influx. An hypothesis could be suggested regarding the effects of ACh on such viscosity changes. The increased synthesis of cyclic AMP is a sort of epiphenomenon that occurs when increased membrane fluidity allows receptors, regulatory component, and adenylate cyclase to interact. This phenomenon is termed "lateral domain redistribution" by Rodbell (1980). In this scheme proposed by Rodbell, emphasis is placed on the GTP-regulatory protein as the transducer rather than on adenylate cyclase, because the changes in phospholipid metabolism depend on GTP.

CONCLUSION

There are many bits of evidence that are consistent with the view that muscarinic inhibition of g_{si} and contractility in avian ventricle are dependent on both reduced activation of adenylate cyclase (pathways I and II in Fig. 9) and antagonism of the effects of accumulated cyclic AMP. Although the experimental evidence points to the incorporation of several reaction pathways for muscarinic inhibition during development of the avian ventricle, a detailed account of how this takes place is lacking.

Acknowledgements

Thanks are due Dr. P. Epstein for critical reading of this manuscript, M. Coutu, P. Hartigan, and C. Skowronek for skillful technical assistance and to F. DiBattista for tireless secretarial help.

REFERENCES

Au TLS, Collins GA, Walker MJA (1980) Rate, force and cyclic adenosine 3′,5′-monophosphate responses to (-) -adrenaline in neonatal rat heart tissue. Br J Pharmacol **69**:601–608

Biegon RL, Pappano AJ (1980) Dual mechanism for inhibition of calcium-dependent action potentials by acetylcholine in avian ventricular muscle: Relationship to cyclic AMP. Circ Res **46**:353–362

Biegon RL, Epstein PM, Pappano AJ (1980) Muscarinic antagonism of the effects of a phosphodiesterase inhibitor (methylisobutylxanthine) in embryonic chick ventricle. J Pharmacol Exp Ther **215**:348–356

Birdsall NJM, Berrie CP, Burgen ASV, Hulme EC (1980) Modulation of the binding properties of muscarinic receptors: Evidence for receptor-effector coupling. *In* Receptors for Neurotransmitters and Peptide Hormones, edited by G. Pepeu, M.J. Kuhar, and S.J. Enna. New York, Raven Press, pp 107–116

Brown BS, Polson JB, Krzanowski JJ, Wiggins JR (1980) Influence of isoproterenol and methylisobutylxanthine on the contractile and cyclic nucleotide effects of methacholine in isolated rat atria. J Pharmacol Exp Ther **212**:325–332

Brown JH (1980) Cholinergic inhibition of catecholamine-stimulable cyclic AMP accumulation in murine atria. J Cyclic Nuc Res **5**:423–433

Cassel D, Pfeuffer T (1978) Mechanism of cholera toxin action: Covalent modification of the guanyl nucleotide-binding protein of the adenylate cyclase system. Proc Natl Acad Sci USA **75**:2669–2673

Clark RB, Salmon DM, Honeyman TW (1980) Phosphatidic acid inhibition of PGE_1-stimulated cAMP accumulation in WI-38 fibroblasts: Similarities with carbachol inhibition. J Cyclic Nucl Res **6**:37–49

Dobson JG JR (1978) Reduction by adenosine of the isoproterenol-induced increase in cyclic adenosine 3′,5′-monophosphate formation and glycogen phosphorylase activity in rat heart muscle. Circ Res **43**:785–792

Endoh M (1980) The time course of changes in cyclic nucleotide levels during cholinergic inhibition of positive inotropic actions of isoprenaline and theophylline in the isolated canine ventricular myocardium. Naunyn-Schmiedebergs Arch Pharmacol **312**:175–182

Frieswick GM, Danielson T, Shideman FE (1979) Adrenergic inotropic responsiveness of embryonic chick and rat hearts. Dev Neurosci **2**:276–285

Galper JB, Klein W, Catterall WA (1977) Muscarinic acetylcholine receptors in developing chick heart. J Biol Chem **252**:8692–8699

Hartzell HC (1979) Adenosine receptors in frog sinus venosus: slow inhibitory potentials produced by adenine compounds and acetylcholine. J Physiol (Lond) **293**:23–49

Hayes JS, Brunton LL, Mayer SE (1980) Selective activation of particulate cAMP-dependent protein kinase by isoproterenol and prostaglandin E_1. J Biol Chem **255**:5113–5119

Hedtke JL, Shideman FE, Goldberg ND (1976) Positive inotropic activity of cholera enterotoxin on the embryonic chick heart. J Pharmacol Exp Ther **197**:27–37

Higgins D, Pappano AJ (1981) Developmental changes in the sensitivity of the chick embryo ventricle to β-adrenergic agonist during adrenergic innervation. Circ Res **48**:245–253

Hirata F, Strittmatter WJ, Axelrod J (1979) β-Adrenergic receptor agonists increase phospholipid methylation, membrane fluidity, and β-adrenergic receptor-adenylate cyclase coupling. Proc Natl Acad Sci USA **76**:368–372

Iijima T, Pappano AJ (1979) Ontogenetic increase of the maximal rate of rise of the chick embryonic heart action potential: Relationship to voltage, time, and tetrodotoxin. Circ Res **44**:358–367

Inui J, Imamura H (1977) Effects of acetylcholine on calcium-dependent electrical and mechanical responses in the guinea-pig papillary muscle partially depolarized by potassium. Naunyn-Schmiedebergs Arch Pharmacol **299**:1–7

Korth M (1978) Effects of several phosphodiesterase-inhibitors on guinea-pig myocardium. Naunyn-Schmiedebergs Arch Pharmacol **302**:77–86

Levy MN (1971) Sympathetic-parasympathetic interactions in the heart. Circ Res **29**:437–445

Lincoln TM, Keely SL (1980) Effects of acetylcholine and nitroprusside on cGMP-dependent protein kinase in the perfused rat heart. J Cyclic Nucl Res **6**:83–91

Linden J, Brooker G (1979) The questionable role of cyclic guanosine 3′:5′-monophosphate in heart. Biochem Pharmacol **28**:3351–3360

Löffelholz K, Muscholl E (1970) Inhibition by parasympathetic nerve stimulation of the release of the adrenergic transmitter. Naunyn-Schmiedebergs Arch Pharmacol **267**:181–184

Löffelholz K, Pappano AJ (1974) Increased sensitivity of sinoatrial pacemaker to acetylcholine and to catecholamines at the onset of autonomic neuroeffector transmission in chick embryo heart. J Pharmacol Exp Ther **191**:479–486

Markowitz C (1931) Response of explanted embryonic cardiac tissue to epinephrine and acetylcholine. Am J Physiol **97**:271–275

McCarty LP, Lee WC, Shideman FE (1960) Measurement of the inotropic effects of drugs on the innervated and noninnervated embryonic chick heart. J Pharmacol Exp Ther **129**: 315–321

Murad F, Chi YM, Rall TW, Sutherland E (1962) Adenylcyclase:III. The effect of catecholamines and choline esters on the formation of adenosine 3′,5′-phosphate by preparations from cardiac muscle and liver. J Biol Chem **237**:1233–1238

Niedergerke R, Page S (1977) Analysis of catecholamine effects in single atrial trabeculae of the frog heart. Proc Roy Soc Lond B **197**:333–362

Pappano AJ (1970) Calcium-dependent action potentials produced by catecholamines in guinea pig atrial muscle fibers depolarized by potassium. Circ Res **27**:379–390

Pappano AJ (1981) Adrenergic receptors and adrenergic mechanisms in the embryonic and fetal heart. *In* Adrenoceptors and Catecholamine Action, edited by G. Kunos. New York, John Wiley and Sons, pp 69–97

Pappano AJ, Carmeliet EE (1979) Epinephrine and the pacemaking mechanism at plateau potentials in sheep cardiac Purkinje fibers. Pflüg Arch **382**:17–26

Polson JB, Goldberg ND, Shideman FE (1977) Norepinephrine- and isoproterenol-induced changes in cardiac contractility and cyclic adenosine 3′:5′-monophosphate levels during early development of the embryonic chick. J Pharmacol Exp Ther **200**:630–637

Purves RD (1978) The Physiology of Muscarinic Acetylcholine Receptors. *In* Cell Membrane

Receptors for Drugs and Hormones: A Multidisciplinary Approach, edited by R.W. Straub, L. Bolis. New York, Raven Press, pp 69–79

Renaud JF, Sperelakis N, LeDouarin G (1978) Increase of cyclic AMP levels induced by isoproterenol in cultured and non-cultured chick embryonic hearts. J Mol Cell Cardiol **10**:281–286

Renaud JF, Barhanin J, Cavey D, Fosset M, Lazdunski M (1980) Comparative properties of the *in ovo* and *in vitro* differentiation of the muscarinic cholinergic receptor in embryonic heart cells. Dev Biol **78**:184–200

Reuter H (1979) Possible regulation of the calcium permeability of cardiac cell membranes by cyclic nucleotides. *In* Advances in Pharmacology and Therapeutics, edited by J.C. Stoclet. New York, Pergamon Press, vol. 3, pp 153–159

Reuter H, Scholz H (1977) The regulation of the calcium conductance of cardiac muscle by adrenaline. J Physiol (Lond) **264**:49–62

Rodbell M (1980) The role of hormone receptors and GTP-regulatory proteins in membrane transduction. Nature **284**:17–22

Ross EM, Maguire ME, Sturgill TW, Biltonen RL, Gilman AG (1977) Relationship between the β-adrenergic receptor and adenylate cyclase: Studies of ligand binding and enzyme activity in purified membranes of S49 lymphoma cells. J Biol Chem **252**:5761–5775

Salomon Y (1979) Adenylate cyclase assay. Adv Cyclic Nucl Res **10**:35–55

Schrader J, Gerlach E, Baumann G (1979) Sites and mode of action of adenosine in the heart: II. Ventricular myocardium. *In* Physiological and Regulatory Functions of Adenosine and Adenine Nucleotides, edited by H.P. Baer, and G.I. Drummond. New York, Raven Press, pp 137–144

Sperelakis N, Schneider JA (1976) A metabolic control mechanism for calcium ion influx that may protect the ventricular myocardial cell. Am J Cardiol **37**:1079–1085

Tsien RW (1977) Cyclic AMP and contractile activity in heart. Adv Cyclic Nucl Res **8**:363–420

Watanabe AM, Besch HR JR (1975) Interaction between cyclic adenosine monophosphate in guinea pig ventricular myocardium. Circ Res **37**:309–317

Watanabe AM, McConnaughey MM, Strawbridge RA, Fleming JW, Jones JR, Besch HR JR (1978) Muscarinic cholinergic receptor modulation of β-adrenergic receptor affinity for catecholamines. J Biol Chem **253**:4833–4836

Discussion

PAES DE CARVALHO: You have discussed the effect of acetylcholine on slow inward current in a tissue that is quite insensitive to acetylcholine. That it is a tissue in which the effect of acetylcholine on the slow inward current is made apparent only when this current is appreciably enhanced by epinephrine led you to suggest that acetylcholine can act through the cyclic AMP system. I am wondering what the situation is in tissues where acetylcholine plays an important regulatory role, such as in the mammalian atrium. It has been shown by Ten Eick et al. (Pfluegers Arch **361**:207, 1976) that in the mammalian atrium acetylcholine will act on the g_K mechanism at concentrations lower than those at which it acts on the slow inward current. Therefore, the action potential can be shortened and the contraction can be consequently weakened by acetylcholine at concentrations where there is no appreciable effect on the slow inward current. On the other hand, data from frog atrium obtained by Giles and Noble (J Physiol **261**:103–123, 1976) suggest that acetylcholine acts at lower concentrations on the slow inward current mechanism than it does on g_K. I ask you, therefore, whether you would expect acetylcholine always to act on the slow inward current indirectly through the cyclic AMP mechanism, or whether in tissues where it plays an important role it could act directly and at a much faster rate on the g_K mechanism at least.

PAPPANO: I would not like to make a case for the atrium by extrapolating data from the ventricle. I am not opposed to the idea that acetylcholine may be acting in atrial muscles through a mechanism different from that in the ventricular preparations we studied.

PAES DE CARVALHO: It seems that in mammalian atrium acetylcholine acts more promptly on g_K than epinephrine or isoproterenol are able to act on the slow inward current. A difference of at least one order of magnitude in time course can be seen for these two effects. I wonder, therefore, what the time course is for the effects of acetylcholine and epinephrine in your preparation. Are they similar?

PAPPANO: The difference that you mention was neatly shown by Otto Loewi (Loewi and Navratil, Pflügers Arch **206**:135, 1924). When you apply simultaneously a muscarinic and an adrenergic substance to the heart, the depressant effect of the muscarinic substance always precedes the enhancing effect of the adrenergic compound. If you block the action of the muscarinic substance, then you see that the onset of the enhancing activity of the adrenergic compound is considerably delayed. This is consistent with a metabolic effect; that is, that adrenaline, acting through cyclic AMP, will require several hundred milliseconds to show a demonstrable action. Now, I agree that the action of acetylcholine on a muscarinic receptor is much faster than this, but still it is not as fast as what we observe for the action of acetylcholine on a nicotinic receptor, where it can act within a fraction of a millisecond or so. In a muscarinic receptor like that studied by Pott (Pfluegers Arch **380**:71, 1979) and by Hartzell (J Cell Biol *86*:6, 1980), acetylcholine takes 30 or 40 msec to act. So, if you compare the effect on muscarinic and on nicotinic receptors, you would be entitled to propose also a metabolic scheme for the muscarinic receptors. I would agree that, in atrium, acetylcholine may be acting more promptly through the potassium conductance mechanism. But this is certainly not true in the ventricle. We have done studies on neonatal rat muscle cells (McCall and Pappano, unpublished observations), and we have also observed the same thing that we observed for the embryonic chick. That is, if you add acetylcholine alone it has practically no effect, and if you add isoproterenol it will speed up the rate of beating. Now, with acetylcholine you will see a depression of the isoproterenol effect, but you will never go below the initial rate observed before isoproterenol. We also studied the calcium uptake in neonatal rat cells, and we found that acetylcholine by itself does not change the calcium uptake, and isoproterenol enhances it. But if you add both acetylcholine and isoproterenol together, the acetylcholine is capable of inhibiting the enhancing action of isoproterenol. Another set of data on this context is obtained from studies that we made of washout of radioactive potassium from neonatal rat cells. If you add isoproterenol, the washout rate increases, as isoproterenol probably acts on some components of the potassium efflux. Acetylcholine by itself has no effect on the potassium washout in the preparations, but if you add both isoproterenol and acetylcholine, in this case acetylcholine is not capable of counteracting the effect of isoproterenol. In these conditions, one might argue that the effect of acetylcholine on heart cells was limited to the slow inward channel or to the calcium channel. Of course, it would be dangerous to extrapolate to the case of the atrial muscle cells. I would not be at all surprised if the situation was different in atrial muscle.

APRIGLIANO: When is the functional innervation established in your tissue?

PAPPANO: You can stimulate an adrenergic nerve and see a change in contraction of embryonic heart by the 16th day, that is 5 days before hatching.

APRIGLIANO: I am wondering whether you can establish a correlation between the arrival of adrenergic innervation and the establishment of your cyclic AMP pathway. You might be able to make a case for the trophic action of innervation on the embryonic cardiac muscle.

PAPPANO: If there is such an influence, we cannot detect it.

LIEBERMAN: I am wondering about the scheme that showed an ATP dependence for the opening and closing of the calcium channel. Would you care to elaborate on this point?

PAPPANO: ATP is needed to provide high energy phosphate for phosphorylation and protein kinases require ATP to phosphorylate membrane protein.

Chapter 19

The Electrophysiological Effects of Cardiac Glycosides on the Isolated Sinus Node of the Rabbit

Felix I.M. Bonke, Gerhard Steinbeck, Maurits A. Allessie, Albert J.C. Mackaay, and Victor A.J. Slenter

In animal as well as in man, slowing of the heart rate is described as the effect of cardiac glycosides. The attribution to an indirect vagomimetic or antiadrenergic effect of the drug is probably correct because Ten Eick and Hoffman (1969) did not find any change in rate in the sinus node of different mammalian species when they tested cardiac glycosides in nontoxic doses after pharmacologic blockade of the influences of autonomic nerves. But, in digitalis-intoxicated patients, often a supraventricular tachycardia can be noted, and injection of high doses of cardiac glycosides into the sinus node artery both in an isolated sinus node preparation (Hashimoto and Kubata, 1974) and in an open-chest dog (James and Nadeau, 1963; Geer et al., 1977) causes an increase in atrial rate. Increased automaticity of the sinus node appears to be the basis for these supraventricular tachycardias, but other mechanisms cannot be excluded. This can only be clarified by using intracellular recordings from sinus nodal fibers under the influence of cardiac glycosides, for no studies, apart from some early observations made by Toda and West in 1966, are available. We will focus in this study on two questions: *(1)* What is the electrophysiologic effect of cardiac glycosides on the isolated sinus node? *(2)* Do cardiac glycosides influence (directly) the sensitivity of sinus node fibers to autonomic transmitters? For both questions, we must study different concentrations of cardiac glycosides.

The Preparation

We used the isolated right atrium of the rabbit. This preparation is suitable for extensive microelectrode study and has been used by us for many years. Furthermore, because other investigators are using this preparation, results of different research groups can be compared.

The preparation includes the sinus node area, the crista terminalis, and the atrial appendage, but not the AV nodal region or the area of the coronary sinus. We removed most of the atrial appendage to reduce the vigor of contraction during the preparation's exposure to cardiac glycosides. The preparation was superfused with a modified Tyrode's solution at a temperature of 37° ± 0.1° C, and the superfusate was gassed with a mixture containing 95% oxygen and 5% CO_2. A detailed description of the preparation and the recording system has been provided in a recent paper by Steinbeck et al. (1980).

As a glycoside, we used ouabain added to the superfusing fluid in concentrations between 10^{-7} and 10^{-6} M.

THE ELECTROPHYSIOLOGIC EFFECT OF OUABAIN ON THE ISOLATED SINUS NODE OF THE RABBIT

In most experiments with 10^{-7} M ouabain added to the superfusate, there was no or almost no effect on rate or rhythm of the isolated right atrial preparation. But, when a concentration 10^{-6} M was used, an increase in rate occurred. Although different preparations reached different rates, in general the response was the same as that shown in Figure 1. The atrial rate increased gradually and after a certain time (15 to 25 min) the rhythm became irregular (although the beat-to-beat intervals differed by not more than 50 msec) until a period of more or less constant fast rate was reached. Thereafter, irregularity of rhythm appeared again, but with great differences in the beat-to-beat interval. Finally, total arrest occurred (not shown in the figure). Comparing the rate just before the "final arrhythmias," starting with the rate under control conditions, we found that ouabain in a toxic concentration (10^{-6} M) caused an increase in rate from about 2.5 to 4.5 Hz (in 30 experiments the control interval changed from 394 ± 43 to 229 ± 26 msec; mean ± SD).

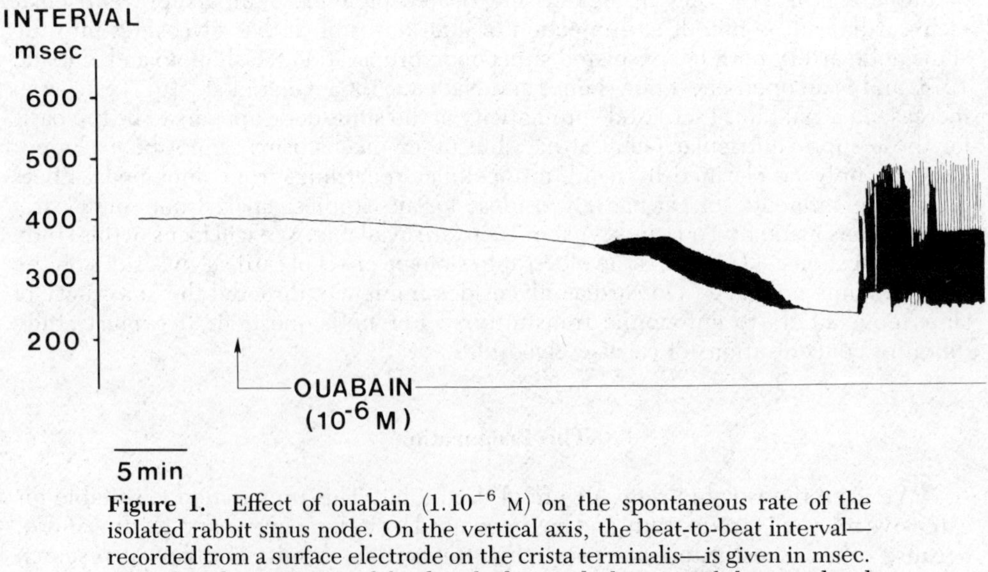

Figure 1. Effect of ouabain (1.10^{-6} M) on the spontaneous rate of the isolated rabbit sinus node. On the vertical axis, the beat-to-beat interval—recorded from a surface electrode on the crista terminalis—is given in msec. After the administration of the drug had started, the interval shortened and after a period of slight irregularities (beat-to-beat variations less than 50 msec) a "ouabain-induced sinus tachycardia" occurred. This was followed by severe irregularities and finally the preparation stopped beating (not shown).

There are three possible causes for this "ouabain-induced sinus tachycardia: *(1)* an increase of the intrinsic rate of the dominant pacemaker in the sinus node, *(2)* an induction or triggering of an ectopic pacemaker that is faster than the original one, and *(3)* a release of catecholamines from vesicles in nerve terminals in the sinus node area. To exclude the third possibility, we investigated the effect of ouabain (10^{-6} M) on the isolated sinus node with and without propranolol. Therefore, a bolus of epinephrine was added to the tissue bath, via a separate infusion system, in such a concentration that the cycle length decreased by at least 100 msec. Then propranolol was added to the superfusate in a concentration sufficient to abolish the effect of the bolus of epinephrine almost completely; that is, an interval change of at most 10 msec was acceptable. (In this way we tried to keep the concentration of propranolol as low as possible to prevent the membrane-stabilizing effect of the drug which could influence our results.) Subsequently, ouabain was also added to the superfusate in a concentration of 10^{-6} M. In seven experiments with a propranolol concentration between 0.2 and 0.5 mg/liter, the rate of the isolated right atrium increased by the same amount under the influence of ouabain (10^{-6} M) as it did under control conditions, that is, without propranolol (the interval changed from 370 ± 25 to 231 ± 12 msec, $N = 7$). Thus, the toxic effect of ouabain on the rate of the isolated sinus node is not mediated via liberation of catecholamines.

To investigate whether the group of dominant pacemaker fibers in the sinus node would keep their dominance when under the influence of a toxic concentration of ouabain, we tried to make a long-lasting impalement of a dominant pacemaker fiber. This is very difficult, however, because the microelectrode has to be kept inside the fiber during a long period (more than 30 min), whereas the contractility of the preparation increases enormously during this period because of the positive inotropic effect of the cardiac glycoside. In some experiments, we could attain this goal. Figure 2 gives a representative example. In the upper panel of this figure, a recording of the transmembrane potential from a sinus node fiber located very close to the dominant pacemaker fibers (less than 250 μ from the fiber discharging the earliest in this preparation) is shown, together with the reference electrogram from the crista terminalis. The upstroke of the action potential preceded activation of the crista terminalis by 28 msec during the control period. After the preparation had been exposed for 27 min to ouabain in a concentration of 5×10^{-7} M, and the impalement of the fiber was still perfect, the beat-to-beat interval had decreased from 375 to 340 msec, and activation of the fiber and the crista terminalis now coincided in time (middle panel of Fig. 2). During further exposure to the drug, the rate increased further, and the upstroke of the action potential occurred even later than the activation of crista terminalis did (in the lower panel, the electrogram preceded the upstroke of the action potential by 9 msec). In the lower panel, this fiber and the neighboring fibers now are discharged from another site in the sinus node (or perhaps even from a site outside the node). Thus, ouabain caused a shift in the location of the dominant pacemaker.

To determine where the pacemaker shifts to, we had to make an accurate map of the spread of activation within the sinus node and the atrium under normal conditions, as well as when the preparation was under the influence of ouabain. Because it is not possible to make enough simultaneous recordings with microelectrodes from the area of the sinus node, we were able only to construct an accurate map of the spread of activation when rate and rhythm were constant and with subsequent impalements with one single microelectrode made under stable conditions.

This was done without too much difficulty under control conditions, but during exposure to ouabain the period of the "ouabain-induced tachycardia" (just before the final arrhythmias occurred, as shown in Fig. 1) last long enough only in some experiments to permit this procedure to be followed. In eight experiments, we were able to

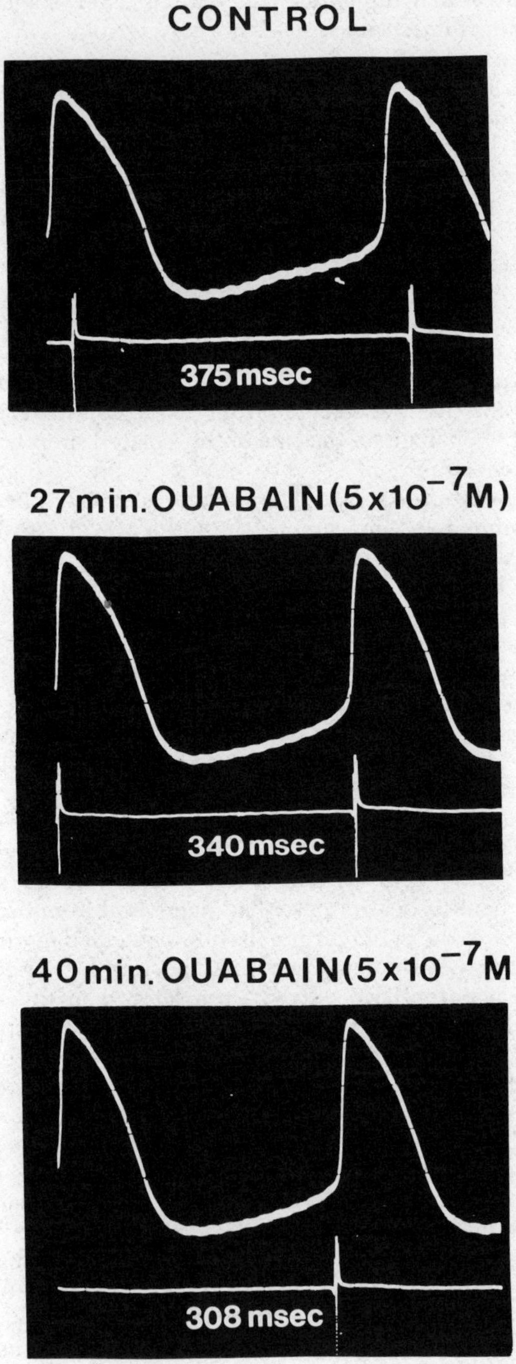
CONTROL
375 msec
27 min. OUABAIN (5x10^{-7}M)
340 msec
40 min. OUABAIN (5x10^{-7}M)
308 msec

do this, and Figure 3 shows one example. The map on the left shows the spread of activation during normal sinus rhythm, and the dominant pacemaker is located about 1 mm from the border between crista terminalis and sinus node. Under the influence of ouabain (in this experiment in a concentration of 8×10^{-7} M), the map at the right side was made, which shows that the dominant pacemaker shifted towards the sinoatrial border although it was still within the sinus node area. Although the activation pattern during the exposure to ouabain usually could not be determined as accurately as it could be during control conditions because of the short period of stable rhythm and the difficulty of making good impalements due to the vigorous contractions of the atrium, in all eight experiments a pacemaker shift towards the sinoatrial border could be demonstrated. The exact site at the sinoatrial border to which the pacemaker shifted varied from preparation to preparation and was either towards the superior vena cava, or towards the inferior vena cava, or somewhere in between.

Thus, ouabain in a toxic dose causes an acceleration of impulse formation within the sinus node, not because the original dominant pacemaker in the center of the node is accelerated, but because fibers at the sinoatrial border are influenced in such a way that they become dominant. Figure 4 may be useful in explaining this phenomenon. The microelectrode was impaled under control conditions in a fiber located between the site of the dominant pacemaker in the center of the node and the crista terminalis, (that is, in the sino-atrial border). In the top left panel, the action potential recording is shown together with a reference electrogram from the crista terminalis. After a long exposure to ouabain, a depolarization could be recorded in this fiber, together with a steepening of the diastolic depolarization and a smooth transition from the diastolic into the systolic depolarization. This figure suggests that this fiber either became one of the group of the dominant pacemaker fibers or was located very close to the group of fibers that, under the influence of ouabain, assumed dominance. It might be argued that the change in the slope of the diastolic depolarization in the bottom left panel, compared with the top left panel, is caused by the shift of the pacemaker towards the impaled fiber, and the change is thus based merely on a stronger electrotonic influence. But the panels at the right show that during atrial pacing the slope of the diastolic depolarization under ouabain is obviously steeper than it is under control conditions. The reason for this difference in sensitivity to ouabain remains uncertain.

Figure 2. Pacemaker shift induced by ouabain in a toxic concentration. Recording of the time-course of the transmembrane potential of a fiber located less than 250 μ away from the earliest discharging pacemaker fibers under control conditions together with a unipolar surface electrogram recorded from the crista terminalis. The oscilloscope was triggered at the level of 50% of the amplitude of the action potential (upper trace). Before the drug was administered the beat-to-beat interval was 375 ms. The drug itself had almost no influence on the configuration of the action potential, but after 27 min the spontaneous rate was faster (interval 340 msec) and the time difference between the action potential (at 50% level of the upstroke) and the intrinsic deflection of the complex of the crista terminalis was only 1 msec, whereas this latency was 28 msec under control conditions. The microelectrode was kept in the fiber and the lower panel shows that after 40 min of drug administration, the crista terminalis is activated earlier than the impaled fiber (the oscilloscope starts after the complex); therefore at this moment the impaled fiber is no longer involved in pacemaking. Vertical calibration at the right side of the lower panel indicates 50 mV. *(Reproduced with permission of the American Heart Association from Steinbeck et al., Circ. Res.* ***46****:406, 1980).*

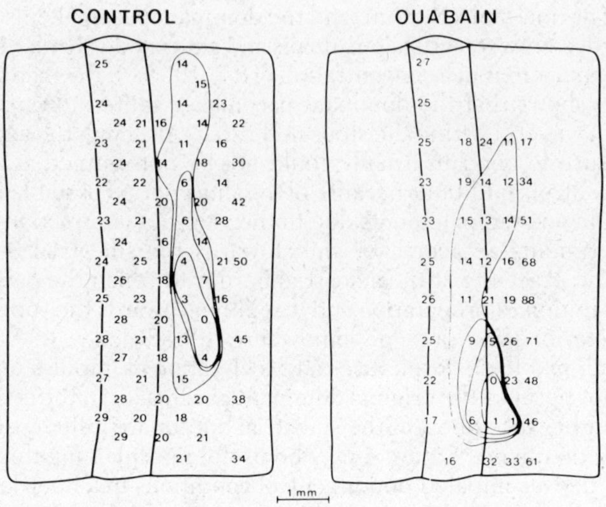

Figure 3. Map of the spread of activation in the sinus node area and the crista terminalis under normal conditions (left side) and during the administration of ouabain in a concentration of 8×10^{-7} M (right side). The map on the right side was made within a period of 6 min, during which the rapid rhythm was stable and there were no irregularities (the administration of ouabain had lasted 1 hour at that time). During control, the cycle length was 340 ms and constant. A total of 61 sites was explored consecutively by the microelectrode; during this period, 10 surface electrograms were recorded continuously from the crista terminalis (interelectrode distance of 1 mm) with an electrode brush. The earliest discharge of a fiber in the area of the sinus node in relation to the crista terminalis is taken as zero. The moment of activation of all other impaled fibers (the moment the upstroke of the action potential reached 50% of its amplitude) is related to this zero reference. These activation times are plotted in the diagrams, and isochronic lines are constructed 5 ms, 10 ms, and 15 ms after 0. In such a way, a reasonable indication is offered for the spread of the impulse from the dominant pacemaker site through the sinus node toward the crista terminalis. In the period during which the "ouabain map" was made, the beat-to-beat interval was almost constant (195–210 ms) and we were able to impale 35 sites with the microelectrode. Together with the 10 surface electrograms, the right map was constructed therefrom. Obviously, the dominant pacemaker site has shifted caudally and toward the sinoatrial border. (Reproduced with permission of the American Heart Association from Steinbeck et al., Circ. Res. **46**:406, 1980).

Purely phenomenologically, it can be concluded that a toxic concentration of ouabain directly influences the sinus node (of the rabbit) in such a way that fibers in the sinoatrial border are depolarized to a greater extent than are fibers in the center of the node, and therefore these border fibers can reach a higher "intrinsic rate of impulse formation" than can other sinus node fibers and thus will assume dominance of the node.

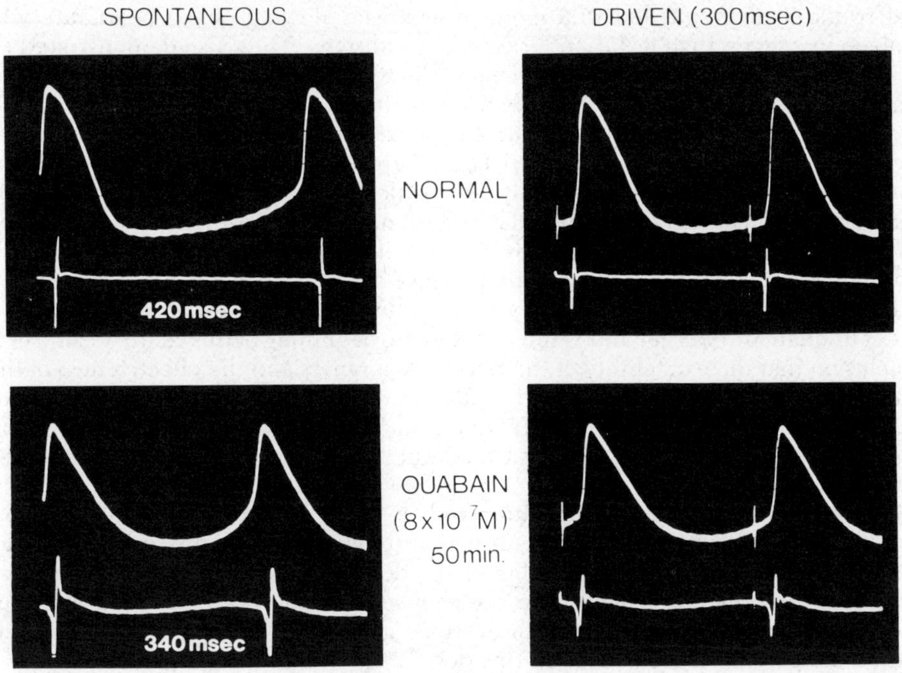

Figure 4. Effect of ouabain on phase 4 depolarization. In the left top panel, the voltage-time course of the transmembrane potential of a latent pacemaker fiber is shown in the upper trace with a unipolar surface electrogram from the crista terminalis (lower trace). During control, the spontaneous interval was 420 ms as shown in the left top panel. The right top panel shows the same impalement under artificial drive of the atrium at an interval of 300 ms. After 50 min of exposure to ouabain in a concentration of 8×10^{-7} M, the fiber (same impalement as above) showed a decrease of maximum diastolic potential, decrease of action potential amplitude, and an increase of the slope of diastolic depolarization; the spontaneous interval has decreased to 340 ms (left bottom panel). These changes are also readily seen when the same impalement before and after ouabain is compared under the same atrial drive interval of 300 ms (right top and bottom panel). Vertical bar: 50 mV. *(Reproduced with permission of the American Heart Association from Steinbeck et al., Circ. Res.* **46***:406, 1980).*

THE INFLUENCE OF CARDIAC GLYCOSIDES ON THE SENSITIVITY OF SINUS NODE FIBERS TO AUTONOMIC TRANSMITTERS

In animal as well as in man, cardiac glycosides will slow the heart rate, and this effect, because it is partly abolished by atropine, is considered to be vagal in origin. Several hypotheses have been advanced to explain this vagal effect: *(1)* sensitization of the heart to vagal activity, *(2)* central vagal stimulation, and *(3)* sensitization of the carotid sinus.

Gaffney et al. (1958) demonstrated in the open-chest dog (vagotomized so that no central vagal influences on the heart could be present) that stimulation of the peripheral trunk of the vagus led to a more pronounced slowing of the heart rate when ouabain was given than it did under control conditions. They also demonstrated that ouabain sensitized the heart to acetylcholine in the heart-lung preparation of the dog. Also in studies with the isolated right atrium of the rabbit, ouabain, in a concentration between 10^{-7} and 10^{-6} M, increased the sensitivity of the SA node to exogenous acetylcholine (Toda and West, 1966). These latter studies, however, were done at a temperature of about 30° C; recently, it was demonstrated that the position of the dominant pacemaker fibers in the isolated sinus node of the rabbit is strongly temperature dependent (Bouman et al., 1978; Mackaay et al., 1980). Therefore, we decided to incorporate into this study an evaluation of the effect of ouabain on the ACh sensitivity of the isolated rabbit sinus node at a temperature of between 37 and 38° C.

Although Rothberger and Winterberg in the beginning of this century came to the conclusion that the excitability of the nervi accelerantes and the effectiveness of their stimulation appeared to undergo no change as a general rule under the influence of digitalis (cited by Cushny, 1925), Méndez et al. (1961) found that in the dog, with an open chest and denervation of the heart, adrenergic cardiac acceleration was inhibited by cardiac glycosides.

Figure 5 was taken from these latter studies. It shows the dose-response curves for the chronotropic effect produced by adrenaline (epinephrine) on the sinus node before and after the administration of a cardiac glycoside. From the lower panel of this figure, two conclusions can be drawn. The catecholamine-induced change in heart rate is lower after the administration of the cardiac glycoside, and the cardiac glycoside caused an increase in heart rate in this dog.

Although this study of Mendez et al. (1961) is explicit, we decided to extend our studies and investigate the effect of ouabain on the catecholamine sensitivity of the isolated sinus node of the rabbit, both because Mendez et al. used a rather high dose of glycosides given in a bolus injection and because we prefer the isolated preparation to the denervated heart in the open-chest dog.

THE EFFECT OF OUABAIN ON THE CHOLINERGIC RESPONSES IN THE ISOLATED RABBIT SINUS NODE

The isolated right atrium of the rabbit was superfused with normal Tyrode's solution, and by an infusion system carbamylcholine was added in several concentrations. We added the drug only during limited periods; the responses therefore are not steady-state values because no steady drug concentration was reached in these short periods. Because the flow of Tyrode's solution was kept constant, responses to the drug infusions were reproducible. The advantage of this procedure is that several "concentrations" can be tested within a relatively short time, whereas for the aim of our study we were more interested in the comparison of the responses with and without ouabain than we were in quantification of the responses.

In Figure 6 the results of such an experiment are shown. Sequentially increasing doses of carbamylcholine (CCh) were tested. For example, the addition of CCh 10^{-7} g/ml, caused a change of the beat-to-beat interval of about 200 msec. We then added ouabain to the Tyrode's solution in a concentration of 10^{-7} M. This concentration of the drug had a clear positive inotropic effect and almost no effect on rate (this is in agreement with the study of Toda and West, 1966). It seems reasonable to suppose that

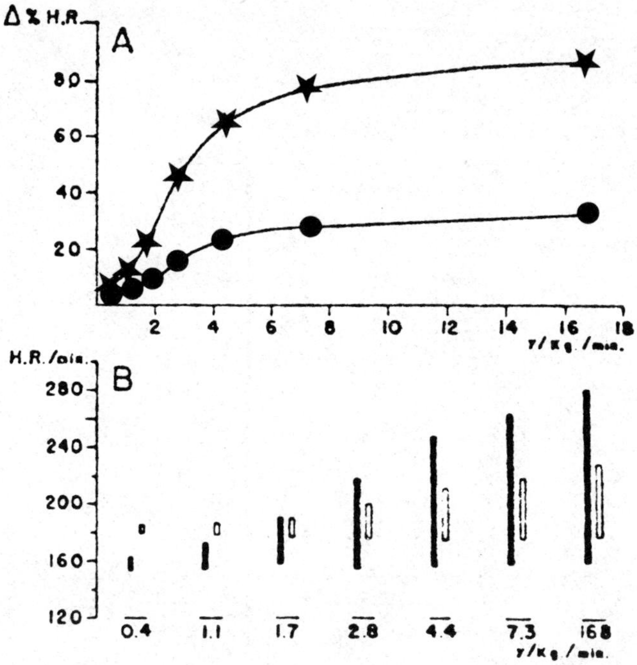

Figure 5. Dose-response curves of the chronotropic effect produced by adrenaline on the sinus node before (stars) and after (closed circles) the administration of 60% of the lethal dose of acetyldigitoxin to a dog with a denervated (surgically) heart.

In A, the increase of the heart rate is expressed as percentage of the basal frequency (ordinate) whereas the dose of adrenaline used is given in μg per kg body weight per min on the abscissa. The curve with the filled circles is obtained 20 min after the administration of the acetyldigitoxin.

Since the basal frequency is influenced by the cardiac glycoside itself, the absolute values of the heart rate are given in B. The solid bars indicate the heart rate in beats per min under control situations and the peak values of the rate during adrenaline administration. The open bars indicate basal and peak heart rate after acetyldigitoxin. Note the increase of the basal heart rate under influence of the cardiac glycoside. *(Reproduced from Mendez et al., J. Pharmacol. Exp. Ther.* **131**:*191, 1961; with permission of the authors and the publishers).*

under this condition the dominant pacemaker has not shifted from the center of the node towards the sinoatrial border and that the same group of fibers dominates the node both during the administration of ouabain and under control conditions. The infusion of carbamylcholine during exposure of the preparation to ouabain obviously caused a greater effect on rate than it did when under control conditions.

Therefore, ouabain in a nontoxic concentration (no effect on impulse formation; positive inotropic effect) enhances the sensitivity of the isolated sinus node to cholinergic substances.

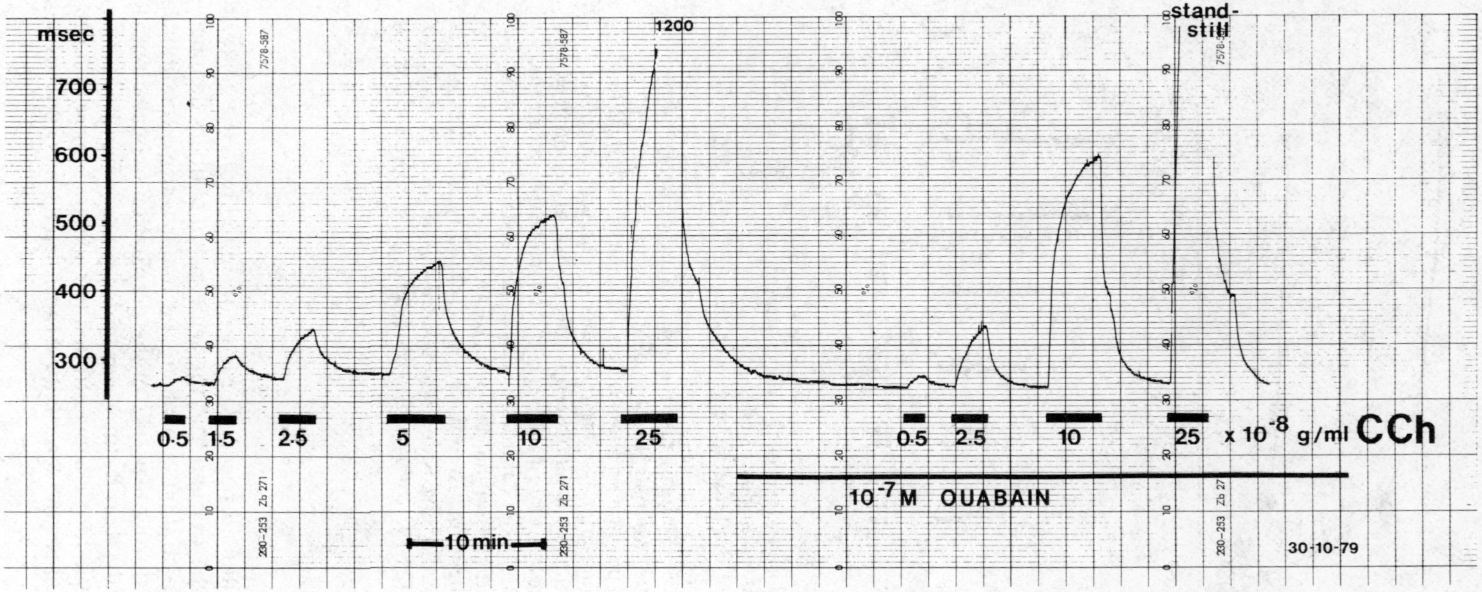

Figure 6. Cholinergic responses of the isolated sinus node of the rabbit under control conditions and under influence of a non-toxic concentration of cardiac glycosides.

By means of an infusion pump carbamylcholine (CCh) was added to the superfusing Tyrode's solution in different concentrations. The infusion was continued only during a short period and therefore the cholinergic responses never reached a steady state; however, the procedure resulted in reproducible responses.

During drug administration, two concentrations of CCh were not tested, viz. 1.5 and 5×10^{-8} g/ml. A concentration of 25.10^{-8} g/ml CCh caused a slowing of rate (interval 1200 ms), whereas the same concentration brought the sinus node to complete silence if ouabain was administered simultaneously.

It is obvious that the cholinergic responses are stronger if the sinus node is under the influence of ouabain.

THE EFFECT OF OUABAIN ON THE ADRENERGIC RESPONSES IN THE ISOLATED RABBIT SINUS NODE

In a series of experiments, we determined the dose-response curve for adrenaline in the isolated right atrium of the rabbit. In Figure 7, for each adrenaline concentration tested, the increase in the spontaneous rate is plotted as a percentage of the maximal effect of the drug. After the administration of ouabain in a nontoxic concentration (10^{-7} M), the procedure was repeated. As shown in Figure 7, the cardiac glycoside did not influence the sensitivity of the sinus node to adrenaline. We then studied the effect of a higher concentration of ouabain. This, however, presented us with the problem that both adrenaline and ouabain, in a concentration of 10^{-6} M, cause an increase in rate. This is illustrated in Figure 8. We used the drug-infusion technique again, and at the moment indicated by an arrow during 30 sec, adrenaline was infused into the tissue bath in a concentration such that the beat-to-beat interval decreased by about 100 msec. After repetition of this procedure, we added ouabain (10^{-6} M) to the Tyrode's

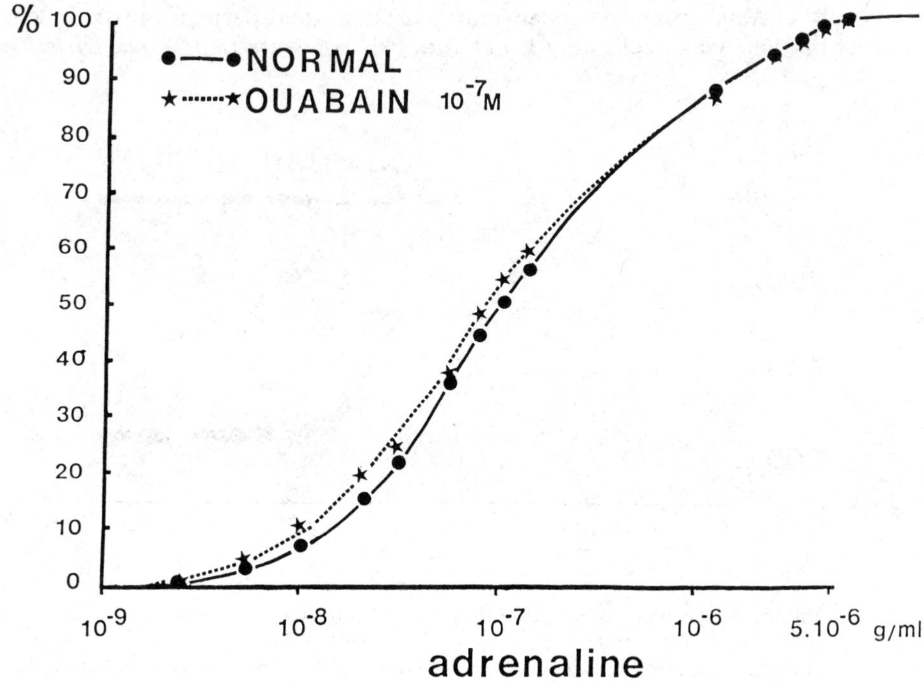

Figure 7. Dose-response curves of the chronotropic effect produced by adrenaline on the isolated sinus node of the rabbit with and without administration of ouabain in a non-toxic concentration. On the ordinate the effect of adrenaline on the beat-to-beat interval is given in percentages. Since during ouabain administration the basic cycle length was the same as during control, whereas in both cases the maximal effect, i.e. the shortest cycle length, was also the same, we might have used on the ordinate also absolute values instead of percentages, but this was not exactly the case in all experiments. The dose-response curve under control conditions (filled circles and continuous line) coincides almost with the curve under ouabain (stars and interrupted line).

solution. A ouabain-induced tachycardia occurred as described in the first part of the present study (see also Fig. 1). Administration of the same amount of adrenaline as during the control situation resulted in a moderate decrease in the beat-to-beat interval. Interpretation of these results, however, is seriously hampered by the limited rate of spontaneous impulse formation in fibers of the sinus node. If the rate is increased because of the effect of ouabain in a toxic concentration, the range between this ouabain-induced beat-to-beat interval and the minimal interval (maximal rate) is small and the "adrenaline effect" never can be the same as it is under control conditions.

Although we used very high concentrations of adrenaline, the rate of the isolated sinus node of the rabbit never exceeded 6 Hz (shortest interval in ten preparations was between 166 and 196 msec, with a mean value of 178 msec. Simultaneous administration of toxic doses of ouabain did not alter the maximal rate of the isolated sinus node.

The adrenaline response, that is, the change in cycle length in milliseconds, of the ouabain-intoxicated sinus node obviously was reduced compared with the control situation as shown in Figure 8. This reduction can be explained, at least in part, by the dependence of the adrenaline response on the preceding cycle length, namely, the shorter the preceding cycle length the smaller the adrenaline response (Op 't Hof, University of Amsterdam, personal communication), and perhaps in part by one or more of the following explanations: *(1)* The toxic concentration of ouabain causes a

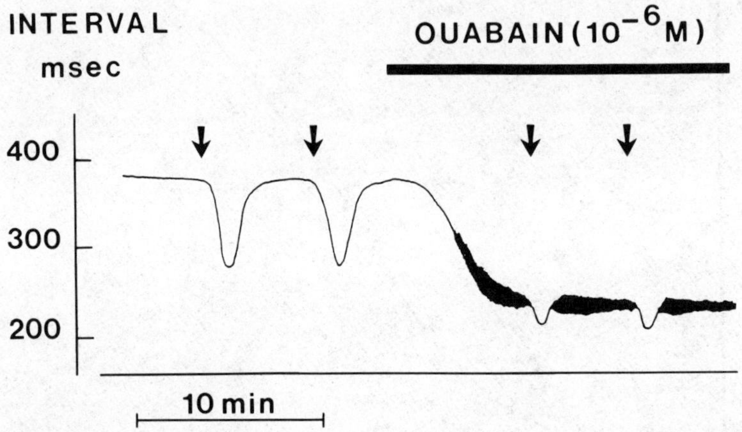

Figure 8. Effect of the administration of adrenaline—given in a bolus infusion into the tissue chamber—under control conditions and during simultaneous addition of ouabain in a toxic concentration. At the ordinate the beat-to-beat interval is given in ms.

At the moment indicated by an arrow the infusion of adrenaline was started and continued for 30 seconds. This resulted in a shortening of the interval by about 100 ms—A second infusion had the same effect. Then ouabain administration was started and at the time the drug had caused an obvious "ouabain-induced tachycardia" (interval about 230 ms), again an infusion of adrenaline was given (the same concentration and during 30 seconds again). This resulted in a shortening of the interval by 22 ms (26 ms during the second infusion). Thus the change in interval caused by adrenaline was much smaller than under control conditions.

shift of the dominant pacemaker from the center of the sinus node towards the sinoatrial border, and these fibers are less sensitive to catecholamines than are the fibers in the center of the node; thus, the reduced adrenaline sensitivity is a secondary effect and not caused by the cardiac glycoside itself. *(2)* Ouabain diminishes the adrenaline sensitivity of the fibers of the sinoatrial border but has no or little influence on the fibers in the center of the node; thus, the reduced adrenaline sensitivity can only be noticed when fibers of the sinoatrial border have assumed dominance of the sinus node. *(3)* In toxic concentrations, ouabain diminishes the sensitivity of all sinoatrial fibers.

To study the first possibility, we did a series of experiments in which we tried to determine separately the adrenaline sensitivity of the border zone and the center of the sinus node. Therefore, we had to make a cut through the sinus node, and such a procedure can easily damage the preparation. Another problem was that the division of the sinus node into a border zone and a central area of the node (or according to Bleeker et al. [1980], among others, a transitional zone and the compact node) is arbitrary and is very difficult to make without the help of microscopic studies. Therefore, we investigated the isolated sinus node very carefully by means of numerous subsequent impalements with a microelectrode. The criteria we used to separate "border fibers" from "central fibers" were that the transition from diastolic depolarization to the upstroke of the action potential had to be sharp and that the upstroke of the action potential had to have a dV/dt max of at least 10 V/sec, and, of course, that the fiber had to be located at the sinoatrial border. After we had made an electrophysiologic "division" of the sinus node, we administered adrenaline in a concentration that would decrease the spontaneous beat-to-beat interval by about 100 msec (in most experiments, a concentration of 6×10^{-7} M was used). Then we mapped the activation pattern of the sinus node again. Under the influence of adrenaline, the dominant pacemaker shifted, in a caudal direction. Then, we divided the preparation into a central nodal preparation and a "transitional" preparation (the sinoatrial border together with crista terminalis and the right atrial appendage) by means of a very fine pair of scissors. Finally, the adrenaline responses of both preparations were determined using the same concentration of adrenaline as used before partition of the sinus node.

As indicated in Figure 9, we made a cut through the sinus node along the interrupted line, and although there is no sharp border between the transitional zone and the compact area of the node, we tried to make this partition in a way such that the "central nodal preparation" (on the right side of the interrupted line in Fig. 9) would contain almost exclusively compact nodal fibers. In this experiment, the spontaneous beat-to-beat interval of the intact sinus node was 370 msec. After the partition, the central nodal preparation beat with an interval of 360 msec, whereas the "transitional" preparation had an interval of 384 msec. The latter preparation showed an adrenaline response of −34 msec (the interval changed from 384 to 350 msec), whereas in the central nodal preparation the response was −100 msec (interval changed from 360 to 260 msec), and this was the same as the response of the preparation before the partition was made (when the interval changed from 370 to 270 msec).

From this and other experiments, it can be concluded that fibers at the sinoatrial border are less sensitive to adrenaline than are fibers in the central nodal area, and this conclusion is in favor of the first hypothesis mentioned.

With the same experimental protocol, we are now testing the second hypothesis. Before a partition is made the preparation is exposed to ouabain in a nontoxic concentration (10^{-7} M), and then the adrenaline response is measured. Thereafter, the partition is made, and the adrenaline response of the preparation is measured. At this moment, however, results are not available.

A more detailed study of the third possibility is one of our future projects.

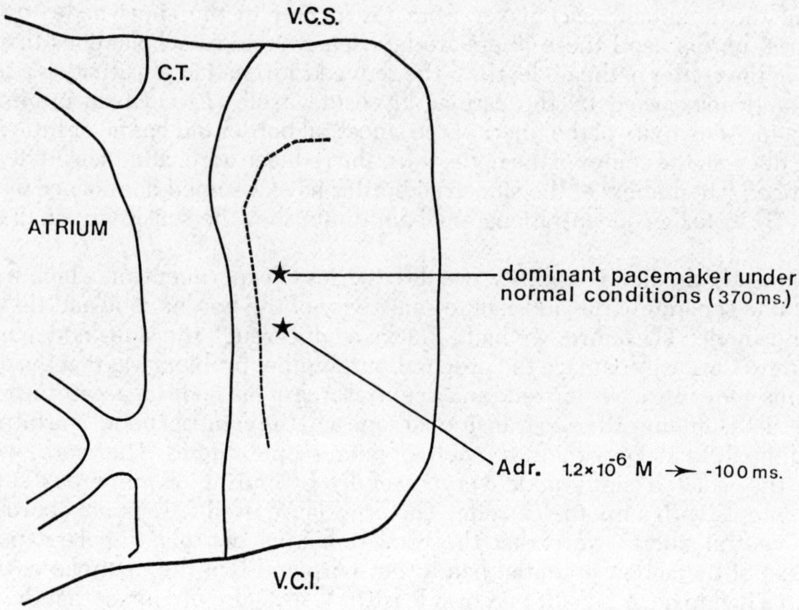

Figure 9. Schematic representation of the procedure followed in the experiment of 16-9-1980. The activation pattern was mapped under normal conditions and after administration of adrenaline to the superfusing fluid. The site of the dominant pacemaker shifted about 1 mm in the direction of the vena cava inferior (v.c.i.); under both conditions the site of the dominant pacemaker was located in the compact nodal area. Thereafter the compact node was separated from the rest of the preparation by making a cut along the interrupted line using a pair of scissors; from the caudal end of this line the incision was made parallel to the crista terminalis (CT) whereas at the cranial end the incision was lengthened in the direction of the septum. V.C.S. = vena cava superior. See text for further description.

CONCLUSION

Ouabain in a nontoxic concentration enhances the cholinergic response of the isolated sinus node, whereas the adrenergic response is not influenced. We could not prove that the sensitivity to catecholamines of sinus node fibers is diminished if cardiac glycosides are administered in a toxic concentration as was concluded by Mendez et al. (1961) for the dog heart in situ.

REFERENCES

Bleeker WK, Mackaay AJC, Masson-Pévet M, Bouman LN, Becker AE (1980) Functional and morphological organization of the rabbit sinus node. Circ Res **46**:11–22

Bouman LN, Mackaay, AJC, Bleeker WK, Becker AE (1978) Pacemaker shifts in the sinus node: effects of vagal stimulation, temperature and reduction of extracellular calcium. In The Sinus Node. Structure, Function, and Clinical Relevance, edited by FIM Bonke. The Hague-Boston-London, Martinus Nijhoff, p 245–257

Cushny AR (1925) The Action and Uses in Medicine of Digitalis and Its Allies. London, Longmans, Green and Co., p 112

Gaffney TE, Kahn JB, Van Maanen EF, Acheson GH (1958) A mechanism of the vagal effect of cardiac glycosides. J Pharmacol Exp Ther **122**:423–429

Geer MR, Wagner GS, Waxman M, Wallace AG (1977) Chronotropic effect of acetylstrophanthidin infusion into the canine sinus nodal artery. Am J Cardiol **39**:684–689

Hashimoto K, Kubota K (1974) Positive chronotropic effect of ouabain in the excised and blood-perfused canine SA node preparation of the dog. Naunyn Schmiedebergs Arch Pharmacol **281**:357–370

James TN, Nadeau RA (1963) The chronotropic effect of digitalis studied by direct perfusion of the sinus node. J Pharmacol Exp Ther **139**:42–52

Mackaay AJC, Bleeker WK, Op 't Hof T, Bouman LN (1980) Temperature dependence of the chronotropic action of calcium. Functional inhomogeneity of the rabbit sinus node. J Mol Cell Cardiol **12**:433–443

Méndez C, Aceves J, Méndez R (1961) Inhibition of adrenergic cardiac acceleration by cardiac glycosides. J Pharmacol Exp Ther **131**:191–198

Steinbeck G, Bonke FIM, Allessie MA, Lammers WJEP (1980) The effect of ouabain on the isolated sinus node preparation of the rabbit studied with microelectrodes. Circ Res **46**: 406–414

Ten Eick RE, Hoffman BF (1969) Chronotropic effect of cardiac glycosides in cats, dogs, and rabbits. Circ Res **25**:365–378

Toda N, West TC: The influence of ouabain on cholinergic responses in the sinoatrial node. J Pharmacol Exp Ther **153**:104–113

Discussion

HOFFMAN: As a pharmacologist, I find it difficult to judge different sensitivities at different sites if an analog is used instead of a natural transmitter. It may be the case, for instance, that the density of distribution of cholinesterase is higher in the part of the node where most vagal terminals are located, so that if you use carbachol instead of acetylcholine you would not see what would happen to acetylcholine once it gets to these receptors. The same may be true for catecholamines. If the uptake of norepinephrine by nerve terminals is as important as we think it is, then you might see differences between effects of norepinephrine, epinephrine, and isoproterenol during exposure to digitalis, as digitalis might inhibit this uptake. For these reasons I find difficult to judge how drugs affect the response of the heart to liberated transmitters if you do not use these transmitters in your study.

BONKE: I share your concern. We also used acetylcholine in our studies, and the effect was the same as it was with carbamylcholine. We never tested norepinephrine instead of epinephrine, but I will do it as soon as I am back home.

PAES DE CARVALHO: I am wondering about the mechanism of the variations in cycle length observed during ouabain intoxication. Is that an actual variation of the pacemaker-firing frequency or is it a sign of varying sinoatrial block?

BONKE: During the first phase of ouabain intoxication, there is only an acceleration of the rate, and conduction is not disturbed. When slight arrhythmias occur, there might be an alternation of dominancy between a pacemaker in the center of the sinus node and a "new" pacemaker in the periphery (transitional zone); we were not able to prove this hypothesis, and it is possible that conduction disturbances also play a role in this phenomenon. The conduction is severely disturbed during the final arrhythmias, causing intranodal (sinoatrial), and even intraatrial conduction block. In some experiments, we also followed the change in rate and rhythm during the recovery of ouabain intoxication (after the administration of the drug was stopped), and then the intraatrial conduction block disappeared within a short time, whereas sinoatrial block sometimes remained for more than half an hour. In these cases, we recorded with a microelectrode a faster rhythm in the sinus node than we did in the atrium, and the relation could be 4:3, 3:2, or even 2:1. Finally, conduction was restored in almost all preparations.

Chapter 20

Characteristics of Impulse Propagation in the Mammalian Atrioventricular Node

Carlos Méndez

In the normal mammalian heart, once an impulse reaches the bundle of His, the electrical activity travels quickly through the specialized conducting system. The Purkinje network rapidly distributes the impulse to the ventricular mass, and the activation of all parts of the ventricular muscle, although not simultaneous, occurs within a short interval. This degree of synchronization favors an effective ventricular contraction. On the other hand, the delay between the contraction of the atria and the ventricles is relatively long; an estimate of it is given by the electrocardiographic P-R interval. In the experimental animal, or in man, the electrograms obtained under normal conditions from the region of the bundle of His show that approximately half of the P-R interval corresponds to propagation across the atrioventricular (AV) node. Accordingly, conduction through this small structure is rather slow (Hoffman and Cranefield, 1960; Méndez and Moe, 1972 and Cranefield, 1975).

The delay provided by the AV node, added to the conduction time required for an impulse to travel through the ventricular specialized tissues, allows atrial contraction to further increase ventricular filling. Therefore, under normal conditions, an important function of the AV node is to provide an extra delay that allows a more effective ejection of blood into the arteries.

Episodes of fast atrial activity are frequently found in the clinic. In these situations, the AV node fulfills another major function. Because of its low margin of safety for propagation, the node of Tawara acts as a filter when the atrial rate is high. Thus, during atrial fibrillation a large number of impulses are blocked in the AV node. This "filter" property is essential for the survival of individuals who have rapid atrial arrhythmias.

In this chapter, emphasis will be placed on: *(1)* the nature of AV nodal action potentials, *(2)* the mechanism of AV nodal propagation, and *(3)* the properties responsible for the "filtering" characteristics of the AV node.

Unless otherwise stated, the experiments described in the following sections were performed on isolated preparations of the rabbit heart.

Supported, in part, by grant 1504 from PNCB of CONACyT, México.

THE NATURE OF AV NODAL ACTION POTENTIALS

Transmembrane Potentials

AV nodal transmembrane potentials are characterized by: *(1)* a low resting potential, *(2)* a low rate of the depolarization phase of action potentials, *(3)* a clear overshoot of the regenerative responses, and *(4)* a duration falling between the action potentials of the atrial muscle and the action potentials of the bundle of His fibers.

The now classical subdivision of the AV region into the three zones (AN, N, and NH), proposed by Paes de Carvalho and De Almeida (1960), is still very useful for communication purposes. As these authors pointed out, the boundary between zones is ill defined, as well as the transition between the atrial fibers and the AN region and between the NH region and the His bundle. But the cells included in the N zone clearly have the lowest resting potentials (approximately −60 mV), and the same is true of the maximal rate of rise of the transmembrane action potential (5 to 20 V/sec); the overshoot remains essentially the same in the three regions (approximately +20 mV), and the duration of action potentials increases progressively from the atrium to the bundle of His (Hoffman and Cranefield, 1960; Paes de Carvalho et al., 1969; Méndez and Moe, 1972; Benítez et al., 1973; Cranefield, 1975).

The Ionic Basis of AV Nodal Potentials

Paes de Carvalho (1966) and Paes de Carvalho et al. (1966, 1969) were the first to suggest that typical AV nodal cells lack a rapid Na^+ channel and that the slow upstroke of AV nodal action potentials is due to a marked decrease in K^+ conductance and the presence of a small inward current.

In cardiac tissues other than nodal tissue, once the fast Na^+ channel is blocked, the presence of adrenergic agents can restore activity characterized by the low rate of rise and slow conduction of the action potentials (Engstfeld et al., 1961; Aceves and Erlij, 1967; Carmeliet and Vereecke, 1969; Pappano, 1970). Parallel to these findings, use of the voltage-clamp technique disclosed the ionic nature of the slow inward current. The slow channel, TTX insensitive, permits, when activated, the passage of Ca and Na ions. This subject will be extensively covered by other participants in this Symposium.

From the point of view of this chapter, it is necessary to mention that Rougier et al. (1969) and Vassort et al. (1969) proposed that the slow inward current, insensitive to TTX but blocked by Mn ions, is responsible for the upstroke of AV nodal potentials. Their proposal was based on the work of Lenfant et al. (1968). These latter authors showed that in the sinoatrial node (SA node), which to a degree resembles the AV node, TTX had no effect, whereas Mn ions suppressed the activity of that structure.

With this background, Zipes and Méndez (1973) showed that TTX does not change either AV nodal potentials or their propagation but that Mn ions in concentrations ranging from 1 to 3 mM, although not decreasing the upstroke of atrial action potentials, did cause complete block at all levels in the AV node.

The observations of Zipes and Méndez (1973) received partial support from the work of Wit and Cranefield (1974) and were fully confirmed and extended by Akiyama and Fozzard (1979). Furthermore, Zipes and Fischer (1974) showed, in intact hearts, that agents that block the slow channel, such as Mn ions, lanthanum, verapamil, and D-600, when injected into the lumen of the artery supplying the AV region, also cause complete AV nodal block.

Zipes and Méndez (1973) concluded that only the slow channel is responsible for the upstroke of N action potentials. De Ceretti et al. (1971), with improved perfusion techniques, found, however, an initial fast Na^+ component in the depolarization limb of AV nodal action potentials, although their records may correspond to the findings in transitional cells in which Paes de Carvalho et al. (1966) found an initial fast upstroke not affected by acetylcholine and presumably caused by the participation of the fast Na^+ channel.

Because the resting potential of AV nodal cells is rather low (−60 mV in the N region), a fast Na^+ channel may exist, but it may be inactivated to a considerable degree at the above-mentioned membrane potential. Shigeto and Irisawa (1974) showed that hyperpolarizations induced by passing current through a suction electrode cause an increase in the dv/dt of AV nodal potentials. These results suggest that the cells explored had fast Na^+ channels that were partially inactivated.

Very recently, Noma et al. (1980) have been able to use the voltage-clamp in isolated small segments of the rabbit AV node. Their results indicate that the inward current responsible for regenerative responses is exclusively provided by the TTX insensitive slow Ca^{2+} and Na^+ channel. Spatial voltage uniformity was adequate in their study, yet in their preliminary paper, the holding potential was −40 mV. This would exclude any possible participation of a fast Na^+ channel, for it would be inactivated.

In unpublished experiments, we have repeated in our laboratory the experiments of Shigeto and Irisawa (1974). Instead of using suction electrodes, we used broken micropipettes whose tips (heat polished) had an internal diameter of 100 to 200 μm. These electrodes were filled with Tyrode's solution and were placed in close contact with the bundle of His. A suitable polarizing system permitted hyperpolarization or depolarization at will of the NH region and its neighboring N cells. The preparation was driven at a constant rate (atrial stimulation). The results were conclusive: hyperpolarizations of varying magnitude of N cells or neighboring NH cells caused a *decrease* of their maximal rate of depolarization. On the other hand, small depolarizations (up to 10 mV) had negligible effects; only stronger depolarizations decreased the maximal dv/dt. Figure 1 illustrates typical results. The curve relating $\dot{V}_{max}$ to diastolic membrane potential has an asymmetrical bell shape. Its maximum seems to correspond to the normal (unpolarized) diastolic potential of the N cell studied. Small hyperpolarizations decreased $\dot{V}_{max}$; small depolarizations had negligible effects; larger hyperpolarizations or depolarizations caused a marked decrease in $\dot{V}_{max}$. These results agree with Hoffman's (1961) observations. That hyperpolarizations did not increase $\dot{V}_{max}$ indicates that typical AV nodal cells do not have fast Na^+ channels that might be inactivated to a considerable degree by the low resting potential. The observations of Zipes et al. (1973) remain valid because large depolarizations decrease $\dot{V}_{max}$.

I emphasize that in cells located in the AN region (perhaps transitional cells) we obtained the same results as those reported by Shigeto and Irisawa (1974). It remains to be seen at what level the AV nodal cells lose any trace of fast Na^+ channels.

THE NATURE OF AV NODAL PROPAGATION

Nonelectrical Propagation

Investigators interested in the electrophysiology of the AV node have assumed, in general, that propagation through the AV node is electrical in nature.

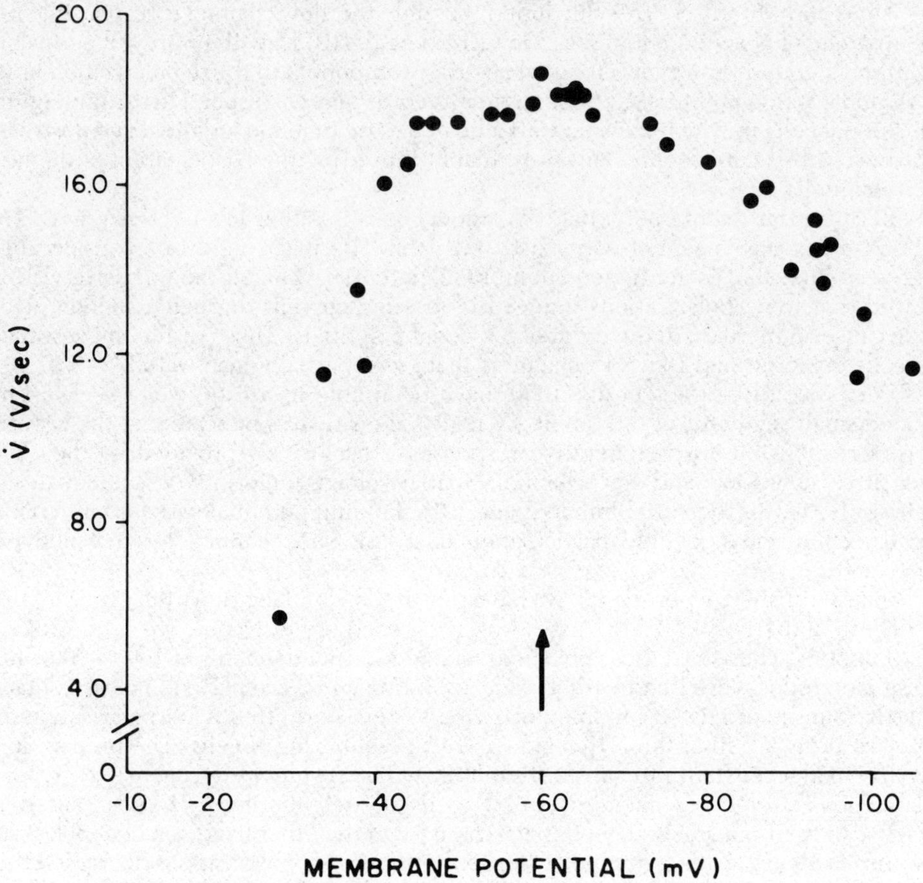

Figure 1. Relation between the maximal rate of rise ($\dot{V}_{max}$) of an N cell (ordinate) and the take off potential (abscissa). The arrow indicates the unpolarized resting potential (Méndez and Hernández, unpublished observations).

Pollack (1976) has seriously challenged this assumption. He observed that sodium fluorescein (mol. wt., 332 daltons) introduced intracellularly diffuses readily from the injected site to neighboring cells in the atrium, ventricle, Purkinje strands, and His bundle. The passage of the dye between N cells, however, was estimated to be at least three orders of magnitude lower than it was between cells of the other tissues studied. These results are backed by some electron microscopic studies that indicate a scarcity of gap junctions in N cells (James and Sherf, 1968; De Felice and Challice, 1969). If this is strictly correct, electrical propagation across the node would be practically impossible: current flow between nodal cells would be negligible, and the physiological stimulus (the action potential of N cells) would be poor because of its small amplitude and its slow rate of rise.

Because of the above-mentioned reasons, Pollack (1976) proposed that the physiologic stimulus is the stretch provided by the contraction of the immediately proximal cells. Evidence for electrical propagation through the AV node, however, is strong (see below).

Although I am not qualified to criticize the above-mentioned studies, I can make some suggestions that may be appropriate. As Pollack has noted (1976), the tip size of microelectrodes must be a compromise between minimization of cell trauma and ability to pass dye iontophoretically. Thus, for some cardiac cells, the size of the microelectrode tips might be adequate, but nodal cells have rather small dimensions, and upon penetration some damage could occur. If this were the case, leakage of the dye to the external medium would take place. Furthermore, extracellular Ca^{2+} leaking into the cell might cause partial decoupling. This is only a possibility, but further studies should clarify this point.

Electron microscopy is a very powerful tool. Mazet and Cartand (1976), however, have pointed out that: "intercellular junctions show a great variation in morphology. Therefore, it is not readily apparent which type of junctional organization might be considered responsible for the existence of intracellular communications and electrotonic coupling." These authors showed that in frog atrial tissue subjected to the freeze-fracture technique "the gap junctions were limited to the presence of circular profiles of 9 nm particles which very seldom form small geometrically packed aggregates." I am not proposing, of course, that the same situation prevails in the mammalian AV node. But, again, further studies might provide a definitive answer.

Electrical Propagation through the AV Node

For cardiac tissues to have propagation of an electrical nature, the following must be shown: *(1)* the cells must be electrically excitable, *(2)* the intercellular connections must have relatively low resistance to current flow, that is, electrotonic spread between neighboring cells must be apparent, and *(3)* the current provided by the active tissue must be large enough to excite more distal elements.

The first two requirements are amply fulfilled in AV nodal cells; the third condition is supported only by indirect evidence. Unfortunately, the AV node does not permit repeating the observations made by Barr et al. (1965) on atrial trabeculae.

Merideth et al. (1968) showed that cells in three regions of the AV node can be stimulated with intracellular current pulses. When these pulses were brief (approximately 5 msec) the current needed to initiate an action potential was rather high. The same occurs, however, in a functional syncytium such as ventricular muscle. In relatively large preparations of this tissue, the average intracellular threshold current is 1.3×10^{-6} A. When the dimensions of the preparation are reduced, the threshold current decreases almost two orders of magnitude (Méndez and Martínez-Palomo, 1974). The reason for this phenomenon is implicit in Noble's (1966) review. Therefore, although the dimensions of the AV node are relatively small, the same is true of the cells that form the structure.

Figure 2 illustrates that a pulse applied intracellularly in an N cell (lower part of the figure) causes an action potential that propagates in both directions and eventually emerges in atrial tissue and in the bundle of His. According to Pollack's hypothesis (1976), only the impaled cell should have responded, and it seems difficult to accept that in a structure that has a small margin of safety for propagation, the stretch caused in neighboring cells by the contraction of a single cell would have activated the whole AV node. A more plausible interpretation is that the pulse depolarized the impaled cell and its neighbors sufficiently to enable the small front wave of activation to propagate in all directions.

In the previous statement, it is implicit that significant electrotonic interactions do take place between N cells. In isolated preparations, it is not difficult to cause blockage between the N and NH regions. Under these conditions, the distal elements

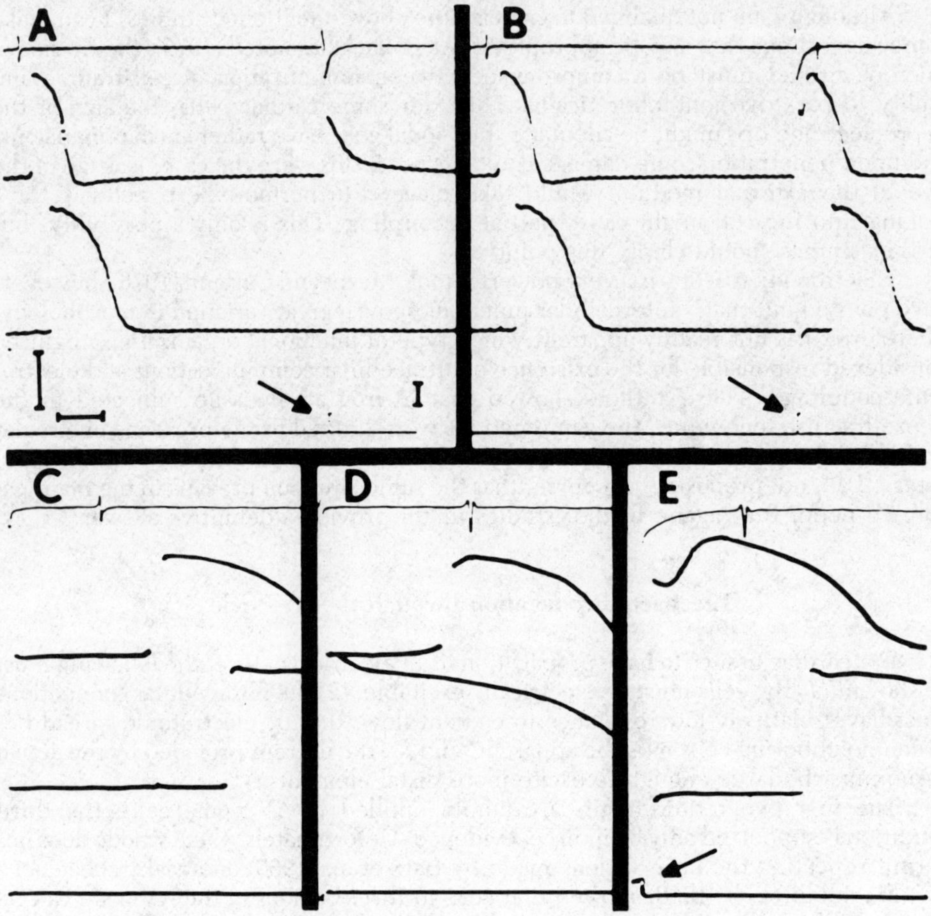

Figure 2. Intracellular stimulation of an N cell. In all panels the upper trace corresponds to an atrial electrogram; the second trace shows the transmembrane potential of an N cell, the same microelectrode was used to pass current and to record the transmembrane potential. The 3rd trace shows the activity recorded from the bundle of His. The lower trace indicates the magnitude of the intracellular current pulse (arrows). In A the current pulse did not reach threshold. In B threshold was attained and propagation reached the atrium and the bundle of His. Panels C, D, and E show at the faster sweep speed the sequence of events during normograde propagation (C), retrograde propagation initiated in the bundle of His (D) and when a threshold intracellular pulse was delivered to the N cell (E). The left vertical calibration corresponds to 50 mV; the horizontal calibration corresponds to 100 msec in A and B and to 20 mV in C, D and E. The calibration at the lower right corner of panel A corresponds to 1×10^{-6} A (Merideth et al., 1968).

that do not fire show subthreshold depolarizations. This might suggest electrotonic spread between active and inactive regions; yet, other explanations are possible.

Low-resistance intercellular connections are known to exist in some cardiac tissues. In these cases it is easy to obtain a reversible conduction block. When this happens there is a marked potential difference between the proximal active segment and the inactive distal tissue. Accordingly, local circuits provide depolarizing current to the inactive segment, but the same current returns to the active site; this current acts as an external anode and hastens the repolarization of the active response. Because the membrane resistance during the plateau is rather high (Weidmann, 1951), the duration of action potentials of the active site can decrease considerably. On the other hand, during discontinuous propagation, once the distal elements fire, the potential difference between both segments not only disappears but reverses its polarity. At that moment a marked hump appears during the plateau of the proximal action potentials, lengthening their duration. Figure 3 shows the sequence of events obtained in sheep Purkinje fibers using the sucrose-gap technique. The lower right section of the figure illustrates the experimental arrangement; it must be emphasized that an external bridge electrically connected compartments 1 and 3. At the beginning of the experiment, the three compartments were perfused with oxygenated Tyrode's solution. Activity initiated in compartment 1 (proximal segment) propagated readily to the distal segment of the fiber located in compartment 3 (panel A of the figure). Between A and B, the solution flowing through compartment 2 was switched to an isotonic sucrose solution. The substitution was not immediate, but as the latter solution replaced the Tyrode's solution the delay between the activity registered between proximal and distal segments increased significantly (panels B and C). As previously described, as soon as the distal segment fired, a hump appeared in the proximal action potential, and its duration was increased. Once the sucrose solution had completely replaced the Tyrode's solution, conduction block occurred and the proximal action potential was considerably reduced in duration; only a subthreshold depolarization was recorded from the distal segment (panel D). At this stage, bidirectional block was established. When only the proximal segment was stimulated, a brief action potential could be recorded from the same segment. Here, the reverse was true: when only the distal segment was stimulated, conduction block occurred, and only a brief action potential was recorded from the other segment. But, properly timed stimulation of both ends of the fiber permitted the simultaneous arrival of action potentials at both ends of the sucrose gap. The magnitude and configuration of both action potentials were relatively similar, and under these conditions current flow between compartment 1 and 3 was negligible. The end result was that on both sides of the gap normally long-lasting potentials were recorded. Therefore, the brief action potentials obtained during conduction block are the result of electrotonic interactions, and the same can be said of the changes in configuration observed during discontinuous propagation.

Essentially the same results as these described above can be obtained in the AV node. Figure 4 illustrates this point. The atrium was driven at a regular basic rate; after each eight basic responses, a stimulus was introduced at different intervals through the same pair of stimulating electrodes. In each panel of the figure, the upper trace shows an atrial electrogram recorded close to the upper node; the second trace corresponds to the transmembrane potential of an N cell, and the lower trace shows the activity of a distal NH cell. In panel A, the interval between the last basic response and the premature response (A_1-A_2) was relatively short. The premature activity clearly did not engage the distal NH cell. The most striking feature of the N response was its short duration. In panel B, the A_1-A_2 interval was increased. Successful propagation to the NH region occurred, but the N-NH interval was long, 38 msec. The corresponding N response shows a marked hump on its repolarization limb, and its duration was considerably longer than it was in A. In panel C, the A_1-A_2 interval was longer, the N-NH interval was 31 msec, and a notch appeared close to the peak of the N response. Accordingly, it was apparent that discontinuous propagation still prevailed. For the basic responses, the N action potentials did not show a notch, and the N-NH interval was considerably shorter.

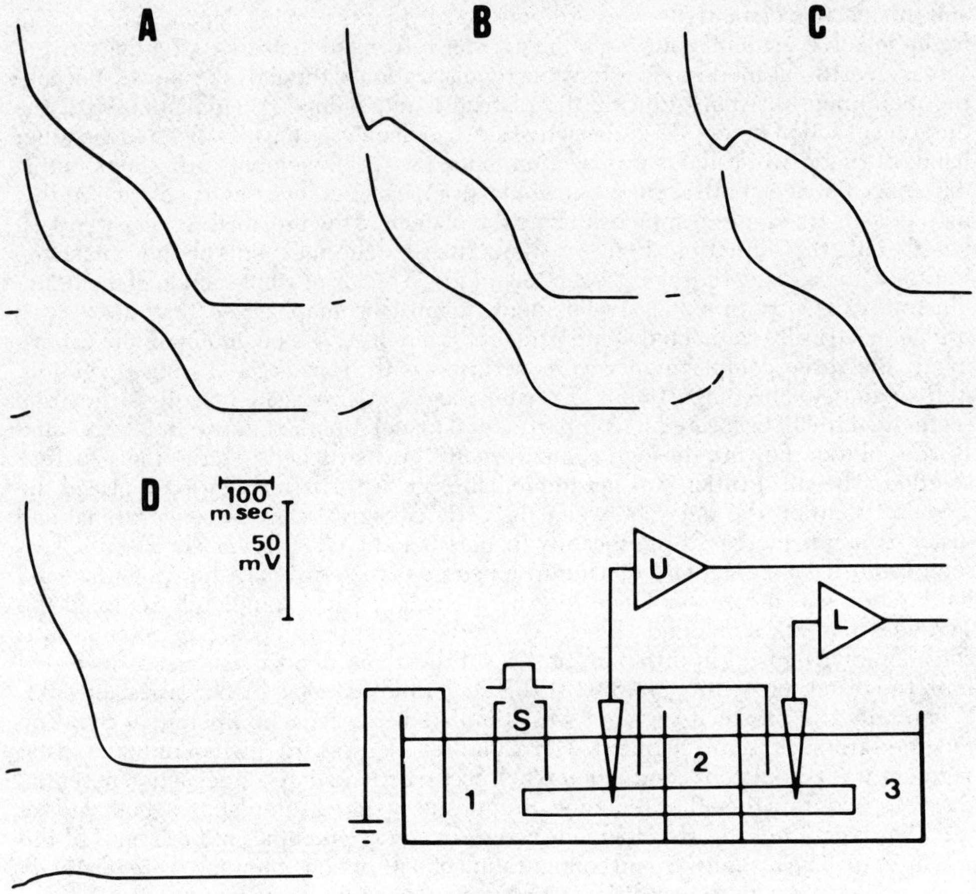

Figure 3. Delayed propagation and conduction block obtained in sheep Purkinje fibers by means of the sucrose-gap technique. The lower right hand diagram corresponds to the experimental arrangement. S, corresponds to the location of the stimulating electrodes. U, corresponds to the upper transmembrane potential record and L to the lower. A conducting bridge connecting compartments 1 and 3 is shown. At the beginning of the experiment, compartments 1, 2 and 3 were perfused with Tyrode's solution; the corresponding action potentials are shown in panel A. Between A and B an isotonic sucrose solution was perfused through compartment 2. For explanation see text (Méndez, unpublished observations).

The similarity between Figures 3 and 4 allows us to assume that electrotonic interactions occur at the level of N cells. Further evidence that electrotonic influences do take place in AV nodal cells was provided by the work of De Mello (1977). By means of a suction electrode applied to the AN region of the rabbit AV node, the author found a space constant of 0.4 mm (approximate).

Finally, the voltage-clamp studies of Noma et al. (1980) show that contiguous nodal cells have low resistance intercellular connections; if not, proper spatial uniformity of voltage would have been impossible.

Because of its location in the heart and its morphology, it has not been possible, until now, to prove or disprove that propagation through the AV node is electrical in

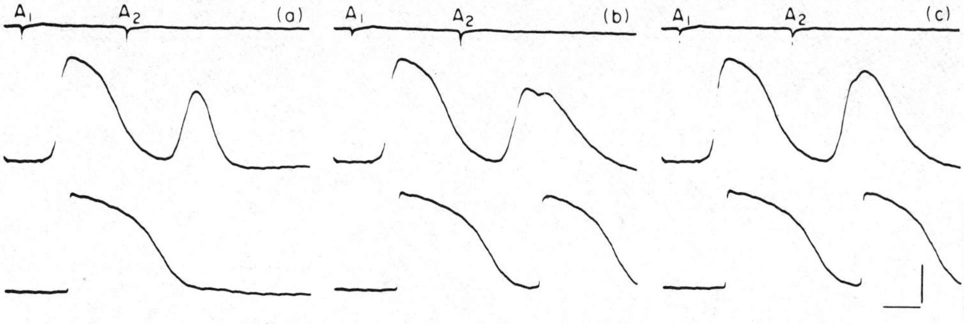

Figure 4. Dependence of action potential configuration of an N cell on the characteristics of propagation. Upper trace: atrial electrograms; middle trace: transmembrane potential of an N cell; lower trace: transmembrane potential of a distal NH cell. Calibrations: 50 msec and 25 mV. For explanation, see text (Méndez and Moe, 1966).

nature. In other words, it has not been possible to perform, in the AV node, experiments similar to those reported by Barr et al. (1965) in frog atrial trabeculae.

Nevertheless, two observations deserve consideration. Propagation through the AV node may be rendered quite critical when the driving atrial rate is high. Under these conditions, two situations may be encountered: *(1)* critical 1:1 propagation may be obtained; *(2)* a large number of impulses may be blocked in the node with occasional propagation.

In the first case, a small hyperpolarization of AV nodal cells causes complete block. Figure 5 shows typical results. The hyperpolarizing pulses were delivered to the region of the bundle of His. When pronounced conduction block took place betwen the N and NH regions, a small depolarization permitted full propagation. Figure 6 illustrates this point.

These phenomena can be readily explained if it is accepted that propagation is electrical and if the N action potentials result exclusively from the activation of the slow channel. Thus, depolarizations should bring the resting potential closer to the threshold potential of the slow channel (approximately −40 mV). On the other hand, hyperpolarizations should cause the opposite effect.

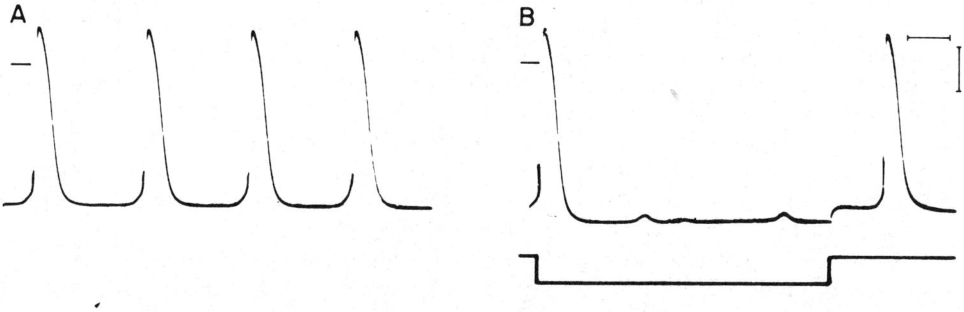

Figure 5. Complete AV block caused by a hyperpolarizing current. A: control. B: same NH cell during the passage of a hyperpolarizing pulse (lower open rectangle). Observe that the pulse started at the peak of the first action potential and while present, two subthreshold depolarizations were recorded. Calibrations: 200 msec and 20 mV (Méndez, 1980).

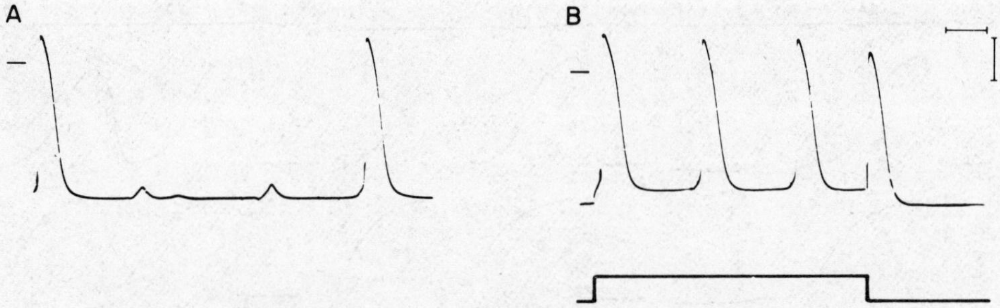

Figure 6. Facilitation of propagation caused by a depolarizing pulse. A: control; notice the subthreshold depolarizations recorded from a proximal NH cell. The lower open rectangle in B shows the initiation and termination of the depolarizing pulse. Observe in B that propagation was restored. Calibrations: 200 msec and 20mV (Méndez, 1980).

It remains to be answered why conduction through the AV node, even under normal conditions, is so slow (0.003 m/sec). Two major factors seem to be involved. In the first place, the nodal potentials are characterized by their small amplitude and by their slow rate of depolarization; this constitutes a poor physiologic stimulus. In the second place, De Mello (1977) attributes slow conduction in nodal tissues to the small space constant (430 μm). Based on the apparent scarcity of nexuses reported in electron microscopic studies and on the results obtained by Pollack (1976), De Mello suggested that "the main reason for the small space constant of the nodal fibers seems to be a high junctional resistance." If this were the case, the spatial voltage homogeneity found by Noma et al. (1980), in their voltage-clamp study, would be hard to explain. Whatever the cause of the small space constant found in nodal tissue, this factor must contribute to slow propagation.

THE "FILTERING" ACTION OF THE AV NODE

The functional refractory period of the AV node is defined as the shortest interval between two His responses propagated from the atrium. As already mentioned, the His action potentials are considerably longer than the AV nodal potentials are. But, the minimum interval between two His responses propagated from the atrium is longer than is the duration of the basic His action potential (Méndez et al. 1964). The reason for this phenomenon can be found in the work of Merideth et al. (1968). These authors showed that the recovery of excitability of the AV nodal cells lags behind the repolarization phase of the action potentials. It is therefore possible that the recovery of inactivation (reactivation) of these cells has a long time constant.

In recent experiments in our laboratory, this was found to be the case. The $\dot{V}_{max}$ was taken as an index of the depolarizing current responsible for the upstroke of AV nodal action potentials. Figure 7 illustrates typical results; the preparation was driven at a regular rate. After each eighth basic response, an atrial extrabeat was introduced at different intervals. In each panel, the first transmembrane potential corresponds to the last basic response; the second action potential corresponds to a premature beat. The lower trace shows their corresponding dV/dt. Clearly, as the

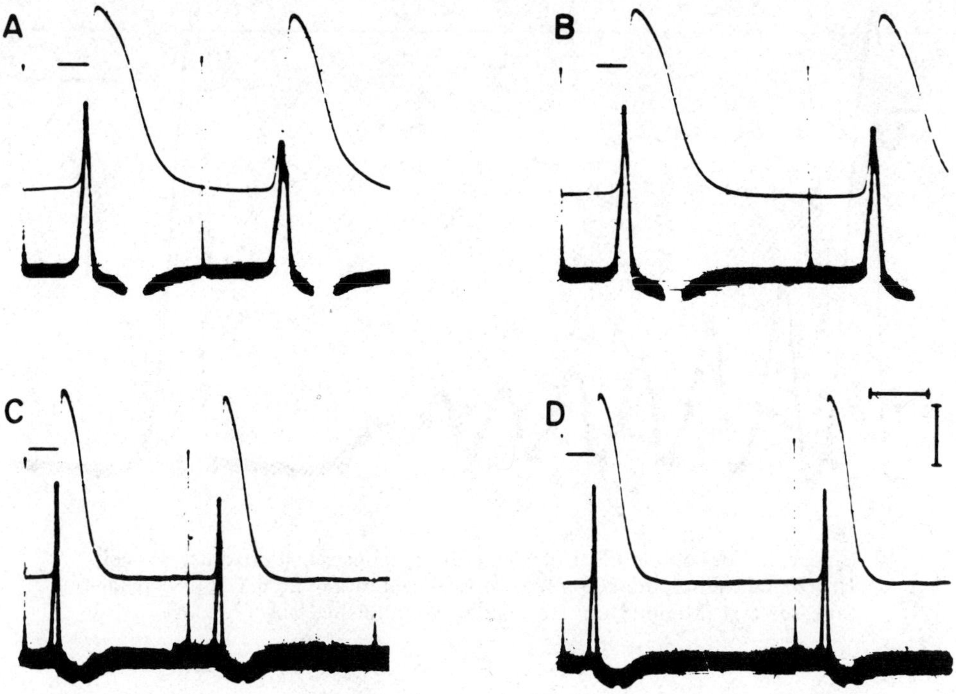

Figure 7. Recovery from inactivation of a distal N cell. Upper trace: transmembrane potentials of the impaled cell; lower trace: differentiated records of the transmembrane potentials. Horizontal calibration: 100 msec for A and B and 200 msec for C and D. Vertical calibration: 20 mV and 5 V/sec. For explanation, see text (Méndez and Hernández, unpublished observations).

interval between the basic response and the premature beat increased, the dV/dt of the premature beat also increased. But this was a slow process. The curve relating the V_{max} to the interval (taken as the time interval between the end of repolarization of the basic response and the moment of appearance of the premature response) seems to follow an exponential course. For N cells, the time constant of the exponential was 120 msec (approximate). This slow recovery from inactivation can explain the "filtering" property of the AV node. In a physiologic system, where the margin of safety for propagation is normally low, a decrease in the effectiveness of the physiologic stimulus can lead to conduction block.

Furthermore, the long time needed for reactivation may be frequency-dependent. This point is still not fully proved, but if this is the case, an explanation for the vague term "fatigue" would be available.

In Figure 8, seven rapid responses were blocked in the AV node. In this figure, the subthreshold depolarizations decreased progressively. This may represent "fatigue" or conduction block occurring closer to the upper node each time. In other experiments, proper timing of the extra beats provided subthreshold depolarizations of the same magnitude. This could imply that conduction block occurred at the same site. If this were the case, the long reactivation time of the last cells that fired would be responsible for the lack of propagation, and the refractory period of more distal cells, which for a long time did not fire, would have nothing to do with the phenomenon.

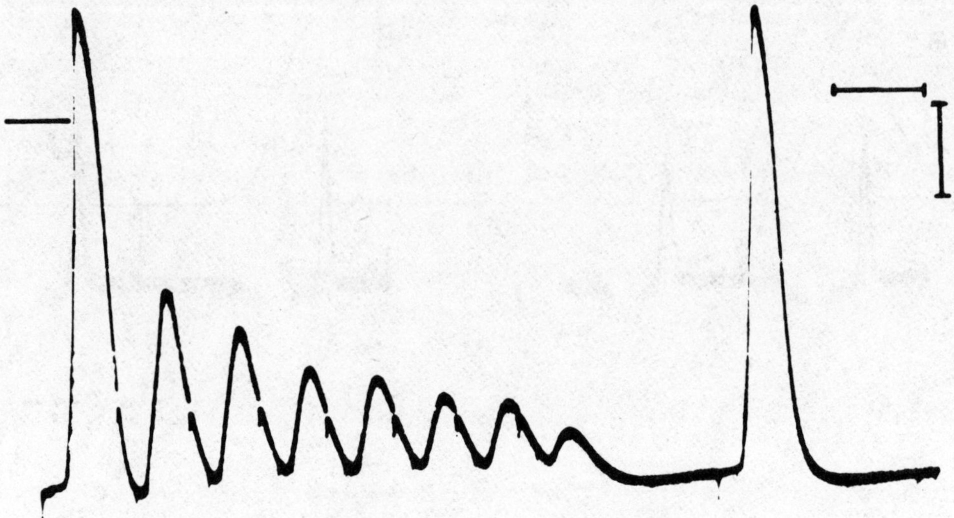

Figure 8. Repetitive block of premature responses in a proximal NH cell. Horizontal calibration: 200 msec; vertical calibration: 20 mV. For explanation, see text (Méndez and Hernández, unpublished observations).

CONCLUSIONS

The experimental data reported in this paper strongly suggest the following: *(1)* The initial depolarization of typical AV nodal cells is provided exclusively by the activation of the slow channel. *(2)* Impulse propagation through the AV node is electrical in nature. *(3)* The slow recovery from inactivation provides the AV node with its "filtering" property.

REFERENCES

Aceves J, Erlij D (1967) Effects of norepinephrine on tissues of the frog heart atrium poisoned by tetrodotoxine. Nature **215**:1178–1179

Akiyama T, Fozzard HA (1979) Ca and Na selectivity of the active membrane of rabbit AV nodal cells. Am J Physiol Cell Physiol **5**:C1–C8

Barr L, Dewey MM, Berger W (1965) Propagation of action potentials and the structure of the nexus in cardiac muscle. J Gen Physiol **48**:797–823

Benítez D, Mascher D, Alanis J (1973) The electrical activity of the bundle of His. The fast and slow inward currents. Pflüg Arch **345**:61–72

Carmeliet E, Vereecke J (1969) Adrenaline and the plateau phase of the cardiac action potential. Pflüg Arch **313**:300–315

Cranefield PF (1975) The Conduction of the Cardiac Impulse, edited by PF Cranefield. Mt Kisco, NY, Futura Publishing Company, Chapter IV

De Ceretti E, Ruiz P, Ponce Zumino A, Parissii IM (1971) Resolution of two components in the upstroke of the action potential in atrioventricular fibers of the rabbit heart. Canad J Physiol Pharmacol **49**:642–648

De Felice LJ, Challice CE (1969) Anatomical and ultrastructural study of the electrophysiological atrioventricular node of the rabbit. Circ Res **24**:457–474

De Mello WC (1977) Passive electrical properties of the atrio-ventricular node. Pflüg Arch **371**:135–139

Engstfeld G, Antoni H, Fleckenstein A (1961) Die Restitution der Erregungsfortleitung und Kontraktions Kraft des K^+-gelähmten Frosch- und Säugeliermyokards durch Adrenalin. Pflüg Arch **273**:145–163

Hoffman BF, Cranefield PF (1960) Electrophysiology of the Heart. New York, McGraw-Hill Book Co, Chapter 5

Hoffman BF (1961) Electrical activity of the atrio-ventricular node. In The Specialized Tissues of the Heart, edited by A Paes de Carvalho, WC De Mello and BF Hoffman. Amsterdam, Elsevier, pp 143–158

James TN, Scherf L (1968) Ultrastructure of the atrioventricular node. Circulation **37**: 1049–1070

Lenfant J, Mironneau J, Gargouil YM, Galand G (1968) Analyse de l'activité électrique spontanée du centre de l'automatisme cardiaque de lapin par les inhibiteurs de perméabilités membranaires. CR Acad Sci Paris, Sér D **266**:901–904

Mazet F, Cartand J (1976) Freeze fracture studies of frog atrial fibres. J Cell Sci **22**:427–434

Méndez C, Han J, Moe GK (1964) A comparison of the effects of epinephrine upon the refractory periods of the AV node and the bundle of His. Naunyn-Schmiedebergs Arch Exp Path Pharmak **248**:99–106

Méndez C, Moe GK (1966) Some characteristics of transmembrane potentials of AV nodal cells during propagation of premature beats. Circ Res **19**:993–1010

Méndez C, Moe GK (1972) Atrioventricular transmission. In Electrical Phenomena in the Heart, edited by WC De Mello. New York, Academic Press, Chapter 12

Méndez C, Martínez-Palomo A (1974) 'Syncytial' nature of ventricular miocardium. Proceedings of the International Union of Physiological Sciences **XI**:81 (abstract)

Méndez C (1980) The slow inward current and AV nodal propagation. In The Slow Inward Current and Cardiac Arrhythmias, edited by DP Zipes, JC Bailey and V Elharrar. Amsterdam, Martinus Nijhoff, Chapter 12

Merideth J, Méndez C, Mueller WJ, Moe GK (1968) Electrical excitability of atrio-ventricular nodal cells. Circ Res **23**:69–85

Noble D (1966) Applications of Hodgkin-Huxley equations to excitable tissues. Physiol Rev **46**:1–49

Noma A, Irisawa H, Kokobun S, Kotake H, Nishimura M, Watanabe Y (1980) Slow current systems in the A-V node of the rabbit heart. Nature **285**:228–229

Paes de Carvalho A, de Almeida DF (1960) Spread of activity through the atrioventricular node. Circ Res **8**:801–809

Paes de Carvalho A (1966) Excitation of the atrioventricular node during normal rhythm. Effects of acetylcholine. In Mechanisms and Therapy of Cardiac Arrhythmias, edited by LS Dreyfus, W Likoff and JH Moyer. New York, Grune and Stratton, pp 341–352

Paes de Carvalho A, Hoffman BF, Langan WB (1966) Two components of the cardiac action potentials. Nature **211**:938–940

Paes de Carvalho A, Hoffman BF, de Paula Carvalho M (1969) Two components of the cardiac action potential. I. Voltage time course and the effect of acetylcholine on atrial and nodal cells of the rabbit heart. J Gen Physiol **54**:607–635

Pappano AJ (1970) Calcium-dependent action potentials produced by catecholamines in guinea pig atrial muscle fibers depolarized by potassium. Circ Res **27**:379–390

Pollack G (1976) Intercellular coupling in the atrioventricular node and other tissues of the heart. J Physiol **255**:275–298

Rougier O, Vassort G, Garnier D, Gargouil YM, Coraboeuf E (1969) Existence and role of a slow inward current during the frog atrial action potential. Pflüg Arch **308**:91–110

Shigeto N, Irisawa H (1974) The effect of polarization on the action potentials of the rabbit AV nodal cells. Jap J Physiol **24**:605–616

Vassort G, Rougier O, Garnier D, Sauviat MP, Coraboeuf E, Gargouil YM (1969) Effects of adrenaline on membrane inward currents during the cardiac action potential. Pflüg Arch **309**:70–81

Weidmann S (1951) Effect of current flow on the membrane potential of cardiac muscle. J Physiol **115**:227–236

Wit AL, Cranefield PF (1974) Effects of verapamil on the sinoatrial and atrioventricular nodes of the rabbit and the mechanism by which it arrests reentrant atrioventricular nodal tachycardia. Circ Res **35**:413–425

Zipes DP, Méndez C (1973) Action of manganese ions and tetrodotoxin on atrioventricular nodal transmembrane potentials in isolated rabbit hearts. Circ Res **32**:447–454

Zipes DP, Méndez C, Moe GK (1973) Evidence for summation and voltage dependence in rabbit atrioventricular nodal fibers. Circ Res **32**:170–177

Zipes DP, Fischer JC (1974) Effects of agents which inhibit the slow channel on sinus node automaticity and atrioventricular conduction in the dog. Circ Res **34**:184–192

Discussion

PAES DE CARVALHO: I am gratified to hear your confirmation that the AV nodal action potential is indeed a pure slow response. As you know, there have been reports claiming that it was not a pure slow response but that it showed a subdued contamination of fast response in its upstroke. It has always seemed to me that these reports of a fast component contamination in the AV nodal action potential were a misinterpretation of data. The electrotonic interaction among AV nodal cells and between these and the atrium in one side and His bundle on the other is indeed fairly intense. Often one does pick up a somewhat faster phase in the upstroke of cells at borders of AV node. This happens only when the cell site is invaded directly from a region of fast activity, as is the case with the AN region in normal conduction and the NH region in retrograde conduction. Such a subdued fast phase is not a local phenomenon due to membrane ionic currents of the cell itself but is rather the electrotonic image of a fast upstroke taking place somewhere else in the neighborhood. Your hyperpolarization experiments show that the existence of a pure slow response in AV nodal cells is not due to inactivation of a fast sodium channel but to its virtual absence, at least in an operational state.

DE MELLO: In relation to your comment that fluorescent dyes do not diffuse from one cell to another within the AV node and the possibility that this might reflect a short space constant, I would like to point out that I have done similar experiments in the sinoatrial node and found no diffusion there either. And yet, we know from electrical studies that both the SA nodal and the AV nodal tissue are composed of electrically coupled cells. I wonder, then, if there may be some other reason for the lack of success with the dye-diffusion experiments. For instance, maybe the junctional channel is narrower in SA and AV nodal cells, or maybe the channel density is smaller. It has been shown by Masson-Pevet (Beeker et al., Circ Res **46**:11–21, 1980) that in the rabbit heart the area of gap junction between sinoatrial nodal cells was ten times smaller than it was between atrial cells. Now, if there is electrical coupling, the question that comes then to my mind is how cells from SA and AV nodes maintain their resting potential at levels that are different from those prevalent in the surrounding atrium and His bundle?

MÉNDEZ: Well, I think that a short enough space constant would permit differences in resting potential. The difference of resting potential among AV nodal cells is not very marked, and at the AN and NH borders there seems to be a transition of resting potentials.

JOHNSON: I am a little bit disturbed by your affirmation that the length constant of the AV node is in the order of half a millimeter. A high longitudinal resistance per unit length would provide a ready explanation for slow conduction in the AV node, but a length constant of 0.5 mm would be far too long to obtain the slowing of conduction that one would predict for the AV node. So if this speaks against high longitudinal resistance as the mechanism for slow conduction in the AV node, what other mechanism do you propose?

MÉNDEZ: I think that one of the reasons for slow conduction is that the slow-response action potential is a very poor physiologic stimulus. It rises slowly, and there is no drop in resistance during its upstroke. So, the action potential is a relatively high-impedance source of current to depolarize the tissue ahead of the wavefront. This situation is radically different from what you see during propagation in atrial muscle, ventricular muscle, and Purkinje fibers, where a strong fast depolarization phenomenon caused by sodium moving into the cell is present. In this last case, the action potential at a given site rises swiftly to complete depolarization and reversal, and as it does so the membrane patch that is producing the inward current becomes a very low resistance source of longitudinal depolarizing current for the tissue ahead. This, I would guess, tends to enhance conduction velocity. On the other hand, in the AV node the conditions for the slow response to move ahead by local circuit interaction between active and inactive segments are so poor that conduction block is rather easy to obtain.

PAES DE CARVALHO: It is certainly possible to create long delays of the order of magnitude seen in the AV node by associating a high longitudinal resistance to a simple fast sodium spike depolarization mechanism. Yet this type of mechanism would still yield a fast upstroke and be sensitive to tetrodotoxin and not to D600. In the AV node, we have slow conduction in the presence of a very slow upstroke. This slow nodal conduction is insensitive to tetrodotoxin and very much sensitive to D600. So, although both are possible mechanisms of slow conduction, in the physiologic condition observed in the AV node the second mechanism is necessarily present.

JOHNSON: I understand what you say, but it's not necessary to postulate that the membrane patches that are coupled by high resistance are necessarily Hodgkin-Huxley-type membranes. They may be operating under some kind of very slow mechanism. But, it is not clear to me that a system formed by slow-response patches simply connected together in a cable arrangement will propagate, at least in the usual fashion.

PAES DE CARVALHO: I agree that coupling resistance must also be an important factor when the current generating mechanism is weak. In this context, the coupling resistance associated with a space constant of 0.5 mm may already pose a significant hindrance to the speed of conduction.

SPACH: About the space constant, I would like to point out that within the dimensions of the AV node it may be perfectly the case that both a slow type of depolarization and an increased longitudinal resistance are involved in slow conduction. One cannot rule out entirely an increased longitudinal resistance by electrical measurements of the type that we have seen reported in the literature. The AV node may be a nonsymmetrical structure so that you might have a longer space constant in one direction than in another. It may be that in the direction in which the depolarization wave progresses the longitudinal resistance is much higher than it is in some other direction.

Chapter 21

Nonuniform Conduction in Cardiac Purkinje Fibers*

Frederick A. Dodge and Paul F. Cranefield

It is well known that a low conduction velocity characterizes cells in two parts of the normal heart, the sinoatrial and atrioventricular nodes. It is also generally accepted that slow conduction in part or all of a pathway can facilitate circus movement of excitation around that pathway. Nodal tachycardia is attributed to circus movement around a pathway in which the necessary delay arises from slow conduction in the AV node. The Wolff-Parkinson-White syndrome is explained by circus movement of excitation around a pathway that contains at least one locus of slow conduction, namely the AV node, and may contain another such locus in the aberrant atrioventricular connection. Slow conduction plays a role not only in causing certain arrhythmias but also in determining certain other features of the normal and abnormal activation of the heart. Sinoatrial delay and AV nodal delay are features of the normal excitation of the heart; a focus of abnormal activity, such as a rhythmically active focus of depolarized fibers, may be connected to the rest of the heart only by slowly conducting fibers. Although slow conduction in those fibers need not directly contribute to the genesis of the arrhythmia it may affect the way in which the focus excites the heart or is prevented from doing so.

Some ten years ago, Hoffman and Cranefield devised techniques to induce slow conduction in segments of Purkinje fibers. In those experiments, a patch of agar containing a high concentration of K^+ was applied to the central segment of a bundle of Purkinje fibers, each end of the bundle remaining exposed to a normal ionic environment. Other experiments were done on preparations in which a branch emerged from the central segment so that the origin of the branch was included in the region depressed by exposure to high $[K^+]_o$. In some experiments, action potentials with slow upstrokes were seen, and a moderate degree of asymmetry was revealed by the conduction velocity differing according to the direction of conduction; smooth, unnotched upstrokes were associated with conduction velocities of or greater than 0.1 m/sec. Experiments on preparations in which there was greater depression of excitability revealed an extraordinarily rich and complex array of phenomena, including

*Supported by USPHS Grant HL-14899

very low-average apparent conduction velocities, of less than 0.05 m/sec, slow and often notched upstrokes, one-way conduction, rate-dependent block, the Wenckebach phenomenon, and the phenomena we called summation and inhibition (Cranefield et al., 1971; Cranefield and Hoffman, 1971).

In our initial interpretation of these phenomena, we pointed out that the depressed excitability and lowered upstroke velocity attributable to the exposure to elevated levels of $[K^+]_o$ could not alone explain our findings; we emphasized the necessity of recognizing that the bundle under study contained several "cells" syncytially interconnected in a way that permitted a complex interaction of abnormal action potentials (cf. Mendez and Moe, 1966; Mendez et al., 1969). We remarked, "The action potentials of cardiac fibers may be made up of two or more components, one of which has a fast rise time and a short duration, the other of which has a slow rise time and a long duration. If this notion is correct and if the slow component can propagate for a short distance in the absence of the fast component, certain of our observations could be explained." We drew attention to the fact that elevation of $[K^+]_o$ alters the permeability of the membrane in a way that increases the electrical load placed on the excited region by the unexcited region (Cranefield et al., 1971, p. 214) and pointed out, with respect to summation and inhibition that, when two impulses approach the center of a depressed fiber from each of its ends, the conditions of electrical loading are very different from those seen when either end alone is excited (Cranefield and Hoffman, 1971, p. 231). We also discussed the ways in which variations in loading and in conduction velocity can cause either shortening or lengthening of the action potential, and pointed out how such changes in duration affect not only the refractory period but also the ability of the action potential to act as a stimulus, and called attention to the effect of low and high intracellular resistance on the interactions between active and inactive segments of the fiber. Finally, we called attention to the possibility that, under abnormal conditions, refractoriness may outlast repolarization.

In the following year (Cranefield et al., 1972), we offered evidence that the slow response can indeed propagate under conditions in which the fast response is absent, and we suggested that under such conditions the slow response might propagate with decrement. We added that although it would be "tempting to regard all of the properties of conduction through a depressed segment as properties of decremental conduction of the slow response," to do so would overlook "the importance of the syncytial nature of Purkinje fibers . . . . We believe . . . that while the presence of the slow response is necessary for the appearance of the phenomena we have described, a full and detailed explanation of them must take into account the syncytial properties of the tissue . . . neither uniform slow conduction nor simple decremental conduction in an unbranched fiber can safely be taken as a model of conduction through a depressed segment of cardiac Purkinje fibers," and said further that "the fast response has a high safety factor of conduction and overrides minor electrical impediments to its spread; the slow response has a low safety factor of conduction and is correspondingly prone to block at branch points or other impediments to forward conduction."

The existence of the slow inward current and the existence of slow channel-dependent, propagated action potentials are now far more widely accepted than they were in the early 1970s, and there has recently been a resurgence of interest in the significance for conduction delays of the inhomogeneities of the cardiac syncytium. It has also been suggested that inhomogeneities and asymmetries of the cardiac syncytium can lead to marked delays in the spread of the cardiac impulse, even when the action potential depends solely on the large and rapidly developing inward currents that arise when the fast channel is maximally activated.

Among the questions we propose to examine are the following: *(1)* What degree of slowing of conduction can occur in an unbranched fiber of uniform properties if the fast channel is blocked but the slow channel remains excitable? *(2)* What degree of slowing of conduction and what kinds of local delays can arise if action potentials dependent on maximal activation of the fast channel encounter regions in which functional or anatomical inhomogeneities characteristic of the normal cardiac syncytium create impediments to propagation? *(3)* What kinds of functional or anatomical impediments to propagation can be created by pathological changes in the heart? And *(4)* what kinds of slow conduction or marked local delays arise when the normal action potential encounters abnormal functional or anatomical impediments to propagation or when the slow response encounters such impediments?

In discussing these questions we will consider the elements that determine the safety factor of conduction and will attempt to relate the safety factor to conduction velocity. An intuitive definition of safety factor that is applicable both to uniform and nonuniform conduction is that the safety factor is the ratio of the stimulating efficacy of the action potential to the minimum stimulus requirement of the unexcited region. In uniform conduction, both the stimulating efficacy of the action potential and the excitability of the unexcited region are determined by the current-voltage relations of the membrane and by its capacitance. Both also depend on the longitudinal resistance; in uniform conduction, however, the source impedance and load impedance depend on r_i in the same way. The safety factor for uniform conduction is therefore independent of r_i. Thus, for a given set of membrane characteristics, we can speak of an "intrinsic safety factor," which is that of a uniform cable that has that given set of membrane characteristics throughout its length.

It has long been recognized that the conduction velocity, the safety factor, and the cable constants are related. If the membrane ionic current is a function only of the membrane potential, and not of time, then those factors can be related by a simple formula (Rushton, 1937). Membrane current is, in general, a function of both time and voltage; when that is so, the conduction velocity and the cable constants are related by a function of the intrinsic safety factor that takes account of the duration of the inward current (Huxley, 1959; Hunter et al., 1975). A straightforward example of why a knowledge of the conduction velocity and the cable constants does not enable us to predict the safety factor is found in the effects of temperature. As shown by Huxley (1959) an increase in temperature, which speeds up all of the permeability changes (including inactivation) but does not affect the cable constants, increases the conduction velocity whereas it decreases the intrinsic safety factor (and can decrease it even to the point of block).

In discussions of nonuniform conduction, it is generally recognized that the shape, rise-time, duration, and amplitude of the action potential may vary, and thus that the amount of current generated at an excited region may vary; it is also generally recognized that the responsiveness or excitability of the extrinsic region may vary. What is less often made explicit is the fact that the current developed at the excited region need not bear a constant or fixed relation to the excitatory current *delivered* to the unexcited region; the ratio between the two can vary with local variations in the cable properties. We must, therefore, consider three influences on the reliability of conduction under nonuniform conditions: *(1)* the action potential of the excited region, considered as a stimulus; *(2)* a "transfer impedance," both as it affects the stimulus generated in the excited region and as it relates it to the stimulus actually delivered to the unexcited region; and *(3)* the "responsiveness" or stimulus requirement of the unexcited region, that is, the minimal movement of charge or current required to excite.

THE ACTION POTENTIAL CONSIDERED AS A STIMULUS

The action potential that arises from a high resting potential in normal cardiac Purkinje fibers has a rapid upstroke followed by a long plateau; regarded as a stimulus, that action potential consists of a large, rapidly developing, but short-lived, low-impedance source of excitatory current, followed by a prolonged, relatively high-impedance source of excitatory current. The slow-response action potential, arising in depolarized fibers, may be regarded as a stimulus that provides, during the upstroke, a relatively small and slowly developing, but comparatively prolonged, source of depolarizing current; the "plateau" of the slow response increases the total duration of the stimulus but does so far less in proportion to the duration of the upstroke than does the plateau of the normal action potential in relation to the fast upstroke. We do not, however, know much about the source impedance characteristics of the slow response.

THE TRANSFER IMPEDANCE

In uniform propagation, the excited region can be regarded as a source of current with a finite source impedance; the cable properties of the unexcited fibers specify an electrical load on that source. In uniform conduction, the excited and unexcited regions are contiguous; in other words, the load acts directly on the source. To separate a transfer impedance from the load placed on the source by the unexcited region is thus artificial. In nonuniform conduction, the flow of current from the source to the unexcited region may be affected by factors other than the cable characteristics of the unexcited region. Under those circumstances, it is useful to introduce the concept of transfer impedance. Under nonuniform conditions, any (or all) of a number of changes can occur that alter the transfer impedance, among them local changes in membrane resistance, changes in fiber diameter (including changes caused by branching or convergence of fibers), and changes in intracellular resistance. Such changes may alter not only the forward spread of excitatory currents but also "load" the excited area in a way that changes the action potential in that area.

EXCITABILITY OF THE UNEXCITED REGION

In uniform conduction with a high safety factor, the conduction velocity is relatively insensitive to small changes in threshold. However, in those cases of nonuniform conduction in which the transfer impedance is so high that the effective stimulus acts only liminally, the strength-duration curve of the tissue becomes crucially important (cf. Katz, 1939; Mendez et al., 1969). The strength-duration curve of Lapicque relates the strength of an applied stimulus to the length of time it must be applied to excite. In classic terms, there is a minimum effective stimulus, the rheobase, which requires a long time to excite. A stimulus weaker than the rheobase will never excite; in general, the stronger the stimulus, the shorter the time required for excitation to appear (latency). In Purkinje fibers, the utilization time of a rheobasic stimulus can be rather long (Dominguez and Fozzard, 1970). When excitation occurs in response to a long, small stimulus, the success or failure of conduction becomes critically dependent on rather small changes in the threshold of the unexcited region, as does the latency.

The excitability of the cardiac fiber and kind of action potential it produces if excited can vary in a remarkably complicated way as a consequence of reducing the resting potential, for example, as demonstrated experimentally with graded elevation of $[K^+]_o$. Moderate elevation of $[K^+]_o$ actually increases conduction velocity in Purkinje fibers, because the effect of moving the membrane potential closer to the threshold potential is not completely counteracted by inactivation of the fast channels (Dominguez and Fozzard, 1970). Greater elevation of $[K^+]_o$ causes progressively greater inactivation, increased leakiness, diminished excitability, and lowered conduction velocity. Still greater elevation of $[K^+]_o$ will bring the membrane potential to a level at which the degree of inactivation is too great to allow propagation based on fast-channel-dependent upstrokes, yet that same membrane potential might be too negative to the threshold potential of the slow response to permit propagation of the slow response. A further elevation of $[K^+]_o$ by bringing the membrane potential close enough to the threshold potential for the slow response, might then allow slow propagation. A still greater increase, accompanied by, among other things, increased leakiness and decreased driving force on the ions that carry inward current, might slow and then arrest propagation. A monotonic increase in $[K^+]_o$ thus might initially increase conduction velocity, then decrease it, then cause block, then restore conduction, then slow it, and finally again cause block.

A COMMENT ON WHAT THEORETICAL MODELS TELL US ABOUT THE MECHANISMS OF SLOW CONDUCTION

For fixed cable constants under conditions where conduction is uniform, theory tells us that an alteration of the membrane characteristics that reduced the maximum upstroke velocity by a factor of 100 would lower the conduction velocity by a factor of 10 (see, e.g., Huxley's (1959) dimensional analysis of the squid axon). The normal propagating action potential in Purkinje fibers has a maximum upstroke velocity typically in the range of 400 to 800 V/sec and a conduction velocity in the range of 2 to 3 m/sec; the slowly propagating action potential evoked by high $[K^+]_o$ and epinephrine has a maximum upstroke velocity of 5 to 10 V/sec and a conduction velocity of 0.1 to 0.15 m/sec. In switching from fast to slow conduction, the observed reduction in conduction velocity by a factor of 20 is quantitatively explained by the reduced upstroke velocity, with an additional factor of 2 arising from the fact that slowly rising waves see a much larger effective membrane capacitance in these fibers (Carmeliet and Willems, 1971). The low upstroke velocity demands that the excited membrane generate only a very small, but long-lasting, net inward ionic current. Indeed, the peak inward ionic current during slow conduction is only about 2% of that required for normal fast conduction.

The theoretical investigation by Lieberman et al., (1973) interprets slow conduction mainly in terms of high internal resistivity arising at the intercellular connections. However, since increasing the internal specific resistivity does not, in itself, reduce the maximum upstroke velocity, we believe that their interpretation cannot explain the slow conduction associated with a very low upstroke velocity, such as that observed in Purkinje fibers exposed to high $[K^+]_o$ and catecholamines, in Purkinje fibers bathed with Na^+-free solutions containing Ca^{2+}, Sr^{2+}, or Ba^{2+}, and in tissues such as the SA and AV nodes (Cranefield and Dodge, 1980).

STRUCTURAL NONUNIFORMITIES

Nowhere in the heart does the structure of the tissue conform to that of a simple uniform cable. Probably the closest electrical approximation to a uniform cable is found in the thinnest Purkinje fibers in which all of the cells that comprise the bundle contact its surface. Because the length of a "cell" is very much less than the characteristic length determined by measurements on the fiber, it is generally assumed that the theory for a uniform cable would be applicable to such fibers, with the added assumption that whatever extra longitudinal resistance might be contributed by intercellular junctions can be lumped with the cytoplasmic resistance to give a higher effective R_i.

We have critically examined this assumption by a simulation in which we introduced leaky septa at 250-μm intervals into a uniform cable of 50 μm diameter that had a characteristic length of 2200 μm. We put squid giant axon-like sodium channels in the membrane, without a voltage-dependent change in potassium permeability, to yield an action potential with an indefinitely long plateau. We set the kinetics of the sodium-conductance change equivalent to those of the squid axon at a temperature of 16.3°C, and we adjusted the density of sodium channels so that the intrinsic safety factor was about four for fast propagation. (Our simulation differs from an essentially similar one of Lieberman et al. (1973) in two details: we designed the membrane characteristics to imitate accurately fast propagation in Purkinje fibers, and we used a spatial increment in the numerical solution of the partial differential equation that was small enough to resolve voltage gradients within each cell.) Cable theory tells us that both the conduction velocity, θ, and the characteristic length, λ, should vary inversely with the square root of the internal resistance, but that the safety factor should not be affected by such changes. As we increased the resistance of the septa in our simulation, we found that θ decreased approximately as predicted over the range in which the resistance of a single septum increased from being negligible to being about 150 times the resistance of the cytoplasm of the "cell"; that is when λ decreased to about one "cell" length. As would be expected, further increases in septal resistance affected the safety factor, and conduction blocked with about a fourfold further increase. Thus, we found a very wide range over which the exponential foot of the action potential and conduction velocity varied in a manner consistent with the assumption that junctional and cytoplasmic resistance could be lumped together so that the theory for a uniform cable could be applied. However, conduction in this model is not strictly uniform. Even when the septal resistance is increased only modestly, to equal that of the cytoplasm of the cell, so that the effective R_i is doubled and the conduction velocity and characteristic length are reduced by 30%, a "cell" is practically isopotential along its length, the conduction delay takes place at each septum, and the maximum upstroke velocity is found to increase towards the limiting value expected from a membrane action potential.

For thicker Purkinje fiber bundles, in which an appreciable fraction of the cells are entirely interior to the surface layer of cells, the electrical behavior of the fiber during fast conduction departs even further from that of a simple uniform cable. We have examined propagation in the model of sheep Purkinje fibers developed by Schoenberg et al. (1975) to rationalize morphometric data with measurements of the cable constants in fibers of varying size. Taking advantage of the axial symmetry of their model, we simulated larger fibers by using two or more parallel, highly interconnected cables (Dodge, 1981). One cable represented columns of surface cells, the others represented columns of interior cells whose external local current was impeded by the thinness of the clefts through which it must flow. Our simulations showed that current for the propagation of the fast impulse is generated only by the surface membrane; excitation of the interior membranes lags behind because of the time required to charge their capacitance through the appreciable series resistance of the clefts. If we made the resistance of the intercellular junctions negligible, then this complex cable behaved essentially like a simple one, and conduction velocity increased approximately with the square root of the diameter of the fiber. But if we made the junctional resistance comparable to the cytoplasmic resistance, the conduction velocity became independent of the fiber diameter, in agreement with the experimental observations of Schoenberg et al. (1975). We explain this result as follows: Even with a very modest junctional resistance, the interior longitudinal current during the fast rising phase is mainly restricted to the surface cells. Change in the internal potential of the interior cells lags behind because of the finite radial coupling resistance; hence, those cells cannot carry much of the longitudial current. This model predicts some features that could be looked for by experiment; namely, it predicts that the foot of the propagating action potential measured in a surface fiber should have a small slow component and that the maximal rate of rise of the internal potential of an interior fiber should be less than half that measured in a surface cell.

In most tissues of the heart, the electrical structure is vastly more complicated. We see thicker fibers branching and thinner branches fusing, with distances between branch points comparable to the electrical characteristic length measured in that tissue. Clearly, such inhomogeneity can greatly affect conduction under appropriate conditions.

INEXCITABLE SEGMENT

In an excitable cell that has no slow channels, a segment can be made inexcitable by adding TTX. In such a segment, the cable properties might be almost unchanged. Khodorov and Timin (1975, pp. 165 ff.) have examined this case for a geometrically uniform "Hodgkin-Huxley axon" containing a segment in which the maximum sodium conductance (g_{Na}) is decreased to 0.1 of its normal value. The active area is loaded by the inexcitable area so that the amplitude and upstroke velocity are diminished as the spike approaches the inexcitable area. In their model, those parameters are reduced by 15% and 30%, respectively, when the action potential is 22.5 mm away from the beginning of the inexcitable area. A mere 17.5 mm into the inexcitable region, a large but purely electrotonic change is seen, some 60 mV in amplitude (as compared with the 90 mV amplitude of the normal spike). Even 30 mm into the inexcitable area the electrotonic spread produces a depolarization about 22 mV in amplitude. Khodorov and Timin did not compute the properties of an axon in which excitable segments both precede and follow the inexcitable segment; so they did not determine how long the inexcitable segment must be to cause block, or what delay might arise if propagation just barely occurs across the inexcitable area. Sharp and Joyner (1980), using the model of ventricular fibers developed by Beeler and Reuter (1977), found that propagation failed when a length of only 0.5 mm was made inexcitable by reducing g_{Na} to zero in fibers whose space constant was 0.6 mm. In cases where propagation barely succeeded, they found conduction delays greater than 10 msec across the blocked region. Although the membrane in their model included slow channels, the assumed density was found to be too low to sustain conduction through a region where fast channels were blocked.

The delay of conduction across a blocked region, illustrated by such simulations, depends crucially upon the excitability characteristics of the specific tissue, but it can be understood, quite simply, in terms of the strength-duration curve for excitation of that tissue. Dominguez and Fozzard (1970) found that a stimulus applied to the end of a healthy Purkinje fiber is rheobasic if it causes a depolarization of about 10 mV. If the plateau, which can provide a long-lasting stimulus, is 70 mV positive to the resting potential, it will produce a 10 mV depolarization at a distance of 1.9 space constants; in other words, excitation could just barely occur beyond a 1.9 λ long inexcitable region with normal cable properties. This indicates that excitation just fails if the segment devoid of excitable channels is about 4 mm long; if the inexcitable segment is marginally shorter, the region beyond it is excited, but with a significant delay. For a rheobasic stimulus, the delay can be at least as long as the membrane time constant, and may be as much as 25 msec (Dominguez and Fozzard, 1970). That delay, over a length of 4 mm, corresponds to an apparent average conduction velocity of 0.2 m/sec. Under those circumstances, the upstroke would be preceded by a long slow "step" but would, judging by the steady-state voltage dependence of inactivation, be only moderately reduced in amplitude and upstroke velocity. An action potential evoked by a rheobasic stimulus applied to a normal Purkinje fiber certainly would not resemble a slow response, even if some additional reduction in amplitude and upstroke velocity arose from the electrical load placed on the action potential by the inexcitable segment. If we envision a segment rendered inexcitable by local elevation of $[K^+]_o$ sufficient, *inter alia*, to decrease membrane resistance by a factor of 4, block would occur over an inexcitable segment less than 2-mm long, but barely successful transmission would occur with about the same delay as that seen when excitation occurs across a longer inexcitable segment of normal length constant, because that delay is determined predominantly by the strength-duration curve.

ISOLATED LOCUS OF UNCOUPLING

An interesting example of the effect on conduction of variations in transfer impedance is found if we examine two normal segments of Purkinje fiber joined by a very short, wholly inexcitable segment that has a very high internal resistance. Such a situation may be envisioned as arising from marked uncoupling throughout an entire cross-section of a bundle. As above, we assume that the plateau is 70-mV positive to the resting potential and that the rheobasic stimulus must depolarize the unexcited segment by 10 mV. The magnitude of the stimulus acting upon the unexcited segment will be determined by the coupling resistance. If the plateau depolarization is seven times the depolarization required to excite and the coupling resistance is six times the input resistance of the unexcited fiber, the stimulus will be rheobasic, and conduction will be delayed by the latency associated with a rheobasic stimulus, perhaps as long as 25 msec for Purkinje fibers. Less marked increases in the coupling resistance will lead to lesser delays, and, on the basis of the shape of typical strength-duration curves, we would expect the delay to decrease approximately in proportion to the coupling resistance. In an experimental model illustrating these principles studied in DeHaan's laboratory, the resistance of the coupling between two aggregates of cultured heart cells was shown to determine the delay in excitation across the junction (Clapham et al., 1980).

The effects on conduction of local and general uncoupling have been investigated theoretically by Lieberman et al. (1973), using a model in which the cable and membrane parameters were chosen to represent their experimental model of strands of cultured heart cells. Several of the points discussed above are illustrated in that paper, but the time scale of the delays in their simulations is somewhat different because the excitability characteristics of their membrane model are significantly different from those measured on Purkinje fibers.

Both in the fiber containing a long inexcitable segment and in the fiber containing a discrete region of marked uncoupling, the excitability of the unexcited region and the amplitude and upstroke velocity of the action potential evoked there are determined by fast-channel properties, whereas the long latency is made possible by the fact that the plateau current becomes part of the stimulus. To the extent that the slow inward current contributes to the plateau, it can be said to play an essential role in the generation of the fairly long conduction delays that can arise across an inexcitable segment or a sharply localized region of marked uncoupling. Sharp and Joyner (1980, Fig. 7 and text p. 412) illustrated this point by a simulation in which a 70 μm long region of very high internal specific resistivity just failed to block conduction and did cause a delay of 15 msec with their standard membrane characteristics, but did block when the amplitude of the plateau was attenuated by reducing the density of slow inward current. A quite different role for the slow inward current will be considered in the next section, in which we will examine the effect on propagation of interposing a segment several length constants long in which there are no excitable fast-channels but in which a propagated slow response can arise.

SEGMENTS OF NORMAL EXCITABILITY CONNECTED BY A SEGMENT CONTAINING ONLY SLOW CHANNELS

A good deal of evidence can be summoned to support the statement that uniform propagation at a conduction velocity of between 0.1 and 0.15 m/sec can occur in cardiac fibers that have a resting potential of −50 to −60 mV and in which the only excitable channel carrying inward current is the slow channel (see Cranefield, 1975). If we envision a bundle of Purkinje fibers 30 mm long, in which the fast upstroke normally conducts at 2.0 m/sec, the upstroke will traverse 30 mm in 15 msec. If the central 10 mm instead conducts a slow response at 0.1 m/sec, propagation through it will require 100 msec, and conduction throughout the entire bundle will require 110 msec; that is, the total conduction time will be increased by 95 msec. Although that degree of slowing is not enough to provide the delay required for reentry, it can play an important role in such abnormalities as the aberrant spread of excitation. If we assume that the slow response cannot readily (if at all) propagate in fibers that have a high resting potential, our model requires each end of the fiber to have a high negative resting potential (−90 to −80 mV) while the central segment has a resting potential of −60 to −50 mV. Among the questions that arise are: *(1)* What kind of transition in resting potential occurs between the segments? *(2)* What peculiarities arise as the fast response enters the depolarized segment, that is, what special features arise when the normal action potential excites the slow response? And *(3)* what special features arise as the slow response emerges from the depolarized segment to excite the normal segment?

No discontinuous change in resting potential can occur in a cable; a gradient of potential determined by the cable properties will always occur. This in turn means that some degree of transition will occur in those characteristics of the excitable channels that are determined by the resting potential (for example, in the degree of inactivation), so that action potentials intermediate in response between the normal action potential and the slow response are to be expected in the transitional region (see Cranefield, 1975, pp. 148−150). It is not easy to evaluate the exact effect of the presence of such transitional action potentials on propagation from a region of high resting potential into a region in which a low resting potential is associated with slow-response activity, but it seems very probable that the fast response can readily stimulate the slow response in the sort of situation we have described. Even if the large current associated with the rapid upstroke should (perhaps because of its brevity) fail to excite the slow response, one would expect the smaller but far longer currents associated with the plateau to do so.

It is altogether less obvious that the slow response can infallibly excite the normal fiber beyond the depolarized segment. The slow response, as mentioned above, has a slow upstroke and generates far less excitatory current than does the fast response. Although the gradient of resting potential from -60 to -50 mV to -90 or -80 mV is one that permits a gradual increase in the availability of fast channels, that same change moves the membrane progressively more negative to the threshold of the slow response. In a region where a "mixed" excitatory response occurs, that is, a region in which both fast and slow channels may contribute inward current it is not immediately obvious whether the increasing availability of the fast channels will compensate for the increasing remoteness of the membrane potential from the threshold potential of the slow response. In this connection we might note that, in a simulation by Sharp and Joyner (1980), the fast response evoked a slow response in a region free of fast channels only if that region was somewhat depolarized, but even under those circumstances the slow response did not excite a fast response beyond the region with no fast channels. To obtain such excitation, Sharp and Joyner had to incease the density of the slow inward current substantially. At least one simulation thus agrees with our surmise that the fast to slow junction can be a region of higher safety factor than the slow to fast junction.

ASYMMETRICAL CONDUCTION

A distinctive feature of many clinically important arrhythmias is that they can be evoked by a critical increase in rate or by a critically timed premature impulse. A similarly distinctive feature of bundles of Purkinje fibers exposed to high $[K^+]_o$ and epinephrine is that such bundles often conduct premature impulses in only one direction and also often display rate-dependent block. In such preparations, a progressive increase in drive rate can convert two-way conduction into one-way block and finally into two-way block. Understanding the mechanisms that give rise to that kind of asymmetry may well shed light on the mechanisms that give rise to rate-dependent arrhythmias in the whole heart.

A well known and robust model for one-way block is that in which the diameter of the excitable cable changes abruptly, as it does at the junction between the axon and the cell body of the motor neuron (cf. Eccles, 1957; Dodge and Cooley, 1973) or at the point at which a small branch emerges from the giant axon (Khodorov and Timin, 1975). Under such circumstances, excitation will always travel from the region of larger diameter to the region of smaller diameter, but, if the diameter changes by a suitably large factor, an impulse traveling in the thin cable will block near the junction because of the increased electrical load imposed on the thin cable. In the critical case in which an impulse traveling in the thin cable barely succeeds in exciting the thick cable, a slight elevation of threshold, caused for example by the impulse arriving in the partially refractory period, will cause block (Coombs et al., 1957). In that model, once the change in diameter has occurred the fiber does not return to its original diameter. In the heart, on the other hand, the kinds of "lesions" that might produce one-way block occur in cables in which the properties are more or less the same on each side of the region through which the asymmetrical conduction occurs. If the abnormalities of that region are symmetrical around its midpoint, then if block occurs it will occur irrespective of the direction of conduction (as it does when the "lesion" is an inexcitable segment, a narrow region of marked uncoupling, or a region capable of generating only the slow response). What is necessary for one-way conduction is the presence of an asymmetrical nonuniformity.

Using a model of a ventricular fiber, Joyner (1981) has examined several kinds of asymmetrical nonuniformities. He found a range of asymmetrical gradients in g_{Na} or in leakage conductance which would produce one-way block, but that range was so narrow that a slight change would produce either two-way conduction or two-way block. Joyner obtained more robust models of one-way block by using asymmetrical gradients in cell diameter or R_i. The minimum change in diameter that gave rise to one-way conduction was a gradual doubling of diameter over a distance in excess of several length constants, followed by an abrupt return to the original diameter. It is doubtful that changes of this kind are characteristic of the cardiac syncytium. There are regions at which the diameter changes more or less gradually, namely regions where one sort of fiber joins another sort (SA node–atrium, atrium–AV node, AV node–His bundle, Purkinje fiber–ventricle), but none of those changes terminates in an abrupt return to the original diameter, a return that is crucial to the production of one-way block in the proposed model. Nor do such changes in diameter seem likely to result from elevation of $[K^+]_o$ or from hypoxia.

Joyner also obtained a robust model of one-way block in a model in which a gradually developing asymmetry in longitudinal resistance was simulated. The minimum change in R_i needed to obtain one-way block in that model was a linear increase over a length of several space constants, to 11 times the normal value, followed by an abrupt return of R_i to its original value. It would be surprising to us if that degree of increase in uncoupling, abruptly terminating in a return to normal coupling, were to exist in normal or even in hypoxic fibers.

In one sense, therefore, Joyner's results suggest both that the normal, high-safety-factor action potential is not readily blocked and that it cannot readily be made to conduct asymmetrically either by plausible changes in the density of fast channels or by plausible changes in the cable properties. Yet the phenomena in question are easy to obtain both in the AV node and in Purkinje fibers exposed to high $[K^+]_o$ or made hypoxic.

On the other hand, we agree with Joyner that an abrupt increase in electrical loading relative to the source impedance is a plausible cause of block and that an anatomical heterogeneity is a logical place to look for such a change. In our opinion, however, only if the action potential is a relatively weak stimulus, and the unexcited area is not easily excited, will plausibly small changes in membrane resistance, cell diameter, or intercellular coupling produce block. And, just as smaller changes in those factors would be needed to cause block, so would smaller degrees of asymmetry in those changes be required to produce one-way block.

It is well known that a certain degree of nonuniformity in the wave front can be detected in bundles of normal Purkinje fibers (Anderson et al., 1970; Spach et al., 1971; Myerburg et al., 1973). As we discuss in more detail below, all that is needed to produce a great exaggeration in that nonuniformity is to excite the bundle prematurely, thus causing an impulse that is a less effective stimulus to propagate, through the same anatomical heterogeneities, in fibers of elevated threshold. An equivalent lowering of the stimulating efficacy of the action potential and increase in the threshold of unexcited areas might well result from exposure to high $[K^+]_o$ or hypoxia.

Hypoxia seems more likely than does elevation of $[K^+]_o$ to cause uncoupling (Wojtczak, 1979); both, however, lead to depolarization with its concomitant effects of diminishing or abolishing the excitability of fast channels and of creating circumstances favorable to the appearance of the slow response—that is, for the replacement of an action potential that normally propagates with a high safety factor by one that presumably travels, under the best of conditions, with a significantly lower safety factor. The conduction disturbances that cause the earliest arrhythmias of myocardial infarction may, for example, result from the marked and irreversible uncoupling seen as the cells die; even under those circumstances the same things that cause uncoupling seem very likely to cause depolarization and its concomitant changes in the excitatory currents and thresholds. However, those kinds of one-way and rate-dependent block that are stable or those experimental kinds that are readily reversible (as in the Purkinje fiber exposed to high $[K^+]_o$ or in the AV node exposed to acetylcholine) seem more likely to result from abnormal action potentials and decreased excitability interacting with preexisting anatomical impediments, and less likely to depend on the appearance of new anatomical impediments.

PREMATURE IMPULSES

In the normal AV node or in Purkinje fibers depolarized by exposure to high $[K^+]_o$, a premature impulse may block at some distance into the conduction pathway; if prolongation of refractoriness blocks or slows the conduction of the next impulse, the prior impulse is said to have undergone "concealed conduction" (Langendorf and Pick, 1956). Under certain circumstances, premature excitation can unmask asymmetries as it does when a premature impulse travels more readily in one direction than in the other. In some experimental situations, unidirectional block of a premature impulse sets up a necessary condition for the initiation of circus movement, namely one-way conduction around the circuitous pathway (Cranefield, 1975; Wit and Cranefield, 1978).

In cardiac fibers, the premature action potential can have a low amplitude and a low upstroke velocity (cf. Kao and Hoffman, 1958). Recovery of excitability is not uniform, because fibers quite near one another can differ markedly in their degree of repolarization. Because a premature impulse travels with a low safety factor, one might expect it to be further slowed or blocked by impediments that have little or no effect on the spread of a normal action potential. Such impediments are unavoidable in syncytial structure containing thick and thin bundles. An impulse that blocks at some points and not at others will necessarily travel along a more circuitous path, further reducing its apparent conduction velocity. An interesting example of this is found in the effect of prematurity on the degree of longitudinal dissociation of a new-born impulse in a false tendon (Myerburg et al., 1973). Punctate, barely threshold stimulation of a canine false tendon or a bundle branch can give rise to a wave of excitation that spreads longitudinally in a nonuniform way, presumably because of a paucity of transverse connections. However, as Myerburg states, "this nonuniformity of the wave of excitation became progressively less marked as a function of distance, and at about 10-mm distal to the site of stimulation, the wave of propagation was almost perfectly uniform across the longitudinal axis." On the other hand, even in a bundle where little or no dissociation of the wavefront appears in response to the regular driven impulse or to a late premature impulse, it is easily evoked by increasing the prematurity of the stimulus; moreover, the more premature is the impulse, the greater is the dissociation of the wavefront. Myerburg suggested that because the lateral connections have a higher r_i than do the longitudinal fibers, a premature and therefore "weakly propagating impulse could be delayed or blocked selectively at the points of higher resistance, thus dissociating the longitudinally-oriented elements from one another."

Myerburg's interpretation calls attention to the interaction between an impulse of low intrinsic safety factor and preexisting impediments to conduction. Premature excitation creates a "weakly propagating impulse;" it also occurs at a moment when that impulse will meet not only preexisting anatomical impediments but also varying degrees of refractoriness created by the heterogeneity of recovery from the effects of the previous impulse.

SUMMARY AND CONCLUSION

Although we have made simulations of a limited kind (see above and see Cranefield and Dodge, 1980) and have found the simulations made by Joyner (Sharp and Joyner, 1980; Joyner, 1981) both useful and thought-provoking, we hesitate to draw definitive conclusions from simulations based on models that represent no more than some small part or some special feature of the complex array of characteristics that we have discussed in this chapter.

Presumably precise simulations, based on the Hodgkin-Huxley axon, have imitated in nerve a remarkable number of phenomena similar to those that we have observed in cardiac Purkinje fibers exposed to high $[K^+]_o$ and epinephrine, such as summation and inhibition at branch points, true reflection, concealed conduction of a reflected impulse revealed by prolongation of the repolarization limb with block of the next antegrade impulse, and other complex changes (see Khodorov and Timin, 1975). Similarly precise simulations on models of the cardiac action potential are vastly more difficult, not only because of the geometrical complexities of the cardiac syncytium, but also (cf. Sharp and Joyner, 1980) because of the gaps in our knowledge of the nature and characteristics of the time- and voltage-dependent currents that generate the cardiac action potential and because of the great difficulty of modeling small but possibly critical changes in the resting potential and the plateau potential attributable to rate- and rhythm-sensitive changes in accumulation or depletion of K^+ or in the level of electrogenic sodium extrusion.

We will be confident that we have attained a reasonably complete understanding of normal and abnormal conduction in the heart when we can simulate propagated action potentials that reproduce all of the features obtainable in experiments in which action potentials are evoked at varying rates, from different resting potentials, and at varying degrees of prematurity. Our detailed knowledge falls far short of providing the information needed to perform such a simulation. The present article calls attention to four particular factors about which we need much more precise information before realistic simulations can be made. They are *(1)* the nature of the pre-existing anatomical heterogeneities (see Clerc, 1976; Weingart, 1977), *(2)* a detailed empirical description of how the responsiveness of the fast channels is modulated by resting potential and by premature excitation, *(3)* a more detailed empirical description of the voltage- and time-sensitivities of the slow channels, and *(4)* the extent and degree of local variations in intercellular junctional resistance.

We do, nevertheless, suspect that the kinds of features of nonuniform slow conduction seen in Purkinje fibers exposed to high $[K^+]_o$ and epinephrine depend, as we suggested in 1971, on interactions between abnormal action potentials and structural and geometrical asymmetries, whether normally present or exaggerated by the experimental conditions. And we suspect such a combination of causes will eventually be found to explain most conduction that has a velocity of less than 0.1 m/sec, shows slow upstrokes, notched upstrokes, and one-way block or rate-dependent block.

REFERENCES

Anderson GJ, Greenspan K, Bandura JP, Fisch C (1970) Asynchrony of conduction within the canine specialized Purkinje fiber system. Circ Res **27**:691–703

Beeler GW, Reuter H (1977) Reconstruction of the action potential of myocardial fibres. J Physiol **268**:117–210

Carmeliet E, Willems J (1971) The frequency dependent character of the membrane capacity in cardiac Purkinje fibres. J Physiol (Lond) **213**:85–93

Clapham DE, Shrier A, DeHaan RL (1980) Junctional resistance and action potential delay between embryonic heart cell aggregates. J Gen Physiol **75**:633–654

Clerc L (1976) Directional differences of impulse spread in trabecular muscle from mammalian heart. J Physiol (Lond) **255**:335–346

Coombs JS, Curtis JR, Eccles JC (1957) The interpretation of spike potentials of motoneurones. J Physiol **139**:198–231

Cranefield PF (1975) The Conduction of the Cardiac Impulse. Mt Kisco, NY, Futura Publishing Co

Cranefield PF, Dodge FA (1980) Slow conduction in the heart. In The Slow Inward Current and Cardiac Arrhythmias. DP Zipes, DC Bailey, V Elharrar (eds). The Hague, Nijhoff, pp 149–171

Cranefield PF, Hoffman BF (1971) Conduction of the cardiac impulse. II. Summation and inhibition. Circ Res **28**:220–233

Cranefield PF, Klein HO, Hoffman BF (1971) Conduction of the cardiac impulse. I. Delay, block and one-way block in depressed Purkinje fibers. Circ Res **28**:199–219

Cranefield PF, Wit AL, Hoffman BF (1972) Conduction of the cardiac impulse. III. Characteristics of very slow conduction. J Gen Physiol **59**:227–246

Dodge FA (1981) Cellular connections and propagation in cardiac Purkinje fibers. Biophys J (in press)

Dodge FA, Cooley JW (1973) Action potential of the motorneurone. IBM Res Develop **17**: 219–229

Dominguez G, Fozzard HA (1970) Influence of extracellular K^+ concentration on cable properties and excitability of sheep cardiac Purkinje fibers. Circ Res **26**:565–574

Eccles JC (1957) The Physiology of Nerve Cells. Baltimore, Johns Hopkins University Press

Hunter PJ, McNaughton PA, Noble D (1975) Analytical models of propagation in excitable cells. Prog Biophys Molec Biol **30**:99–144

Huxley AF (1959) Ion movements during nerve activity. Ann NY Acad Sci **81**:221–246

Joyner RW (1981) Mechanisms of unidirectional block in cardiac tissues. (in press)

Kao CY, Hoffman BF (1958) Graded and decremental responses in heart muscle fibers. Am J Physiol **194**:187–196

Katz B (1939) Electric Excitation of Nerve. London, Oxford University Press

Khodorov BI, Timin EN (1975) Nerve impulse propagation along nonuniform fibers. Prog Biophys Molec Biol **30**:145–184

Langendorf R, Pick A (1956) Concealed conduction. Further evaluation of a fundamental aspect of propagation of the cardiac impulse. Circulation **13**:381–399

Lieberman M, Kootsey JM, Johnson EA, Sawanobori T (1973) Slow conduction in cardiac muscle. A biophysical model. Biophys J **13**:37–55

Mendez C, Moe GK (1966) Some characteristics of transmembrane potential of AV nodal cells during propagation of premature beats. Circ Res **19**:993–1010

Mendez C, Mueller WJ, Merideth J, Moe GK (1969) Interaction of transmembrane potentials in canine Purkinje fibers and at Purkinje fiber-muscle junctions. Circ Res **24**:361–372

Myerburg RJ, Nilsson K, Befeler B, Castellanos A, Gelband H (1973) Transverse spread and longitudinal dissociation in the distal A-V conducting system. J Clin Invest **52**:885–895

Rushton WAH (1937) Initiation of the propagated disturbance. Proc Roy Soc. B **124**:210–243

Schoenberg M, Dominguez G, Fozzard HA (1975) Effect of diameter on membrane capacity and conductance of sheep cardiac Purkinje fibers. J Gen Physiol **65**:441–458

Sharp GH, Joyner RW (1980) Simulated propagation of cardiac action potentials. Biophys J **31**:403–423

Spach MS, Barr RC, Serwer GS, Johnson EA, Kootsey JM (1971) Collision of excitation waves in the dog Purkinje system: extracellular identification. Circ Res **29**:499–511
Weingart R (1977) The actions of ouabain on intercellular coupling and conduction velocity in mammalian ventricular muscle. J Physiol (Lond) **264**:341–365
Wit AL, Cranefield PF (1978) Reentrant excitation as a cause of cardiac arrhythmias. Am J Physiol **235**:H1–H17
Wojtczak J (1979) Contractures and increase in internal longitudinal resistance of cow ventricular muscle induced by hypoxia. Circ Res **44**:88–95

Discussion

LIEBERMAN: I would like to remind you that, in 1973, I, along with Sawanobori, Johnson, and Kootsey published in Biophysical Journal a paper that precedes the Joyner model and that emphasizes the importance of longitudinal resistance in slowing of conduction. Also, there have been other published papers in which the effect of hypoxia or anoxia are interpreted by an increase in longitudinal resistance. These conditions may increase intracellular free calcium and, as a secondary effect, may decrease and eventually eliminate intercellular coupling. We might then expect from these conditions an initial slowing of conduction and an eventual block.

CRANEFIELD: I agree that longitudinal resistance can become important in the slowing of conduction. But, in your 1973 article, if I am not mistaken, you did have to slow the upstroke of the action potential to obtain the desired degree of slowing of conduction; that is to say, the increase in longitudinal resistance alone did not produce the desired degree of slowing. In my view, it is precisely when you have a slow upstroke, generating a weak source of axial current, that the longitudinal resistance may become critical. That may be what happens in the AV node and is an example of what I called, in my talk, a geometrical impediment to conduction. The longitudinal resistance becomes of critical importance to the production of slow conduction and block only when you already have an abnormal action potential propagating with a low safety factor.

SPACH: In relation to your last comment, I would like to recall what I presented in my paper in which conduction block was seen first in the longitudinal fast propagation direction instead of the transverse direction of a sheet of atrial fibers. This was obtained when we made the action potential have a decreased safety factor by stimulating it at the earliest possible portion of repolarization. What we observed was that conduction block occurred first in the direction of a low longitudinal resistance and only later in the direction of higher longitudinal resistance. So this is a bit of a problem, especially regarding what you said about Myerburg's results. According to these, we should expect, in my case, a block first in the transverse direction, and we obtained exactly the opposite. Essentially the same result was obtained with action potentials made critical by increased extracellular potassium. Both the premature and the K^+-depressed action potentials were departing from voltages between −60 and −70 mV. Second, what you pointed out is a need for an increased complexity at the microscopic level! As for the site of block, we think what most commonly happens is block at the transition from low to high axial resistivity, similar to the computer simulation of Lieberman et al. (Biophys J **13**:37, 1973), rather than at the site of transition from high to low axial resistivity, as in the simulation of Sharp and Joyner (Biophys J **31**:403, 1980). According to the latter, blockade happens when the action potential emerges from a localized area of increased longitudinal resistance, which is equivalent to a situation in which you have a sudden increase in surface area of activated membrane, or a branch. In cardiac muscle, on the other hand, you seem to have block as you enter the high longitudinal resistance region, not when you emerge from it. This is consistent with the simulation of Lieberman et al., which shows that the higher the longitudinal resistance, the easier it is to get block, but if you slow axial current otherwise, you don't.

CRANEFIELD: You make three interesting points. The first refers to Myerburg's results. He himself called attention to the bundles within the Purkinje fibers that remained entirely isolated over rather long distances in some of his experiments. This was seen more easily in his case because he was using highly punctate stimulation. The second point concerns the block seen when the action potential emerges from a small-diameter fiber into a large-diameter fiber. This will cause one-way block. To get two-way block, we might envision a situation in which the impulse goes from a fiber of large diameter into one of small diameter and then into a fiber of large diameter. Similarly, in a situation in which conduction through a segment depends only on slow-response activity you might get block in either direction. But in both cases, although block will occur no matter which way the impulse travels, it will occur at a different point depending on the direction of conduction (that is, at the point where the diameter increases or at the point where slow response activity has to excite the fast response). The block occurs at the "far end" in each case. This might give rise to some interesting properties in a syncytium. The third point concerns the 1973 Lieberman et al. paper. Increasing longitudinal resistance will not decrease the upstroke velocity of the action potential. Actually the opposite should happen. It is not at all clear to me how slow conduction in the AV node can be explained by increased longitudinal resistance alone. That would not give you a slow upstroke. It is not clear to me how you can reduce upstroke velocity from 500 to 10 V/sec just by increasing longitudinal resistance.

LIEBERMAN: It might be the case that the slow upstroke you observe in the AV node is, for instance, an electrotonic reflection of fast activity elsewhere.

CRANEFIELD: That may be possible. On the other hand, in our original experimental model, in which we had a localized segment exposed to elevated potassium and epinephrine, conduction was slowed as upstroke velocity decreased and yet no increase in longitudinal resistance was expected to occur, at least in the opinion of those who work with intercellular coupling. That this preparation very rapidly reverted to normal behavior when reexposed to normal solutions is another indication that propagation slowing is not mediated by an increase in longitudinal resistance.

PAES DE CARVALHO: I would like to add something to Lieberman's comments on the possibility that the slow action potential observed in the AV node is an electrotonic reflection of fast activity occurring somewhere else. To project an electrotonic image along a cable, we must keep some time and voltage relationship with the source signal, so that increasing delays are associated with decreasing amplitudes. In the AV node, action potentials are very slow and appear at perfectly discrete times. If they were an electrotonic reflection, to get that much delay we would have a very diminished amplitude, which is not observed. In conclusion, I would like to say that I am sure that changes in longitudinal resistance must be very critical, both for slowing and blockade of propagation in a region like the AV node where the excitatory current is so weak. But, we should not take the argument as far as to negate the existence of a slow response because there one would get into trouble with an extensive amount of evidence, both electrophysiologic and pharmacologic, that show that the slow action potentials are indeed a peculiar entity, and not just some sort of modification in intensity and velocity of a simple sodium spike.

LIEBERMAN: I agree that one point does not exclude the other.

JOHNSON: If we were to do those simulations again, we would not choose a Hodgkin-Huxley membrane. We would perhaps use our fast Na^+ channel kinetics for heart muscle, which is faster than that shown originally for squid, and we would add to it the small, slowly inactivating current that is about 100 times smaller and slower than the initial fast sodium current. This small current would be responsible for the slow response in presence of tetrodotoxin. There is an argument about whether this is sodium or calcium, but no one disagrees that there is a slow inward current. We find now that it inactivates a good deal faster than we thought. Originally, it was thought to inactivate in about 100 msec, and now this time is coming down to about 10 msec. Isenberg, in single cells, got a similar value for the time constant of inactivation for this slow current.

CRANEFIELD: I look forward to seeing your new simulation and to learning what the action potential shapes will turn out to be.

HOFFMAN: With respect to Dr. Spach's comments, I think it is not easy to generalize that in heart muscle the block occurs when the propagating impulse enters the area of difficulty. We may have the impression that this is so, but it is not necessarily correct. Whether the impulse blocks at the entrance or at the exit of a region of difficulty in conduction depends on how the passive and active characteristics are changing at each boundary.

CRANEFIELD: I agree. It is precisely for this reason that modeling can be misleading in mimicking conduction difficulties and block in heart muscle. We do not know in heart how to model precisely the behavior of active and passive characteristics in terms of spatial distribution and in terms of their response to situations like changed stimulus shapes and premature impulses. Until we know all this we must be very careful when extrapolating from model to reality in heart muscle.

Chapter 22

Excitability and Propagation of Slow Responses in Rabbit Atrium Partially Depolarized by Added K^+ and Ba^{2+}*

Masako Oya Masuda, Marilene de Paula Carvalho and Antonio Paes de Carvalho

The invasion of a slow response zone by a normal action potential is an important matter as it happens in the AV node during normal heart activation and presumably also in regions of myocardium that become partially depolarized under abnormal conditions. We have studied the phenomenon by creating a slow-response segment in a long (about 1 cm) strip of otherwise normal left atrium from the rabbit heart.

We created a slow-response zone by means of a partial depolarization, which was obtained by increasing the K^+ concentration of the Tyrode's solution in the presence of Ba^{2+} (TKBa solution). Ba^{2+} decreases resting potassium conductance and seems to be able to flow inward through the slow channel, both of which effects increase the channel depolarizing capability.

This chapter is divided into three parts. In the first part, we describe the general aspects of the slow response obtained in the TKBa solution. In the second part, we study the stimulation of slow responses by normal propagated action potentials. In the third part, some characteristics identified in the previous section are analyzed in a preparation in which slow responses are stimulated by current pulses directly applied to TKBa-treated preparations.

METHODS

Rabbits, each weighing about 1.5 kg, were killed by a cervical blow. The heart was rapidly excised, and strips of pectinate muscles were dissected from the left atrial roof.

*Supported by grants from the Conselho de Ensino para Graduados (CEPG-UFRJ), Conselho Nacional de Desenvolvimento Científico e Tecnológico (SEPLAN/CNPq) and Financiadora de Estudos e Projetos (SEPLAN/FINEP).

In those experiments in which the slow response was stimulated by a normal propagating action potential, a long (about 1 cm) atrial strip, as homogeneous as possible, was mounted in a chamber in which three serially arranged liquid compartments were created with the aid of thin rubber partitions. The partitions were perforated in such a way as to fit snugly around the strip, thus avoiding gross leakage between compartments. In the present case, the center and one of the extremities of the preparation were bathed in normal Tyrode's solution while the other extremity was bathed in a modified solution (TKBa). The normal Tyrode's composition is the following: 137 mM NaCl, 2.7 mM KCl, 0.5 mM $MgCl_2$, 2.7 mM $CaCl_2$, 12 mM $NaHCO_3$, 1.8 mM NaH_2PO_4, and 6.0 mM glucose. It was bubbled with 95% O_2 and 5% CO_2, at 33 to 35° C (pH, 7.2). The solution (TKBa) used to depress normal excitability, hence creating conditions for slow response to be the only electrical response, was obtained from the normal Tyrode's solution by increasing KCl to 12.7 mM, reducing $CaCl_2$ to 0.5 mM, and adding 1 mM $BaCl_2$.

As current pulses are applied to the normal region, a normal propagated action potential invades the depressed region and there stimulates a propagating slow response. In experiments requiring the slow response to be directly stimulated by current pulses, atrial strips were placed in a single chamber, the whole preparation was bathed in TKBa, and the stimuli were applied directly to its surface.

Intracellular and extracellular recordings were made through conventional methods. (For more details in Methods, see Masuda [1976]; Paula Carvalho [1977]; and Masuda and Paes de Carvalho [1982].)

RESULTS AND DISCUSSION

Characterization of the TKBa Slow Response

In 1961, Engstfeld, Antoni, and Fleckenstein stated that the simple addition of adrenaline to the perfusing solution makes it possible to reestablish excitability in pieces of myocardium that have been depolarized by an increase of extracellular potassium concentration. But, the action potentials thus observed exhibit a very slow time course and bear a remarkable similarity to action potentials of SA and AV nodes (Paes de Carvalho et al., 1959; Hoffman et al., 1959). Since then, this kind of activity, known as the slow response, has been evoked by a number of procedures. All share the common features of inactivating or blocking the fast, TTX-sensitive sodium conductance and enhancing the depolarizing capability of the slow inward current, either by means of its pharmacologic stimulation or by the simultaneous reduction of outward currents (Cranefield, 1975).

The first aspect that drew our attention to the study of the TKBa slow response was that smooth, typical, slow responses were observed in only about 65% of the preparations. The remaining 35% displayed irregularly shaped slow responses with notches and even with two peaks (Masuda, 1976; Paula Carvalho, 1977).

To determine parameters for describing the slow-response action potential, data for 19 impalements displaying typical, smooth time courses were selected from nine different experiments, and the following values were established: amplitude, 49.6 ± 1.6 mV (mean ± SEM); duration (measured at 90% repolarization), 395.5 ± 19.7 msec; maximum rate of depolarization, 1.6 ± 0.3 V/sec.

The resting potential was carefully checked in eight cells (no DC shift was observed during impalement and withdrawal) and ranged between −40 and −60 mV. Tetrodotoxin (1 μg/ml) had no effect on this slow response whereas D-600 (1 μg/ml), $MnCl_2$ (5 mM), and acetylcholine (15 μg/ml) blocked it completely. Also the stimulation threshold was at least 10 times higher for the propagated slow response than it was for the normal action potential (Paula Carvalho, 1977).

To determine conduction velocity, we established successive recording sites along a uniform pectinate muscle, and we plotted the delay at each recording site against the distance along the preparation. In four experiments, conduction velocity varied between 0.04 and 0.08 m/sec. This kind of determination was not possible in some preparations, especially those in which odd-shaped slow responses were recorded more frequently, because no linear relationship existed between the distance along the long axis of the preparation and the activation delays. We do not know yet how this kind of pattern is generated, but the anatomical nonhomogeneity of the preparation seems to play an important role in determining this kind of behavior. Even though it seemed to us that further investigation on this point would be extremely interesting, we performed all our experiments with strips from the roof of the atrium characterized by homogeneous parallel bundles of pectinate muscle. Almost all of them were displaying smooth, regularly propagating slow responses.

INVASION OF THE TKBa REGION BY A NORMAL PROPAGATING WAVEFRONT

General Aspects

In this section we consider how a normal wavefront stimulates a slow response. Figure 1 shows typical records simultaneously obtained from the three compartments as the preparation was driven at 1 Hz by stimuli applied to the end of the preparation immersed in normal Tyrode's solution. The activity in this normal extremity (right compartment) was monitored by extracellular recordings (lower trace). Transmembrane potentials were recorded from the tissue in the central (upper trace) and left (middle trace) compartments. In Figure 1A, the three compartments were perfused with normal Tyrode's solution. The surface record in the normal (right) compartment shows the expected fast biphasic deflection. Normal action potentials could be recorded from the middle and left compartments.

Figure 1B shows recordings at the same extracellular and intracellular sites after perfusing the left compartment for 20 min with TKBa. The two other chambers were kept in normal Tyrode's solution throughout. Both the extracellular recording of the right compartment and the intracellular recording of the middle chamber are comparable to the corresponding records shown in Figure 1A (notice the reduced sweep speed in Fig. 1B). In the test (left) compartment, the resting potential is reduced (not shown in figure), and the time course of the action potential is completely different from that displayed by a normal action potential. Note that activity takes much longer to appear and has a much lower rate of depolarization and amplitude. In other words, it is a typical slow response, as previously described (Cranefield, 1975).

The above data show that the three-compartment chamber used in our experiments allows a rather sharp boundary to be established between a normal and a depressed region in such a way that a normal wavefront can stimulate the slow response.

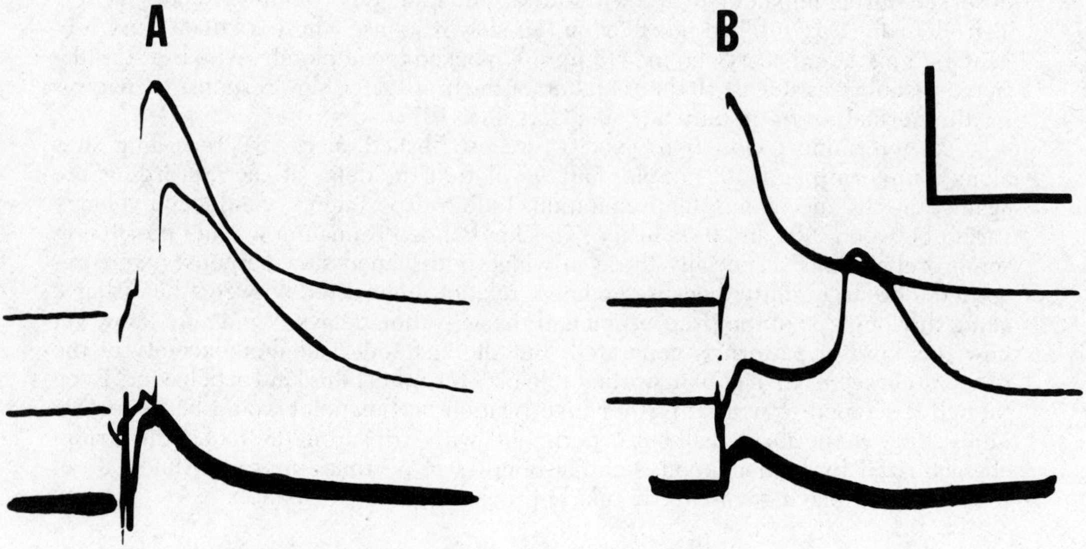

Figure 1. Potentials recorded in the three chambered bath. Upper trace, intracellular recording from a cell in the middle chamber; middle trace, intracellular recording from a cell in the left (test) compartment; lower trace, extracellular recording from the right (normal) compartment. *A*, The three compartments were perfused by normal Tyrode's solution. Calibration: vertical, 60 mV for intracellular recordings; horizontal, 100 ms. *B*, 20 minutes after the left compartment had been perfused with TKBa. Calibration: vertical, 60 mV for the intracellular recordings; horizontal, 200 ms. (Figs. 1–3 and 5–7 reproduced with permission from Circ Res 50:419–427, 1982.)

Effect of Cycle Length on Slow Response Activity Stimulated by Normal Propagation

Figure 2 shows the behavior of a TKBa-perfused region when invaded by a normal propagating wavefront, stimulated at different frequencies. The experimental arrangement was the same as it was in Figure 1, except that activity from the middle chamber was not monitored. The upper trace, a surface electrogram of the normal region, did not change significantly throughout the experiment. The lower trace, a recording of the TKBa slow response, was obtained from the same cell throughout the experiment.

A change in cycle length brought about remarkable changes in the slow-response behavior. In Figure 2A, the preparation was stimulated at 1.25 Hz (cycle length 800 msec). The superposition of two successive cycles indicates the occurrence of a 2:1 block of the slow response. This kind of behavior is ascribed to fatigue and is frequently observed in the AV node, as well as in artificial slow responses. In Figure 2B, a lower rate (1 Hz; cycle length, 1000 msec) reversed the 2:1 block. Propagation from the normal to the depressed region became slower, and the depolarization rate of the slow response decreased as a consequence of the 1:1 conduction. In fact, when compared with Figure 2A, the slow response has actually undergone an increase in frequency. In Figure 2, C–E, propagation into the slow response zone improved and dV/dt increased. That no further differences are visible is evidence of the absence of fatigue at these frequencies. As the frequency was lowered to 0.31 Hz (cycle length, 3200 msec)

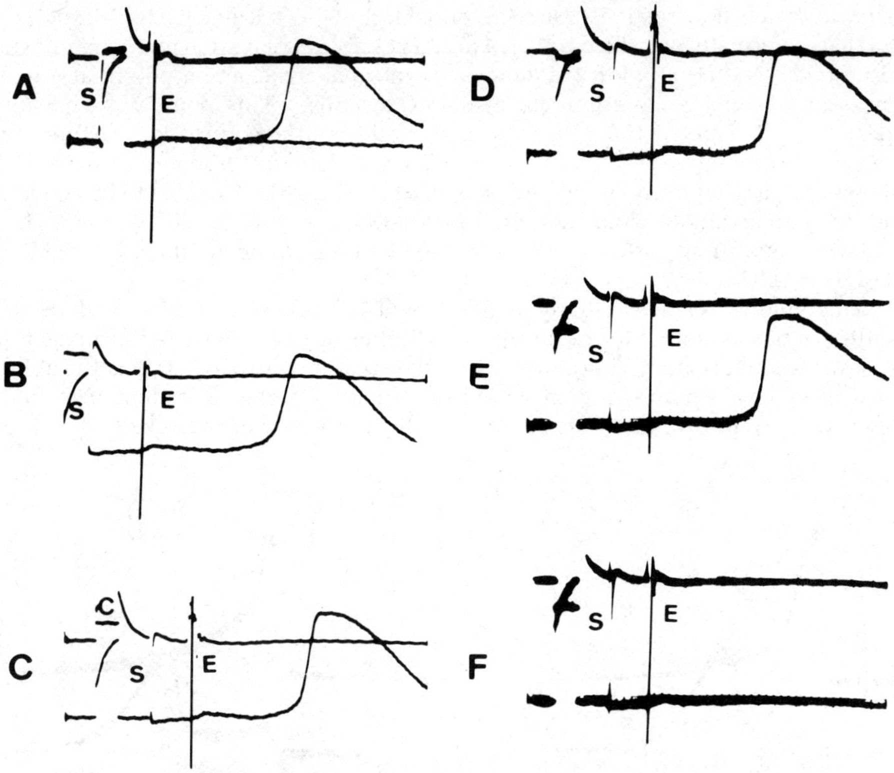

Figure 2. Effect of cycle length on slow response. Upper trace in all panels is an extracellular recording from the normal chamber. Lower trace is TKBa slow response in the test compartment. Microelectrode was kept in the same cell throughout the experiment. S = stimulus artifact, E = activity in the normal region, C = calibration (50 mV for intracellular potential and 50 ms). Cycle length was increased from *A* to *F*: *A*, 800 ms; *B*, 1000 ms; *C*, 1300 ms; *D*, 1600 ms; *E*, 2000 ms; *F*, 3200 ms.

in Figure 2F, the normal action potential was no longer able to stimulate the slow response. This could be due either to failure of slow-response excitation at the boundary between normal and depressed tissue (entry block) or to slow-response conduction block within the depressed region.

Both the high-frequency conduction block, caused by fatigue, and the low-frequency block were consistently observed in all experiments. Therefore, a limited frequency range exists in which a normal action potential can stimulate slow responses at a sustained 1:1 ratio. This range varies in different preparations from a top limit of 0.63 to 2.5 Hz to a bottom limit of 0.13 to 0.4 Hz.

Shape of Invading Action Potential and Low Frequency Block of Slow Responses

As stimulation frequency is lowered, the atrial action potential plateau decreases in amplitude and duration (Hoffman and Suckling, 1954; Gibbs and Johnson, 1961; Paula Carvalho, 1972). On the other hand, the excitability of partially depolarized tissue, in which slow responses are the only form of electrical activity, is much lower than that of normally polarized tissue. Thus, a possible explanation for the result shown in Figure 2F is that, at a low frequency, the normal atrial action potential was not a source strong enough to stimulate the slow response. This point was checked by experiments in which action potentials recorded from the central compartment were taken as representative of the actual waveshape invading the test compartment. Figure 3 shows that, as frequency decreased from 0.33 Hz *(A)* to 0.13 and 0.11 Hz, the normal (middle compartment) action potential plateau became progressively lower. In this particular experiment, a slow response was evoked at frequencies down to 0.13 Hz and failed at 0.11 Hz.

This kind of result is clearly suggestive of the importance of the shape of the invading action potential for determining whether or not activity will propagate into the slow response region. Therefore, it would be reasonable to expect that the ability to invade the slow response region would be equally affected by other experimental manipulations altering the plateau. Two such situations were checked.

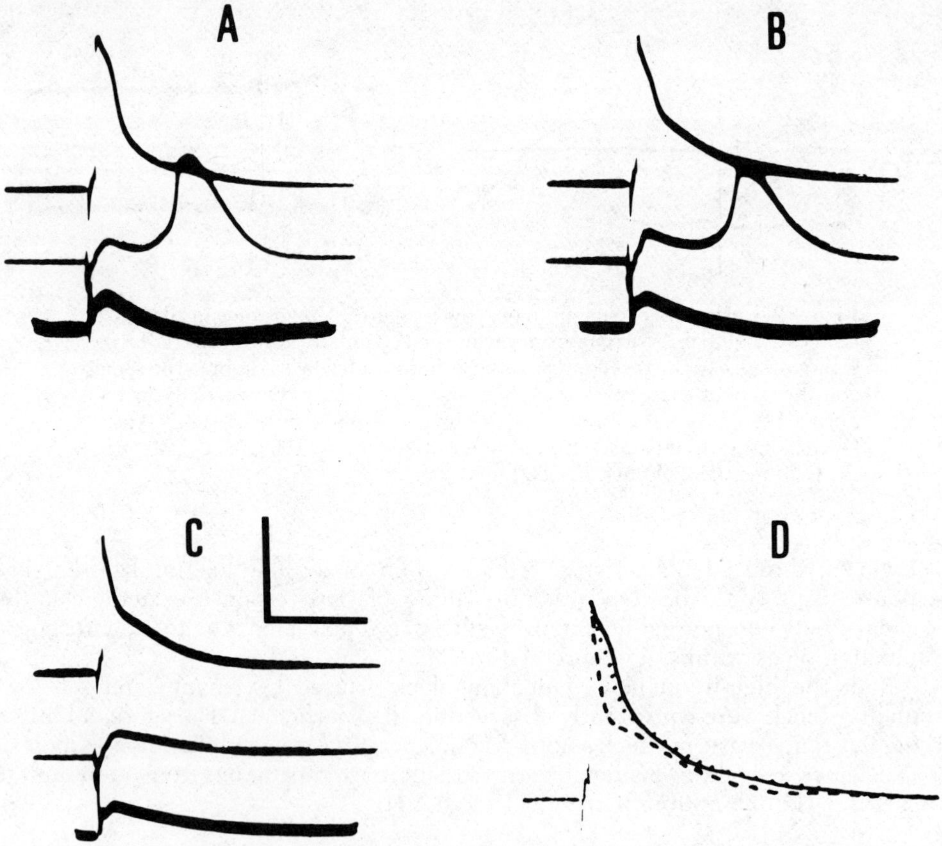

Figure 3. Influence of the invading action potential shape on the stimulation of slow responses. Upper trace, intracellular recording from the middle chamber. Middle trace, intracellular recording from the TKBa chamber. Lower trace, extracellular recording from the control chamber. *A*, 0.33 Hz; *B*, 0.2 Hz; *C*, 0.1 Hz; *D*, superimposition, *A* ——— *B* ···· *C* ---- . Calibration, 60 mV (intracellular recording) and 200 ms.

The effect of acetylcholine (ACh) is a typical situation under which the plateau of normal atrial action potential is reduced. Figure 4 shows the results of an experiment in which ACh was added to the middle chamber in a final concentration of 20 μg/ml, which is enough to block the plateau of normal atrial action potential (Hoffman and Cranefield, 1960).

After the application of ACh, slow-response stimulation by normal propagated activity became critical. The irregularly shaped slow response in Figure 4B indicates the appearance of a slight wavefront asynchrony. Excitation difficulty became more pronounced, in Figure 4C, where at first the only sign of activity was a depolarization of

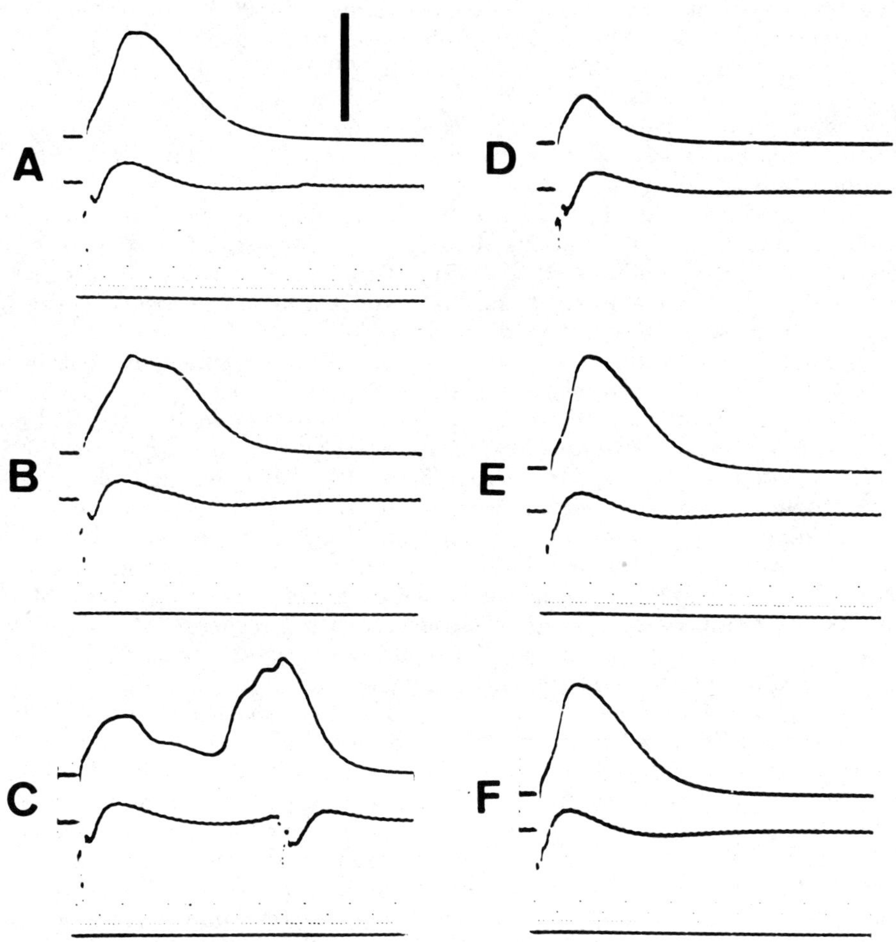

Figure 4. Effect of acetylcholine in the middle chamber. Upper trace, intracellular recording from the TKBa chamber. Middle trace, extracellular recording from the control chamber. Lower trace, time calibration: 100 ms. Between *A* and *B*, acetylcholine was added to the middle chamber. *B*, *C* and *D*, subsequent cycles after application of the drug. Observe rebound to the normal region in *C*. *E*, after acetylcholine washout. *F*, sixth cycle after application of D-600 to the middle chamber. Vertical calibration bar: 50 mV.

small amplitude that could be interpreted as a simple electrotonic reflection of the activity in neighboring regions. But, slow-response activity, which had been started or recirculated somewhere in the TKBa region, reached the recording site once again and propagated backwards to the normal chamber (as shown by the surface electrogram). Figure 4D shows that stimulation of slow response in the TKBa chamber stopped by the sixth cycle after ACh was applied.

To determine whether such blockade of the slow response is due to the shortening of the normal action potential induced by ACh or to its leakage into the TKBa chamber (which would cause direct inhibition of the slow response), we applied D-600 to the middle chamber in a final concentration of 1 μg/ml in the same experiment. In presence of leakage of D-600, slow response would certainly be blocked while in absence of leakage no change is to be expected since D-600 has only a minor effect on the normal action potential. The result was that no change in the slow response was observed throughout the application of D-600 (see Fig. 4F).

Therefore, we came to the conclusion that the application of acetylcholine, by shortening the duration of the normal action potential, makes it unable to stimulate slow responses at a frequency at which, under normal conditions, it would be an effective stimulus.

It is now important to ascertain whether changes in the time course of the invading action potential are the sole determinant of success in the excitation of a slow response in the TKBa-depressed area. To test this point, we used the fact that early extrasystoles often show a longer and higher plateau than the basic cycle response (Gibbs and Johnson, 1961; Edmands et al., 1966).

Figure 5 shows results of such an experiment. Normal action potentials from the middle chamber and the corresponding slow responses from a cell in the TKBa region were recorded. In panel A, the preparation was stimulated at 1.25 Hz, and normal action potentials with a well-developed plateau were seen to propagate into the TKBa region, eliciting a slow response at each cycle. Panel B shows that when the same preparation was stimulated at a lower frequency (0.2 Hz) slow responses were no longer stimulated. Concomitantly, the characteristic low-frequency depression of the normal AP plateau was observed. At this point, an extra pulse was coupled to each basic drive at an interval of 450 msec, and successive cycles were recorded. Figure 5C shows the first cycle of paired stimulation. Observe that the response AP_2 to the second stimulus has roughly the same time course as the normal action potential in panel A does. But, although the action potential in panel A propagated into the TKBa region and elicited a slow response, AP_2 in panel C failed to do so. Instead, it only induced a subthreshold depolarization with a larger amplitude and longer duration than did the one induced by the first action potential of the pair (AP_1). At the second paired cycle, the subthreshold depolarization caused by AP_2 increased even further and eventually led to a delayed slow response (panel D). In other experiments, a slow response was stimulated only between the third and fifth cycles after paired stimulation was started. Meanwhile, a progressive increase in the amplitude and duration of the subthreshold depolarization was seen to occur from cycle to cycle. As a consequence, the delay in the appearance of the slow response after AP_2 was much longer in the second cycle than it was when the preparation was stimulated at a higher rate (see panel A). Eventually, the delay became stabilized within a few cycles (three to six cycles); in panel E, the slow response was stimulated with a steady delay after each AP_2.

Note that in all cases, the plateau in AP_1 was very much lowered. In fact, the cycle length at 0.2 Hz was so long (5 sec) that the application of the paired stimulus S_2 did not alter the shape of AP_1 in the following cycle (compare panels B and C).

The results in Figure 5, C–E, indicate that, once the preparation becomes quiescent, a simple restoration of the time course of the stimulating action potential is

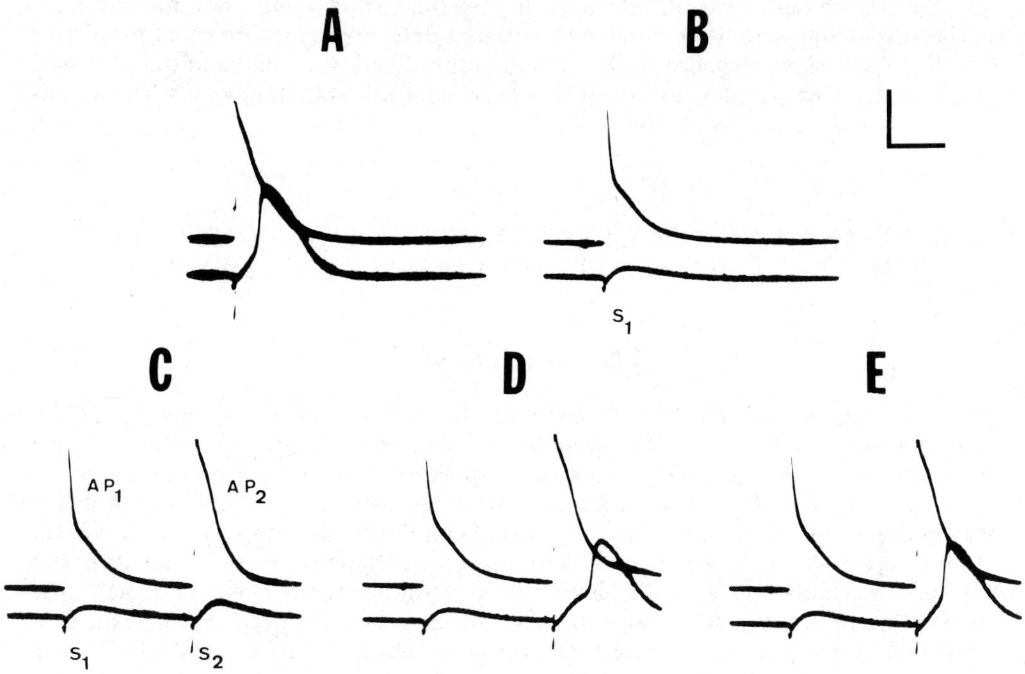

Figure 5. Effect of paired stimulation. Intracellular recording from the central chamber (upper trace) and TKBa chamber (lower trace). Microelectrodes kept in the same cells from *A* to *E*. *A*, stimulation at 1.25 Hz showing normal action potential and slow response. *B*, at 0.2 Hz, slow response is not stimulated by AP_1. *C*, *D* and *E* are subsequent sweeps after the onset of paired stimulation. Calibration: 40 mV for upper trace and 20 mV for lower trace. Horizontal, 200 msec.

not enough to ensure its propagation into the depressed region. It takes a few cycles for an action potential with a well-developed plateau to effectively stimulate the slow response area. Also, interestingly, the extra pulses generate subthreshold depolarizations that increase in amplitude and duration from cycle to cycle until they become able to stimulate slow responses. Under such circumstances, the slow response first appears after a considerable delay, but this delay becomes progressively shorter until it reaches a steady value, which persists for all the following cycles. It is as if the first extra pulses, though unable to stimulate a slow response, induce some kind of excitability enhancement. Such enhancement would persist and accumulate from one cycle to the next until a level was reached at which the slow response threshold could be reached by a normal action potential wavefront.

We could therefore suggest that the subthreshold depolarization is actually a measure of the excitability of the slow response at that moment, although in a large preparation like ours this could be masked by electrotonic reflections of slow responses occurring around that region. Cukierman and Paes de Carvalho (1982), working under almost perfect space-clamp conditions, showed results very similar to those described in this section and ascribed them to an excitability characteristic of TKBa depressed tissue.

So, at this point, we could conclude that the time course (amplitude and duration) of the stimulating action potential is essential in determining its ability to propagate into the TKBa slow-response region. On the other hand, we could add that rate and rhythm also seem to play an essential role in determining whether a stimulus can effectively induce a slow response.

RATE AND RHYTHM DEPENDENCY OF THE EXCITABILITY OF ELECTRICALLY STIMULATED SLOW RESPONSES

Low Frequency Block

Slow-response excitation seems to be affected both by the rate and rhythm and by the time course of the normal action potential. To further distinguish between these two influences, we perfused a whole strip of left atrial roof, as homogeneous as possible, in a single chamber bath and stimulated it directly by current pulses in such a way as to permit independent manipulation of amplitude, duration, and frequency of stimuli. We took special care to make sure that conduction problems did not affect the results. To achieve this goal, we chose only structurally homogeneous preparations. Also, recordings were made at two different sites of each preparation. The first (proximal) site was as close as possible to the stimulating electrode (within 100 μm or less); the second (distal) electrode was placed far from the stimulating point but on the same muscle bundle, so that conduction problems could be easily detected from the delay between the activation of the two points.

Figure 6 shows results obtained in a typical experiment. The upper trace is the recording from the proximal electrode, and the lower trace is that from the distal electrode. Panel A shows records obtained as the preparation was driven at 1 Hz (cycle length, 1 sec), with pulses of 34 V and 10 msec (read at the output of the type 2533 Devices stimulator). Under this condition, the slow response was stimulated at all cycles. When the frequency was lowered to 0.5 Hz (cycle length, 2 sec), the amplitude and duration of the stimulus remaining the same; the slow response was no longer stimulated (panel B). Although this condition was maintained for at least 5 min, slow responses did not reappear (low frequency block).

If stimulus duration was next increased from 10 to 15 msec and frequency maintained at 0.5 Hz (cycle length, 2 sec), the slow response reappeared (Fig. 6C). Three minutes later (Fig. 6D), stimulus duration was restored back to 10 msec. In successive cycles, the delay between the stimulus artifact and the slow response in the proximal microelectrode increased progressively until it finally disappeared completely at the sixth cycle. It seems as though, in time, the depressed tissue became progressively less excitable, down to a point where the electrical pulse was no longer sufficient to stimulate the slow response. As long as nothing was altered, the preparation stayed quiescent. In Figure 6E, stimulus amplitude was increased from 34 to 37 V, duration and frequency remaining the same. The slow response was again stimulated.

Even though the delay between stimulus artifact and slow response in the proximal recording site increased progressively during successive cycles, no significant change was observed in the conduction time between the proximal and the distal points. This observation gives support to the fact that the low frequency block, at least when one is dealing with a structurally uniform preparation, is actually related to slow-response excitability and not to the conduction process.

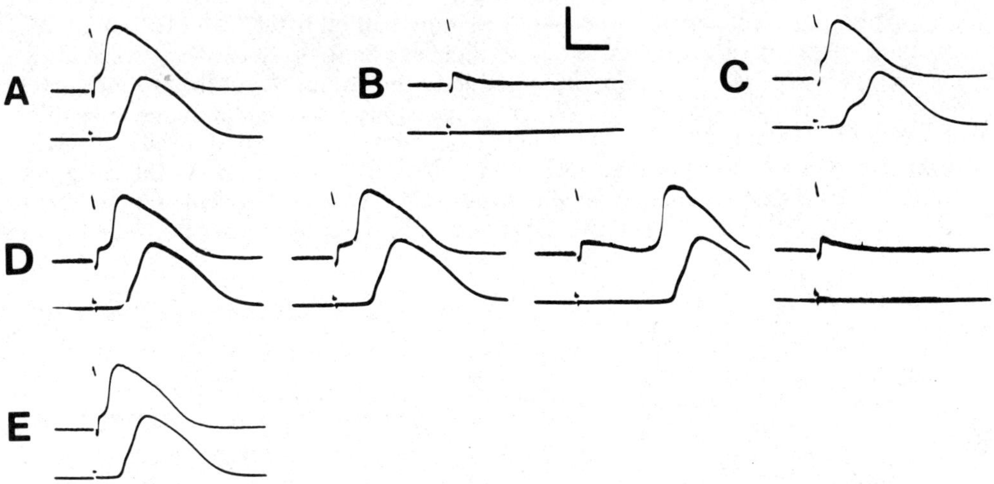

Figure 6. Effect of duration, amplitude and frequency of direct electrical stimulation on the slow response. A whole strip of left atrial muscle was perfused by TKBa and stimulated by current pulses, with varying frequencies, amplitude and duration. Records were made from two different cells, along the propagation pathway. The stimulation parameters were as follows: *A*, 1 Hz (T = 1 s); St = 34 V × 10 ms. *B*, 0.5 Hz (T = 2 s); St = 34 V × 10 ms. *C*, 0.5 Hz (T = 2 s); St = 34 V × 15 ms. *D*, 0.5 Hz (T = 2 s); St = 34 V × 10 ms. *E*, 0.5 Hz (T = 2 s); St = 37 V × 10 ms. Calibration: vertical, 40 mV; horizontal: 50 ms.

Also, once a preparation was effectively stimulated at a given frequency, a sudden reduction in the duration or amplitude of the stimulating pulse did not lead to a sudden cessation of the slow response (Fig. 6). It usually took several cycles for the slow response to disappear, as if a sudden stimulus reduction caused a progressive decrease of excitability. Again, it is as if a sufficiently strong stimulus enhances the excitability and, the cycle length being short enough for the next cycle to come before this enhanced state disappears, excitability builds up to a steady, higher level at which the slow response is stimulated at every cycle. As the stimulus is reduced, such enhancement also decreases, causing a progressive decrease of membrane excitability, until the process stabilizes at a new, lower, level. If this level is too low for a given duration, amplitude, and frequency of stimulus, the slow response is no longer stimulated. After cessation, slow responses can be readily reestablished by increasing any of the three parameters above. An increase in frequency reduces the delay between two successive cycles and decreases the delay of the enhanced state, whereas an increase in duration or amplitude increases enhancement in each cycle.

The results in Figures 5 and 6 demonstrate the interplay among these four stimulation parameters: duration, amplitude, rhythm, and frequency.

High Frequency Block

It has been mentioned already that when the slow response is stimulated by a normal action potential above a certain frequency, let's say 1 Hz, conduction block appears. One example is the 2:1 block shown in Fig. 2A. In this section, we describe conduction blocks observed in preparations fully bathed in TKBa and stimulated by current pulses directly applied to one of their extremities. Recordings were always made from two cells, one as close as possible to the stimulus and the second further away on the same muscle bundle. When the preparations were stimulated at frequencies around 1 Hz (as in Fig. 7A), recordings from both sites indicated, in all cycles, slow responses of about the same normal amplitude and time course. As the frequency increased, the first change to be observed was the delay between the two sites. Observe that, although at 1 Hz (Fig. 7A) there was a delay of 78 msec between the two

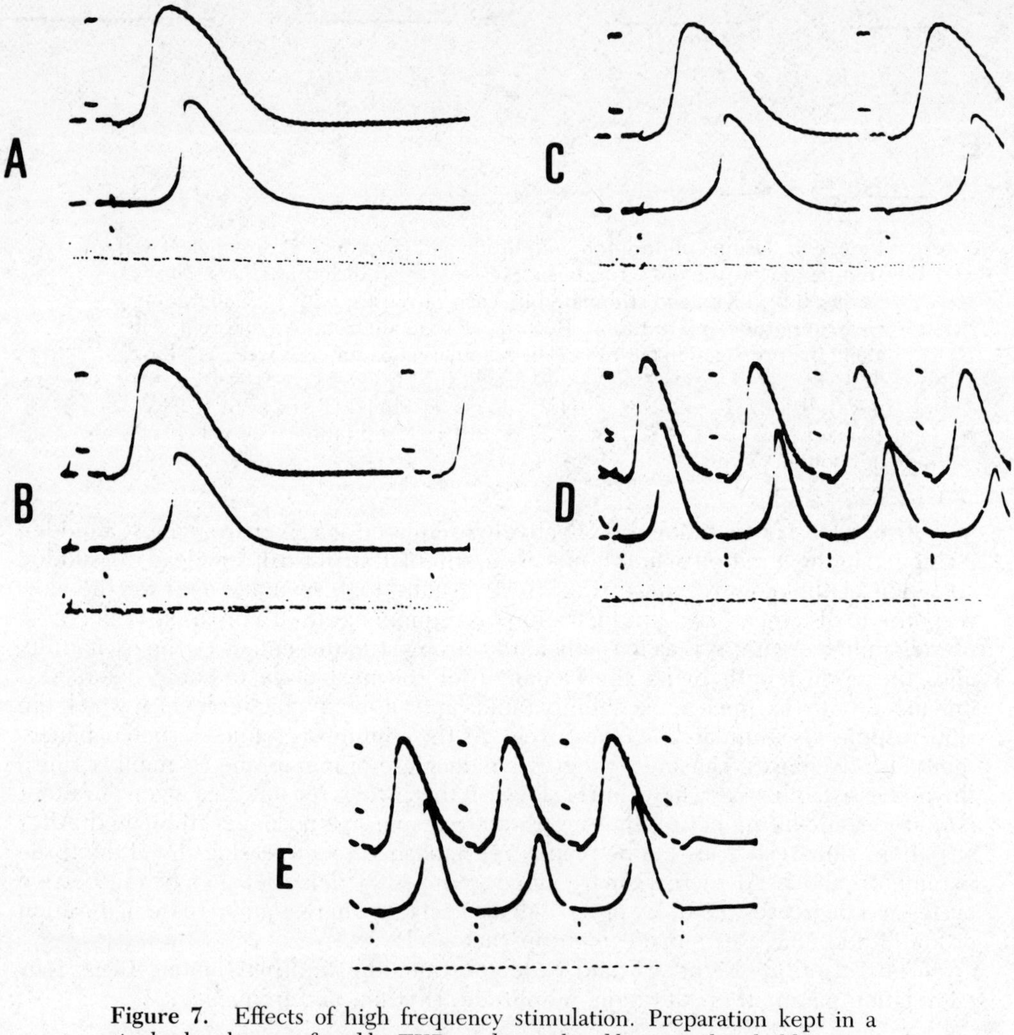

Figure 7. Effects of high frequency stimulation. Preparation kept in a single chamber, perfused by TKBa and stimulated by suprathreshold rectangular pulses applied through a small pipette. Records obtained from two different cells, one as close as possible to the point of stimulation, the second, away from the first, on the same strand of fibers. *A*, preparation stimulated at 1 Hz; *B*, at 1.25 Hz; *C*, 1.67 Hz and *D* and *E*, at 2 Hz. All pictures taken from the same penetrations. Calibration: vertical, 50 mV and horizontal, 100 ms for the larger distance between successive points, in the lower trace of each figure.

slow responses (measured at 50% depolarization), at 1.67 Hz (Fig. 7C), this delay increased to 115 msec. At each frequency, however, the delay stabilized at a constant value for all cycles. As frequency was increased further, fatigue became even more pronounced. Figure 7D shows that the delays between the activation times of the two sites were much longer at a higher rate than they were at a lower rate and also that they varied cumulatively from cycle to cycle. The amplitude of the slow response in the second site decreased from cycle to cycle, until the response was barely able to reach the distal recording site by the fourth cycle. Figure 7E, which is a continuation of the situation in panel D, shows a progressive conduction delay that ended up with the fourth stimulus being too early to stimulate a slow response even in the proximal site.

Paes de Carvalho and Almeida (1960) and Paes de Carvalho (1961; 1966) had already described precisely this same behavior for the AV node. This effect has been attributed to the extremely slow recovery of excitability exhibited by the AV node action potential (Merideth et al., 1968).

Figure 8 shows an experiment similar to that of Merideth et al. (1968). The experimental arrangement was the same as it was in Fig. 7, except that the stimulus in this case was barely threshold. The preparation was driven at a low rate (0.1 Hz) and an extra stimulus (S_2) with the same intensity and duration but with different delays from the basic stimulus was applied. Observe that, in Figures 8, A and B, when S_2 was applied during the slow response itself, no activity was induced, as expected. In Figure

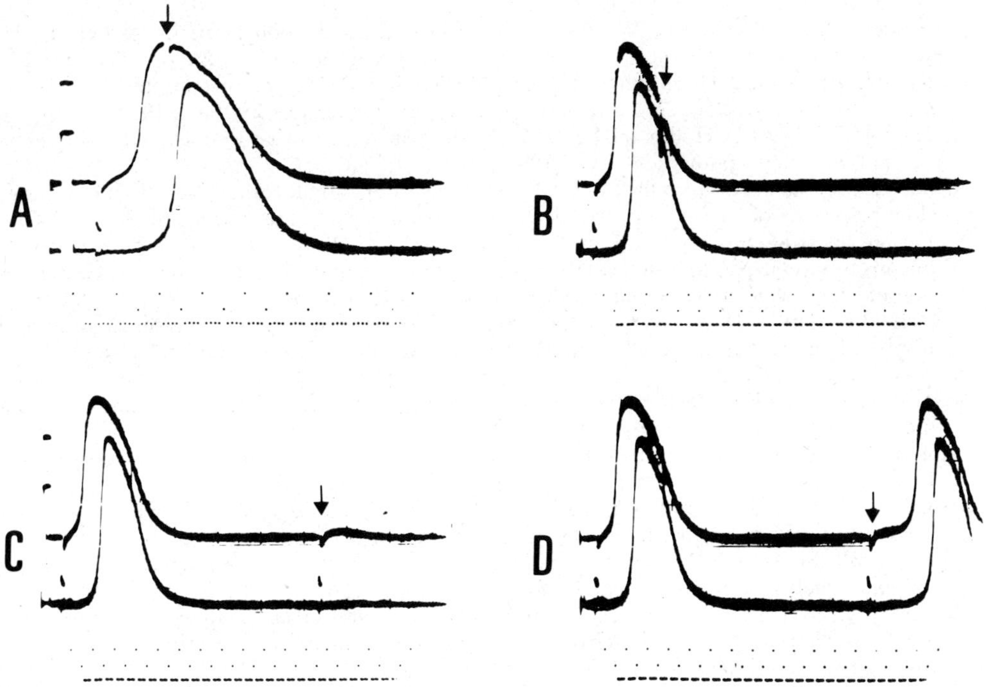

Figure 8. Relative refractory period of the slow response. Experimental conditions as in Figure 5, except stimulus intensity which was, in this case, nearly threshold. Preparation driven at a basic frequency of 0.1 Hz (T = 10 s). An extra stimulus S_2, with the same characteristics as the basic stimulus, is applied with different delays as indicated by arrows. In *A*, S_2 was applied 170 ms after S_1; in *B*, 330 ms; in *C*, 1200 ms and in *D*, 1300 ms. Calibration: 50 mV and 100 ms.

8C, S_2, applied 1200 msec after S_1, was still unable to elicit a new response. Only when S_2 was applied 100 msec later was it able to induce a slow response.

Our conclusion, therefore, is that the high frequency block is mainly due to the slowness of recovery of excitability after a slow response has been induced. Thus, unlike the low frequency block, which does not depend on the presence of the slow response, the high frequency block is intimately associated with the previous occurrence of a slow response in that tissue.

REFERENCES

Aronson RS, Cranefield PF (1973) The electrical activity of canine cardiac Purkinje fibers in sodium free calcium rich solutions. J Gen Physiol **61**:786–808

Carmeliet E, von Bogaert PP (1969) Strontium action potentials in cardiac Purkinje fibers. Arch Int Physiol Biochim **77**:134–135

Carmeliet E, Vereecke J (1969) Adrenaline and the plateau phase of the cardiac action potential. Pflüg Arch **313**:300–315

Cranefield PF (1975) The Conduction of the Cardiac Impulse. Mt Kisco, NY, Futura Publishing Company

Cranefield PF, Hoffman BF, Paes de Carvalho A (1959) Effects of acetylcholine on single fibers of the atrioventricular node. Circ Res **7**:19–23

Cranefield PF, Hoffman BF, Wit AL (1971*a*) Block of conduction in partially depolarized cardiac Purkinje fibers induced by an α-adrenergic agent. Nature New Biology **234**:159–160

Cranefield PF, Klein HO, Hoffman BF (1971*b*) Conduction of the cardiac impulse: I. Delay, block and one way block in depressed Purkinje fibers. Circ Res **28**:199–219

Cranefield PF, Wit AL, Hoffman BF (1972) Conduction of the cardiac impulse, III. Characteristics of very slow conduction. J Gen Physiol **59**:227–246

Cukierman S, Paes de Carvalho A (1982) Frequency dependent excitability of "membrane" slow responses of rabbit left atrial trabeculae in presence of Ba^{2+} and high K^+. J Gen Physiol (in press)

Edmands R, Greenspan K, Fisch C (1966) Effect of cycle length alteration upon the configuration of canine ventricular action potential. Circ Res **19**:602–610

Engstfeld G, Antoni H, Fleckenstein A (1961) Die Restitution der Erregungsfortleitung und Kontraktionskraft des K^+-gelähmten Frosch-und Säugetiermyokards durch Adrenalin. Pflüg Arch **273**:145–163

Gibbs CL, Johnson EA (1961) Effect of changes in frequency of stimulation upon rabbit ventricular action potential. Circ Res **9**:165–170

Hoffman BF, Cranefield PF (1960) Electrophysiology of the Heart. New York, McGraw Hill Book Co

Hoffman BF, Paes de Carvalho A, de Mello WC, Cranefield PF (1959) Electrical activity of single fibers of atrioventricular node. Circ Res **7**:11–18

Hoffman BF, Suckling EE (1954) Effect of heart rate on cardiac membrane potentials and the unipolar electrogram. Am J Physiol **179**:123–130

Janse MJ, van Capelle FJL, Freud GE, Durrer D (1971) Circus movement within the AV node as a basis for supraventricular tachycardia as shown by multiple microelectrode recording in the isolated rabbit heart. Circ Res **28**:403–414

Lenfant J, Mironneau J, Gargouil YM, Galand G (1968) Analyse de l'activité électrique spontannée du centre de l'automatisme cardiaque de lapin par les inhibiteurs de perméabilités membranaires. C R Acad Sci (D) (Paris) **266**:901–904

Lewartowski B, Czarnecke M, Zielinski A (1969) Adaptation pattern of cellular action potentials of rabbit atria to the changes in rate and rhythm of stimulation. Acta Physiol Acad Sci Hung **36**:335–341

Mascher D (1970) Electrical and mechanical responses from ventricular muscle fibers after inactivation of the sodium carrying system. Pflüg Arch **317**:359–372

Mascher D, Peper K (1969) Two components of inward current in myocardial muscle fibers. Pflüg Arch **307**:190–203

Masuda MO (1976) Excitação e propagação da resposta lenta em miocárdio. PhD thesis presented to Universidade Federal do Rio de Janeiro

Masuda MO, Paes de Carvalho A (1982) Rate and rhythm dependency of propagation from normal myocardium to a Ba^{2+}, K^+ induced slow response zone in rabbit left atrium. Circ Res **50**:419–427

Matsuda K, Hoshi T, Kameyama S (1958) Action of acetylcholine and adrenaline upon membrane potential of the atrioventricular node. (Tawara) Tohoku J Exptl Med **68**:16

Méndez C, Moe GK (1966) Some characteristics of transmembrane potentials of AV nodal cells during propagation of premature beats. Circ Res **19**:993–1010

Méndez C, Moe GK (1972) Atrioventricular transmission. In Electrical Phenomena in the Heart, edited by WC de Mello. New York, Academic Press, pp 263–291

Merideth J, Méndez C, Mueller WJ, Moe GK (1968) Electrical excitability of atrioventricular nodal cells. Circ Res **23**:69–85

Paes de Carvalho A (1961) Cellular electrophysiology of the atrial specialized tissues. In The Specialized Tissues of the Heart, edited by A Paes de Carvalho, WC de Mello, BF Hoffman. Amsterdam, Elsevier, pp 115–130

Paes de Carvalho A (1964) Uma hipótese dualista do potencial de ação cardíaco: experimentos introdutórios. Thesis presented to Universidade Federal do Rio de Janeiro

Paes de Carvalho A (1966) Excitation of the atrioventricular node during normal rhythm. Effects of acetylcholine. In Mechanism and Therapy of Cardiac Arrhythmias, edited by LS Dreifus, W Likoff, JH Moyer. New York, Grune & Stratton, pp 341–352

Paes de Carvalho A, Almeida DF (1960) Spread of activity through the atrioventricular node. Circ Res **8**:801–809

Paes de Carvalho A, Hoffman BF, Carvalho MP (1969) Two components of the cardiac potential. I. Voltage time course and the effect of acetylcholine on atrial and nodal cells of the rabbit heart. J Gen Physiol **54**:607–635

Paes de Carvalho A, de Mello WC, Hoffman BF (1959) Electrophysiological evidence for specialized fiber types in rabbit atrium. Am J Physiol **196**:483–488

Paula Carvalho M (1972) Influência da frequência de estimulação sobre a forma do potencial de ação cardíaco. MS thesis presented to Universidade Federal do Rio de Janeiro

Paula Carvalho M (1977) Propagação da resposta lenta no miocárdio: bloqueios de condução. PhD thesis presented to Universidade Federal do Rio de Janeiro

Discussion

WEIDMANN: It's nice to have a heart with a memory. What about the possibility that the memory is adrenaline released by the electrical stimulus? The obvious experiments to perform to clear this question would be to use propranolol and see if the memory is still there.

MASUDA: Catecholamine release is certainly one possibility if we consider the direct stimulation experiments shown here. But, we should not expect an adrenaline release to influence much when the stimuli are weak (1.5 × threshold) and applied to the normal end of the preparation several millimeters away from the site of slow-response recording. For this reason, I do not believe that the "memory" effects shown here are caused by a local release of adrenaline. I wanted to point out that we also have obtained slow responses in left atrium immersed in 20 mM K^+ with adrenaline, and the memory effects are still there. In this case, you have just so much epinephrine in the bath that probably whatever you might release with a weak stimulation from nerve terminals may not make much of a difference.

BONKE: The results of your experiments with a three-compartment chamber did not show any electrotonic reflection of the slow response on the action potential recorded in the middle "normal compartment." I wonder how far within the depressed compartment were you recording the slow response.

MASUDA: The recording was performed between 5 and 10 mm away from the middle chamber in the experiments to which you refer. You are correct in noticing that the slow response, at this distance, is not electrotonically reflected in the normal middle compartment.

BONKE: Is the slow-response action potential really resulting from propagation through the middle chamber? To clarify this, you have to make recordings close to the boundary between the "depressed" and the middle compartment.

MASUDA: We have indeed obtained records of slow responses very near (less than 0.5 mm) the partition that separates the middle from the test chamber. Samples of such records are shown in Figures 4 and 5. Note that the action potential that propagates through the middle chamber sets up a local subliminal response in the depressed tissue at the entrance of the test chamber. The full slow-response arises from this subliminal response after a delay that depends both on action potential shape and repetition rate. There is, therefore, some degree of hesitation at the entrance of the slow-response zone. As to the propagation of the slow response in the test compartment, it proceeds with apparent homogeneity along a given muscle bundle (apparent conduction velocity, 0.04 to 0.08 m/sec). Dr. Paula Carvalho (1977), however, has shown in her Ph.D. thesis that considerable delays can occur among adjacent bundles, sometimes creating opportunities for reentry within the depressed region.

JOHNSON: If the propranolol experiment proposed by Weidmann still leaves you with a memory effect, I would like to recall a paper that Gibbs, Tille, and I published a long time ago on the plateau phase of the rabbit ventricular action potential. We were able to show that the plateau configuration depended very much on the previous history of excitation in that particular preparation. We can be pretty sure in that case that there was some sort of a memory there. Actually, that paper was entitled "An example of information retention in heart muscle."

CARMELIET: Let us accept the thesis that there is a memory effect. Do you have any working hypothesis as to what that memory is? Is there no change in membrane potential, for instance?

MASUDA: There is at short stimulus intervals a summation of subthreshold responses. Cukierman will show that clearly in his talk. But the memory effects I am talking about here are very long effects that take seconds to disappear. We have, at the moment, no guess as to its nature.

CRANEFIELD: My question is addressed to Carmeliet. Did you not see strontium action potentials that built up gradually as you started stimulating them?

CARMELIET: Yes, this is correct, and I think that Pappano has also seen a similar effect. But like Dr. Masuda, I have no idea as to what this may be due.

Chapter 23

Slow Response Excitation: Dependence on Rate and Rhythm*

Samuel Cukierman and Antonio Paes de Carvalho

Much evidence points toward the existence of two distinct depolarizing mechanisms in cardiac cell electrogenesis (Paes de Carvalho et al., 1966; 1969). The first mechanism, related to phase O (Weidmann, 1955), is a fast Na^+-dependent electrogenesis that may be blocked either pharmacologically by tetrodotoxin (Hagiwara and Nakajima, 1966) or inactivated by relatively low resting potentials (Weidmann, 1955). The second one is considered to be partially responsible for the plateau of normal cardiac action potentials and for the whole action potential in SA and AV nodes. This slow inward current (Beeler and Reuter, 1970; New and Trautwein, 1972; Reuter, 1973) has rather different kinetics from phase O electrogenesis and is not affected by tetrodotoxin, but can be blocked by drugs such as D-600 (see Cranefield, 1975) that do not primarily affect the rapid initial Na^+ current.

Under appropriate conditions it is possible to obtain tetrodotoxin-insensitive propagated action potentials (slow responses) in a variety of cardiac tissues (Cranefield, 1975). Among such conditions are the inactivation and/or block of the Na^+-dependent rising phase and the stimulation of slow inward channels. Several treatments have been used for slow-response excitation (Cranefield, 1975). In this study, we used 1 mM Ba^{2+} and an increased extracellular K^+ concentration (10 mM) in Tyrode's solution (TKBa solution). Ba^{2+} is known to substitute for Ca^{2+} in transporting charges across excitable membranes (Reuter, 1973); also, it has a blocking effect on g_K (Sperelakis et al., 1967; Hermsmeyer and Sperelakis, 1970), increasing membrane resistance and decreasing the resting potential. Both effects facilitate slow-response excitation.

In large ribbons of rabbit atrial tissue, TKBa slow responses propagated with the expected decrease in conduction velocity (around 0.05 m/sec) and exhibited peculiar excitable characteristics (Masuda, 1976; Paula Carvalho, 1977; Masuda and Paes de Carvalho, 1982). Those studies suggested that slow response excitability depends on pacing frequency. Also, previous excitation history was considered important in terms of eliciting the slow response. Such results could not be clearly interpreted in the large atrial preparations used in their studies, as it has been difficult to ascertain whether

*Supported by CEPG/UFRJ, SEPLAN/CNPq and SEPLAN/FINEP, Brazil.

such peculiarities are related to the excitability properties of slow response or to possible interferences connected with conduction disorders.

We developed a preparation (Cukierman, 1978; Cukierman and Paes de Carvalho, 1982), the isolated rabbit left atrial trabecula, that, when immersed in TKBa solution, can generate "membrane" slow responses. In the absence of propagation, we studied the frequency-dependence of slow response excitability. In this chapter, we discuss some of these properties.

METHODS

Small (2- to 3-mm-long, 0.4- to 0.8-mm-wide) atrial trabeculae were dissected free from the rabbit left atrium. One end of the trabecula was fixed to the bath's floor. The other end was held onto a glass suction electrode (internal tip diameter, 0.6 mm) filled with normal or modified (TKBa) Tyrode solution. The suction electrode was connected to a DC-isolated stimulator unit by means of an Ag/AgCl wire. The stimulating circuit was closed by means of an Ag/AgCl electrode immersed in the bath. Current was measured as the voltage drop across a known resistor and was displayed on a dual-beam oscilloscope (Tektronix 565). Conventional KCl-filled glass capillary microelectrodes (DC resistance: 15 to 20 MΩ) were used for recording intracellular potentials. The recordings were referenced to bath earth. To measure the preparation length constant, transmembrane passive electrotonus were obtained differentially between an intracellular and a similar extracellular microelectrode. The extracellular microelectrode was positioned as close as possible to the intracellular one so that no voltage deflections would be obtained from the neighboring extracellular space when the intracellular microelectrode was withdrawn. Microelectrodes were led through Ag/AgCl interfaces to input capacitance-compensating preamplifiers. All the recordings were displayed on the oscilloscope, and photographs were taken of the screen.

The following solutions were used: *normal Tyrode's solution*, composed of 137 mM NaCl, 2.7 mM KCl, 2.7 mM $CaCl_2$, 0.5 mM $MgCl_2$, 12 mM $NaHCO_3$, 1.8 mM NaH_2PO_4, and 6 mM dextrose; and a *high K^+, Ba^{2+} Tyrode's solution (TKBa)*, composed of 129.7 mM NaCl, 10 mM KCl, and 1 mM $BaCl_2$, with other constituents unaltered. These solutions were bubbled with 95% O_2 and 5% CO_2 and then warmed to allow a final bath temperature of 35 to 36° C. The pH was 7.1 to 7.2. The bath was continuously perfused at a rate of 3 ml/min.

RESULTS

Electrophysiological Characteristics of Left Atrial Trabeculae in Normal Tyrode's and TKBa Solutions

In normal Tyrode's solution, under the suction electrode method of stimulation, action potentials propagated with the usual velocities of 0.65 ± 0.20 m/sec (N=14) (mean ± SD, and N being the number of experiments). The amplitude and configuration of the action potential were similar to those previously described in rabbit atrial tissue (Hoffman and Cranefield, 1960). Length constant measurements obtained with subliminal pulses in isolated left atrial trabeculae indicated a value of 1.10 ± 0.19 mm (N=9) (Cukierman and Paes de Carvalho, 1982).

On changing from normal Tyrode's to TKBa solution, the following electrical parameters were altered: *(1)* The resting potential decreased from −80.3 ± 5.1 (*N*=20) to −55.0 ± 2.3 mV (*N*=15). *(2)* The total action potential amplitude decreased from 104.2 ± 7.7 (*N*=20) to 60.2 ± 3.4 mV (*N*=15). *(3)* The action potential duration (measured at half amplitude) increased from 28.1 ± 11.6 (*N*=20) to 83.7 ± 18.7 msec (*N*=15). The action potential obtained in TKBa solution (slow response) was also of a different quality from that present in normal Tyrode's solution: it was insensitive to tetrodotoxin (10 μg/ml) and could be readily abolished by D-600 (3 μg/ml) or acetylcholine (10 μg/ml) (Cukierman, 1978).

Figure 1, A and B, shows pairs of simultaneous recordings of stimulated TKBa slow responses in different trabeculae. In each panel, the upper trace corresponds to the current pulse, the two middle traces are intracellular recordings from different cells (interelectrode distance, 2.0 mm in Fig. 1A, 1.2 mm in Fig. 1B), and the bottom trace is the high-gain voltage difference between the two intracellular records. As shown, slow response upstrokes occurred at the same time at different points along the trabecula. This result was consistently observed in all trabeculae studied and was found to be independent of stimulus characteristics (intensity, duration, and pacing frequency). No extracellular potential changes were detected on the surface of these trabeculae during slow response activity. Both findings suggest that the preparation behaves in a uniform way, that is, the entire trabecula develops an upstroke simultaneously. No conduction velocity measurements could be made, and the trabecular slow response can therefore be regarded as a "membrane" action potential.

The passive response to a subliminal current pulse indicated no electrotonic decay along different trabeculae. Because of this space uniformity, we could not measure in these preparations any length constant, and so we assumed it to be much longer than the preparation length (Cukierman and Paes de Carvalho, 1982). The spatial homogeneity of the preparation when immersed in TKBa solution makes it suitable for studies of the basic excitable mechanisms of the slow response.

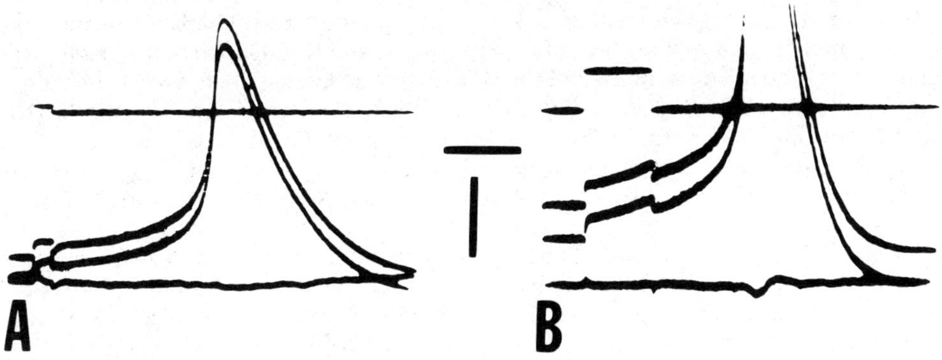

Figure 1. "Membrane" slow responses from different trabeculae (*A* & *B*). Upper trace is current pulse, middle traces are slow response recordings from two different cells (interelectrode distance 2.0 mm for *A* and 1.2 mm for *B*) and lower trace is the difference record between the two simultaneous intracellular potentials. Calibration: horizontal (50 ms, *A*; 100 ms, *B*); vertical (20 mV, *A*; 7.7 mV, *B*); difference record: 8.7 mV (*A* & *B*); current strength (90 μA, *A*; 35 μA, *B*).

Stimulus Requirements for Slow Response Activity

Excitability is usually described by means of strength-duration curves. In normal Tyrode's solution, the rheobase and chronaxie for stimuli that depolarize the suctioned portion of the trabecula typically have values of 3.1 μA and 0.9 msec, respectively; under this condition (with a suction pipette as a cathode), charge requirements have been found to be less than they are with reverse polarity (Cukierman and Paes de Carvalho, 1982).

Slow response excitation requires stronger stimuli. In rested (quiescent for 30 to 40 sec) preparations immersed in TKBa solution, rheobase and chronaxie increase almost ten times. The condition under which stimulation requirements are least however, is the hyperpolarization (suction pipette as anode) of the suctioned portion of the trabecula. This condition leads to slow response excitation because it depolarizes in a spatially uniform way the larger portion of the preparation outside the suction pipette (Cukierman and Paes de Carvalho, 1982). Depolarization of the suctioned portion of the trabecula can stimulate slow response activity only through anodal-break excitation at the free segment of the trabecula.

Effects of Stimulation Frequency on Slow Response Excitability

Figure 2 illustrates what happens to slow response activity when the frequency of stimulation is altered. The middle traces on panels A to C show that as pacing frequency is reduced (from 1 Hz in Fig. 2A to 0.33 Hz in Fig. 2C), with the strength and duration (not shown) of the stimulus remaining the same, the stabilized slow-response (after two to three stimulation cycles) latency increases. The bottom trace, which corresponds to the first time derivative of the slow response, indicates that the decrease in stimulation frequency is followed by an increase in the maximum rate of rise (dV/dt). Panels D to F show that the peak dV/dt is not related to latency itself but to stimulation frequency. Here, slow-response latency was altered by reducing current strength (from D to F) at the same pacing frequency of 1 Hz. Peak dV/dt is shown to be unaltered. Figure 2 shows that the slow-response upstroke is not initiated from a stable resting potential. All panels show a small depolarizing step, similar to a diastolic depolarization, that mediates between the stimulus and the slow response itself. This depolarizing step is a determinant of the slow-response latency, because no difference in the slow-response voltage threshold is observable. We call this depolarizing step the *subliminal response.* Figure 2 also shows that the shortening of slow-response latency at higher frequencies is not due to an enhancement of the slow-response depolarizing mechanism, as the slow-response upstroke velocity is shown to decrease in this condition.

Figure 3, A and B, shows that frequency-dependent phenomena occur at the onset of stimulation in a preparation that has been previously rested for 60 sec. In panel A, the upper trace corresponds to the current pulse and the lower trace to superimposed intracellular recordings during the first four successive stimulation cycles. As shown, latencies shortened progressively until a minimum stable value was obtained after four to eight cycles. This behavior is the *latency adaptation phenomenon.* Also shown, the upward inflection leading to the upstroke of the slow-response occurred at the same voltage in all cycles. What seemed to vary from cycle to cycle was the subliminal response, a shortened latency being a direct consequence of the temporal evolution of the subliminal response. Up to a certain cycle number, determined by the stimulation frequency, the subliminal response became faster cycle after cycle, bringing the membrane potential to the slow-response threshold voltage earlier. Figure 3B, which shows data for another preparation, shows that the decrease in latency during

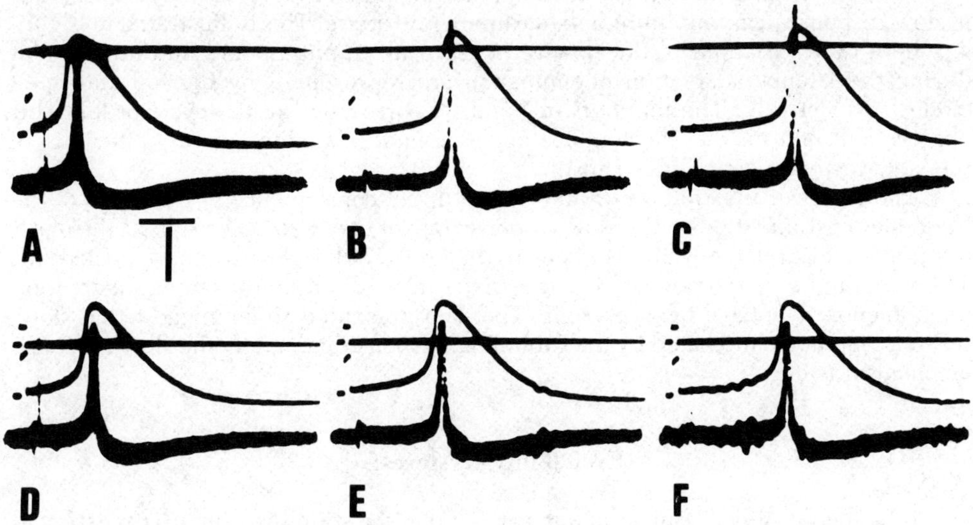

Figure 2. Relationship between pacing frequency and slow response latency and upstroke velocity. The upper trace is the current pulse (only for *D*, *E* & *F*), the middle trace is the intracellular recording and the lower trace is the first time derivative of the intracellular recording. *A*, *B* & *C*: maintaining the same current strength (not shown), the pacing frequency is altered from 1 Hz (*A*) to 0.5 Hz (*B*) and 0.33 Hz (*C*). *D*, *E* & *F*: same pacing frequency (1 Hz), but current strength is reduced from *D* to *F*. Calibration: horizontal, 90 ms; vertical, 35 mV, 1.8 V/s and 800 μA.

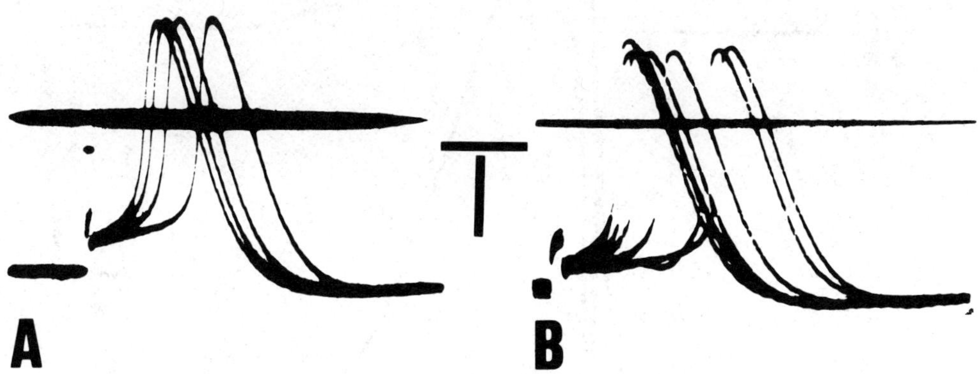

Figure 3. Intracellular recordings during latency adaptation phenomena in two different preparations (*A* & *B*). Calibration: horizontal, 200 ms; vertical, 20 mV and 200 μA (only for *A*).

the latency adaptation phenomenon does not always progress monotonically. Sometimes oscillations in latency occurred, even though this was a rare event. As shown, the second and third cycles developed upstrokes at longer intervals, compared with the first cycle.

The latency adaptation phenomenon is accompanied by a cycle-to-cycle decrease in slow-response peak amplitude and maximum rate of rise. This is illustrated in Figure 4, where time variations of the slow-response peak amplitude and maximum dV/dt during the latency adaptation phenomenon are represented by the full and open circles, respectively. The numbers in Figure 4 correspond to the cycle order. This observation confirms that shortened latencies are not related to a greater efficiency of the slow-response gating mechanism.

The behavior illustrated in Figure 4 is a direct consequence of the effect of the frequency of stimulation on the slow-response rate of rise (Fig. 2, A to C). At the onset of stimulation at relatively low frequencies (below 0.17 Hz), slow-response peak dV/dt and peak amplitude did not vary in successive cycles. Even so, the latency adaptation phenomenon may have been present. The data presented so far suggest that slow-response latency is mediated by the subliminal response and not by the slow-response mechanism itself.

Excitability Hysteresis

It has been noticed (Paula Carvalho, 1977) that the stimulus strength necessary to bring the rested atrial preparation into activity (I_{To}) is higher than what would be necessary to maintain activity after adaptation to a given rate ($I_{T\infty}$). This observation

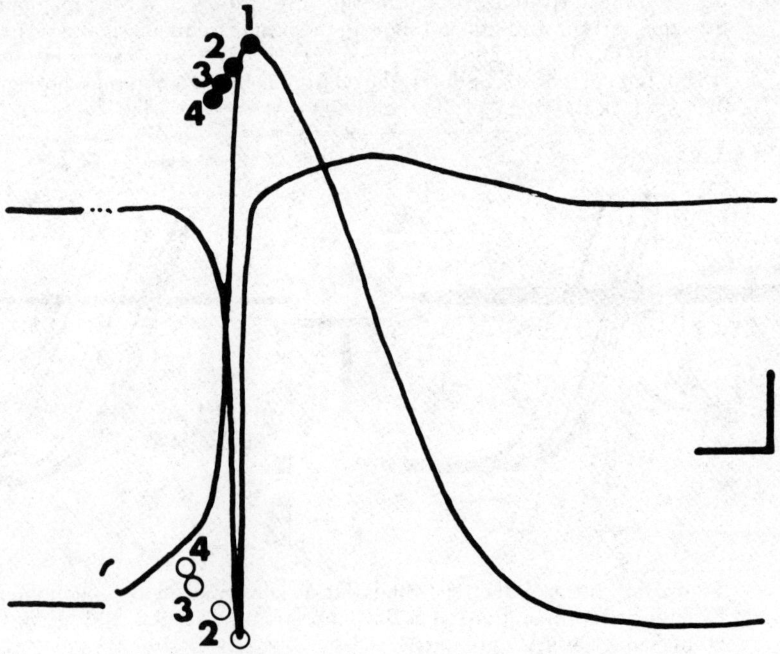

Figure 4. Slow response amplitude and dV/dt during latency adaptation phenomenon. Stimulation frequency: 0.67 Hz. Open and full circles are maximum dV/dt and slow response peak amplitude respectively. Numbers correspond to cycle sequence. Calibration: horizontal, 50 ms; vertical 10 mV and 1.0 V/s.

also applies to "membrane" slow responses, as illustrated in Figure 5. In all panels, the upper trace is the stimulus; and the lower trace, the intracellular potential. Panels A and B illustrate the determination of I_{To}. Once the preparation had completed its latency adaptation under I_{To} at 1 Hz (panel B), we observed that stable slow responses could be elicited with smaller stimuli (panels C and D). In E, the slow response finally disappears. Panel F shows that I_{To} is unaltered (compare with panel A) after a 60-sec resting period. We call this phenomenon *excitability hysteresis*. It can also be demonstrated by appropriate changes of stimulus duration only. During the course of a progressive decrease in stimulus amplitude, no alteration in the slow-response form or amplitude could be observed. But, the amplitude and the time to peak of the subliminal response increased as current strength decreased, causing an increase in slow-response latency (Fig. 5, C and D).

It was shown in Figure 2 that on increasing stimulation frequency, slow-response latency and subliminal-response rate of rise also increase. On the other hand, excitability hysteresis (lower threshold in beating preparations) was attributed to the hysteretic behavior of the subliminal response. If both phenomena reflect an increase of subliminal response, one may predict that the intensity of excitability hysteresis will depend on stimulation frequency. One of the experimental protocols designed to test this hypothesis was as follows. I_{To} was determined for the rested preparation by means of a very low pacing frequency (0.087 Hz). The preparation was then allowed to beat for 30 sec under a given test frequency. After this period, current strength was decreased gradually until the minimum current yielding stable slow-response activity ($I_{T\infty}$) was found. The procedure was then reapplied with another test frequency after a 90-sec

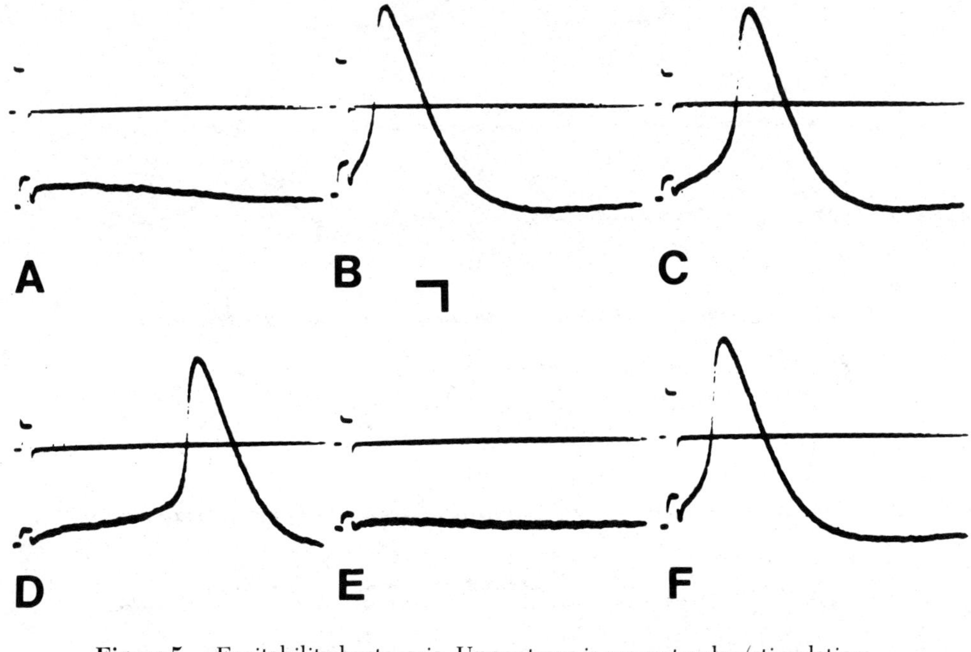

Figure 5. Excitability hysteresis. Upper trace is current pulse (stimulation frequency, 1 Hz) and lower trace corresponds to intracellular recordings. All panels correspond to recordings from the same cell. Calibration: horizontal, 50 ms; vertical, 10 mV and 300 μA.

period of quiescence. This process is illustrated in Figure 6. Columns A, B, and C differ in the test frequency used during the 30-sec period (A is at 0.5 Hz; B, at 0.25 Hz; C, at 0.17 Hz). The first row shows I_{To} after a 90-sec resting period. The second row shows stabilized slow responses (at the end of a 30-sec test period) stimulated with I_{To} at different frequencies. Row three shows stabilized slow responses with current pulse of approximately 0.9 I_{To}. The fourth row exhibits only subliminal responses as the stimulus was adjusted to just below $I_{T\infty}$. Notice that *(1)* I_{To} (row 1) remained constant throughout the experimental procedure; *(2)* the hysteresis phenomenon became more pronounced as test frequency increased (compare current records in the fourth row); *(3)* slow-response latency varied inversely with test frequency (see rows 2 and 3); *(4)* two superimposed subliminal responses occurred (see panel B4), with the second and third cycles occurring after the current strength was decreased slightly below $I_{T\infty}$. The subliminal response that was once effective in slow-response excitation now decreased in amplitude and time course to a steady low level that was incapable of triggering a slow response. This slight decrease of the current strength to a point below $I_{T\infty}$ did not lead to a prompt disappearance of the slow response. One or two cycles with progressive lengthening in slow-response latency occurred (not shown) before the subliminal response (a decrease in amplitude and time course) caused excitation failure, and in another few cycles, this subliminal response reached a steady low level.

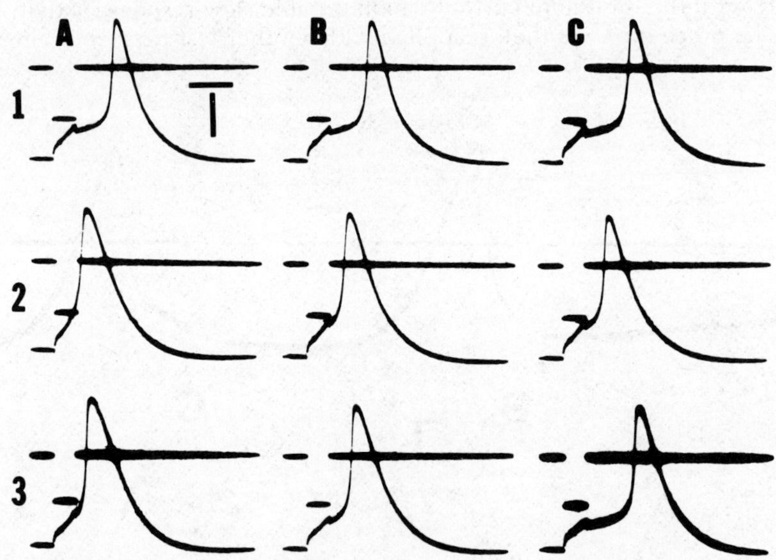

Figure 6. Relationship between excitability hysteresis and stimulation frequency. Upper and lower traces correspond to current pulse and intracellular recordings respectively. Calibration: horizontal, 100 ms; vertical, 20 mV and 35 μA.

The experimental procedure used above enabled us to draw a family of steady-state strength-duration curves, one for each stimulation frequency ($I_{T\infty}$-duration plot), as illustrated in Figure 7. The uppermost curve (full circles) was obtained at a low pacing frequency (0.087 Hz). This curve is equivalent to the rested strength-duration curve (I_{To}-duration plot) because no hysteresis is observable under this pacing frequency. The three other curves were determined for three different frequencies (open circles denote 0.17 Hz; squares, 0.25 Hz; and triangles, 0.5 Hz). Downward displacement of $I_{T\infty}$-duration curves occurs when the testing frequency increases. This suggests an increase in slow-response excitability, because a less stimulating charge is necessary at higher rates for sustaining slow response activity. In other words, the excitability hysteresis ratio ($I_{T\infty}/I_{To}$) approaches unity as pacing frequency decreases.

If the hysteresis phenomenon is attributable to the subliminal response, it should be possible to demonstrate temporal summation of subthreshold stimuli at certain time intervals. The rationale behind this is that a subthreshold pulse would create a subliminal response reflecting a state of increased excitability. If this is true, a second even weaker test pulse would add its effect to this state of increased excitability and trigger a slow response. This is illustrated in Figure 8. Panel A shows that a single subthreshold stimulus (0.78 I_{To}) applied at a frequency of 0.125 Hz evokes only a subliminal response. In this experiment, a second weaker test pulse (0.5 I_{To}) applied within less than 140 msec of the first one achieved slow-response excitation. Two different time delays between pulses are illustrated in panel B (50 msec) and C (125

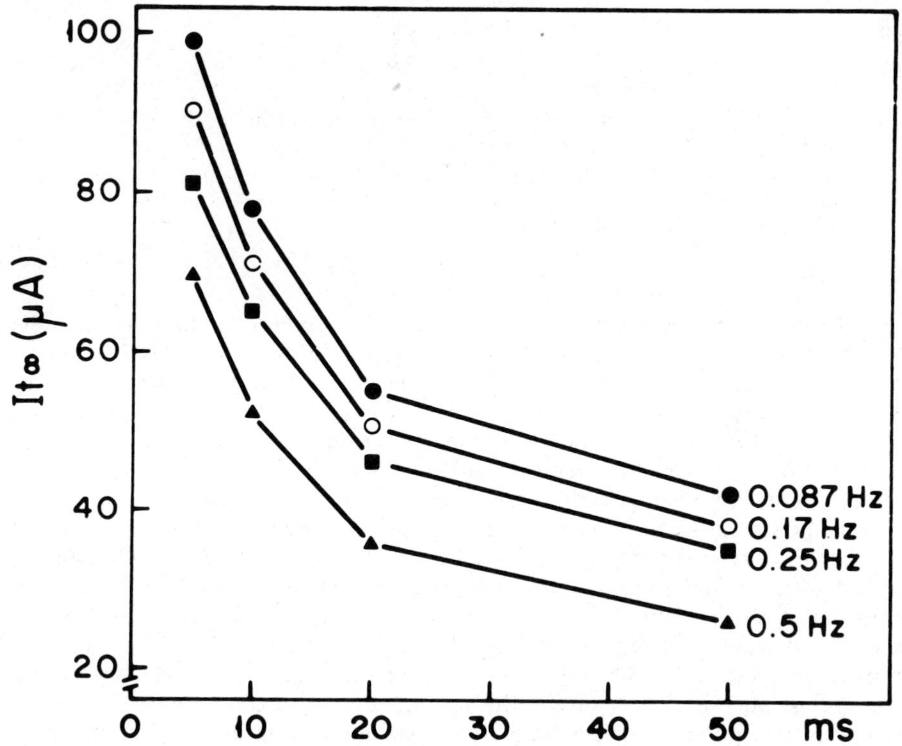

Figure 7. Strength-duration curves obtained at different stimulation test frequencies following experimental protocol of Fig. 6.

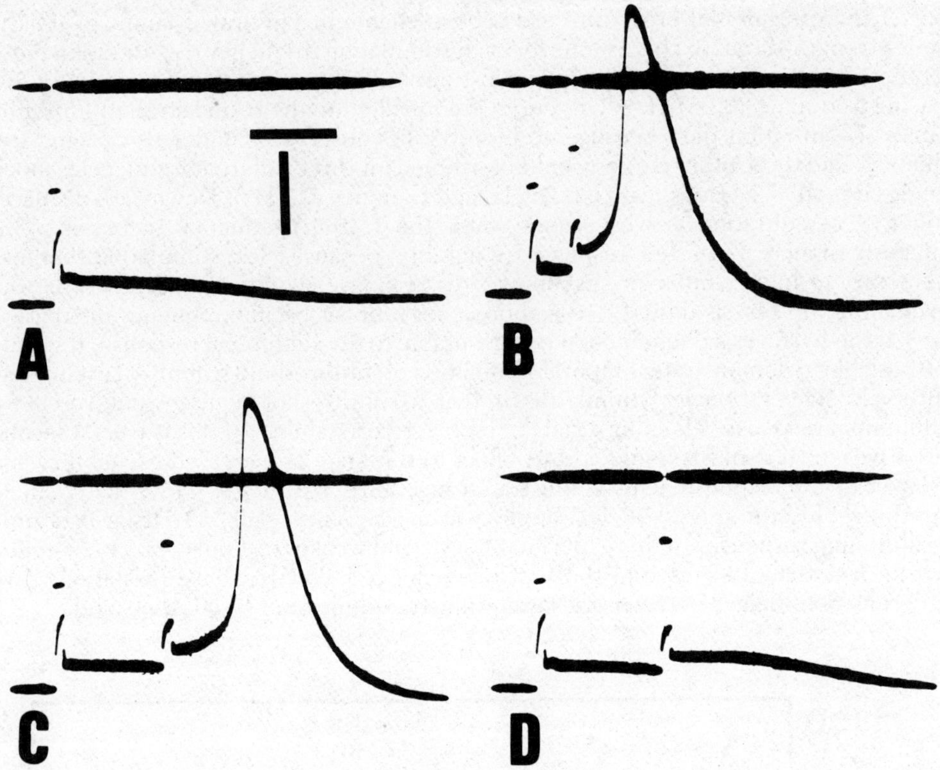

Figure 8. Slow response excitability enhancement by paired pulse stimulation. Upper and lower traces are current pulse and intracellular recording respectively. Basic frequency: 0.125 Hz. First and second pulses have a strength of 0.78 I_{To} and 0.50 I_{To} respectively. Calibration: horizontal, 100 ms; vertical, 20 mV and 185 μA.

msec). In panel C, the slow response latency (in relation to the second pulse) is increased as compared with panel B, indicating some loss in excitability due to the longer delay between pulses. In panel D (time interval between pulses, 140 msec) slow-response excitation no longer occurs. But, slow-response excitation may reappear when the amplitude of the first and/or the second pulse increases (not shown in figure).

Paired pulse-stimulation experiments may give the impression that the state of increased slow-response excitability is restricted to the time during which the subliminal response exists, much in the same way as temporal summation of subthreshold responses in nerve. We observed, however, that a state of increased excitability is manifest well beyond the duration of the subliminal response. This is a necessary conclusion of experiments in which excitability enhancement can be demonstrated from cycle to cycle at frequencies below 1 Hz and down to 0.33 Hz. The long duration of the enhanced state can also be shown in Figure 9. In each panel, the upper trace is the stimulus, and the lower one is the intracellular recording. Rows 1 and 2 show continuous low speed pen recordings from the same cell with different subthreshold current pulses (0.80 I_{To} and 0.85 I_{To}, respectively). Columns A, B, and C represent three different stimulation frequencies (0.33, 0.5, and 1 Hz, respectively). Between subsequent panels in each row, the preparation was allowed to rest for 60 sec. Panel A_1

shows that a stimulation frequency of 0.33 Hz did not stimulate slow responses. As stimulation frequency was increased, slow-response activity appeared on the 16th cycle (B_1 and C_1 in Fig. 9). Slow responses were obtained at all stimulation frequencies (row 2) as current strength was slightly increased.

Figure 10 shows, at an expanded sweep rate and from another preparation, the temporal evolution of the subliminal responses. The upper trace shows the stimulus current that was kept constant throughout. The lower trace shows the intracellular recording. Panel A displays the first three stimulation cycles after a 40-sec resting period. Panel B shows that the subliminal response increased in amplitude, rate of rise, and duration after nine successive cycles. Both panels show that the subliminal response is followed by an after-hyperpolarization. This after-hyperpolarization increased in amplitude from A to B. Finally, panel C (three stimulation cycles after the end of B) shows that subliminal response was now effective for slow-response stimulation.

The results of experiments are consistent with the idea that a cumulative increase in slow-response excitability may occur during successive stimulation cycles. The degree of accumulated enhancement does not seem to have an electrical representation, but it becomes manifest as a facilitation of the subliminal response to stimuli. It

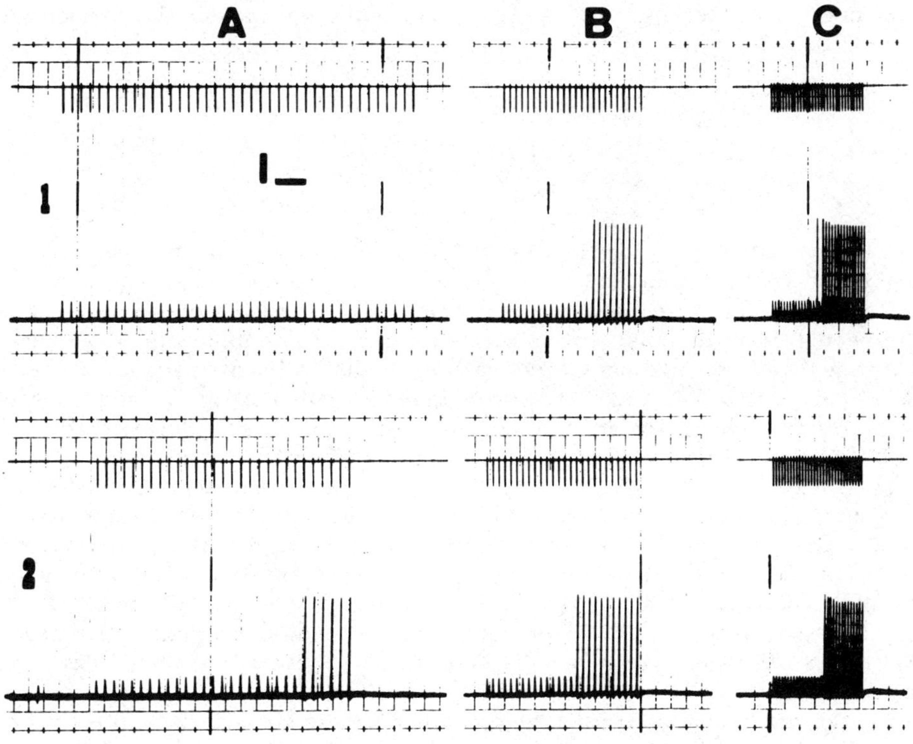

Figure 9. Cumulative slow response excitability enhancement. In each row, upper trace is the stimulus (0.80 I_{T_0} and 0.85 I_{T_0}, rows 1 & 2 respectively) and lower trace corresponds to intracellular recordings. *A*, *B* & *C* are three different stimulation frequencies (0.33, 0.5 and 1.0 Hz respectively). Calibration: horizontal, 10 ms; vertical, 15 mV and 120 μA.

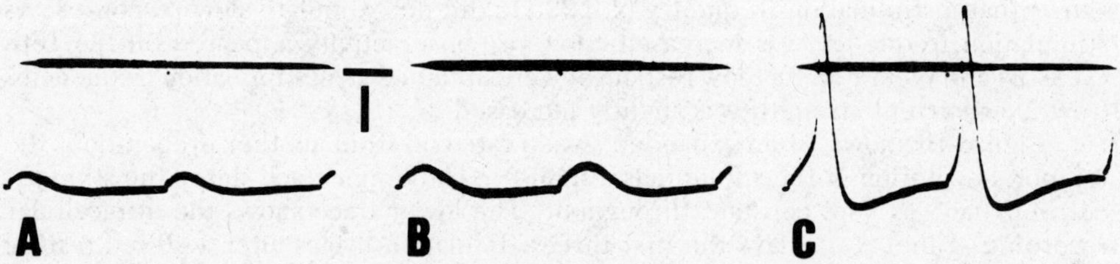

Figure 10. Cumulative slow response excitability enhancement. Upper and lower traces correspond to stimulus (0.75 I_{T_0}) and intracellular recording respectively. Panels *A*, *B* & *C* represent three different moments after the beginning of stimulation (*A*, first three cycles after a 60 second resting period; *B*, 6 cycles after *A*; *C*, 3 cycles after *B*). Stimulation frequency, 1.0 Hz. Calibration: horizontal, 300 ms; vertical, 30 mV and 70 μA.

is also apparent that excitability enhancement is related to the stimulus-subliminal-response phenomenon, as cycle-to-cycle enhancement occurs even in the absence of a successful slow response. In addition to this, the peak amplitude of subliminal response may oscillate in the course of a long train of stimuli (Figs. 9 and 10), introducing some degree of uncertainty as to the exact moment the firing of a slow response will occur.

DISCUSSION

Isolated atrial trabeculae in TKBa solution display synchronously activated slow responses. This is caused by a significant increase in the length constant of the preparation (Cukierman and Paes de Carvalho, 1982). Such a finding is not totally unexpected. In several different preparations, Ba^{2+} blocks g_K, leading to an increase in resting membrane resistance (Sperelakis et al., 1967; Hermsmeyer and Sperelakis, 1970). This effect is followed by a decrease in resting potential (Antoni and Oberdisse, 1965). Our observations of "membrane" slow responses caused by an increased length constant may well be explained by this blocking effect. In 1 mM Ba^{2+} Tyrode's solution, we have also noted automatic activity, as did Antoni and Oberdisse (1965). This automaticity could be suppressed by an increase in the extracellular K^+ concentration (TKBa solution). For this reason, the above procedure was applied, because in 1 mM Ba^{2+} Tyrode's solution slow responses were present, but could not be elicited at will (Cukierman, 1978).

TKBa slow responses have been studied under conditions permitting propagation (Masuda, 1976; Paula Carvalho, 1977; Masuda and Paes de Carvalho, 1982). Under such conditions, electrotonic interactions during slow-response activity are often present owing to conduction disorders. Slow-response characterization is thus difficult. The spatial uniformity of membrane voltage during slow-response electrogenesis obtained in our preparation eliminates such interferences. We believe that the intracellular potential and its dV/dt do indeed represent genuine properties of the slow response.

The "membrane" slow response is shown here to be a grossly stereotyped, all-or-nothing action potential. It has a threshold voltage around −35 mV, a value that is in general agreement with the voltage threshold for the slow inward current (Beeler and Reuter, 1970; New and Trautwein, 1972). The peak amplitude and dV/dt of the slow response are influenced by the stimulation frequency, showing a depression at higher frequencies. It is thought that this depression may be related to the slow recovery of the gating mechanisms responsible for the slow response upstroke.

Slow inward current is known to inactivate (New and Trautwein, 1972). But, we have observed no decrease in peak dV/dt of slow responses that arise at the end of prolonged subliminal responses, which keep the membrane at a voltage range near the slow-response threshold for several hundred miliseconds. No accommodation to slowly rising stimuli was ever observed. Either inactivation is absent at this voltage range or it has a rate constant well in excess of the times involved in the subliminal response.

Slow responses always arise from a low-voltage depolarizing step, the subliminal response. When stimulus characteristics (strength, duration, cycle length) are suitable, the subliminal response triggers the slow response. We have no irrefutable evidence that the subliminal response is generated by a mechanism different from the slow response gating mechanism. In fact, D-600 and acetylcholine affect both responses (Cukierman, 1978). Slow-response behavior as a function of stimulating frequency and rhythm is, however, just opposite to that observed for the subliminal response. When pacing frequency is high, slow-response "fatigue" (loss of amplitude and dV/dt) is observable. Yet, under these conditions, slow-response latency tends to be minimal because of an improved subliminal response.

The subliminal response behaves in a complex way. Its effectiveness in stimulating a slow response depends not only on the characteristics of the stimulus voltage and the time course, but also on the previous excitation history of the tissue. It seems that the preparation has some sort of memory that vanishes with a very long time constant ($t_{\frac{1}{2}}$, around 4 sec). In this sense, it displays excitability hysteresis, frequency-dependent latency, and latency-adaptation phenomena. At low stimulation frequencies, a stronger stimulus will be necessary for the subliminal response to trigger the slow response. At higher stimulation rates, a less intense stimulus will suffice in leading the subliminal response to the slow-response firing voltage in the same preparation. Enhancement of slow-response excitability is, therefore, translated into an enhancement of the subliminal response, in terms of its peak amplitude and time in reaching the slow-response threshold.

On the other hand, although the subliminal response to a fixed stimulus is a good indicator of the enhanced slow-response excitability, it is certainly not the primary cause of this condition. Excitability enhancement is demonstrable at cycle lengths well above the subliminal response's duration. Although subliminal response is an indicator of the enhanced state of slow-response excitability, the experiments shown in Figures 9 and 10 suggest that other factors may contribute towards defining the level of slow response excitability. These figures show that oscillations in subliminal responses occur during a train of identical successive stimuli. Except for strength, duration, and rate of stimulus, we cannot clearly identify, at present, the other factors that control the subliminal response. The enhanced excitable state is not necessarily translated into changes of intracellular potential that we can measure precisely. We often observed, however, that the subliminal response is diminished in amplitude during after-hyperpolarizations following slow responses or subliminal responses themselves. This could just mean that these after-hyperpolarizations are mediated by increases in g_K that lower membrane resistance and thus shunt the subliminal response.

TKBa slow responses driven at rates above 1 Hz shows definite signs of "fatigue" (see also Cranefield, 1975). Even below 1 Hz, peak dV/dt of slow responses is seen to decrease with increasing rates of drive. Although we still do not know what the mechanism of fatigue is, it is quite clear that a fully developed, efficient, slow response can only be obtained within a certain frequency range, the lower limit of which is determined by the temporal relationship between the stimuli. This is the same conclusion reached by Masuda et al. (see Chapter 22) in their study of propagation of activity from normal to TKBa-depressed myocardium.

Work on digitalis-induced after-depolarizations (Ferrier et al., 1973) and oscillatory after-potentials (see Fig. VI−12 from Cranefield, 1975; Hiraoka et al., 1979) suggest some analogies between these phenomena and the TKBa subliminal response. Both after-depolarizations and oscillatory after-potentials increase with the number of previous beats in a train. They are also larger at a higher stimulating frequency. These increased oscillations are often seen to trigger trains action potentials. It has been suggested that an increase in intracellular Ca^{2+} is associated with the transient inward current responsible for the after-depolarizations (Kass et al., 1978). On the other hand, the subliminal response hyperpolarizes a few milivolts (see Fig. 10) beyond the resting potential when its peak amplitude reaches a sizable value. This may be related to the presence of Ca^{2+}-dependent K^+ channels in the heart (Isenberg, 1975). All these points of similarity seem to us to constitute enough circumstancial evidence to support the possibility that subliminal responses, after-depolarizations, and oscillatory prepotentials share a common phenomenologic basis.

REFERENCES

Antoni H, Oberdisse E (1965) Elektrophysiologische Untersuchungen über die Barium-induzierte Schriftmacheraktivität im isolierten säugetier Myokard. Pflüg Arch **284**:259−272

Beeler GW, Reuter H (1970) Membrane calcium current in ventricular myocardial fibres. J Physiol **207**:165−190

Cranefield PF (1975) The Conduction of the Cardiac Impulse. Mount Kisco, NY, Futura Publishing Company

Cukierman S (1978) A resposta lenta em trabécula atrial isolada. MSc thesis presented to Instituto de Biofísica, Universidade Federal do Rio de Janeiro

Cukierman S, Paes de Carvalho A (1982) Frequency dependent excitability of "membrane" slow responses of rabbit left atrial trabeculae in presence of Ba^{2+} and high K^+. J Gen Physiol 79 (in press)

Ferrier, GR, Saunders JH, Méndez C (1973) A cellular mechanism for the generation of ventricular arrhythmias by acetylstrophantidin. Circ Res **32**:600−609

Hagiwara S, Nakajima S (1966) Differences in Na and Ca spikes as examined by application of tetrodotoxin, procaine and manganese ions. J Gen Physiol **49**:807−818

Hermsmeyer K, Sperelakis N (1970) Decrease in K^+ -conductance and depolarization of frog cardiac muscle produced by Ba^{++}. Am J Physiol **219**:1108−1114

Hiraoka M, Okamoto Y, Sano T (1979) Effects of Ca^{2+} and K^+ on oscillatory afterpotentials in dog ventricular muscle fibers. J Mol Cell Cardiol **11**:999−1015

Hoffman BF, Cranefield PF (1960) Electrophysiology of the Heart. New York, McGraw-Hill Book Co

Isenberg G (1975) Is potassium conductance of cardiac Purkinje fibres controlled by Ca_i^{2+}? Nature **253**:273−274

Kass, RS, Lederer WJ, Tsien RW, Weingart R (1978) Role of calcium ions in transient inward currents and aftercontractions induced by strophantidin in cardiac Purkinje fibres. J Physiol **281**:187−208

Masuda MO (1976) Excitação e propagação da resposta lenta no miocárdio. D.Sc. thesis presented to Instituto de Biofísica, Universidade Federal do Rio de Janeiro.

Masuda MO, Paes de Carvalho A (1982) Rate and rhythm dependency of propagation from normal myocardium to a Ba^{2+}, K^+-induced slow response zone in rabbit left atrium. Circ Res **50**:419−427

New W, Trautwein W (1972) The ionic nature of slow inward current and its relation to contraction. Pflüg Arch **334**:24–38

Paes de Carvalho A, Hoffman BF, Carvalho MP (1969) Two components of the cardiac potential. I. Voltage time course and the effect of acetylcholine on atrial and nodal cells of the rabbit heart. J Gen Physiol **54**:607–635

Paes de Carvalho A, Hoffman BF, Langan WB (1966) Two components of the cardiac action potential. Nature **211**:938–940

Paula Carvalho M (1977) Propagação da resposta lenta no miocárdio: bloqueios de condução. D.Sc. thesis presented to Instituto de Biofísica, Universidade Federal do Rio de Janeiro.

Reuter H (1973) Divalent cations as charge carriers in excitable membranes. Prog Biophys Mol Biol **26**:1–43

Sperelakis N, Schneider M, Harris EJ (1967) Decreased K^+ conductance produced by Ba^{2+} in frog sartorius fibres. J Gen Physiol **50**:1565–1585

Weidmann S (1955) The effect of the cardiac membrane potential on the rapid availability of the sodium-carrying system. J Physiol **118**:348–360

Discussion

DE MELLO: I wonder if your frequency effects can be explained by the summation of subthreshold phenomena. Some time ago, Hoffman and also Noble showed that this type of summation can exist. I think that, particularly when you have a partially depolarized preparation, electrotonic phenomena can play a very important role in reaching threshold voltage. My second question is, what is the difference in level between the threshold stimulus for a fast response and a slow response? Is there a big difference?

CUKIERMAN: We do not think that we can explain the results by a simple summation of subthreshold or subliminal phenomena. This summation certainly exists at short stimulus intervals. But we have shown here that longer time effects, such as those observed at a frequency of 30 cycles/min or less, must be phenomena that exist well beyond the duration of the subliminal response or of any voltage alteration due to the preceding cycle. The longest subliminal responses obtained in this high potassium-barium medium are of the order of a few hundred milliseconds only. As to the second question, the answer is yes, there is a large difference between threshold stimulus intensity for fast and slow responses. You generally need a much larger and longer stimulus to elicit slow response. Both rheobase and chronaxie are increased about ten times in high potassium, barium Tyrode solution.

BROWN: As I heard your presentation, I was reminded of the early days of calcium currents when Hagiwara and Nakajima showed that you needed to add EGTA inside the barnacle muscle fiber to get a calcium spike. This turned out to be due to two different causes. First, that calcium inside inactivates the calcium channel, and second, that calcium inside activates an outward potassium channel. Now, in your case if you take into consideration that barium blocks the potassium channel and that barium can readily traverse the Ca channel, at each beat, then you have a setting for results of the type you showed here. As you present the cell with barium, it blocks the potassium channel and facilitates the inward current through the slow channel so that you eventually are able to get a slow response. This response is going to depend on frequency and on the kinetics of barium entry into the cell and uptake in the cell. There would be a number of ways in which you could test this hypothesis. For instance, you could try temperature changes, as you would expect the barium uptake to be extremely dependent on temperature, with a Q_{10} of 3 or so. Another suggestion is that you might use mitochondrial poisons, which should also affect the cycle-length effect.

CUKIERMAN: First, I would like to say that in our preparation we have added barium into a Tyrode solution containing 10 mM K^+ and 2.7 mM Ca^{2+}. Ca^{2+} and Ba^{2+} are therefore simultaneously present. I presume Ca^{2+} is still playing its physiologic role and its kinetics are not appreciably altered. Now, as to your suggestion that the results might be explained by some sort of kinetic effect between barium accumulation in the cell and its effect on the membrane, I am not quite clear on how this should come about. The effect is opposite to the intracellular calcium-dependent slow channel inactivation and potassium activation: as we increase the stimulation frequency, slow response excitation is improved. Besides, I would like to point out that the upstroke velocity and amplitude of the slow response itself is little sensitive to frequency, with a relationship that is in the opposite direction of what is needed for the memory effect; that is, upstroke velocity and amplitude decrease as cycle length is shortened. It seems that the secret for the memory effect resides rather in the subliminal response that leads to the slow response. As to your other suggestions, we have tried temperature effects, and there was a very marked temperature dependence for the slow response and its excitability. Actually, this response cannot be elicited in temperatures below 30° C. There is information from our laboratory, as well as from others, that metabolic poisons and hypoxia do inhibit the appearance of slow response.

CARMELIET: I would like to point out that although in your experiments the effects were obtained in the presence of barium, in other situations, like in the presence of catecholamines, you see very similar phenomena. The same result can also be seen in chloride-free solutions. Omitting the chloride is just enough to make these effects appear.

RAMÓN: Could you tell me if these slow responses do actually propagate?

CUKIERMAN: In the conditions of the present experiment, they do not propagate; they are "membrane" action potentials. But, in larger preparations, as shown before by Masuda in the previous paper, these responses do propagate at the usual slow response rate of 0.01 to 0.05 m/sec, which is about the same rate at which natural slow responses propagate within the atrioventricular node.

Chapter 24

Are Arrhythmias Caused by Automatic Impulse Generation?

Brian F. Hoffman and Kenneth H. Dangman

Perhaps because the normal rhythm of the heart results from the automaticity of cells in the sinoatrial node, it is tempting to assume that at least some abnormal rhythms, including those arising at ectopic sites, also can result from automatic impulse generation in one or another type of cardiac fiber. There is no doubt that, under conditions that do not seem to be distinctly abnormal, many different cell types in the heart can generate what appear to be automatic impulses; thus, automaticity can be considered a normal property of a number of types of specialized cardiac cells. These cells include the specialized atrial fibers of rabbit heart (Paes de Carvalho et al., 1959), the canine atrial plateau fibers (Hogan and Davis, 1968), atrial fibers near the coronary sinus ostium (Wit and Cranefield, 1977), and fibers of the His-Purkinje system in canine and ungulate hearts. Also, there is adequate evidence from experiments on cardiac tissues studied in vitro to demonstrate that both many of the specialized cardiac cell types (Hauswirth et al., 1969; Noble, 1975; Cranefield, 1975) and also the muscle fibers of the atria (Brown et al., 1976) and ventricles (Imanishi and Surawicz, 1976; Katzung and Morgenstern, 1977) can generate impulses automatically if, because of experimental intervention, the maximum diastolic potential (MDP) fails to attain a sufficiently negative value. It seems reasonable in this regard to speak of *normal automaticity*, a usual property of many of the different specialized cell types in the heart, and also *abnormal automaticity*, the mechanism causing spontaneous impulse generation by both specialized and nonspecialized fibers when they are partially depolarized. The general question that we wish to examine is whether either or both of these mechanisms cause arrhythmias of the human heart in situ and, if they do, can the operation of one or the other be identified with certainty. The question is of some importance because the answer might have bearing on the design and use of antiarrhythmic drugs.

Abnormal cardiac rhythms also can be generated by other mechanisms. For the most part, these rhythms can be categorized as resulting from triggered activity (Cranefield, 1975, 1977) or reentrant excitation (see Wit and Cranefield, 1978). Triggered activity typically is the result of early or delayed after-depolarizations (Crane-

Original studies described here were supported by grants HL-12738 and HL-24354-02 from the NHLBI, NIH.

field, 1975). Reentrant excitation is the result of either some form of circus movement or of reflected activity (Antzelevitch et al., 1980; Wit et al., 1972a; 1972b). The distinction between triggered and automatic rhythms is not always clear. Indeed, for some experiments on what we have called abnormal automaticity it might be more precise to speak of triggered repetitive activity because the apparently automatic discharge was induced during regular or spontaneous activity. The only satisfactory test of automatic activity is a demonstration of the spontaneous resumption of rhythmic action potentials after a sufficiently long period of quiescence. In this sense the only action potential which can be defined as automatic is the first one of a series. We believe that this restraint imposes an unnecessary hindrance and will, therefore, be somewhat arbitrary in the use of the terms "automatic" and "triggered." For example, in Figure 1, we show the transmembrane potentials recorded from a bundle of canine cardiac Purkinje fibers during superfusion with standard Tyrode's solution ($[K^+]_o$ = 4.0 mM) and after addition of $BaCl_2$ in an amount sufficient to provide a concentration of Ba^{2+} of 0.5 mM (see Reid and Hecht, 1967). The record shows a progressive decrease in MDP and a concomitant increase in the slope of phase-4 depolarization with the gradual emergence of a stable rhythm. During this rhythm, each action potential appears to result from the preceding phase-4 depolarization. Because the effect of Ba^{2+} is uniform over the preparation and the space constant is considerably increased, all cells demonstrate similar and almost simultaneous changes in transmembrane potential. If the barium-induced repetitive activity is arrested, as by drug application, on washing out the drug, spontaneous activity reappears. The rhythm thus satisfies the stipulated test for automaticity.

In other cases, the demonstration that impulse generation is automatic is not always easy. Records from diseased human atrium (Bush et al., 1971; Hordof et al., 1976) and infarcting canine ventricle (Friedman et al., 1973; Lazzara et al., 1973) often show regularly repeating action potentials that appear to result from phase-4 depolarization in cells with a reduced MDP. At times the apparently automatic focus is surrounded by zones of complete entry and exit block, and in this case it may be

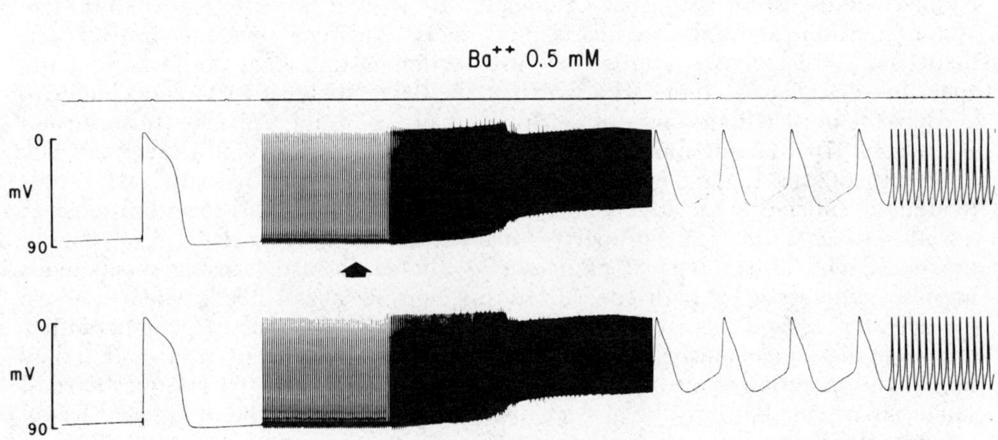

Figure 1. Transmembrane potentials recorded from two sites in a bundle of canine Purkinje fibers; records are obtained with a pen recorder that does not reproduce rapid transients. Control records, at the left, are obtained at fast and slow paper speed during regular stimulation in control Tyrode's solution. At the arrow the superfusate is changed to one containing Ba^{2+}, 0.5 mM. Note the decrease in MDP and development of abnormal automaticity with similar transmembrane action potentials at both sites.

reasonable to assume that the activity has not been triggered by impulses propagating from adjacent fibers. Also, it may be possible to apply the stop-start test. Most records of apparently automatic activity recorded from preparations of diseased human atrium or infarcting canine ventricle, however, show evidence of electrical coupling between the automatic focus and the remainder of the preparation. Because data is available only for the fiber from which we are recording, the possibility cannot be excluded that the first (apparently automatic) impulse was caused by some change in membrane potential in another fiber. Indeed, the onset of automatic activity might even result from a decrease in the effectiveness of electrical coupling between the fiber under study and other fibers that have a higher resting potential. In either case, the first recorded action potential would not be automatic, and all subsequent action potentials thus might have been triggered.

Within these limits, the question that we wish to examine is whether or not we can determine for the heart in situ that an abnormal rhythm is caused by automatic impulse generation, and, if so, whether the automatic impulse generation is due to a normal or an abnormal mechanism. For many years, different groups of investigators studying isolated preparations of cardiac tissue, the hearts of experimental animals in which arrhythmias had been induced, and the arrhythmic human heart have tried to develop sets of rules that might discriminate between automatic and reentrant rhythms. More recently, similar tests have been proposed for triggered rhythms (see Rosen, Chapter 25; Rosen et al., 1980). To separate automatic rhythms and those caused by reentry, two tests have been applied most consistently. Overdrive pacing at a rate higher than the intrinsic rate has been used to identify an automatic rhythm; if, after the end of the rapid pacing, the intrinsic rhythm is suppressed and gradually returns to its control rate (post-overdrive suppression) the rhythm is assumed to be automatic. For such a rhythm, premature impulses cause no, or only transient, perturbations (see below). In the case of a reentrant mechanism, on the other hand, premature impulses occurring at the correct time in the cycle typically initiate or terminate the arrhythmia (Bigger and Goldreyer, 1970; Wellens et al., 1974), typical overdrive suppression is not demonstrated, but overdrive can terminate the rhythm.

These responses to overdrive and to premature impulses are typical for automatic and reentrant rhythms, but a number of exceptions have been described. Also, most of the data was accumulated before triggered activity was generally appreciated. In an attempt to simplify matters, we will consider only sustained rhythms, that is, those that last for a number of impulses, and will not deal with extrasystoles or occasional ectopic impulses. These, too, can result from automaticity, reentry, or triggering, and each mechanism can have similar manifestations. For example, several recent studies (Jalife and Moe, 1976, 1979) have shown that when an automatic parasystolic focus is coupled to the heart by a segment manifesting entry but not exit block, electrotonic interactions across this segment will modify the time of discharge of the automatic focus in a predictable manner. In general, an impulse arriving at the site of block early during phase 4 of the automatic focus will delay discharge, whereas one occurring late during phase 4 will cause the action potential to occur prematurely. These effects are similar to those exerted by current pulses (Weidmann, 1951). Because of this electrotonic interaction, the frequency of occurrence and timing in the cycle of the ectopic impulses will be a function of the basic heart rate, as may be the case for either reentrant or triggered impulses.

Even for sustained rhythms, the identification of the underlying mechanism by use of overdrive or premature stimulation presents some problems. As stated, the normal automatic rhythm is suppressed by overdrive and only reset by premature impulses, whereas the reentrant rhythm is initiated and terminated by premature impulses and does not show overdrive suppression. The behavior of abnormal automatic foci has not been described. Unfortunately, triggered rhythms also show a dependence on imposed alterations in rate and rhythm. Like a reentrant rhythm, a triggered rhythm can be started and stopped by a properly timed premature impulse (see Rosen, Chapter 25). Also, both reentrant rhythms and triggered rhythms can be initiated by rapid pacing. Like a normally automatic focus, the source of the triggered rhythm can be suppressed by overdrive (see Gadsby, Chapter 13 and Fig. 6). There is evidence that a reentrant rhythm can be entrained; that is, pacing at a rate higher than the initial rate due to reentrant excitation can, on termination of pacing, be shown to have accelerated the reentrant rhythm. It is not unreasonable to assume that some triggered rhythms might show similar behavior. Even the canine sinus node at times responds to overdrive by marked acceleration (Chan and Gliklich, unpublished observation). In this case, and probably in other cases, it is possible that the mechanism causing the initial rhythm has been replaced by another mechanism that causes the faster rhythm. Because of these and other complexities, we will not examine any or all tests in detail.

Rather, we will present some data that presumably characterize automatic rhythms and discuss these in relation to characterization of normal and abnormal automaticity. We will comment briefly on the likelihood that induced changes in rate and rhythm can generate sufficiently precise rules to identify mechanisms for arrhythmias of the in situ heart. Then, we will consider briefly whether the effects of selected pharmacologic agents and the use of improved techniques to record electrical activity from the in situ heart can help discriminate among the more probable causes of arrhythmias.

EFFECTS OF OVERDRIVE

The effect of overdrive on rhythms that almost certainly are automatic is well known. In the conscious dog or human, if the atria are paced at a rate sufficiently faster than the normal sinus rate, the phenomenon of overdrive suppression typically is observed at the end of the period of pacing. In this case, overdrive suppression consists of a usually modest increase in the cycle length of the resumed sinus rhythm (the returning cycle); typically, thereafter, the sinus rate gradually returns to its control value. In unipolar electrograms recorded directly from the vicinity of the sinus pacemaker (Fig. 2) (Cramer et al., 1977, 1978; Hariman et al., 1980a) one can show that overdrive suppression and particularly the prolonged returning cycle, are associated with a decrease in the diastolic slope of the sinus node electrogram. This presumably reflects in large measure a decrease in the slope of phase-4 depolarization of the automatic pacemaker cells (Cramer et al., 1977). Overdrive suppression is not the only possible consequence of overdrive on sinus node function. Under different conditions, the returning impulse may be generated at another site, and at times overdrive may be followed by a more rapid, rather than a transiently slower, rhythm. The rapid rhythm may result from reflexes that accelerate the sinus pacemaker or from initiation of another mechanism for impulse generation. Nevertheless, typically the normally automatic canine and human sinus nodes show overdrive suppression.

Other rhythms that almost certainly result from normal automaticity of His bundle and Purkinje fibers are the idioventricular rhythms present in animals and humans with chronic heart block. In the conscious resting dog with chronic surgically induced heart block, the ventricular rate ranges from 40 to 60 beats/min, and, if block is in the upper His bundle, the configuration of the electrocardiogram suggests that

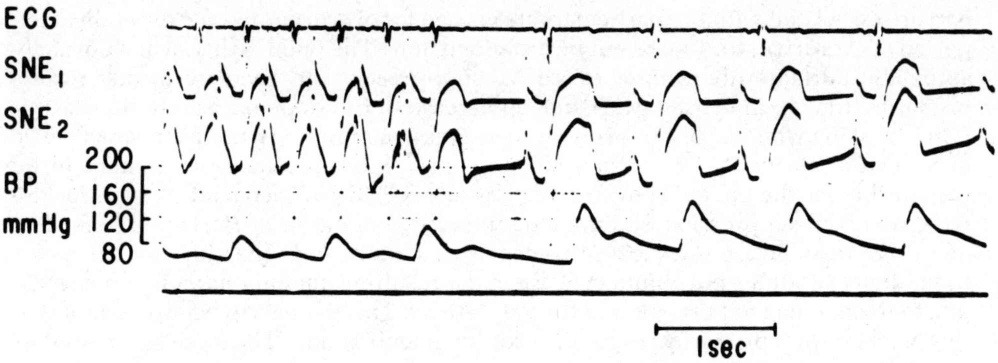

Figure 2. Effects of overdrive pacing on unipolar electrograms from the *in situ* canine sinus node. Traces from above downward are the ECG, unipolar electrograms from two sites over the sinus node and a tracing of systemic arterial pressure. After termination of pacing the trace labeled SNE_2 shows, for the returning cycle, a depressed diastolic slope and clear upstroke slope. For subsequent complexes the steepness of the diastolic slope increases with shortening of the sinus cycle length. (Chan and Gliklich, unpublished record).

impulses originate in the proximal portion of the His-Purkinje system. The rate of this rhythm responds in the expected way to changes in automatic tone. Presumably, the rhythm results from normal automatic impulse generation in specialized fibers of the conducting system. In the conscious dog, after a period of reasonably rapid ventricular pacing, this rhythm typically demonstrates marked overdrive suppression, whereas premature impulses cause only a resetting of the rhythm. As in the case of sinus rhythm, under some experimental conditions, such as tests made soon after interruption of the His bundle, overdrive may be followed by a more rapid rhythm, the so-called "overdrive enhancement" (Vassalle et al., 1976; 1977). Nevertheless, if tests are made at a sufficient interval after induction of heart block, even when the cycle length for ventricular pacing is as short as 250 msec, overdrive suppression is obtained.

So far, we have established that certain rhythms of the in situ heart, rhythms that we assume result from normal automaticity, typically demonstrate overdrive suppression. Before asking if this test can identify automatic rhythms with certainty, or can discriminate between normal and abnormal automaticity, we will look into the mechanism for overdrive suppression of normally automatic fibers.

The phenomenon of overdrive suppression of automatic impulse generation has been examined by recording transmembrane potentials from isolated preparations of sinoatrial node and Purkinje fibers (Vassalle, 1970). The isolated Purkinje fiber preparation probably is a reasonable model for the study of overdrive suppression of normal automatic firing since, until recently, it has been the subject of most studies on the ionic basis for normal automatic impulse generation by cardiac fibers. The phenomenon has been analyzed in some detail by Vassalle and his colleagues (Vassalle, 1970; Vassalle et al., 1976), and the findings need be summarized only briefly. At the onset of overdrive, especially if the rate is high, frequently there is some decrease in MDP. But if the cycle length is not too short, during overdrive MDP then increases above the control value. On cessation of overdrive, the slope of phase-4 depolarization is decreased. Both variables, MDP and slope of phase 4, only gradually return to their control values. There are many variations on this typical pattern, and these for the most part are associated with the particular rate chosen for overdrive and the duration of the period of overdrive; they need not be examined now. The point is that, when normally automatic Purkinje fibers show overdrive suppression, the decrease in rate results primarily from an increased MDP and a decrease in the slope of phase-4 depolarization. In asking whether or not overdrive suppression might be a unique characteristic of normal automaticity, it is important to consider the mechanisms thought to be responsible for the effects of overdrive. Vassalle (1970, 1976) concluded that, for the most part, the suppression of automatic impulse generation in Purkinje fibers after overdrive resulted from increased transport of sodium and potassium by the membrane-bound sodium-potassium-ATPase and a resulting augmented outward current due to the unequal net transport of the two cations. There seems to be little doubt that this mechanism is primarily responsible for the phenomenon. The increase in number of action potentials per unit of time during overdrive results in a net gain of sodium by the fiber, and the increase in intracellular sodium activity stimulates the pump. Overdrive suppression can be abolished if the pump is poisoned by digitalis, and indeed, it may be replaced by overdrive enhancement. The net gain in sodium has been demonstrated through the use of intracellular sodium-selective electrodes (Deitmer and Ellis, 1978) and other methods (Eisner and Lederer, 1980a), and the electrogenic nature of the pump in heart fibers has been demonstrated clearly (Gadsby and Cranefield, 1979a; 1979b; Eisner and Lederer, 1980b).

Besides this mechanism for overdrive suppression, a few additional factors should be considered. For Purkinje fibers studied in vitro, and probably for other cardiac tissues studied in vitro, during rapid activation there is not only an increase in sodium activity inside the fiber, but also an increase in potassium activity just outside the fiber (Baumgarten and Isenberg, 1977; Kunze, 1977; Cleeman and Morad, 1979; Kline et al., 1980; DiFrancesco et al., 1980). The magnitude of this change will, of course, depend on the fine structure of the tissue and be quite prominent if much of the sarcolemma faces narrow clefts. The change in the potassium concentration just outside the sarcolemma might influence the rate of automatic impulse generation by any or all of several mechanisms: by increasing conductance for outward potassium current, by influencing the sensitivity of the pump to a change in $[Na^+]_i$, and by changing the current-voltage characteristics of the membrane across which the pump current flows. Also, when active transport has been augmented sufficiently, the active uptake of K^+ from clefts may decrease $[K^+]_o$, and this in turn can modify both the value of the MDP, the slope of phase-4 depolarization, and the passive current-voltage characteristics of the membrane. These effects all may contribute to the magnitude and duration of overdrive suppression of normally automatic pacemakers; nevertheless, the net effect is reasonably consistent.

To simplify matters, we will assume that normally automatic cells in the His Purkinje system typically show overdrive suppression because of augmented pump current. We then must ask if the same mechanism operates in the sinus node and if fibers firing because of abnormal automaticity can be expected to show similar or different responses to overdrive. Even though the abnormally automatic cells most likely have a pump that can be stimulated by changes in intracellular sodium concentration, it might be that for these cells the effects of overdrive would differ from those shown for normally automatic cells. For instance, abnormal automaticity typically is observed when maximum diastolic potential is reduced. If the maximum diastolic potential has been reduced sufficiently in Purkinje fibers, the fast inward channel will be largely inactivated and the automatic action potentials thus will result largely from depolarizing current in slow inward channels. If this is the case, because the slow inward current is primarily a calcium current, overdrive might not directly increase $[Na^+]_i$ by very much, and the usual stimulus to the pump would not be present.

Alternatively, if the net sodium influx for an action potential is reduced in an abnormally automatic focus, a greater number of driven impulses might be needed to provide a sufficient increment in $[Na^+]_i$. Finally, even if there were no appreciable inward sodium current during the paced slow responses, these responses might cause an increase in intracellular calcium concentration. That increase, through sodium-for-calcium exchange at the sarcolemma, might augment $[Na^+]_i$ and provide the necessary stimulus to increase electrogenic pumping. Also, an increase in $[Ca^{2+}]_i$ might increase sarcolemmal K^+ conductance and either slow impulse generation or increase MDP and stop it. These considerations suggest that, for a given period of overdrive at a given rate, the magnitude of overdrive suppression may be a function of the maximum diastolic potential in the automatic cells. Also, because the effects of overdrive are complex, as noted above, the relationship between the rate and duration of overdrive and the degree of suppression of automatic impulse generation need not reflect only augmented electrogenic pumping.

To obtain data relating to these questions, we have examined the relationships between the rate and duration of overdrive and the extent of overdrive suppression by using normally automatic Purkinje fibers and also two different experimental models of abnormal automaticity. One is a preparation in which Purkinje fibers are partially depolarized by exposing them to Tyrode's solution containing a low concentration of Ba^{2+} (see Fig. 1); and the other, a preparation of subendocardial fibers from 24-hour infarcts in canine hearts (see Fig. 7).

When one contrasts the response of Purkinje fiber preparations with automatic activity and normal maximum diastolic potentials to that of preparations in which abnormal automaticity has been induced by exposure to Ba^{2+} or by acute infarction, short periods of overdrive have quite different effects. In the normally polarized fibers, overdrive suppression is prominent, and for short periods of pacing the extent of depression frequently is related to the rate of overdrive. In abnormally automatic fibers in which MDP is less than -60 mV, overdrive at similar rates and for similar times causes almost no overdrive suppression. For fibers with intermediate values of MDP (-60 to -80 mV), the degree of overdrive suppression also is intermediate (Figs. 3–5). When the effect of the duration of a period of overdrive at a fixed rate is evaluated, the results show that for abnormally automatic fibers with maximum diastolic potentials of approximately -55 mV, a sufficiently long period of overdrive can cause very marked overdrive suppression. This overdrive suppression seems to be due at least in major part to activation of the sodium pump and an electrogenic outward current, because inhibition of the pump by a sufficient concentration of ouabain largely abolishes the post-overdrive slowing.

One might assume that these characteristics of normally and abnormally automatic foci would help differentiate between these mechanisms in the case of the in situ heart. Some preliminary evidence bearing on this has been provided by Ilvento et al. (1981). They studied dogs in which heart block had been induced by injecting formalin into the vicinity of the common Bundle. They tested the effects of overdrive both 24 hours and 1 to 2 weeks after heart block had been induced. When tests were made at sufficiently long intervals after surgical intervention, the control idioventricular rhythm was slow and overdrive had its usual effect. Soon after surgery, however, when the ventricular rhythm was rapid, overdrive suppression was not demonstrated after pacing for 15 sec at cycle lengths between 1000 to 250 msec. In some of these latter experiments, overdrive caused acceleration of the fast rhythm, as noted also by Vassalle. Unfortunately, the duration of the period of overdrive was not varied systematically for the fast rhythm.

The results described for effects of overdrive on normal and abnormal automaticity in isolated preparations of Purkinje fibers suggest that there are quantitative

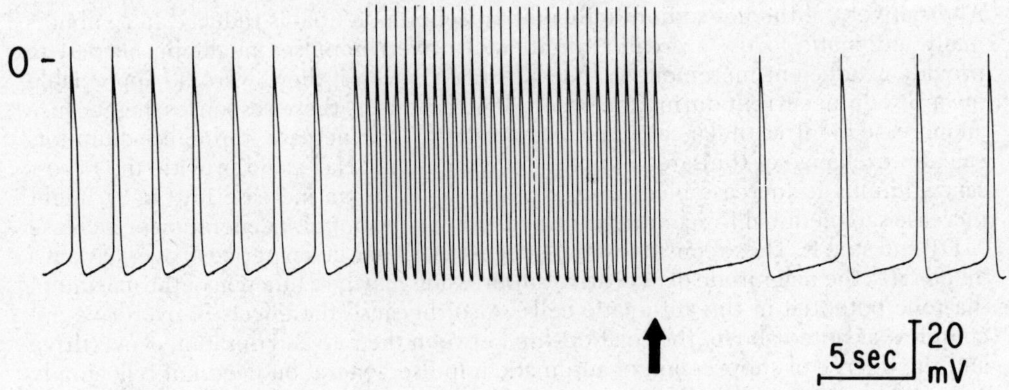

Figure 3. Effects of overdrive on normal automaticity (MDP = −80 mV) in isolated Purkinje fibers. Fifteen seconds of overdrive stimulation at a cycle length of 500 msec; last stimulated beat shown by arrow. Control cycle length 2150 msec, recovery cycle 5400 msec. Zero reference potential at upper left, time and voltage calibrations at lower right.

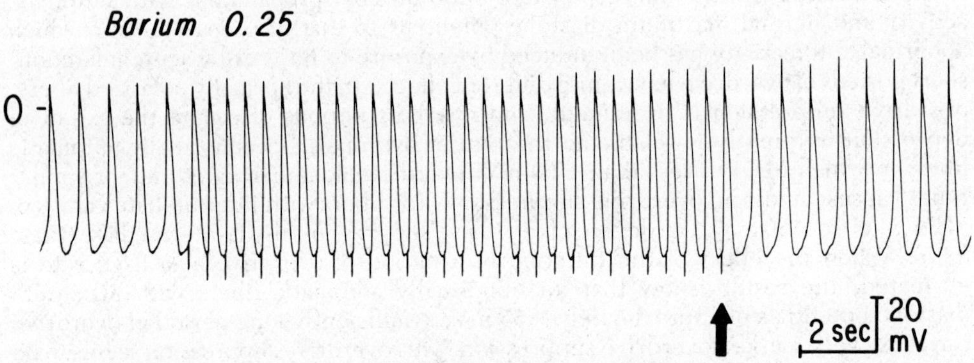

Figure 4. Effects of overdrive on abnormal automaticity (MDP = −52 mV). Fifteen second period of overdrive stimulation in barium-treated Purkinje fiber (0.25 mM $BaCl_2$ added to Tyrode's superfusate). Cycle length 500 msec, last stimulated beat shown by arrow. Control cycle length 810 msec, recovery cycle 790 msec. Zero potential shown at upper left, time and voltage calibrations shown at lower right.

differences in response, but that, in general, overdrive at the proper rate and for a sufficient time should be followed by slowing of automatic impulse generation. On the other hand, it is likely that rhythms caused by delayed after-depolarizations also may be slowed or terminated after a period of rapid impulse generation. Figure 6 shows records from canine Purkinje fibers obtained from an infarcting dog heart; the fibers beat arrhythmically. It appears as though the first few impulses in each group are automatic and result from phase-4 depolarization. As the rate increases, however, a triggered rhythm apparently due to delayed after-depolarizations is initiated. During the rapid triggered rhythm, maximum diastolic potential increases until one after-

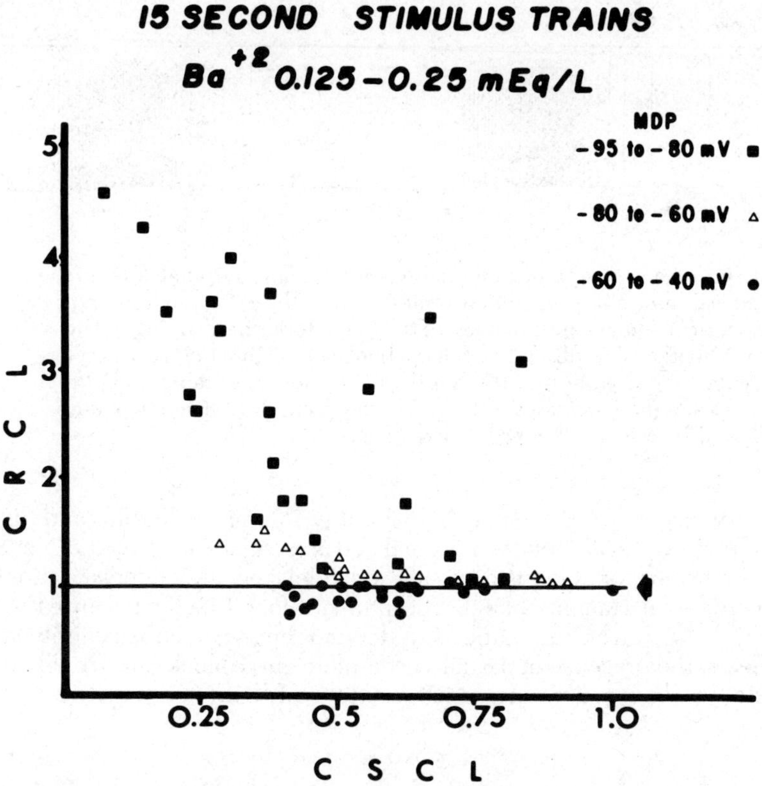

Figure 5. Effects of 15 second periods of overdrive on automatic activity. Responses grouped according to MDP of pacemaker prior to overdrive train: (1) Normal automaticity (squares) in untreated Purkinje fibers or fibers treated with very low concentrations of $BaCl_2$ (0.025 to 0.05 mM), all having MDPs of −80 to −95 mV. (2) Purkinje fibers with intermediate MDPs (−60 to −80 mV) after treatment with barium (0.125 mM) shown by triangles. (3) Data from fibers with abnormal automaticity (MDP = −40 to −60 mV in $BaCl_2$ of 0.125 or 0.25 mM concentration in Tyrode's solution) shown by circles. Corrected recovery cycle length (CRCL, obtained by dividing recovery cycle length by spontaneous cycle length prior to overdrive) plotted against corrected stimulus cycle length (CSCL, obtained in the same manner). Points falling above a CRCL of 1 (horizontal line shown by arrow) indicate overdrive suppression, points falling below this line show overdrive enhancement. Stimulus rates of 2 to 2.5 times control spontaneous rates (CRCL less than 0.5) seem to allow discrimination between abnormal automaticity and normal automaticity.

depolarization fails to initiate an action potential; a pause then ensues. From records of this sort, we would assume that for triggered rhythms caused by delayed after-depolarizations, overdrive might exert effects similar to those described for normal and abnormal automatic rhythms. Indeed, Gadsby (see Chapter 13) recently has described similar effects of overdrive on triggered rhythms initiated in canine coronary sinus fibers and provided evidence that suppression of impulse generation was caused by augmented electrogenic pumping.

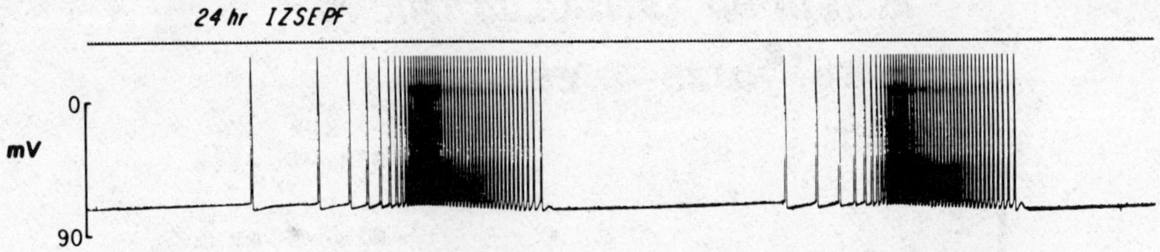

Figure 6. Transmembrane potentials recorded from a Purkinje fiber in the subendocardium of a preparation removed from the infarcting region of a canine heart 24 hours after ligation of the left anterior descending coronary artery. Note that slow phase 4 depolarization leads to initiation of an accelerating automatic rhythm; the rhythm then becomes quite rapid, MDP first decreases and then increases, the rhythm slows and the last action potential is followed by a delayed afterdepolarization.

In summary, use of overdrive may help identify automatic rhythms and, in some cases, may help discriminate between normal and abnormal automaticity. Nevertheless, triggered rhythms, or at least those caused by delayed after-depolarizations, can respond to overdrive in a manner like that of automatic foci. Finally, because the effect of the imposed rhythm on an automatic focus depends on the electrical coupling of the focus to the heart, the presence of partial or complete entry block can strongly modify the response of an abnormally automatic focus to overdrive.

EFFECTS OF SINGLE PREMATURE EXTRASYSTOLES

As we have mentioned, techniques to produce single extrasystoles have been used to investigate the properties of automatic foci in the heart. Such techniques have been widely used in clinical studies to examine the function of the sinus node (Strauss et al., 1973, Bigger and Strauss, 1973, Reiffel, 1979), and also to study idioventricular pacemaker activity (Klein et al., 1973). Experiments on both intact hearts and isolated preparations have indicated that automatic rhythms are only transiently affected by single extrastimuli; if the rhythm is started or stopped by a single extrastimulus, it is attributed to some other mechanism, such as reentry or triggered activity.

Clinical studies on the sinus node pacemaker have tended to indicate that an automatic rhythm may respond in one of three ways to a single extrasystole, according to its timing in the atrial diastolic period (Bigger and Strauss, 1973). Very early premature stimuli (delivered during the first 30% of the diastolic period) may produce an interpolated beat. That is, the first spontaneous beat following the forced (premature) beat will occur at a cycle length of about 70% of the basic spontaneous cycle length. Thus, the "conjoined" cycle length (the "forced" cycle length plus the returning cycle length) will approximately equal the basic spontaneous cycle length. This interpolation phenomenon can be explained by positing entrance block into the sinus node, presumably in the perinodal fibers, which results in "protection" of the sinus pacemaker and allows its activity to continue unimpeded.

Single extrasystoles applied during the middle of the atrial diastolic period (that is, covering the segment between the times when 30% and 75% of the diastolic period has elapsed) produce conjoined cycles that are shorter than the sum of two basic cycles.

That is, the premature impulse is thought to invade the sinus node and discharge it. Normal pacemaker activity then proceeds and results in a returning cycle that begins and ends prematurely with respect to the anticipated normal cycle of activity. Thus, the conjoined cycle is shortened. Such responses are used to estimate the sinoatrial conduction time, by assuming *(1)* that the sinoatrial and atriosinus conduction times are equal, and *(2)* that discharge of the sinus node cells results in "reset" of the pacemaker, which subsequently fires at the control basic cycle length.

If single extrasystoles are evoked during the final 25% of the diastolic period, a third type of response can be elicited. These late extrasystoles are thought to block in the perinodal fibers, as they collide with the wavefront emerging from the sinus node that has been generated by the "next" sinus impulse. The extrasystole thus prevents the spontaneous sinus node impulse from invading the atrium, but it does not discharge the pacemaker itself. The pacemaker site, which has not been perturbed, then produces a "normal" atrial beat after the expected interval (the conjoined cycle is twice the basic atrial cycle length). This produces a "compensatory pause," or a slightly lengthened returning cycle, following the extrasystole.

Most clinical studies of sinus node function necessarily make the assumptions mentioned above. These assumptions may not be valid. In studies on isolated right atrial-sinus node preparations from the rabbit, it has been found that most of the premature impulses that "reset" the sinus node also transiently alter the spontaneous cycle length of the pacemaker fibers. Bonke et al. (1969) reported that the sinus node returning cycle was lengthened following an extrasystole, and that this was caused by a decrease in the slope of phase-4 depolarization, a shift in the pacemaker site within the node, or both. Klein et al. (1973) found that premature extrasystoles elicited during midcycle produced no change or slowing of the subsequent returning cycle of the sinus node. In contrast, early atrial premature depolarizations shortened the sinus node's returning cycle, but lengthened the atrial returning cycle, reflecting an increase in the sinoatrial conduction time. Thus, the data obtained from isolated tissues suggest that studies of sinus node function in intact hearts that depend only on atrial stimulation and the recording of atrial activity should be interpreted with caution. Explicit insights into the response of the in situ sinus node to extrastimulus or overdrive protocols awaits the application of extracellular potential recording techniques to the in situ heart.

Much less is known of the effects of single extrasystoles on ventricular pacemaker activity. It has been reported that, in patients with complete heart block, extrasystoles occurring late in the basic cycle (following the T wave of the last idioventricular beat) generally increased the length of the returning cycle. Following extrasystoles elicited during the T wave, the returning cycle is shorter than the basic cycle in about 95% of the cases (Klein et al., 1973). Studies on isolated Purkinje fibers (Klein et al., 1972) are compatible with these clinical findings. Late extrasystoles (elicited during phase 4) often shifted the pacemaker site and resulted in increased maximum diastolic potentials and a decreased slope of phase-4 depolarization during the returning cycle. Early extrasystoles, which were defined as those with upstrokes occurring during phase 3, tended to shorten the returning cycle. Generally, this shortening of the returning cycle could be explained by a decrease in the duration of the premature action potential. The slope of phase 4 during the returning cycle did not change consistently after these early premature extrasystoles. Occasionally, pacemaker shifts and transient acceleration of the automatic rate occurred following these early stimuli.

Recently, we have studied the effects of single extrasystoles on normal and abnormal automatic activity in isolated preparations of canine Purkinje fibers. In fibers demonstrating normal automaticity, we confirmed the findings of Klein et al. (1972) that extrasystoles during phase 4 provoked returning cycles that were longer than the control spontaneous cycle lengths were. Exceptions were noted when stimuli of high strengths or excessive duration were used during experiments conducted on two different preparations. In these experiments, decreases in spontaneous cycle length (of the returning cycle and often for the next few beats) occurred following application of a single stimulus either early or late during phase 4. This effect presumably was due to catecholamine release, because the acceleration of automatic rate was blocked by exposure to propranolol (2×10^{-7} M). We also studied the effects of impulses initiated at various times during phase 4 on fibers showing abnormal automaticity following exposure to barium (0.15 to 0.25 mM) and having MDP's in the range of −40 to −60 mV. In general, the returning cycle was identical to the control (spontaneous) cycle length. In about 20% of cases, the length of the returning cycle deviated from control values by more than 2% but less than 10%, and in about 3% of the cases, the returning cycle length deviated from control by 10 to 20%. These variant responses were not related to the timing of the premature stimulus in diastole. The results of similar experiments on preparations from 24-hour infarcts showing abnormal automatic activity were far more variable. Either shortening, lengthening, or no change of the returning cycle relative to the control cycle could occur. Returning cycle lengths could be as much as 130% of the control value, but generally if lengthening occurred, the cycle length did not increase by more than 10%. In some preparations, decreases in cycle length occurred, but the returning cycle length was never less than 88% of control values. As in the case of barium-induced abnormal automaticity, the effects of the extrasystoles on the returning cycles did not appear to be related to the timing of the stimulus in diastole. Also, as in the experiments on the barium-treated fibers, the effects of extrasystoles on abnormal automaticity in the infarcted preparations were transient. Control cycle lengths were restored within 2 to 3 beats after the extra beat.

These results show that abnormally automatic foci generally resemble normally automatic pacemakers in their response to single premature impulses. Although there are some differences between them, the major contrast of responses to single premature impulses is between automatic and reentrant or triggered rhythms.

LOCAL ELECTROGRAMS

Unipolar electrograms can be used, under appropriate conditions, to demonstrate the type of change in the transmembrane potential that is the basis for impulse generation. In the case of the sinus node studied in vitro, during sinus rhythms the extracellular electrogram recorded from the pacemaker cells in the sinus node shows deflections that reflect phase 4 depolarization and phase 0 of the transmembrane action potential (Fig. 7) (Cramer et al., 1977; 1978). Because these extracellular potential changes are quite small, as well as quite characteristic, the electrogram can be used both to demonstrate the presence of automatic impulse generation and to localize, rather precisely, the pacemaker. When the heart rate is slow enough to prevent an admixture of the diastolic and upstroke slopes with T and U waves, the same sort of electrograms can be recorded from the in situ canine and human (Hariman et al., 1980a; 1980b; Reiffel et al., 1980) sinus nodes from either the epicardial or endocardial surfaces of the right atrium. These findings suggest that it might be possible to identify automatic rhythms of the in situ heart by recording characteristic electrograms. Very likely the method can be used to discriminate between ectopic impulse generation on one hand and reentrant excitation on the other. The method, however, will not discriminate between normal and abnormal automaticity and is limited in its ability to differentiate between automatic and triggered rhythms. In studies on the canine

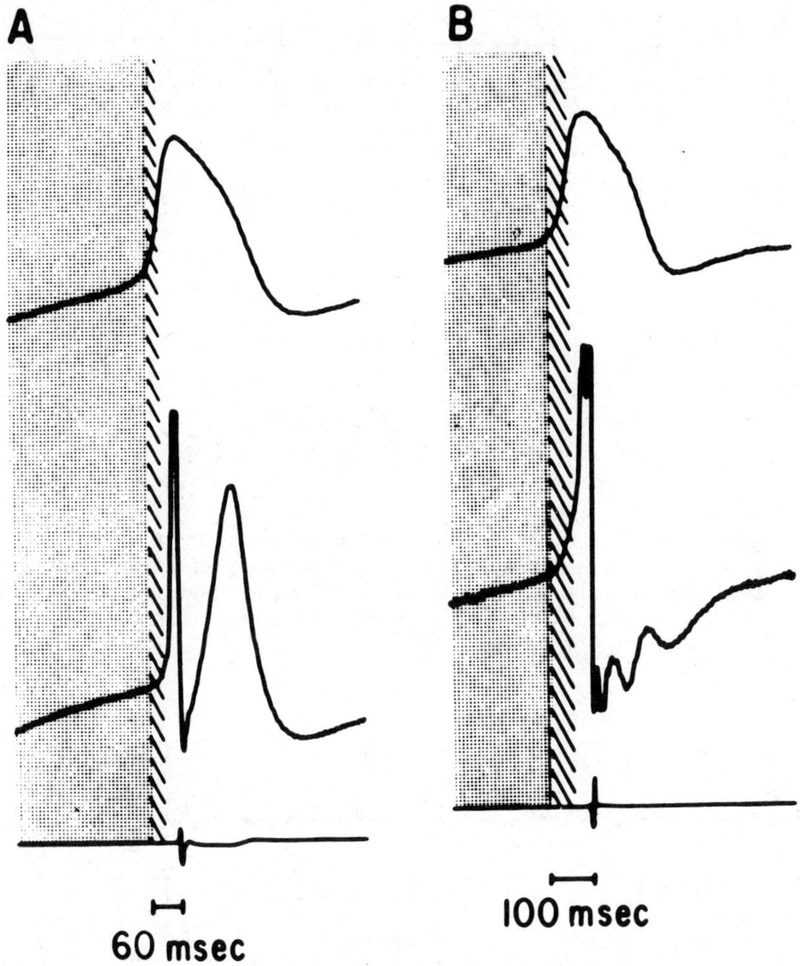

Figure 7. Transmembrane action potentials (top traces) and a unipolar extracellular electrogram (middle traces) recorded from the pacemaking region of the sinus node in two isolated preparations of canine right atrium. The stippled area shows the temporal relationship between the diastolic slope of the electrogram and phase 4 depolarization in the record of transmembrane potential; the cross-hatched area shows the temporal correspondence between the upstroke slope in the electrogram and phase 0 of the transmembrane potential record. A bipolar extracellular electrogram from right atrium is the bottom trace.

coronary sinus in vitro, unipolar extracellular electrograms that demonstrate the delayed after-depolarizations typical of this tissue can be recorded (Fig. 8). When the after-depolarizations are initiating a sustained rapid rhythm, the electrogram resembles that recorded from a rapid automatic focus; only at the beginning and end of the burst of triggered activity can the extracellular potential change caused by the delayed afterdepolarization be identified.

Some comment on unipolar electrograms resulting from early after-depolarizations (EAD) is warranted (Fig. 9).

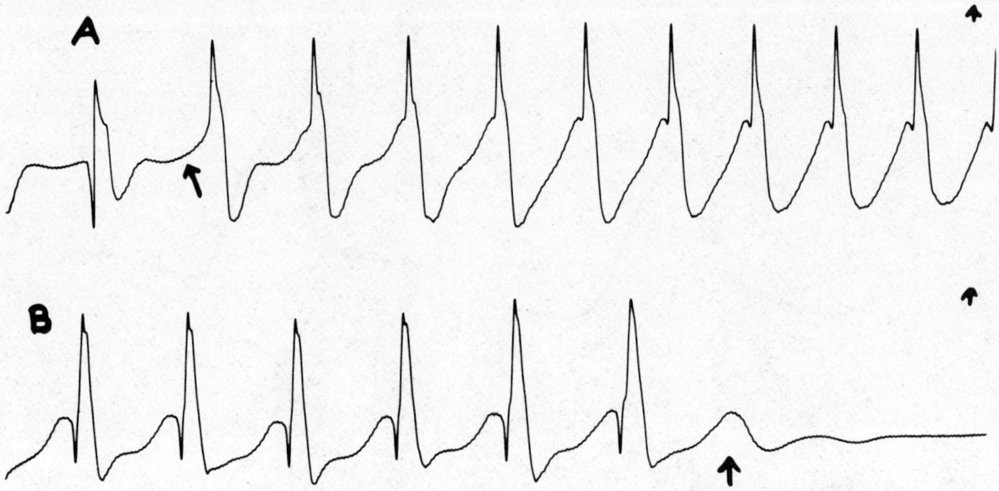

Figure 8. Records of delayed afterdepolarizations and triggered rhythm recorded from an isolated preparation of canine coronary sinus through a unipolar extracellular electrode. The afterdepolarization is seen clearly only at the onset and offset of the triggered rhythm (arrows) (unpublished record, M. Cramer and A.L. Wit).

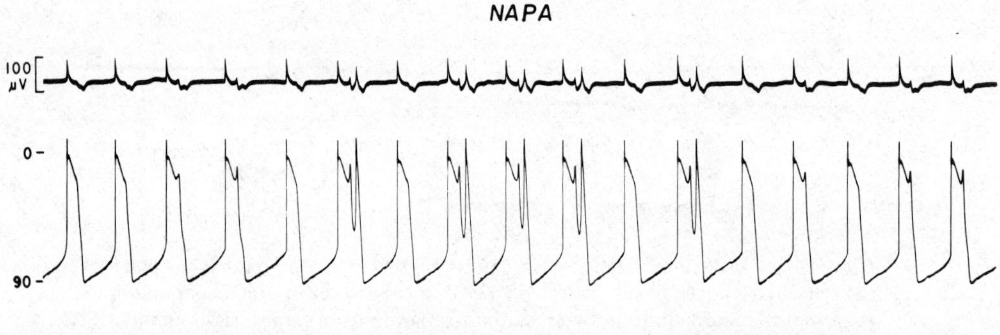

Figure 9. Simultaneous tracings of transmembrane potential and unipolar extracellular electrogram recorded from an isolated preparation of canine Purkinje fibers after exposure to N-acetylprocainamide. The early after-depolarizations developed after some action potentials give rise to clear deflections in the electrogram. Calibrations are shown in the figure.

For isolated preparations of Purkinje fibers, one or two early after-depolarizations (EAD) occurring after each Purkinje fiber action potential cause clear and characteristic deflections in the electrogram (Fig. 9). If the EAD's set up a sustained rhythm, however, the changes in transmembrane potential resemble those recorded from an abnormally automatic focus, and thus it seems unlikely that during this rhythm the local electrogram would show any unique characteristics.

In summary, the unipolar electrogram can be useful in identifying automatic rhythms, as opposed to those caused by delayed after-depolarizations, only if records are obtained from the proper location at the onset and offset of the triggered rhythm. Electrograms should be helpful in differentiating between ectopic impulse generation and reentry, but there is no reason to assume that normal and abnormal mechanisms for automatic impulse generation necessarily would result in differing electrograms.

THE EFFECTS OF DRUGS

If the changes in sarcolemmal ionic conductances responsible for normal automaticity differ from those underlying abnormal automaticity, then chemicals might be found to influence one but not the other mechanism for impulse generation. Also, chemicals or drugs might help discriminate between rhythms caused by abnormal automaticity and those caused by delayed after-depolarizations (DAD) or by EAD's. At the outset, this approach has several limits. The net transmembrane ionic current that causes either phase-4 depolarization or DAD is small; thus, any reasonable increase in outward current would strongly modify impulse generation. Similarly, the changes in membrane potential that underlie both abnormal phase-4 depolarization and DAD are voltage-dependent (as is the case for normal automaticity), and thus an increase in outward current causing a more negative MDP also might modify the mechanism for impulse generation (Vassalle et al., 1977; Imanishi and Surawicz, 1976). In spite of these problems, some possibly useful information can be obtained by considering carefully defined examples.

First, we can consider differences in response to drugs of normally automatic Purkinje fibers and Purkinje fibers generating abnormal automaticity when MDP is less than −60 mV. One might assume that the ionic basis for phase-4 depolarization differed between the two examples. Unfortunately, the cause of phase-4 depolarization in either case is somewhat uncertain (see Cohen, Chapter 16; Pappano and Carmeliet, 1979). Nevertheless, the assumption still can be tested. We have tried to do this in part by using drugs that differ in their effects on the transmembrane potentials of Purkinje fibers. One drug that shows some promise is ethmozin, a new antiarrhythmic agent (Danilo et al., 1977; Morganroth et al., 1979) that reduces $\dot{V}_{max}$ of phase 0 like lidocaine but does not modify the slope of normal phase-4 depolarization. In contrast, ethmozin is quite effective in slowing or terminating abnormal automatic rhythms in Purkinje fibers exposed to Ba^{2+} or in the ischemic endocardium of infarcting canine hearts (Dangman and Hoffman, 1978). Lidocaine, on the other hand, decreases the slope of phase-4 depolarization in normally automatic Purkinje fibers but not in Purkinje fibers generating abnormal automaticity (Allen et al., 1978; Dangman and Hoffman, 1978). Obviously, other effects of these agents also might modify the rate of impulse generation. For example, ethmozin will slow impulse generation in normally automatic Purkinje fibers, apparently by causing a shift in threshold potential (Dangman and Hoffman, 1981). Nevertheless, studies on ventricular rhythms in dogs with complete heart block seem to support the suggestion provided by studies on normal and abnormal automaticity in vitro. Ilvento (Ilvento et al., 1981) showed that, 24 hours after production of heart block, rapid idioventricular rhythms were slowed by ethmozin but not by lidocaine; 1 week or more later, slow idioventricular rhythms were slowed by lidocaine but not by ethmozin.

A similar approach to discriminating between normal and abnormal automaticity might depend on the ionic current responsible for generating the action potential upstroke. In fibers (other than the SA node) with a normal MDP, this current would depend on fast inward channels, whereas in partially depolarized fibers (MDP < -60 mV), the upstroke would depend mainly on current in slow inward channels. We have attempted to look for drugs that might take advantage of this difference by testing several slow-channel blocking drugs. In vitro, both verapamil and nifedipine slow or stop abnormal impulse generation in Purkinje fibers exposed to Ba^{2+} and in fibers from 24-hour infarcts. Nifedipine has almost no effect on normal phase-4 depolarization in Purkinje fibers (Dangman and Hoffman, 1979; 1980), and verapamil has only a small effect (Danilo et al., 1980). If, when given to intact animals, nifedipine and verapamil do not cause excessive release of catecholamines, they may provide an additional means to test for abnormal automaticity.

Pharmacologic tests, like other tests, are more likely to be effective in discriminating between normal and abnormal automaticity when MDP in the abnormally automatic focus is quite low. With intermediate values of MDP, the effects of drugs might be difficult to predict. Also, there is little reason to hope that the drugs evaluated so far can discriminate between rhythms caused by abnormal automaticity or those caused by DAD. DAD's in Purkinje fibers, when caused by digitalis intoxication, are decreased in amplitude by a wide variety of antiarrhythmic drugs (Rosen and Danilo, 1980), including those that act primarily on fast or slow inward channels.

CONCLUSIONS

The distinction we have made between normal and abnormal automaticity, which depends on the level of MDP, obviously is inappropriate because the sinus node, the normally automatic pacemaker of the mammalian heart, generates impulses from a low MDP and shows many of the characteristics of our abnormally automatic Purkinje fibers. If we fully understood the ionic mechanisms for automatic impulse generation in sinus node, in normally polarized and partially depolarized specialized fibers, and in partially depolarized muscle fibers, a more reasonable classification might be possible. Nevertheless, it seems likely that some automatic rhythms result from phase-4 depolarization in normal specialized fibers and some from phase-4 depolarization in partially depolarized fibers that may or may not be specialized.

Because, among apparently automatic rhythms of the in situ heart, there are differences in responses to electrical stimulation and drugs, and because these responses often resemble those obtained for in vitro preparations, which show normal or abnormal automaticity, it probably is permissible to assume that both mechanisms can be the cause of arrhythmias. Further studies in which data are obtained for responses to selected patterns of stimulation and to selected drugs and in which records of local electrograms are obtained may provide the means to definitely identify each of these mechanisms and clearly differentiate them from triggered activity caused by afterdepolarizations.

REFERENCES

Allen JD, Brennan FJ, Wit AL (1978) Actions of lidocaine on transmembrane potentials of subendocardial Purkinje fibers surviving in infarcted canine hearts. Circ Res **43**:470–481

Antzelevitch C, Jalife J, Moe GK (1980) Characteristics of reflection as a mechanism of reentrant arrhythmias and its relationship to parasystole. Circulation **61**:182–191

Baumgarten CM, Isenberg G (1977) Depletion and accumulation of potassium in the extracellular clefts of cardiac Purkinje fibers during voltage clamp hyperpolarization and depolarization. Pflüg Arch **368**:19–31

Bigger JT, Jr, Goldreyer BN (1970) The mechanism of supraventricular tachycardia. Circulation **42**:673–688

Bigger JT, Jr, Strauss HC (1973) The evaluation of sinoatrial node function in man. MCV Quarterly **9**:77–85

Bonke FIM, Bouman LN, van Rijn HE (1969) Change of cardiac rhythm in the rabbit after an atrial premature beat. Circ Res **24**:533–544

Brown HF, Clark A, Noble SJ (1976) Identification of the pacemaker current in frog atrium. J Physiol **258**:521–545

Bush HL, Jr, Gelband H, Hoffman BF, Malm JR (1971) Electrophysiological basis for supraventricular arrhythmias. Arch Surg **103**:620–625

Cleemann L, Morad M (1979) Extracellular potassium accumulation in voltage-clamped frog ventricular muscle. J Physiol **286**:83–111

Cramer M, Hariman RJ, Boxer R, Hoffman BF (1978) Electrograms from the canine sinoatrial pacemaker recorded in vitro and in situ. Am J Cardiol **42**:939–946

Cramer M, Siegal M, Bigger JT, Jr, Hoffman BF (1977) Characteristics of extracellular potentials recorded from the sinoatrial pacemaker of the rabbit. Circ Res **41**:292–300

Cranefield PF (1975) The Conduction of the Cardiac Impulse. Mt Kisco, NY, Futura Publishing Company

Cranefield PF (1977) Action potentials, afterpotentials and arrhythmias. Circ Res **41**:415–423

Dangman KH, Hoffman BF (1978) The effects of EN-313 on abnormal automaticity in canine cardiac Purkinje fibers. Circulation **57/58**:11–104

Dangman KH, Hoffman BF (1979) The effects of nifedipine on abnormal automaticity in canine cardiac Purkinje fibers. Circulation **60**:II–209

Dangman, KH, Hoffman BF (1980) Effects of nifedipine on electrical activity of cardiac cells. Am J Cardiol **46**:1059–1067

Dangman KH, Hoffman BF Effects of ethmozin on automatic and triggered impulse initiation in canine cardiac Purkinje fibers. Circ Res (Submitted, 1981)

Danilo P, Langan WB, Rosen MR, Hoffman BF (1977) Effects of the phenothiazine analog, EN-313, on ventricular arrhythmias in the dog. Eur J Pharmacol **45**:127–139

Danilo P, Hordof AJ, Reder RF, Rosen MR (1980) Effects of verapamil on electrophysiologic properties of blood superfused cardiac Purkinje fibers. JPET **213**:222–227

Deitmer JW, Ellis D (1978) The intracellular sodium activity of cardiac Purkinje fibers during inhibition and re-activation of the Na-K pump. J Physiol **284**:241–259

DiFrancesco D, Noma A, Trautwein W (1980) Separation of current induced by potassium accumulation from acetylcholine-induced relaxation current in the rabbit S-A node. Pflüg Arch **387**:83–90

Eisner DA, Lederer WJ (1980a) Characterization of the electrogenic sodium pump in cardiac Purkinje fibers. J Physiol **303**:441–474

Eisner DA, Lederer WJ (1980b) The relationship between sodium pump activity and twitch tension in cardiac Purkinje fibers. J Physiol **303**:475–494

Friedman PL, Stewart JR, Wit A (1973) Spontaneous and induced cardiac arrhythmias in subendocardial Purkinje fibers surviving extensive myocardial infarction in dogs. Circ Res **33**:612–626

Gadsby DC, Cranefield PF (1979a) Electrogenic sodium extrusion in cardiac Purkinje fibers. J Gen Physiol **73**:819–837

Gadsby DC, Cranefield PF (1979b) Direct measurement of changes in sodium pump current in canine cardiac Purkinje fibers. Proc Natl Acad Sci **76**:1783–1787

Hariman RJ, Hoffman BF, Naylor RE (1980) Electrical activity from the sinus node region in conscious dogs. Circ Res **47**:775–791

Hariman RJ, Krongrad E, Boxer RA, Bowman FO, Malm JR, Hoffman BF (1980b) Methods for recording electrograms of the sinoatrial node during cardiac surgery in man. Circulation **61**:1024–1029

Hariman RJ, Krongrad E, Boxer RA, Weiss MB, Steeg CN, Hoffman BF (1980c) Method for recording electrical activity of the sinoatrial node and automatic atrial foci during cardiac catheterization in human subjects. Am J Cardiol **45**:775–781

Hauswirth O, Noble D, Tsien RW (1969) The mechanism of oscillatory activity at low membrane potentials in cardiac Purkinje fibers. J Physiol **200**:255–265

Hogan PM, Davis LD: Evidence for specialized fibers in the canine right atrium. Circ Res **23**:387–396

Hordof A, Edie R, Malm J, Hoffman B, Rosen M (1976) Electrophysiologic properties and response to pharmacologic agents of fibers from diseased human atria. Circulation **54**: 774–779

Ilvento JP, Provet J, Danilo P, Rosen MR An electrophysiologic and pharmacologic study of fast and slow idioventricular rhythms in the dog. Circ Res (Submitted, 1981)

Imanishi S, Surawicz B (1976) Automatic activity in depolarized guinea pig ventricular myocardium. Circ Res **39**:751–759

Jalife J, Moe GK (1976) Effects of electrotonic potentials on pacemaker activity of canine Purkinje fibers in relation to parasystole. Circ Res **39**:801–809

Jalife J, Moe GK (1979) A biologic model of parasystole. Am J Cardiol **43**:761–772

Katzung BO, Morgenstern JA (1977) Effects of extracellular potassium on ventricular automaticity and evidence for a pacemaker current in mammalian ventricular myocardium. Circ Res **40**:105–111

Klein HO, Cranefield PF, Hoffman BF (1972) Effect of extrasystoles on idioventricular rhythm. Circ Res **30**:651–665

Klein HO, Singer DH, Hoffman BF (1973) Effects of atrial premature systoles on sinus rhythm in the rabbit. Circ Res **32**:480–491

Kline RP, Cohen I, Falk R, Kupersmith J (1980) Activity-dependent extracellular K^+ fluctuations in canine Purkinje fibers. Nature **286**:68–71

Kunze DL (1977) Rate-dependent changes in extracellular potassium in the rabbit atrium. Circ Res **41**:122–127

Lazzara R, El-Sherif M, Scherlag BJ (1973) Electrophysiological properties of canine Purkinje cells in one-day-old myocardial infarction. Circ Res **33**:722–734

Morganroth J, Pearlman AS, Dunkman WB, Horowitz LN, Josephson ME, Michelson EL (1979) Ethmozin: A new antiarrhythmic agent developed in the USSR. Efficacy and tolerance. Am Heart J **98**:621–628

Noble D (1975) The Initiation of the Heartbeat. Oxford, Clarendon Press

Paes de Carvalho A, deMello WC, Hoffman BF (1959) Electrophysiological evidence for specialized fiber types in rabbit atrium. Am J Physiol **196**:483–488

Pappano AJ, Carmeliet EE (1979) Epinephrine and the pacemaking mechanism at plateau potentials in sheep cardiac Purkinje fibers. Pflüg Arch **382**:17–26

Reid JA, Hecht HH (1967) Barium-induced automaticity in right ventricular muscle in the dog. Circ Res **21**:849–855

Reiffel JA (1979) Principles and applications of electrophysiologic testing of sinus node function. Cardiovasc Med **4**:97–111

Reiffel JA, Gang E, Gliclich J, Weiss MB, Davis JC, Patton JN, Bigger JT (1980) The human sinus node electrogram: A transvenous catheter technique and a comparison of directly measured and indirectly estimated sinoatrial conduction time in adults. Circulation **62**: 1324–1334

Rosen MR, Danilo P (1980) Effects of tetrodotoxin, lidocaine, verapamil and AHR-2666 on ouabain-induced delayed afterdepolarizations in canine Purkinje fibers. Circ Res **46**:117–124

Rosen MR, Fisch C, Hoffman BF, Danilo P, Lovelace DE, Knockel SB (1980) Can accelerated atrioventricular junctional escape rhythm be explained by delayed afterdepolarizations? Am J Cardiol **45**:1272–1284

Strauss HC, Saroff AL, Bigger JT, Jr, Giardina EGV (1973) Premature atrial stimulation as a key to the understanding of sinoatrial conduction in man. Circulation **67**:86–93

Vassalle M (1970) Electrogenic suppression of automaticity in sheep and dog Purkinje fibers. Circ Res **27**:361–377

Vassalle M, Cummins M, Castro C, Stuckey JH (1976) The relationship between overdrive suppression and overdrive excitation in ventricular pacemakers. Circ Res **38**:367–374

Vassalle M, Knob RE, Cummins M, Lara GA, Castro C, Stuckey JH (1977) An analysis of fast idioventricular rhythm in the dog. Circ Res **41**:218–226

Weidmann S (1951) Effect of current flow on the membrane potential of cardiac muscle. J Physiol **115**:227–236

Wellens HJJ, Lie KI, Durrer D (1974) Further observations on ventricular tachycardia as studied by electrical stimulation of the heart: Chronic recurrent ventricular tachycardia and ventricular tachycardia during acute myocardial infarction. Circulation **49**:647

Wit AL, Cranefield PF (1977) Triggered and automatic activity in the canine coronary sinus. Circ Res **41**:435–445

Wit AL, Cranefield PF (1978) Reentrant excitation as a cause of cardiac arrhythmias. Am J Physiol **235**:H1–H17

Wit AL, Cranefield PF, Hoffman BF (1972a) Slow conduction and reentry in the ventricular conducting system. II. Single and sustained circus movement in networks of canine and bovine Purkinje fibers. Circ Res **30**:11

Wit AL, Hoffman BF, Cranefield PF (1972b) Slow conduction and reentry in the ventricular conducting system. I. Return extrasystole in canine Purkinje fibers. Circ Res **30**:1

Discussion

I. COHEN: Robin Falk, Richard Kline, and I have recently performed voltage-clamp studies with trains of repetitive depolarizations in which the membrane was depolarized for 50 msec every 100 msec. We saw that when the holding potential was −80 mV there was a large pump current following a 2-min train. Then, when we repeated the same protocol using a holding potential of −55 mV, from which we think the fast sodium inward current is almost totally inactivated, we saw little pump current after the same 2-min train. When tetrodotoxin was added during the experiments from a −80 mV holding potential, it also eliminated the majority of the pump current that was seen. This, therefore, supports the idea that there may be a different expectation of the results of overdrive suppression experiments from a high or a low resting potential.

HOFFMAN: I am reassured about the pump experiments. But I wonder if even during overdrive at low resting potential there isn't enough increase in the intracellular sodium, perhaps owing to an exchange of calcium for sodium, to turn on the Na-K pump. I say this because even though most of the time, let us say 90% of the time, we get results that agree with your data, there still is a small percentage of experiments in which we do not.

CARMELIET: Concerning your barium model showing that depolarized Purkinje cells do not exhibit overdrive suppression, I would like to add that the absence of overdrive suppression can also be demonstrated in a Purkinje fiber immersed in a high-potassium solution containing adrenaline. A major difference between these two models is that the potassium conductance is severely shut off in the barium model.

HOFFMAN: Yes, that is true. But we see no particular difference between the Purkinje fiber depolarized by potassium and that depolarized by barium. Yet, in either case, sometimes you can show overdrive suppression at a low resting potential.

CARMELIET: Does that not surprise you? I would expect no overdrive suppression in the case of an increased extracellular potassium and adrenaline.

HOFFMAN: Well, it may be that there is enough accumulation of potassium outside cells to provide another mechanism for overdrive suppression.

JOHNSON: I think the situation here is rather complicated. It all depends on what happens to the Na^+-K^+ electrogenic transport. I think you can explain both instances of presence or absence of overdrive suppression depending on what you do to the transport system.

HOFFMAN: I agree it is complicated, I just hope Gadsby can explain it all to me some day.

SOMMER: Could you specify what you mean by specialized fibers?

HOFFMAN: I call specialized fibers those that show one or more unique characteristics in the transmembrane potentials. I would include in this category fibers from the sinoatrial and atrioventricular nodes that show only slow responses. I would also include the specialized atrial fibers and the His-Purkinje system that can show pacemaker activity under physiologic conditions. As an extension, I would add the fibers deep into the coronary sinus that can generate after-depolarizations; the fibers of the coronary sinus ostium that show automatic activity, and also the fibers in the canine and human AV valve that show delayed after-depolarizations and can originate triggered rhythms. So, by specialized fibers, I mean a large group that obviously is not homogeneous. I think we can define them as specialized fibers in a functional sense. We can say that there are structural differences associated with this specialization. Now, we have no idea of whether these structural changes are sufficient to serve as criteria for morphologic differentiation, or even if these changes are in any way associated with functional specialization.

SOMMER: At the present state of the art of structural analysis, we can do no more than acknowledge clear structural differences between a few cell populations in the atrium, such as between the common atrial and nodal cells, and between atrial cells with and without transverse tubules.

PAES DE CARVALHO: I would like to ask Dr. Sommer if he disagrees with Dr. James's characterization of specialized fibers within atrial muscle.

SOMMER: Yes, I disagree in the following sense. Any attempt at correlating electrophysiologic records obtained from atrial cells suffers the constraint that recordings made from one cell reflect the electrical activity of an electrically coupled network of such cells rather than that of a single cell. Therefore, the anatomical identification of so-called specialized cells lacks an independent rigorous correlate, unless such specialized cells form a more or less insulated large network as, for example, the bundles of Purkinje cells in the ventricle, or the nodal cells. We, as many before us, have not been able to confirm the existence in the atrium of tractlike accumulations of cells that can, by any rigorous anatomical cellular criterion, be separated, safely, from the rest of the common atrial cells. But I should like to point out (about which more is in our written contribution to this symposium) that our laboratory always has taken, and still is taking, James's notion of specialized tracts quite seriously. After our recent studies, we are not persuaded that there is a predilection for identifiable tracts of atrial cells without transverse tubules, the latter being typical for conduction cells in the ventricles. But, a study is yet needed of bundles of atrial muscle cells that may be distinguished by tight apposition, which, as we have shown earlier, greatly influences the electrical properties of cardiac cell networks; such bundles may be preferentially located in certain regions of the atrium.

Chapter 25

Delayed Afterdepolarizations and Clinical Arrhythmogenesis

Robert F. Reder and Michael R. Rosen

Until recently, clinical cardiac arrhythmias were thought to result from abnormalities of conduction, or automaticity, or both (Rosen and Hoffman, 1973). Recent studies of cellular electrophysiology, however, have led to the recognition of additional mechanisms that may be responsible for clinical arrhythmias. One example is the delayed after-depolarization, which may lead to "triggered activity" (Cranefield, 1977). In this chapter we will discuss the cellular electrophysiologic characteristics of delayed after-depolarizations and explore the relationship between them and certain clinical arrhythmias. To clarify how after-depolarizations differ from other mechanisms responsible for arrhythmias, we shall begin by reviewing briefly both reentry and automaticity.

REENTRY AND AUTOMATICITY

As described classically, reentry requires a site of unidirectional block, slow retrograde conduction, and reemergence of a slowly propagated impulse into normal tissue whose refractory period has terminated (Moe, 1975). Such reentrant circuits can involve well-defined anatomical pathways (as in the Wolff-Parkinson-White syndrome) (Gallagher et al., 1978), or they can involve conduction block and reentry in the distal Purkinje system (Wit et al., 1972) or the atrium (Allessie et al., 1973). The presence of conduction block may be seen in tissues with normally low levels of membrane potential and slow conduction, such as the AV node; or it may result from pathologic depression of conduction in tissues that normally have high levels of membrane potential, such as the Purkinje system. Moe (1975) reviewed a variety of clinical arrhythmias that may be due to reentry, including atrial flutter, atrial fibrilla-

---

Certain of the studies referred to were supported by USPHS-NHLBI grants HL-12738 and HL-07419 and grants from the New York Heart Association.

tion, paroxysmal supraventricular tachycardia, isolated atrial, and ventricular "echo" beats, intraventricular "echo" beats, ventricular flutter, and premature ventricular beats showing fixed coupling. In clinical studies, one of the criteria for reentry is based on the initiation and termination of such rhythms by appropriately timed, premature impulses. The premature impulse is thought to establish or to interrupt the reentrant circuit by altering the refractory periods of the tissues involved. Usually a "window" of appropriately timed, premature impulses can be defined, within which both initiation and termination of the arrhythmia can be elicited (Wellens, 1978). A second criterion used in clinical electrophysiologic studies is the response of an arrhythmia to overdrive pacing. A reentrant rhythm should be interrupted by overdrive stimulation, assuming the drive stimuli penetrate and alter the refractory periods of the tissues in the reentrant circuit. On cessation of overdrive, the arrhythmia should not recur until those conditions that initially brought it about recur, either spontaneously or as a result of electrical stimulation. Alternatively, on some occasions overdrive pacing may initiate a reentrant (presumably) arrhythmia.

The same clinical pacing techniques are used to identify automatic rhythms. The rhythms most readily identified as automatic respond to overdrive in a manner similar to normal isolated Purkinje fibers manifesting normal automaticity (Noble, 1975). That is, in response to overdrive pacing in isolated tissues and in clinical studies, normal pacemakers in the sinoatrial node, atrium, and ventricle show overdrive suppression (Vassalle, 1977). The basis for overdrive suppression appears, in the main, to be an increased electrogenic pumping resulting from the Na^+ entry that is induced by the rapid stimulus rate. For cells of the sinus node, factors such as increased influx of Na^+ or Ca^{++} as well as increased K^+ efflux have been implicated, as has acetylcholine release (Kodama, 1980). Programmed premature stimulation will not result in termination of this type of automaticity, although the automatic focus may be reset by premature depolarizations.

Another type of automaticity has been described in cells with low levels of membrane potential (less than or equal to -60 mV). At these levels of membrane potential, the current responsible for normal pacemaker function presumably is inactivated (Noble, 1975). Abnormal automaticity has been described in canine cardiac Purkinje fibers that have been depolarized by barium or cesium (Dangman and Hoffman, 1981), in experimental myocardial infarction in dogs (Dangman and Hoffman, 1978), and in diseased human atrium (Mary-Rabine et al., 1980). This type of automaticity is different from the normal in that it usually is not overdrive-suppressed. On cessation of overdrive the automatic pacemaker almost immediately assumes its pre-overdrive rate and may at times actually increase in rate (K. Dangman, personal communication). The mechanism and characteristics of this type of event are the subject of Chapter 16 of this volume.

AFTERDEPOLARIZATIONS AND TRIGGERED ACTIVITY

Triggered activity refers to a rhythm whose occurrence depends on a preceding beat or beats to initiate it. In the broadest sense, then, reentry might qualify as a triggered rhythm. However, as described by Cranefield (1977), triggered activity should be considered as resulting from impulse initiation by a single cell or group of cells as the result of an after-depolarization. The presence of unidirectional block and slow conduction needed for the occurrence of reentry are not required here.

Two types of after-depolarizations have been described: early and delayed after-depolarizations (Cranefield, 1977). The former are depolarizing potentials occurring during repolarization of the action potential (at voltages usually less than −50 mV). In studies on isolated tissue, these have been shown to induce repetitive electrical activity. Such after-depolarizations probably result from oscillatory changes in the slow inward current responsible for the plateau. The characteristics of early after-depolarizations and their ability to cause clinical arrhythmias are not well defined at this time; this phenomenon, however, should be considered as a potential arrhythmogenic mechanism.

Delayed afterdepolarizations have been more completely described. These are oscillations that occur following the repolarization of a cell to its maximum diastolic potential (Fig. 1) (Cranefield, 1977). Although early studies noted that oscillatory events occurred in electrical diastole (Segers, 1941; Bozler, 1943), intense investigation of delayed after-depolarizations using microelectrode techniques did not begin until the 1970s (Cranefield, 1973; Davis, 1973; Ferrier et al., 1973; Rosen et al., 1973a; 1973b; Saunders, 1973; Cranefield et al., 1974). In distinguishing the rhythms resulting from delayed after-depolarizations from those induced by normal automaticity, Cranefield (1977) noted that for the former to occur an action potential must be the inciting event. That is, delayed after-depolarizations cannot arise de novo, whereas automaticity can and does. Once they occur, delayed after-depolarizations can cause single premature depolarizations or bursts of tachyarrhythmia (Fig. 2).

Delayed after-depolarizations have been described in a variety of experimental settings. Rosen et al. (1973a; 1974b), Davis (1973), Ferrier et al. (1973), and Saunders et al. (1973) demonstrated delayed afterdepolarizations (also called oscillatory afterpotentials [Ferrier, 1977] in Purkinje fibers in the presence of toxic concentrations of digitalis (Fig. 3). Here, delayed afterdepolarizations and their resultant triggered rhythms supplanted normal phase-4 automaticity. Digitalis-induced delayed after-depolarizations also have been described in canine atrial (Hashimoto and Moe, 1973)

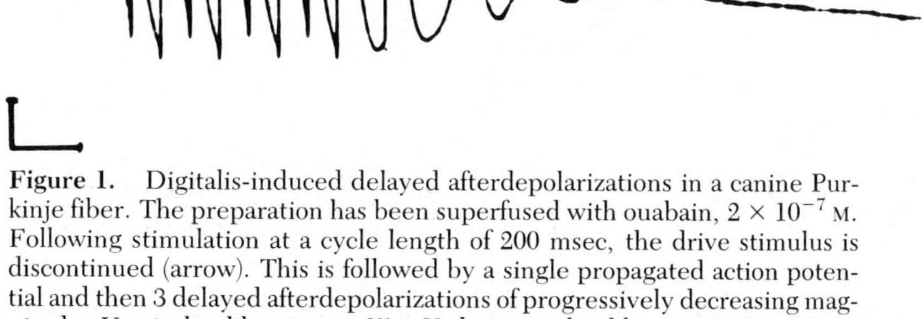

Figure 1. Digitalis-induced delayed afterdepolarizations in a canine Purkinje fiber. The preparation has been superfused with ouabain, 2×10^{-7} M. Following stimulation at a cycle length of 200 msec, the drive stimulus is discontinued (arrow). This is followed by a single propagated action potential and then 3 delayed afterdepolarizations of progressively decreasing magnitude. Vertical calibration = 25 mV; horizontal calibration = 500 msec. (Modified after Rosen, M. and Danilo, P.: Digitalis-induced delayed afterdepolarizations. In *The Slow Inward Current*, edited by Zipes et al., Martinus Nijhoff, 1980, pp. 295–308.)

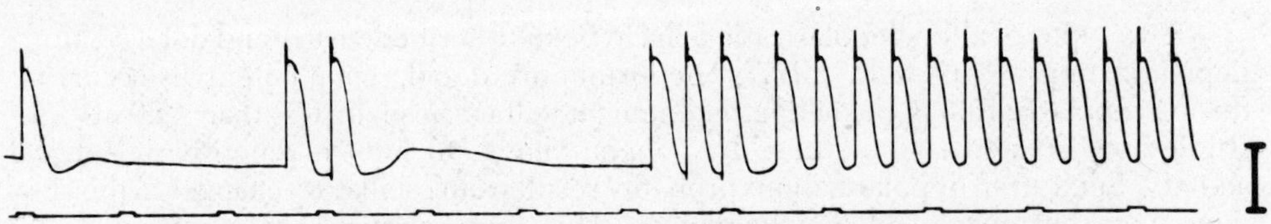

Figure 2. Triggered rhythm induced by delayed afterdepolarizations. A Purkinje fiber bundle has been superfused with ouabain, 2×10^{-7} M. When the drive stimulus was discontinued the preparation was quiescent. Following a single stimulus there is a propagated action potential followed by a small delayed afterdepolarization. Introduction of two stimuli (center) induces a larger delayed afterdepolarization. Introduction of three stimuli (right) results in triggered activity. Time marks = 1 second. Vertical calibration = 50 mV.

and ventricular (Davis, 1973; Ferrier et al., 1973; Rosen et al., 1973a; 1973b; Saunders, 1973) specialized conducting tissue and ventricular muscle (Ferrier, 1976; 1977), and in human atrium (Ferrier, 1976) and ventricle (Rosen et al., 1980a). In the absence of digitalis, delayed after-depolarizations have been demonstrated in canine Purkinje fibers (Fig. 3)(Wit et al., 1973), simian (Wit and Cranefield, 1976), and human (Wit et al., 1977) atrioventricular valvular tissue, canine coronary sinus (Wit and Cranefield, 1977), rabbit right atrium (Saito et al., 1978), and diseased human atrium (Wit et al., 1979a).

An important difference between normal automatic pacemakers and delayed after-depolarizations is seen in the response of both phenomena to overdrive stimulation. As mentioned above, normal pacemakers are overdrive-suppressed. In contrast, when delayed after-depolarizations occur, overdrive stimulation results in an increase in after-depolarization amplitude and a decrease in the coupling interval of the delayed after-depolarization to the drive impulse (Fig. 3). As these events occur, there is an increase in the likelihood that the after-depolarization will reach threshold and initiate an ectopic impulse or train of impulses. Moreover, as overdrive cycle length decreases, the cycle length of any arrhythmia resulting from delayed after-depolarizations also decreases.

Once delayed after-depolarizations induce spontaneous rhythms, these persist for variable periods of time. They may cease suddenly, or their cycle length may increase over several cycles before cessation. Introduction of single or multiple premature stimuli sometimes causes a delayed after-depolarization-induced rhythm to stop (as can occur with reentrant rhythms)(Wit et al., 1979a). But, induced premature impulses also can reset the rhythm or induce a rhythm occurring at an even shorter cycle length.

THE RELATIONSHIP BETWEEN DELAYED AFTERDEPOLARIZATIONS AND CLINICAL ARRHYTHMIAS

Perhaps the most likely delayed after-depolarization-induced arrhythmia is the repetitive ventricular response described for digitalis-intoxicated dogs by Lown et al. (1967) and Hagemeijer and Lown (1970). They sewed epicardial electrodes to the hearts of anesthesized dogs and introduced premature stimuli during the terminal phases of the T wave or during electrical diastole. Prior to digitalis administration,

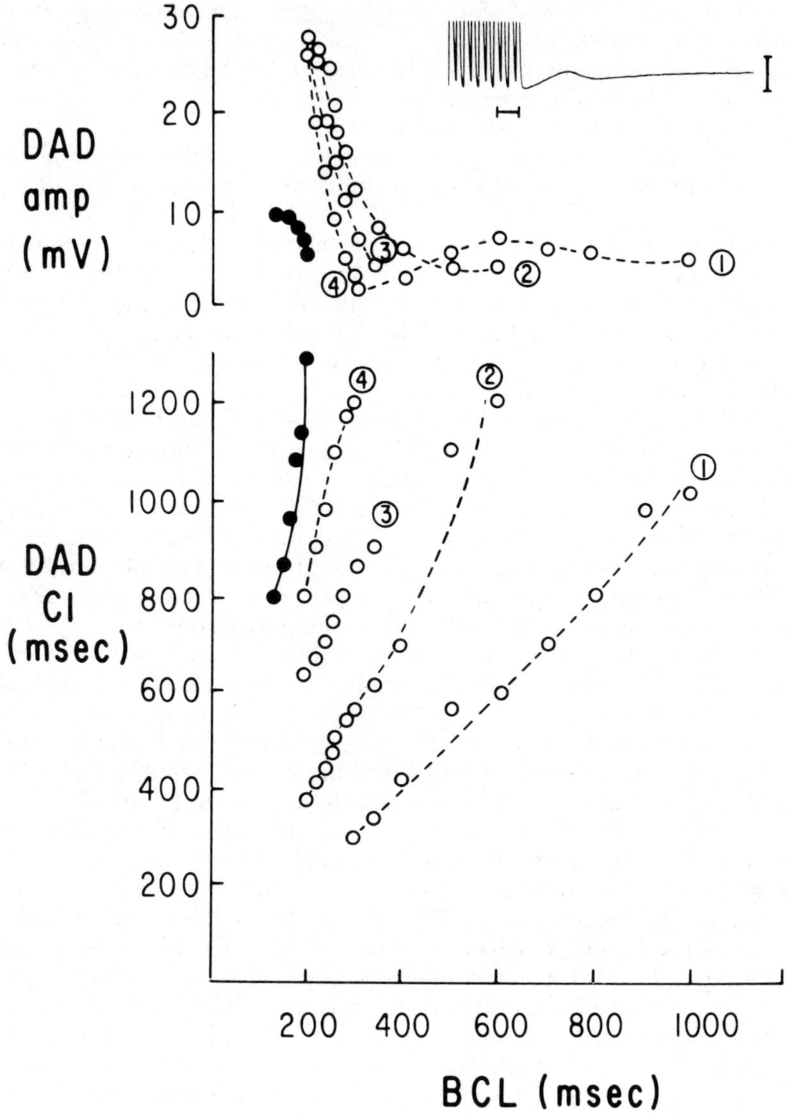

Figure 3. Relationship of basic cycle length (BCL) to amplitude (amp) and coupling interval (CI) of delayed afterdepolarizations in a canine Purkinje fiber. The filled circles indicate delayed afterdepolarizations occurring prior to superfusion with ouabain. These are seen only at very short drive cycle lengths (see insert). The unfilled circles indicate the first 4 delayed afterdepolarizations in sequence that occurred in the preparation after superfusion with ouabain, 2×10^{-7} M (numbered 1–4). Note that as BCL decreases, the coupling interval of the delayed afterdepolarizations also decreases. For the first delayed afterdepolarization in the sequence, peak amplitude is attained at BCL = 600 msec. It then becomes smaller. The second, third and fourth delayed afterdepolarizations all become larger as BCL decreases further. (Modified after Rosen, M.R.: Cellular mechanisms of cardiac arrhythmias. In *Cardiac Arrhythmias: A Decade of Progress*, edited by D. Harrison, G.K. Hall & Co., 1981, pp. 275–303.)

premature stimuli elicited only single ectopic beats. The dogs then were made digitalis-toxic with acetylstrophanthidin. The pacing study was repeated, and it was found that the premature stimulus usually induced several ectopic beats instead of one, and the stimulus amplitude needed to induce the initial ectopic beat decreased. As the animals became more toxic, the arrhythmia became more persistent until ventricular tachycardia ensued. Repetitive ventricular responses were more likely to be induced by premature stimuli early in the cardiac cycle than late in electrical diastole.

The dependence of the repetitive ventricular response on the preceding drive-cycle length, and its occurrence with stimuli of lesser amplitude at greater degrees of digitalis intoxication, parallel the behavior of digitalis-induced delayed afterdepolarizations in cellular electrophysiologic studies. This observation has led to the suggestion that the repetitive ventricular response may be an afterdepolarization-induced arrhythmia (Rosen et al., 1975).

Clinically, it has been more difficult to identify arrhythmias that might be the result of delayed after-depolarizations. Although invasive electrophysiologic techniques have been used to categorize arrhythmias in patients, these rhythms usually are considered to result from reentry or automaticity. To emphasize that a mechanism such as delayed after-depolarizations might equally well or better explain the mechanism of certain clinical arrhythmias, we will refer briefly to a recent study of patients with accelerated atrioventricular junctional escape rhythms (Rosen et al., 1980b). This study made the assumption that if delayed after-depolarizations were the cause of a clinical arrhythmia, then there should be a defineable relationship between the after-depolarization-induced arrhythmia and the dominant preceding heart rate. The basis for the assumption was that delayed after-depolarizations are not likely to induce propagated action potentials at very long cycle lengths because their amplitude is low. However, as cycle length decreases, there is an increasing likelihood that the delayed after-depolarizations will attain threshold and initiate action potentials (see Fig. 3). Therefore, in the clinic one would expect to see few after-depolarization-induced arrhythmias at very slow heart rates (i.e. $\leq$ 60/min), but as heart rate increases, the likelihood of arrhythmias whose basis is the delayed after-depolarization is increased. Based on studies by Ferrier et al. (1973), the peak incidence of such arrhythmias should be at a cardiac cycle length of about 600 msec. In fact, this observation of the cycle-length dependence of an arrhythmia was characteristic of accelerated junctional escape (Rosen et al., 1980b). Another characteristic of clinical arrhythmias resulting from delayed after-depolarizations is that the cycle length of any premature beats preceding the arrhythmia should further condition the cycle length of the arrhythmia; the shorter the cycle length of the premature beat, the shorter should be the cycle length of the subsequent arrhythmia. This, too, occurred in accelerated junctional escape rhythms (Rosen et al., 1980b).

Other clinical arrhythmias, too, can be explained by delayed after-depolarizations although not to the exclusion of other mechanisms. Zipes et al. (1979) and Josephson et al. (1978) have suggested this with respect to certain nonsustained ventricular tachycardias. Both indicated the possibility of a triggered activity as the mechanism, as well as the difficulty in differentiating this from reentry.

Although the above observations are helpful and suggest that accelerated junctional escape rhythms may be explained as well by delayed after-depolarizations as by other mechanisms, certain other characteristics of delayed after-depolarizations hinder our attempts to identify with certainty arrhythmias arising from this mechanism and to differentiate them from arrhythmias arising from other mechanisms. To illustrate, we will refer to Figure 4. This demonstrates the relationship between delayed after-depolarization amplitude, threshold potential, and coupling interval in two

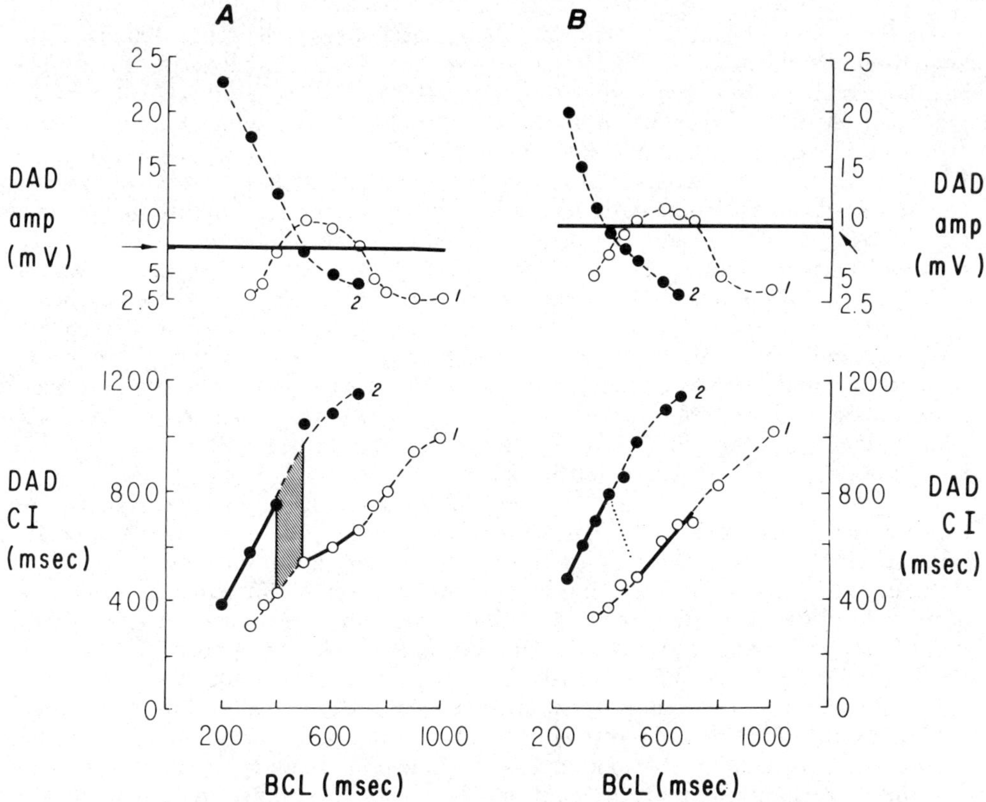

Figure 4. The relationship of DAD amplitude (amp) and coupling interval (CI) to basic cycle length (BCL) in two Purkinje fibers (A and B), each having two delayed afterdepolarizations in sequence. The arrows and horizontal lines identify threshold potential. See text for discussion. (Reprinted by permission of American College of Physicians, from Rosen, M.R. and Reder, R.F.: The role of triggered activity in the genesis of cardiac arrhythmias. *Annals of Internal Medicine*, 94:794–801, 1981.)

Purkinje fiber preparations. In panel A, as drive cycle length decreases, the first delayed after-depolarization that occurs (DAD_1) attains threshold at a cycle length of 700 msec and would be expected to initiate one or a series of triggered action potentials. As drive cycle length decreases, so would the coupling interval of the impulses initiated by the DAD_1. At CL = 500 msec, however, the second delayed after-depolarization (DAD_2) also becomes suprathreshold, and between CL 500 and 400 msec, either the first or the second delayed after-depolarization might initiate an arrhythmia. The resulting arrhythmia occurring between the BCL range of 500 and 400 msec might be very unstable, showing coupling intervals of 400 to 1000 msec (as indicated by the shaded zone) depending on whether the first or second delayed after-depolarization initiated it. At drive cycle lengths less than 400 msec, there again would be a linear decrease in the cycle length of the triggered arrhythmia.

Another possibility is explored in Figure 2B. Here the DAD_1 from drive cycle lengths of about 700 to 500 msec are suprathreshold and would be expected to induce triggered activity. Between 700 and 500 msec, there would be a decrease in the cycle length of the ectopic rhythm, which would approximate the drive cycle length. At 500 msec, there would be a brief "gap," and then at cycle lengths less than 400 msec, the arrhythmia would occur at a frequency approximately twice that of the drive. The "gap" occurs because at cycle lengths between 400 and 500 msec, the DAD_1 now are too small to attain threshold, and the second delayed after-depolarizations in the sequence (DAD_2) are not sufficiently large. Finally at a CL less than 400 msec, the DAD_2 attain threshold and would induce triggered activity at progressively shorter coupling intervals as cycle length decreases. Note that although the coupling interval for the DAD_1 is approximately 450 msec at a drive cycle length of 500, that of the DAD_2 is about 1000 msec. Hence, if one were stimulating a patient's heart electrically and an arrhythmia resulting from delayed after-depolarizations having the characteristics in Figure 4B were occurring, one might see the following: at cycle lengths of 700 to 500 msec, a triggered arrhythmia having progressively shorter coupling intervals approximately equal to the drive cycle length would occur. This would be followed by a "gap" between 500 and 400 msec during which there would be no triggered arrhythmia. Finally at a CL less than 400 msec, an arrhythmia whose cycle length is approximately twice the drive cycle length would be seen.

In reviewing Figure 4, then, we see that delayed after-depolarizations can be expected to give rise to arrhythmias whose cycle lengths depend on the overall drive rate of the preparation (or heart); but, the drive cycle length-coupling interval relationship can be complex. That is, the coupling interval of the arrhythmia may be equal to or a multiple of the basic drive cycle length. As suggested in Figure 4A, the clinical identification of triggered arrhythmias may be hampered by the appearance of chaotic rhythms whose relationship to overdrive pacing is not readily apparent. However, even if the pattern is not chaotic but attains the more orderly relationship suggested in Figure 4B, the differentiation of an afterdepolarization-induced rhythm from one that is reentrant may be difficult, if not impossible. One might argue that the most specific descriptor of reentrant rhythms clinically has been the ability to initiate and to terminate them by appropriately timed premature stimuli. Yet, Moe (1975) and Wit et al. (1979a) have emphasized that this criterion is not specific because delayed after-depolarization-induced rhythms also can be initiated and terminated by single prematures.

A final area of concern is the differentiation of delayed after-depolarization-induced and abnormal automatic arrhythmias clinically. This problem can be understood by referring to Figure 5. Here, in a ouabain-intoxicated Purkinje fiber, overdrive pacing at progressively decreasing cycle lengths is followed by the appearance of an automatic rhythm. Instead of being overdrive-suppressed, this abnormal form of automaticity is overdrive-enhanced. Moreover, not only is the period of quiescence shorter as the overdrive rate increases, but the cycle length of the automatic rhythm itself diminishes slightly. Whether delayed after-depolarizations are occurring concurrently with the abnormal automaticity is difficult to say from this record, although in prior studies we have established that both mechanisms can occur simultaneously in the same cell (Hordof et al., 1978; Mary-Rabine et al., 1980).

CONCLUSIONS

An increasing body of evidence is being marshalled that suggests *(1)* that reentry and overdrive-suppressable automaticity may not be sufficiently diverse in their manifestations to explain all clinical tachyarrhythmias and *(2)* that delayed after-depolarizations and the resultant triggered activity have characteristics that are descriptive of

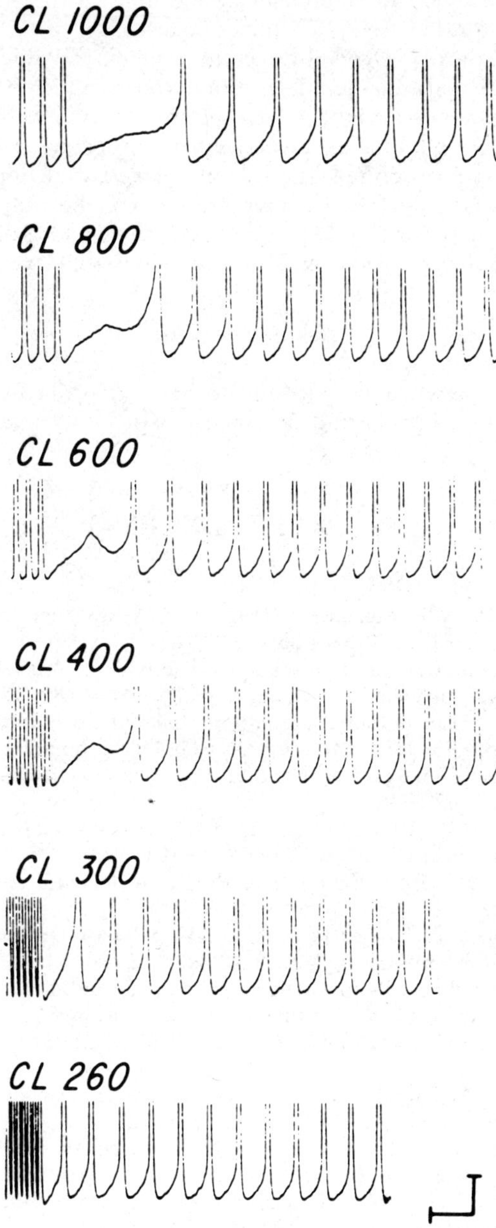

Figure 5. Abnormal automaticity in digitalis-intoxicated Purkinje fiber. As the fiber bundle is driven at progressively shorter cycle lengths, escape time becomes briefer and there is some acceleration of the arrhythmia as well. Vertical calibration 15 mV; horizontal 2 sec. (Reprinted from Rosen and Danilo, *Circ Res* **46**:121, 1980 by permission of the American Heart Association).

at least a part of the spectrum of clinical arrhythmias. At present, it is difficult, if not impossible, to differentiate delayed after-depolarizations from reentry or from abnormal automaticity clinically. Even at the cellular level, the differentiation of abnormal automaticity and delayed after-depolarizations is often sufficiently difficult to make one wonder if both phenomena might not be different manifestations of a single mechanism. It is to be hoped that as investigations proceed and as clinical and basic techniques become more refined, the role of delayed after-depolarizations and other underlying mechanisms for clinical arrhythmias will be defined more specifically. When this occurs, the result should be more precise diagnosis of arrhythmias and more specific and more effective therapy than now is possible.

Acknowledgements

The authors express their gratitude to Mrs. Cynthia Brandt and Ms. Isabella Hewitt for their help in preparing this manuscript.

REFERENCES

Allessie MA, Bonke FIM, Schopman FJG (1973) Circus movement in rabbit atrial muscle as a mechanism of tachycardia. Circ Res **33**:54–62

Bozler E (1943) The initiation of impulses in cardiac muscle. Am J Physiol **138**:273–282

Cranefield PF (1973) Ventricular fibrillation. N Engl J Med **289**:732–736

Cranefield PF (1977) Action potentials, after potentials and arrhythmias. Circ Res **41**:415–423

Cranefield PF, Aronson RS (1974) Initiation of sustained rhythmic activity by single propagated action potentials in canine cardiac Purkinje fibers exposed to sodium-free solution or to ouabain. Circ Res **34**:477–481

Dangman K, Hoffman BF (1978) The effects of EN-313 on abnormal automaticity in canine cardiac Purkinje fibers. Circulation **57** & **58**:II–104 (abstr)

Dangman K, Hoffman BF (1981) Effects of nifedipine on electrical activity of cardiac cells. Am J Cardiol (in press)

Davis LD (1973) Effect of changes in cycle length on diastolic depolarization produced by ouabain in canine Purkinje fibers. Circ Res **32**:206–214

Ferrier GR (1976) The effects of tension on acetylstrophanthidin-induced transient depolarizations and aftercontractions in canine myocardial and Purkinje tissues. Circ Res **38**:156–162

Ferrier GR (1977) Digitalis arrhythmias: role of oscillatory afterpotentials. Prog Cardiovasc Dis **19**:459–474

Ferrier GR, Saunders JH, Mendez C (1973) A cellular mechanism for the generation of ventricular arrhythmias by acetylstrophanthidin. Circ Res **32**:600–609

Gallagher JJ, Pritchett ELC, Sealy WC, Kasell J, Wallace AG (1978) The preexcitation syndromes. Prog Cardiovasc Dis **20**:285–327

Hagemeijer F, Lown B (1970) Effect of heart rate on electrically induced repetitive ventricular responses in the digitalized dog. Circ Res **27**:333–344

Hashimoto K, Moe GK (1973) Transient depolarizations induced by acetylstrophanthidin in specialized tissue of dog atrium and ventricle. Circ Res **32**:618–624

Hordof AJ, Spotnitz A, Mary-Rabine L, Edie R, Rosen MR (1978) The cellular electrophysiologic effects of digitalis on human atrial fibers. Circulation **57**:223–229

Josephson ME, Horowitz LN, Farshidi A, Kastor JA (1978) Recurrent sustained ventricular tachycardia: I. Mechanisms. Circulation **57**:431–440

Kodama I, Goto J, Ando S, Toyama J, Yamada K (1980) Effects of rapid stimulation on the transmembrane action potentials of rabbit sinus node pacemaker cells. Circ Res **46**:90–99

Lown B, Cannon RL, Rossi MA (1967) Electrical stimulation and digitalis drugs: repetitive response in diastole. Proc Soc Exp Biol Med **126**:698–701

Mary-Rabine L, Hordof AJ, Danilo P, Malm J, Rosen MR (1980) Mechanisms for impulse initiation in isolated human atrial fibers. Circ Res **47**:267–277

Moe GK (1975) Evidence of reentry as a mechanism of cardiac arrhythmias. Rev Physiol Biochem Pharmacol **72**:55–81

Noble D (1975) The Initiation of the Heartbeat. Clarendon Press, Oxford, pp 96–98

Rosen MR, Hoffman BF (1973) Mechanisms of action of antiarrhythmic drugs. Circ Res **32**:1–8

Rosen MR, Gelband H, Hoffman BF (1973a) Correlation between effects of ouabain on the canine electrocardiogram and transmembrane potentials of isolated Purkinje fibers. Circulation **47**:65–72

Rosen MR, Gelband H, Merker C, Hoffman BF (1973b) Mechanisms of digitalis toxicity: effects of ouabain on phase 4 of canine Purkinje fiber transmembrane potentials. Circulation **47**:681–689

Rosen MR, Wit AL, Hoffman BF (1975) Electrophysiology and pharmacology of cardiac arrhythmias: IV. Cardiac antiarrhythmic and toxic effects of digitalis. Am Heart J **89**:391–399

Rosen MR, Dangman K, Danilo P, Hoffman B, Hordof A, Mary-Rabine L, Reder R, Reemtsma K (1980a) Electrophysiology of human Purkinje and ventricular fibers. Circulation **62**:III–56

Rosen MR, Fisch C, Hoffman BF, Danilo P, Lovelace ED, Knoebel SB (1980b) Can accelerated atrioventricular junctional escape rhythms be explained by delayed afterdepolarizations? Am J Cardiol **45**:1272–1284

Saito T, Otoguro M, Matsubara T (1978) Electrophysiological studies of the mechanism of electrically induced sustained rhythmic activity in the rabbit right atrium. Circ Res **42**: 199–206

Saunders JH, Ferrier GR, Moe GK (1973) Conduction block associated with transient depolarization induced by acetlystrophanthidin in isolated Purkinje fibers. Circ Res **32**:610–617

Segers M (1941) Le role des potentials tardifs du coeur. Mem Acad R Med Belg Ser II **1**:1–30

Vassalle M (1977) The relationship among cardiac pacemakers: overdrive suppression. Circ Res **41**:269–277

Wellens HJJ (1978) Value and limitation of programmed electrical stimulation of the heart in the study and treatment of tachycardias. Circulation **57**:845–853

Wit AL, Hoffman BF, Cranefield PF (1972) Slow conduction and reentry in the ventricular specialized conducting system. Circ Res **30**:1–22

Wit AL, Fenoglio JJ, Wagner BM, Bassett AL (1973) Electrophysiological properties of cardiac muscle in the anterior mitral valve leaflet and the adjacent atrium in the dog: Possible implication for the genesis of atrial dysrhythmias. Circ Res **32**:731–745

Wit AL, Cranefield PF (1976) Triggered activity in cardiac muscle fibers of the simian mitral valve. Circ Res **38**:85–98

Wit AL, Cranefield PF (1977) Triggered and automatic activity in the canine coronary sinus. Circ Res **41**:435–445

Wit AL, Boyden PA, Gadsby DC, Cranefield PF (1979a) Triggered activity as a cause of atrial arrhythmias. In Cardiac Arrhythmias: Electrophysiology, Diagnosis and Management, edited by OS Narula, Baltimore, Williams and Wilkins, pp 14–31

Wit AL, Fenoglio JJ, Hordof AJ, Reemtsma K (1979b) Ultrastructure and transmembrane potentials of cardiac muscle in the human anterior mitral valve leaflet. Circulation **59**: 1284–1292

Zipes DP, Foster PR, Troup PJ, Pederson DH (1979) Atrial induction of ventricular tachycardia: reentry versus triggered automaticity. Am J Cardiol **44**:1–8

Discussion

FOZZARD: I agree with you that the mechanism you pointed out for triggered arrhythmias does indeed occur, or at least plays a role in certain arrhythmias. I am particularly impressed with your evidence for an accelerated junctional rhythm triggered by a premature ventricular contraction. Most of us are fairly convinced that this is indeed the mechanism, mostly because none of us can think of any other way for it to occur. But, this phenomenon is a sort of clinical curiosity unless one wants to use it as a sign of digitalis toxicity, or some other specific pathologic process. There are, however, some very pressing problems like ventricular tachycardia promoted by digitalis intoxication. This could also be due to a delayed afterdepolarization, although reentry is the standard explanation. Triggered rhythms could occur as well in some of the other instances you failed to go into, such as hypoxia. Now, the standard clinical approach for reentry rhythms is to stimulate with a single premature beat to try to stop the arrhythmia. It was really like throwing a monkey wrench in the works to have this triggered automaticity also with the characteristic that it can be stopped by a single premature beat. There does seem to be some difference, however. For instance, in the typical clinical reentry arrhythmia a single premature beat seems to be able to stop the ventricular tachycardia immediately, whereas in the case of triggered automaticity, at least in the laboratory model, there seems to be one beat or two before the arrhythmia stops after the application of the single premature beat. I wonder if you have exploited this difference to differentiate between these two mechanisms of ventricular tachycardia. One last point I want to make is that most of the arrhythmias or fast rhythms produced in the laboratory are slower than the overdrive that caused them, but most ventricular tachycardias are faster than the rhythms that cause them.

ROSEN: The problem with your suggestion for differentiation between common reentry arrhythmias and triggered ventricular tachycardia is that in triggered rhythms one or two beats do not always appear after the premature beat that stops the arrhythmia. If you do not see several beats after the premature, there may or may not be a triggered rhythm. If you do see several beats after the premature, then, there is a fairly good possibility that there is a triggered rhythm, but this is *not* exclusive of other mechanisms.

WIT: I would like to caution Dr. Rosen when he extrapolates from digitalis-induced delayed after-depolarizations to other situations in which triggered rhythms can be caused. For instance, in our studies on triggered activity of the canine AV valve, we showed that this rhythm could be stopped by a single premature stimulus, and we never observed any impulses after the stimulated impulse. The other difference in this particular example is that triggered activity caused by delayed after-depolarization in atrial tissue is not stopped by any of the antiarrhythmic drugs that are effective in stopping triggered activity caused by digitalis intoxication. In the canine atrial fibers of the AV valve, triggered activity could only be stopped by slow-channel blockers and not by lidocaine or quinidine. So, it may be difficult to extrapolate from the case of digitalis to the case of all possible arrhythmias that are dependent on delayed after-depolarizations.

ROSEN: I fully agree with Andy Wit's comments. One should be very careful in making extrapolations from the digitalis model to other situations such as the atrium, as he has shown.

PAES DE CARVALHO: I have been wondering about the possibility that the delayed after-depolarizations are very much akin to the subliminal response that we see in the barium-depolarized atrial fibers. In all experiments in which drugs were used to depress the excitability of the slow response, we found that the subliminal response is equally depressed. Do you also find that drugs abolishing triggered activity also do abolish the delayed after-depolarizations?

ROSEN: We find that the same drugs that suppress triggered activity also depress delayed after-depolarizations. But different drugs act in very different ways. For instance, verapamil depresses the amplitude of the delayed after-depolarization more at short than at long cycle lengths. With lidocaine, there is uniform depression independent of cycle length. With tetrodotoxin there is an effect that is intermediate between that of lidocaine and that of verapamil. Also, hyperpolarizing the fiber can render the delayed afterdepolarization incapable of eliciting an action potential, as occurs with acetylcholine in atrial muscle.

Chapter 26

Conduction in Ischemic Myocardium

Mechanisms for Arrhythmias in the Early Phase of Myocardial Ischemia

Frans J.L. van Capelle and Michiel J. Janse

The life-threatening arrhythmias that frequently occur within minutes after the onset of myocardial infarction in man can be studied in the laboratory, using as a model an animal heart in which a coronary artery is suddenly ligated. We have used isolated hearts of pigs and dogs for this purpose, and by multichannel recording we have tried to unravel some of the mechanisms contributing to the occurrence of early arrhythmias in acute ischemia.

What are those mechanisms? Both reentry and ectopic automaticity are good candidates. The reentrant nature of fibrillation has been appreciated for a long time (Garrey, 1914), and there is little doubt about the role of reentry in the transition from tachycardia to fibrillation. But the mechanisms underlying single or multiple extrasystoles or the first beats of a spontaneous tachycardia are less certain. Recent literature has emphasized the possible role of ectopic mechanisms in partially depolarized fibers (Cranefield, 1975).

In this context, multichannel DC recording is a useful technique. It permits mapping of the sequence of activation and can therefore be used to identify the origin of ectopic beats. When a complete circuit is mapped, it can also confirm the role of spatial reentry. At the same time, it permits sampling of the extracellular potential distribution, which in turn enables us to estimate the magnitude of the currents of injury and to map their source distribution. These currents are quite strong, and it seems legitimate to speculate about their possible arrhythmogenic effects.

In the present paper, we will first present our experimental results. We will then proceed to speculate about the mechanisms that may be involved, using computer simulations to illustrate some of the underlying ideas. In reality, of course, our notions were as much influenced by the simulations as the other way round. The most important concept emerging from this interaction is that of latent automaticity, the idea being that automaticity may be suppressed but not completely abolished by the influence of surrounding tissue. Under certain circumstances, it may emerge as an overt mechanism and be responsible for the occurrence of arrhythmias. It remains to be established whether latent automaticity will prove to be a useful concept to explain clinical and experimental arrhythmias. In any case, it is an illustration of the heuristic potency of simulation techniques.

EXPERIMENTAL FINDINGS

Methods

The methods have been described elsewhere in more detail (Janse et al., 1980). In essence, hearts of pigs and dogs were isolated and perfused according to the Langendorff technique with a mixture of modified Tyrode's solution and blood. Regional ischemia was produced by clamping the left anterior descending coronary artery. DC extracellular electrograms were recorded simultaneously from 60 epicardial or intramural sites. The electrodes consisted of silk or cotton wicks soaked in isotonic saline. The saline was in contact with a chlorided silver wire, which was connected to a high-impedance unity-gain amplifier. Differential DC amplifiers then measured the potential at each wick with respect to the DC potential of the aortic root. Various electrode arrangements were used: terminals were either spaced regularly on the epicardial surface within a rectangle, the distances between terminals varying between 1.5 and 4 mm, or they had a more irregular configuration that covered a large part of the heart. A high speed A/D converter sampled the signals and wrote them in a ring buffer in the memory of a PDP 11/34 computer. Depending on the aims of the experiment, samples were taken every 1 msec or every 8 msec. During the experiment the signals were monitored and as soon as an event (premature beats, ventricular fibrillation) occurred, a button was pushed causing the contents of the ring buffer (usually 2 sec of signal) to be transferred to a high-speed, digital, tape recorder. The data were analyzed, using an interactive computer program that displayed the signals on a graphic display. Activation moments could be entered using a joy stick. Zero potentials were obtained from control signals, and DC potential values could be obtained at any desired moment of the cardiac cycle.

Transmembrane potentials were recorded from the subepicardium, using floating microelectrodes. A second floating microelectrode, located as closely as possible in the extracellular space, was used as a reference.

Isopotential maps were constructed, using an electrode with regularly spaced terminals. The spatial distribution of current sources (transmembrane current flowing out of the cells) and sinks (current flowing into the cells) could be calculated from the isopotential maps. The spatial distribution was proportional to the second spatial derivative, which was estimated using a relation given by Bickley (1948). To determine the source or sink current at site C, we used the potential values of the eight surrounding terminals:

B_1	A_1	B_2
A_2	C	A_3
B_3	A_4	B_4

The source current i is then given by the relation:

$$i = -\frac{4\sum_{k=1}^{4} V(A_k) + \sum_{k=1}^{4} V(B_k) - 20V(C)}{6\rho L^2}\ (A/m^3)$$

in which V is the DC potential at the terminals, ρ is the specific tissue resistance (we assumed 400 Ω cm), L is the distance between the electrodes in the grid, and 6 is a geometric factor.

Discussion of Results

Within 2 to 6 min following sudden occlusion of the left anterior descending coronary artery, we observed ventricular premature beats in 75% of the cases; runs of 8 or more ectopic beats occurred in 45% and ventricular fibrillation in 32% of the occlusions. The sequence of events associated with this pronounced vulnerability of the heart for rhythm disturbances in acute ischemia is discussed below.

Figure 1 shows transmembrane potentials and local DC electrograms recorded from the subepicardium of the pig heart before and after occlusion of the left anterior descending coronary artery. Zero potentials were obtained when both microelectrodes were in the extracellular space; in the extracellular recordings, the zero potential is the potential of the aortic root. Before occlusion (control), the resting membrane potential was −87 mV; and the action potential amplitude, 105 mV. Note, however, that intracellular potential measurements in the beating heart are known to be less reliable than they are in isolated superfused preparations. In the extracellular signals, the TQ and ST segments were isoelectric. Six minutes after occlusion, the resting potential had decreased to −75 mV, and concomitant reductions in amplitude and upstroke velocity of the action potential were observed. A depression of the TQ segment reflected the loss of resting potential in the extracellular recordings. The velocity of conduction decreased as a result of the depression of the upstroke of the action potential, and this in turn led to a delay in the activation of the ischemic cells, which was evident as a late intrinsic deflection (indicating local active depolarization) in the extracellular tracings (arrow). The decrease in plateau voltage of the action potential betrayed itself in the extracellular complex as a true ST segment elevation. Alternation in the amplitude and the duration of the action potential developed after 6 min (not shown in the figure) and progressed via 2:1 and 4:1 responses until the cell became completely inexcitable after 8 min. The resting potential was then about −50 mV. At this stage, the extracellular complex was completely monophasic with a −12 mV TQ depression and a +25 mV ST elevation. Surprisingly, this phase of inexcitability was transient: action potentials, albeit of low amplitude and short duration, could be recorded again from previously unresponsive cells after about 30 min. This phase was also transient, and after 1 or 2 hours the center of the ischemic zone was inexcitable again, this time for good.

The effects of acute ischemia on the sequence of activation and on the distribution of the extracellular potential during the TQ and ST segments are depicted in Figure 2. Intramural wick electrodes (Janse et al., 1979) were inserted in a row at 4-mm distances in the free lateral wall of the left ventricle starting from the interventricular septum (upper left panel). At each site, extracellular complexes were recorded from the subepicardium and from intramural positions at 4-mm and 8-mm depths. Activation maps and potential distributions in the corresponding transmural section are depicted in the figure. In the control situation, the TQ and ST segments were isoelectric (not shown in the figure). In the other instances the absolute values of TQ depression and ST elevation after coronary occlusion have been added. The resulting maps correspond with the "ST elevation" as recorded with AC amplifiers. Activation patterns and TQ/ST maps are shown at 8 min, 30 min, and 2 hours after coronary artery occlusion for beats that were propagated from the atrium. The transition between zones with a negative and a positive TQ/ST potential corresponds with the electrical border between ischemic and normally perfused myocardium. It is drawn here as a straight line; in reality, it is an irregular jagged plane where peninsulae of normal and ischemic cells intermin-

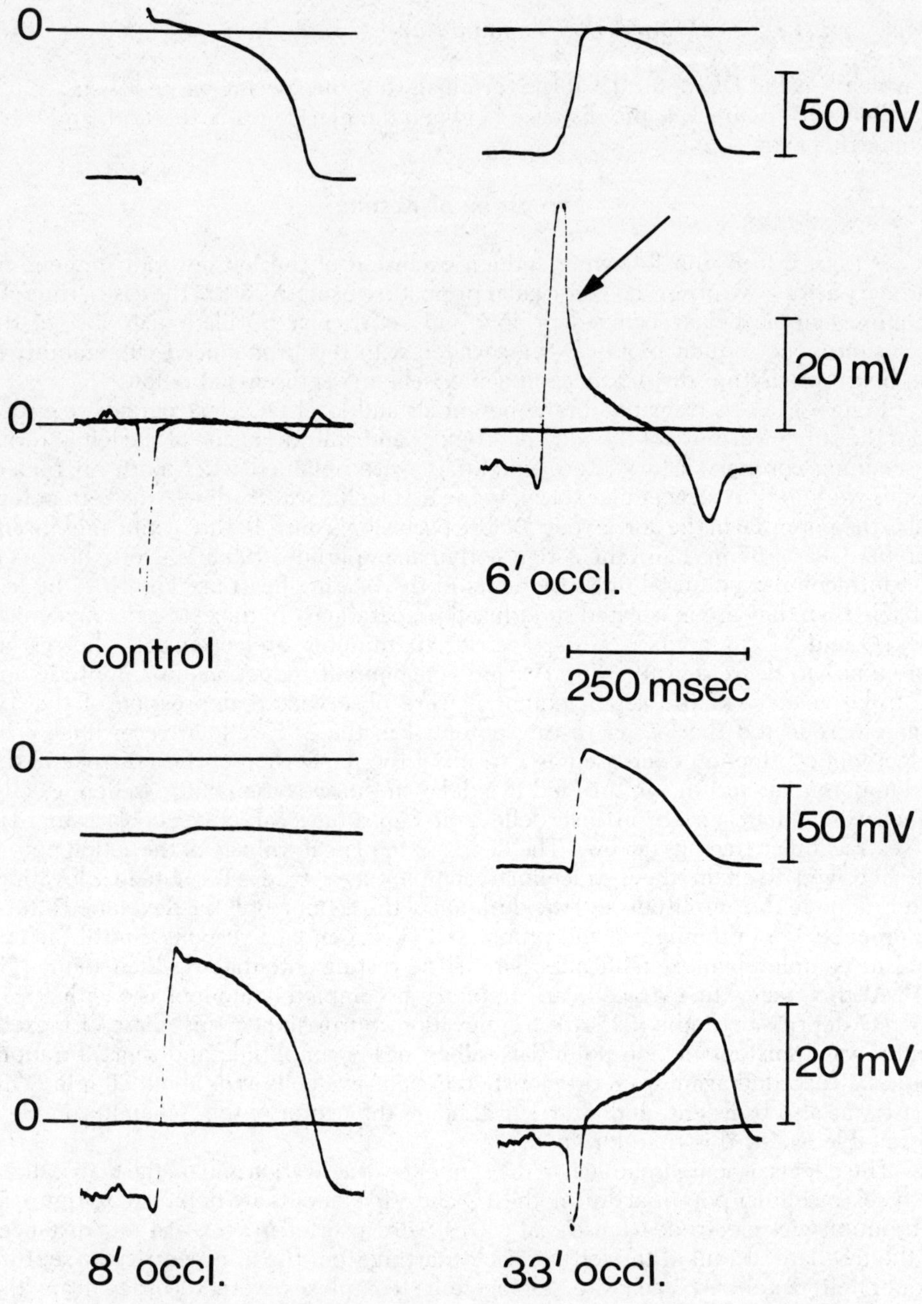

Figure 1. Electrophysiological changes in the isolated perfused pig heart after coronary artery occlusion. Top trace: transmembrane potential, lower trace: local extracellular DC electrogram. Zero potential in the extracellular recording is the potential of the aortic root. Before occlusion TQ and ST segments are isoelectric. After occlusion the TQ segment becomes depressed as a result of the reduction of the transmembrane resting potential. The decrease in plateau voltage of the action potential is reflected in the extracellular signal as an ST elevation. After 8 minutes the action potential has disappeared and the extracellular complex is monophasic. A transient recovery of activity is seen after 33 minutes. (Reproduced with permission from MJ Janse and D Durrer, Ned Tijdschr Geneesk 122:1964,1968,1978.)

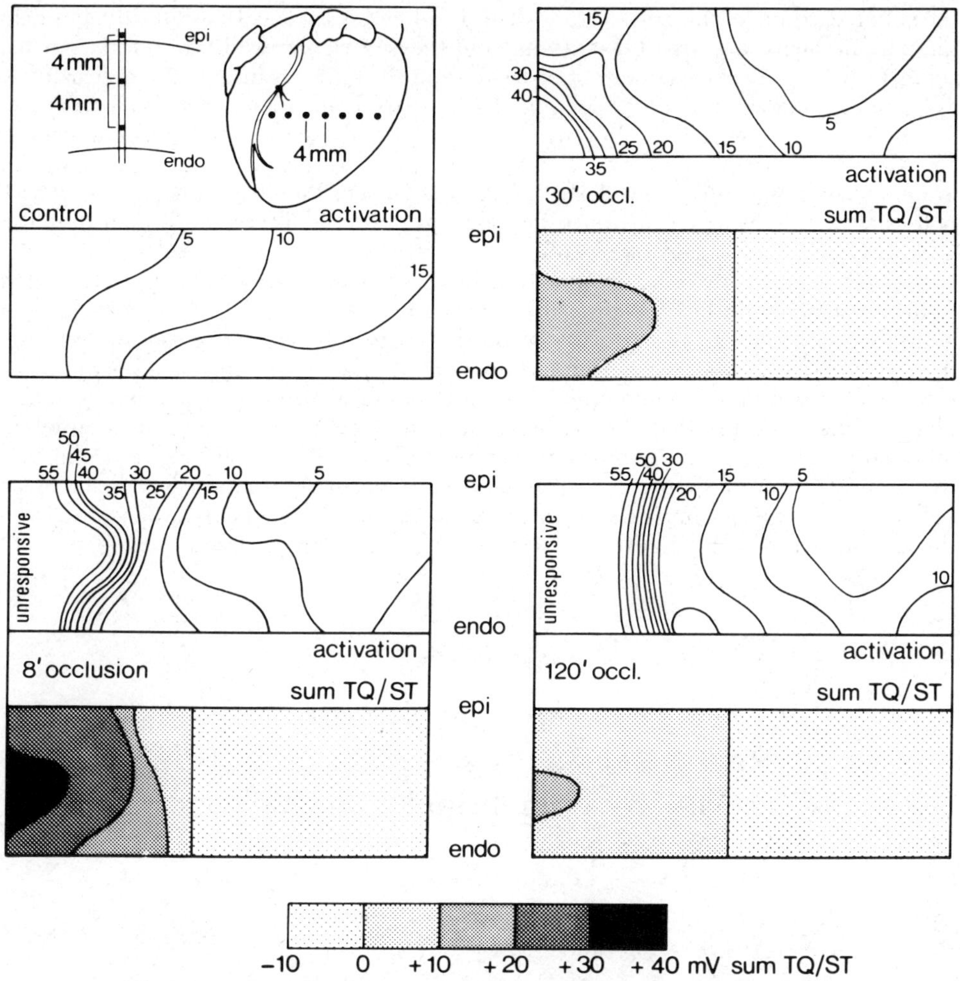

Figure 2. Activation patterns and distribution of the difference between ST and TQ segment potentials in a segment of the left ventricular wall. The segment is represented as a rectangle in which the upper edge is the epicardium and the lower edge the endocardium. Intramural wick electrodes (upper left panel) were inserted in a row and at each site extracellular DC electrograms were recorded from the subepicardium and from intramural sites at 4 mm and 8 mm depth. Eight minutes after coronary occlusion the activation pattern has changed, the velocity of conduction has decreased and the center of the ischemic zone has become unresponsive. A transient recovery of excitability occurs after 30 minutes. After 2 hours, the center is inexcitable again. (Unpublished results by J Cinca and MJ Janse)

gle, despite the fact that in the porcine heart the separation between ischemic and normally perfused cells is sharp (Janse et al., 1979). In the activation maps, isochronal lines separate areas that are excited within 5 msec intervals. In the control situation, activation proceeds from left to right, and the wall segment is depolarized within 20 msec. Eight minutes after occlusion, the activation wave proceeded from right to left, and activity was recorded during a period of 55 msec. The earliest activity was found in the subepicardium of the normal zone. This is related to the fact that Purkinje fibers in the porcine heart, are distributed thoughout the ventricular wall. Therefore, normal activity during sinus beats does not proceed from the endocardium to the epicardium, as in human and canine hearts (Hamlin et al., 1975; Holland and Brooks, 1976). The ischemic center, where the difference between ST and TQ potentials exceeded about 25 mV, was inexcitable. After 30 min, activity had returned to the center of the ischemic zone, which was invaded after about 40 msec. The magnitude of the TQ/ST potentials was reduced. A further reduction was observed after 2 hours, but then the ischemic center was again inexcitable.

Figure 3 shows three selected extracellular DC electrograms that were recorded from an isolated pig heart 3 min after coronary occlusion: "a" was recorded from nonischemic myocardium close to the border (note the isoelectric TQ and ST segments), and "b" and "c" were from ischemic myocardium. The distance between the electrodes was 4 mm. The complexes at electrode b were nearly completely monophasic. This indicates that the tissue under this electrode was almost completely inexcitable. The signals at c show a pronounced alternation of the T wave. Following the deepest T wave, a spontaneous premature beat occurred. In this case, the intrinsic deflection at a was not preceded by an r wave as it was during beats propagated from the atrium (arrow). This figure contains several of the most characteristic features of

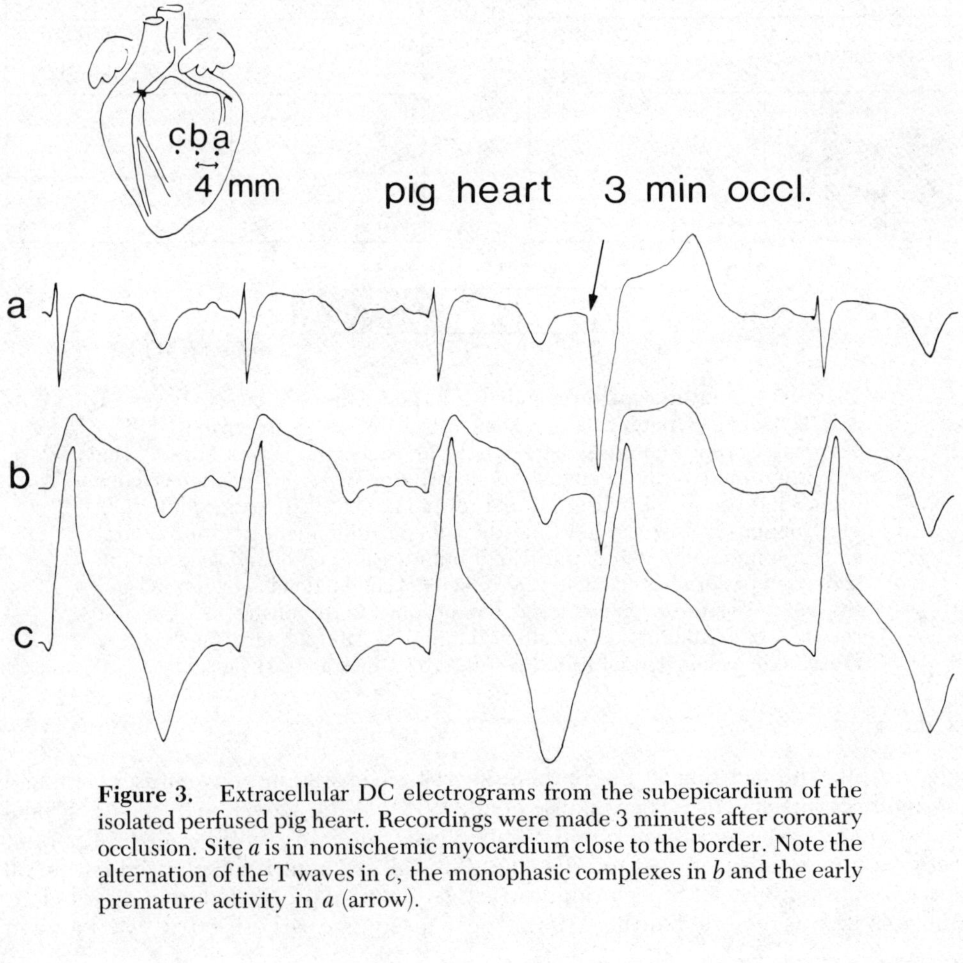

Figure 3. Extracellular DC electrograms from the subepicardium of the isolated perfused pig heart. Recordings were made 3 minutes after coronary occlusion. Site *a* is in nonischemic myocardium close to the border. Note the alternation of the T waves in *c*, the monophasic complexes in *b* and the early premature activity in *a* (arrow).

ventricular premature beats in the acute phase of ischemia: the earliest activity emerged in the nonischemic tissue close to the border zone; a pronounced negative T wave was present in the central ischemic area, indicating delayed repolarization; and finally, a zone of inexcitability was interposed between the nonischemic myocardium and the central ischemic area, which still was showing activity (usually alternating or in the form of 2:1 responses).

Figure 4 shows six selected DC electrograms recorded from sites located 1.5 mm apart. The multiple electrode consisted of 60 terminals, which were arranged in a rectangular grid that covered the area, indicated in the upper right part of the figure. The tracings correspond to the positions a–f indicated in this area. A basic beat, which was propagated from the atrium, was followed by a deep negative T wave in the central ischemic area (sites a–d). Site f, although still in the ischemic area, was close to the border, as is evident from the small amount of TQ depression and ST elevation and from the early intrinsic deflection. Site d was inexcitable, showing a monophasic extracellular complex. The T wave was followed by a spontaneous ventricular premature beat. The DC potential distribution during the T wave is shown in the upper right hand panel. A gradient of 35 mV was seen over a distance of 7.5 mm. The distribution of current sources and sinks occurring at the same moment is depicted in the lower panel. The area was smaller in this case, because the source current could not be calculated at the edge of the grid. The current sources close to the border were about 2 $\mu A/mm^3$. This may be compared with the source current associated with propagation of a broad wavefront through normal myocardium tissue, which has a magnitude of about 5 $\mu A/mm^3$ (Janse et al., 1980). The current of injury across the border just before the emergence of a spontaneous ventricular premature beat thus appears to be about half as strong as the electrotonic currents associated with propagation of activity in the normal myocardium.

Figure 5 shows AC electrograms at two time scales, from intramural electrodes in a dog heart. The recordings were made 5 min after coronary occlusion. In the top trace, which was recorded from the normal subendocardium close to the ischemic border, Purkinje activity can be seen (arrows). The second and third traces, which are from nonischemic endocardial and epicardial sites show only muscle activity. A spontaneous ventricular premature beat (1st extra) initiated a bout of ventricular tachycardia (B), which subsequently degenerated into ventricular fibrillation (C). Purkinje activity preceded myocardial activity both during basic beats (which are propagated from the atrium) and during the initial beats of the tachycardia. Only when ventricular fibrillation had developed did the activity of the Purkinje cells occur later than the depolarization of the adjacent myocardium. During the tachycardia, as well as in basic beats, the activation sequence was from endocardium to epicardium.

Figure 6 shows the sequence of activation during two ectopic beats, occurring after 4 min of regional ischemia. We used a 60-terminal epicardial electrode, and we recorded activity from both ischemic and nonischemic myocardium. Isochronal lines separate areas activated within 20-msec intervals; time zero was arbitrarily chosen. Beat A was the third one of a ventricular tachycardia that eventually degenerated into ventricular fibrillation. Early activity emerged in the nonischemic part, just as it did in the first two ectopic impulses. The electrophysiologic border, defined as the place where the TQ segments of sinus beats become negative, is indicated in B by a dotted line. The ectopic activity invaded the ischemic tissue but was blocked in the central area. Two wavefronts bypassed this area of block and joined on the left side of the area covered by the electrode. The wavefront ending at 120 msec, shown in A, retrogradely invaded the area of unidirectional block and continued at 140 msec, as shown in B. Again two wavefronts circled around a central area of block. The lower wave was blocked at 240 msec, but the upper wave continued. At 300 msec, the recording

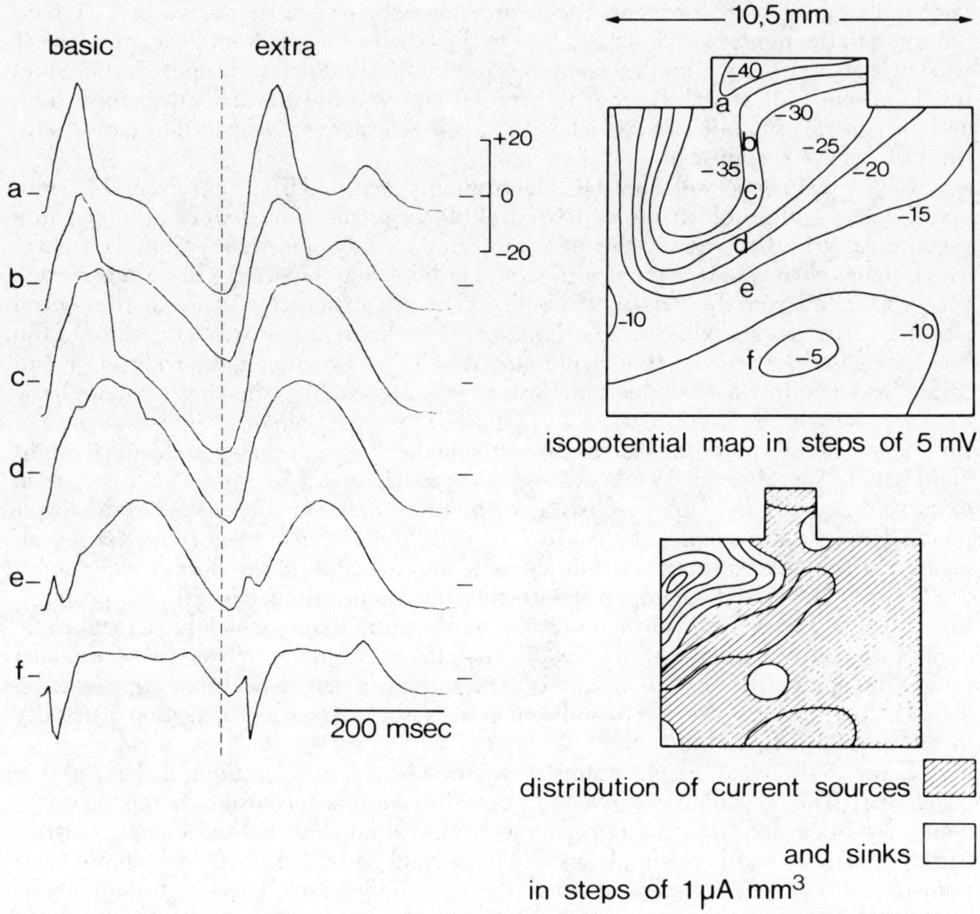

Figure 4. Selected DC electrograms from epicardial sites showing supraventricular (basic) beat and spontaneous ventricular premature beat (extra). Recordings were made 4 minutes after occlusion. Note negative T wave in *a*, *b* and *c*, inexcitability in *d* and earliest premature activity in *f*. In the upper right panel the area is indicated from which 60 DC electrograms were simultaneously recorded from sites 1.5 mm apart. Isopotential lines depict the potential distribution at the times indicated by the dotted line in the tracings. The distribution of the current sources and sinks is depicted in the lower right panel. The area is now smaller since the source current cannot be calculated at the edges of the grid.

ended, and we did not know how the arrhythmia proceeded. When somewhat later a new 2-sec period of recording began, the heart was fibrillating. In Figure 7, the characteristic pattern of activation during ventricular fibrillation is shown. In contrast with the large circus movements present in the early phase of the arrhythmia, multiple wavefronts were now present simultaneously. Again, time zero was arbitrarily chosen. The upper wavelet describes an S shaped pattern during the time depicted in the three panels of Figure 7. The first panel shows it completing a small circus movement counterclockwise around a small area of block, the diameter being about 5 mm. The

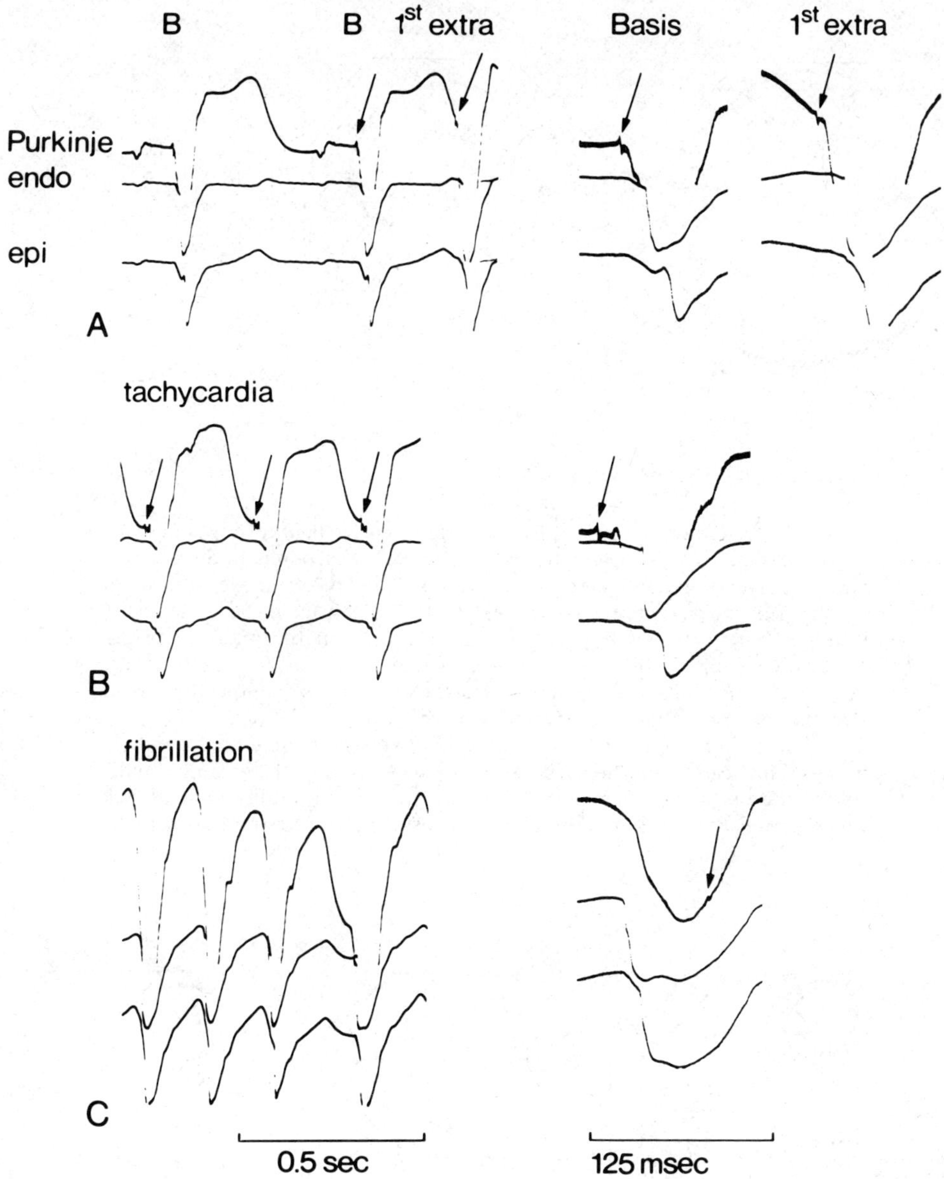

Figure 5. AC recordings of extracellular potentials in the isolated dog heart 5 minutes after coronary occlusion. The signals are shown at two time scales. The top trace is from the nonischemic subendocardium close to the border of the ischemic region. In this tracing Purkinje activity can be seen (arrows). The second and third traces show myocardial activity from the nonischemic subendocardium and subepicardium. In *A* two basic beats *(B)* which are propagated from the atrium are followed by a spontaneous premature beat (1st extra), which initiates a bout of ventricular tachycardia, shown in *B*, and which in turn degenerates into ventricular fibrillation *(C)*. Purkinje activity precedes myocardial activity during basic beats and during tachycardia, but not during ventricular fibrillation.

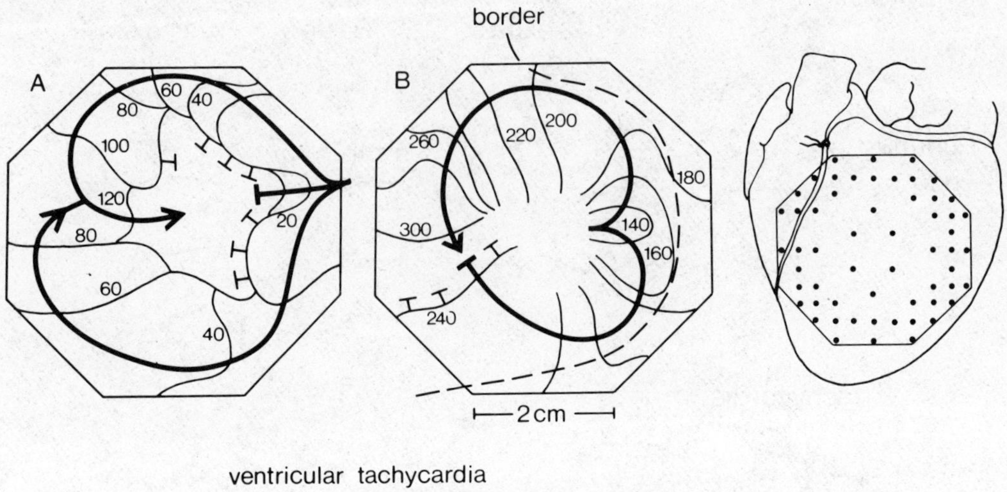

Figure 6. Excitation pattern during two consecutive beats of a spontaneous ventricular tachycardia occurring after 4 minutes of ischemia in the isolated pig heart. The right hand panel shows the multiple DC electrode, sutured to the anterior surface of the ventricles. Dots indicate electrode terminals. Panels *A* and *B* depict the pathway of activation in the area under the electrode. Isochronal lines separate areas activated within 20 msec intervals. Time zero was arbitrarily chosen. Thick lines with arrows indicate general direction of wavefronts, transverse bars indicate conduction block. The dotted line in *B* represents the border between ischemic and normally perfused myocardium. The earliest activity in *A* is found at the nonischemic side of the border. Two wavefronts bypass an area of unidirectional block which (panel *B*) is retrogradely invaded, resulting in reentrant activity.

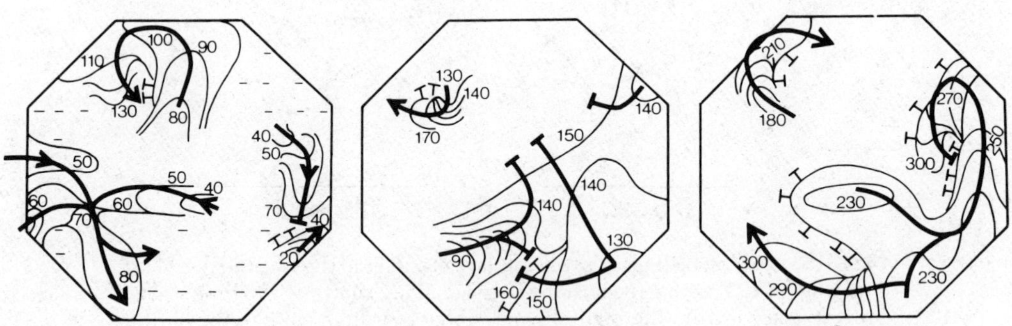

Figure 7. Activation patterns in three successive "beats" of the same arrhythmia as shown in Figure 6, but at a later stage. Multiple wavefronts are present, giving rise to multiple reentry. This fragmentation into multiple reentrant wavelets is characteristic for ventricular fibrillation.

second panel shows it curving to the left, and the third panel shows it forming a clockwise circus movement. But, completed circus movements during fibrillation were the exception rather than the rule. Usually, multiple wavelets followed tortuous paths around temporary islets of conduction block. Sometimes wavefronts collided, sometimes they joined and summated. Areas that show conduction block at one moment could conduct the impulse at the next. By and large, this chaotic activity bears a striking ressemblance to the activation pattern in a computer study by Moe et al. (1964). Compare also Figure 10, which comes from a computer simulation presented in the second part of this chapter.

"Focal" Ectopic Activity

The ectopic impulses that initiate reentrant arrhythmias seem to have a "focal" origin. Our experimental findings from intact hearts concerning the genesis of single or multiple premature beats in the setting of acute ischemia can be summarized as follows: *(1)* the earliest ectopic activity emerges from the nonischemic tissue adjacent to the electrophysiologic border zone, *(2)* very often, a deep negative T wave from the ischemic area precedes the earliest ectopic activity, *(3)* propagating activity apparently does not bridge the gap between the latest activity recorded from the basic beat and the earliest ectopic activity, and *(4)* Purkinje activity precedes myocardial activity in ectopic beats, whenever it is recorded.

Schematically, the anatomical situation can be described as follows: the normal subendocardium, containing strands of Purkinje fibers, is separated by a zone of inexcitable ischemic tissue from the more centrally located ischemic myocardium, showing, for example, 2:1 responses. Every second action potential in the central ischemic area is long and its time of activation is delayed, so that repolarization occurs later than in the normal Purkinje fibers at the other side of the inexcitable border. Electrotonic current flowing through the border zone tends to depolarize the normal Purkinje fibers, where the earliest ectopic activity is observed.

Antiarrhythmic Actions

Theoretically, antiarrhythmic effects can be achieved by influencing either the "focal" or the reentrant component of early ischemic arrhythmias. Because the mechanism of the focal mechanism is not fully known, therapeutic efforts in that direction are largely speculative at present. The position is somewhat better for reentry, because it is clear that the fragmentation into multiple wavelets that leads to fibrillation can occur only when excitability and the velocity of conduction are depressed without having vanished. It is no coincidence that spontaneous ventricular fibrillation does not occur when the majority of the ischemic cells are inexcitable, that is, between 8 and 20 min and again after about 1 hour. It seems likely that the temporary phase of recovery of activity observed in isolated hearts between about 20 and 40 min is related to the delayed phase of arrhythmias occurring at the same period (Kaplinsky et al., 1979).

Lidocaine is known to reduce the incidence of ventricular fibrillation drastically in patients with acute myocardial infarction (Lie et al., 1974) without affecting the incidence of single or multiple ventricular premature beats. The effects of lidocaine on the electrical changes induced by ischemia are shown in Figure 8. Transmembrane potentials and extracellular complexes were recorded from the same site in an isolated pig heart during several occlusions. Each occlusion lasted for 15 min and was followed by a 30-min period of reperfusion, during which the electrophysiologic parameters returned quickly to their control values. In a series of control experiments, four successive occlusions were performed in absence of the drug. It turned out that the second, third, and fourth occlusions were quite comparable with the electrophysiologic changes due to ischemia. They all deviated from the first occlusion, however. Therefore, we used the second occlusion as a control for the experiments in which lidocaine was tested. Lidocaine was then added to the perfusion fluid 15 min before the third occlusion. After 6 min of ischemia (Fig. 8) the fiber was inexcitable in the presence of lidocaine, whereas it still showed a sizable action potential in absence of the drug. In Figure 9, the results of three experiments are pooled. In each heart, the amplitude of the action potentials was measured at the same site during ischemia both in the presence and the absence of lidocaine. Lidocaine clearly accelerated the reduction of the amplitude of the action potential during ischemia. Mapping experiments demonstrated that ventricular premature beats, emerging from the same site of origin as they did during control occlusions, still occurred in the presence of lidocaine.

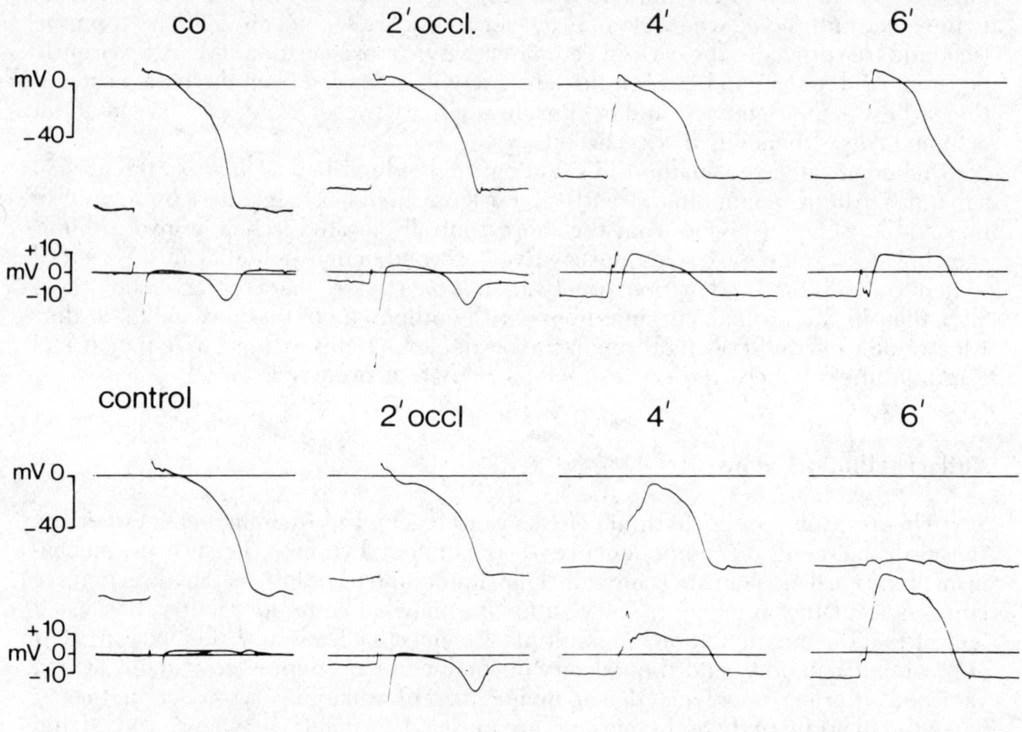

Figure 8. Transmembrane potentials (upper trace) and local DC electrograms (lower trace) before and after coronary occlusion in the presence and absence of lidocaine. Recordings are from the same position in the same isolated pig heart. Upper panel: second occlusion, in the absence of drug (control). Lower panel: third occlusion after a 30-minute reperfusion during which lidocaine was administered. Note absence of response after 6 minutes of ischemia in the presence of lidocaine whereas a sizable action potential is still present at the same stage in the control occlusion. (Unpublished results of R Cardinal and MJ Janse)

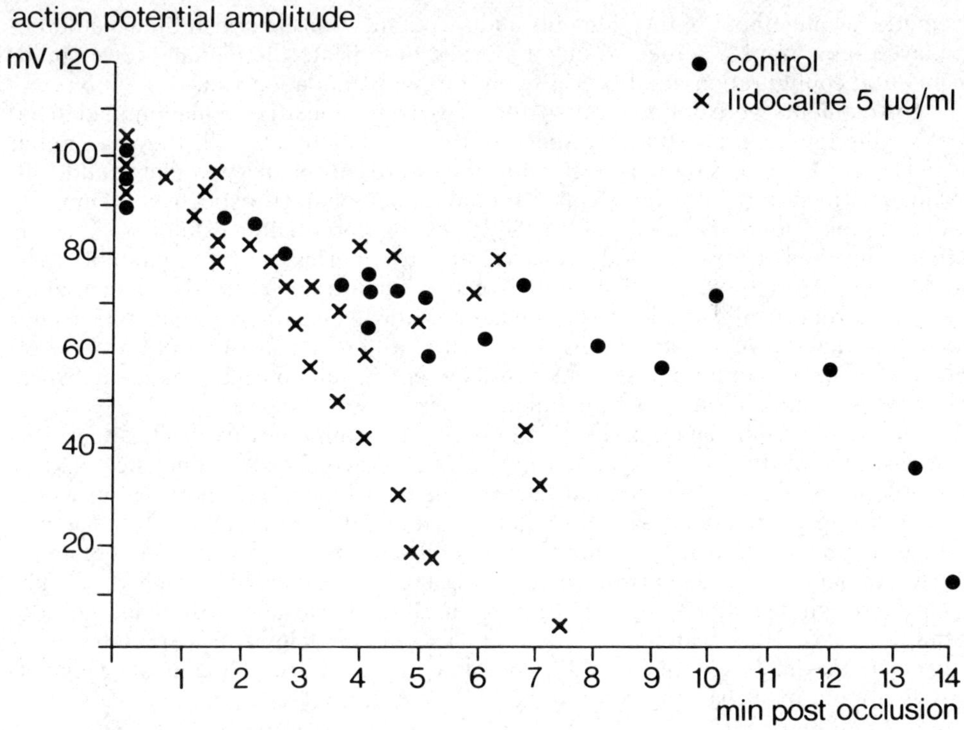

Figure 9. Pooled results of three experiments. Action potential amplitude was measured at the same site in each heart as a function time elapsed after coronary artery occlusion in the presence and absence of lidocaine. The drug accelerates the decline of the amplitude of the action potentials. (Unpublished results of R Cardinal and MJ Janse)

Circus movements around large areas of inexcitable myocardium also still occurred, albeit infrequently. Fragmentation into multiple reentrant wavelets leading to ventricular fibrillation was seen only once in 13 occlusions, as opposed to 8 times out of 13 in the absence of lidocaine (Cardinal et al). Considering the time course of the reduction of the action potential amplitude, it seems reasonable to postulate that the conditions necessary for multiple reentry in the ischemic zone exist when slow conduction is present, coinciding with an action potential amplitude of, say, 40 to 70 mV. Such conditions exist during a much shorter time when lidocaine is present, and therefore the chances for fibrillation to occur are greatly reduced, although not absolutely abolished.

COMPUTER SIMULATION STUDIES

Description of the Model

To study the electrical interaction between excitable elements, we constructed a computer model consisting of an arbitrary number of such elements. A more complete description of the model has appeared elsewhere (van Capelle and Durrer, 1980). The geometric arrangement of the elements and the connections between them could be displayed on a graphic screen. Using a joystick to indicate the elements, we could change the configuration at all times, even during a simulation run.

The elements were defined by two differential equations. The equations had to be kept simple to obtain a reasonable speed of the simulation (after all, they had to be solved for all elements simultaneously), but they were chosen in a way that would still permit us to incorporate the most important physiologic characteristics of heart muscle in our model. Elements could have a stable resting potential or exhibit pacemaker activity; they had an absolute and a relative refractory period, and an excitability that would depend on the take-off potential of the "membrane", steady depolarizing external currents would accelerate pacemakers, while hyperpolarizing currents would slow them down or even stop them. We created a library consisting of a variety of similar elements, and for subsequent multielement simulation runs, elements were extracted from this library, to be coupled in various ways.

Essentially the behavior of the elements was determined by two voltage-current relations. One of these, $i_0(V)$, had a segment of negative chord conductance, and it could therefore depolarize the membrane regeneratively. This was how the upstroke of the action potential of an element was brought about. Subsequently, the inactive voltage-current relation $i_1(V)$ restored the membrane potential to its resting state. The instantaneous voltage-current relation was a weighed average between $i_0(V)$ and $i_1(V)$, the weighing factor Y representing the instantaneous state of excitability of the membrane. We thus had $i(V) = Y\, i_1(V) + (1-Y)\, i_0(V)$, where Y assumed values between 0 (maximal excitability) and 1 (complete inexcitability). The rate of change of the membrane potential was determined by

$$C\, dV/dt = -i(V) + i_{ex}$$

where C was the membrane capacitance and i_{ex} represented the current entering the cell through its connections with other elements (or through an intracellular stimulating electrode). The behavior of Y was controlled by the second equation:

$$T\, dY/dt = Y_{inf}(V) - Y$$

which states that Y would move to its steady-state value Y_{inf} with a rate constant T. $Y_{inf}(V)$ would be an S shaped function of V, assuring that Y would move toward zero (maximal excitability) when V was below the resting potential and to unity when the membrane was sufficiently depolarized.

Reentrant Arrhythmias

It was easy to evoke reentrant arrhythmias in planar sheets consisting of many elements. The main results, which were reported in more detail elsewhere (Van Capelle and Durrer, 1980) can be summarized as follows: *(1)* the center of a circus movement need not be an inexcitable obstacle, *(2)* circus movements could occur in homogeneous sheets consisting of identical elements, and *(3)* multiple vortices could be present in sheets of sufficient magnitude. The example shown in Figure 10 illustrates these findings. A complex reentrant tachycardia was evoked in a square sheet consisting of 529 identical elements. The elements are depicted by small crosses in the left hand panel of Figure 10. Each element was coupled to its immediate neighbors on the same horizontal or vertical row, and all coupling resistances were the same. Isochronal lines depict the progression of the wavefronts during the interval indicated by a horizontal line under the action potentials in the right hand panel. The action potential of trace 6 is noteworthy, because it represents an element that was inexcit-

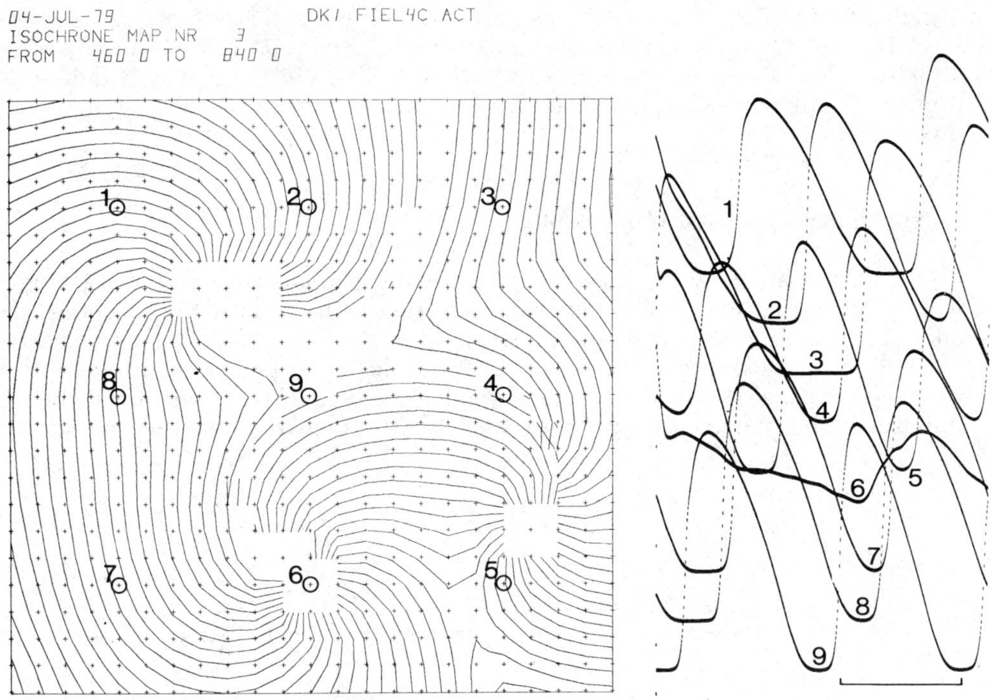

Figure 10. Threefold circus movement arrhythmia in a synthetic sheet consisting of 23 × 23 elements. Left panel: isochronal lines associated with progression of activation wavelets. Distance between isochrones corresponds with 20 time steps. Right panel: action potentials of nine selected elements. Location of elements is depicted in left hand panel. Horizontal line under the tracings indicates time interval of activation map in left hand panel. (By permission of the American Heart Association, Inc. from FJL van Capelle and D Durrer, Circ Res **47**:454–466, 1980)

able during this time interval. This element could therefore serve functionally as an obstacle for reentrant wavefronts: as seen from the isochronal map, it was in the vortex of a circus movement. Three such vortices present at the same time are shown in Figure 10. They were not stable and kept moving more or less freely over the sheet. One of the vortices disappeared a little later, when the activation wave associated with it was blocked near the edge of the sheet, but the other two remained active until the computer was turned off many cycles later. To initiate this particular arrhythmia, we made temporary cuts in the sheet to force the activation wave in a complex reentrant pattern, whereafter the cuts were patched at the appropriate moment.

The question that presents itself at this point is: how can an excitable element serve as the vortex of a circus movement? The answer is that the central elements of the vortex are kept inactivated by depolarizing electrotonic currents that flow from the active "head" of the circulating wavefront (which is spatially close to the center of the circus at all times) to the elements in the vortex. This conclusion is supported by an experimental study on circus movement tachycardias in the rabbit left atrium (Allessie et al., 1977) and a computer study of Gul'ko and Petrov (1972).

It must be pointed out that the elements used in the present simulation study correspond to rather depressed tissue. This is both because of technical reasons (healthy elements requiring much more computer time) and because arrhythmias can be evoked more easily in depressed elements. For multiple vortices to be produced in a planar sheet, the conduction velocity had to be low and the elements quite depressed, a situation which corresponds rather nicely with that in acutely ischemic myocardium.

Latent Automaticity and Cell Coupling

The automaticity of pacemaker elements in the computer model could be modified by varying the amount of coupling between these elements and the nonautomatic ones. An example is given in Figure 11, where the action potentials of a nonpacemaker element (N) and of a pacemaker element (P) are displayed for various values of the coupling resistance. When there was no coupling (panel A), N was silent, and P fired at its intrinsic rate. When the coupling was weak, subthreshold responses became visible

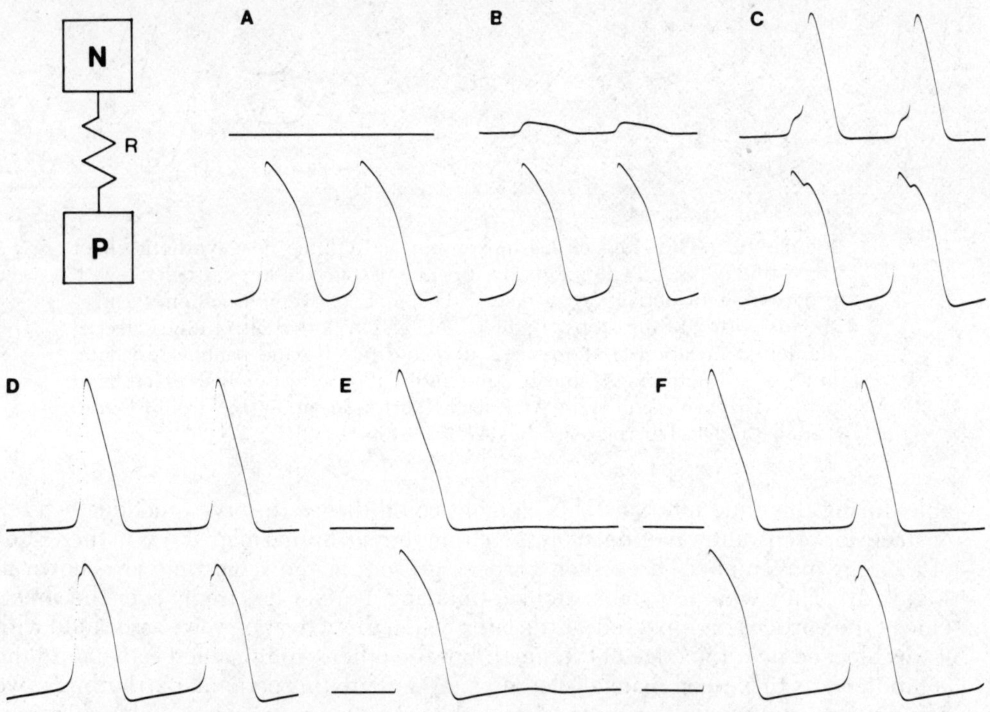

Figure 11. Interaction between a nonautomatic (N) and a pacemaker (P) element. Panel *A*: no coupling present. Element N is silent and P fires at its intrinsic rate. Panel *B*: weak coupling, local responses are present in element N. Panel *C*: marginal conduction, note the "foot" of N and the lengthening of the action potential of P. Panel *D*: strong coupling. The frequency of the ensemble is lower than the intrinsic pacemaker frequency shown in A. Panel *E*: with even tighter coupling the ensemble is silent. Upon stimulation of N the ensemble fires and subthreshold after-oscillations follow the action potential of the pacemaker element. Panel *F*: when a critical amount of coupling is present, sustained automatic activity can be turned on after stimulation of the initially silent ensemble.

in N (panel B), and when the coupling was somewhat tighter these responses reached threshold and element N fired (panel C, note the foot in the trailing action potential and the lengthening of the leading one). The stronger the coupling, the smaller the phase lag between the two, until they fired practically in unison (panel D). The frequency of the ensemble was now much lower than the intrinsic rate of the pacemaker element. The reason was mainly that the nonpacemaker element supplied a hyperpolarizing current to the pacemaker during all or the larger part of its phase 4, thereby counteracting its natural diastolic depolarization. When the coupling was tight enough, as in Figure 11E, the ensemble may have become completely silent. When it was stimulated, a single activation resulted and was followed by subthreshold afteroscillations. Interestingly, when a critical amount of coupling was present, a conditionally stable ensemble resulted, in the sense that overt automaticity could be turned on by a single stimulus (panel F). Incidentally, it could be turned off again in the same way if the stimulus was appropriately timed (not shown).

The behavior of a coupled ensemble depends not only on the value of the coupling resistance, but also on the sizes or total membrane areas of the elements. When differences in size exist, it is intuitively clear that the larger element will tend to dominate the other, and that the action potentials and the electrophysiologic properties of the ensemble, when stiffly coupled, will resemble those of the larger element. If the pacemaker element in an ensemble such as that presented in Figure 11 is large enough, it cannot be stopped by the nonautomatic cell. In that case, tight coupling only results in an increasing resemblance between the action potentials of both elements, until it becomes impossible to tell from the recordings which element is the pacemaker and which is the nonautomatic element (not shown).

Modeling Inexcitable Tissue

We created a special type of element to mimic some of the properties of ischemic tissue. Ischemic heart cells lose their resting potential and become inexcitable. We therefore omitted the regenerative inward current $i_0(V)$ in these elements, and we adjusted the resting potential to zero. In this way, we obtained completely depolarized and completely inexcitable elements, which essentially constituted a leakage pathway to the extracellular space through an RC filter. When coupled to normal elements they tended to depolarize and inactivate them. The depolarizing current involved might be compared with a current of injury. This current was able to turn on overt automaticity in cases where latent pacemaker activity was present. This is illustrated in Figure 12. In the upper panel, an ensemble consisting of a nonpacemaker element (N) and a pacemaker element is shown. The action potential was that of the pacemaker. The automaticity of the ensemble was latent: only after stimulation did an action potential ensue, followed by a subthreshold afterdepolarization. When an "ischemic" element (I) was added (lower panel) overt automaticity was restored.

Interaction Across an Area of Bidirectional Block

Inexcitable elements also were used to create an area of partial or total conduction block. The mechanism of such a block was different from the one encountered in Figure 11 panel B; in the present case conduction failed because of local loss of excitability rather than because of the existence of a high resistance barrier for the conduction of the impulse. Because in our experiments the border zone appeared to be completely inexcitable when extrasystoles emerged from its healthy side, we created

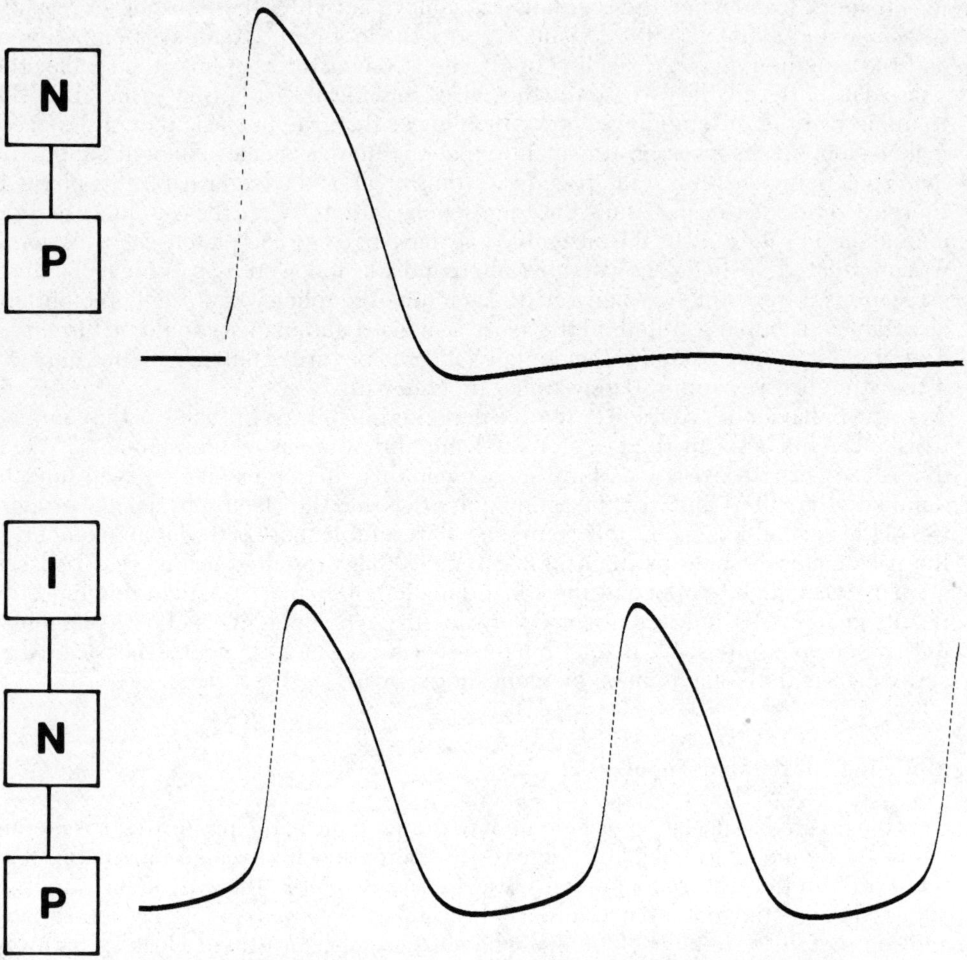

Figure 12. Influence of a depolarized element on latent automaticity. Upper panel: action potential of pacemaker element (P) in an ensemble with latent automaticity. The nonpacemaker element (N) is stimulated, resulting in an action potential followed by subthreshold oscillatory activity. Lower panel: spontaneous activity following attachment of an "ischemic" element (I).

an area of bidirectional block, using an inexcitable element to represent the border. We were interested to see whether activity at one side of a similar gap could modify activity at the other side. That such is the case is illustrated in Figure 13.

Elements 2–4 in Figure 13 formed an inexcitable gap. Element 3 was completely inexcitable because of its lack of regenerative current; its resting potential was somewhat negative because it was passively polarized by its neighbor elements 2 and 4. Conversely, the latter were partly depolarized by currents flowing from element 2, although elements 1 and 5 partially counteracted this effect. As a result, elements 2 and 4 are largely inactivated. They were therefore considered to be part of the inexcitable gap in the present context. A long string of excitable elements connected both sides of

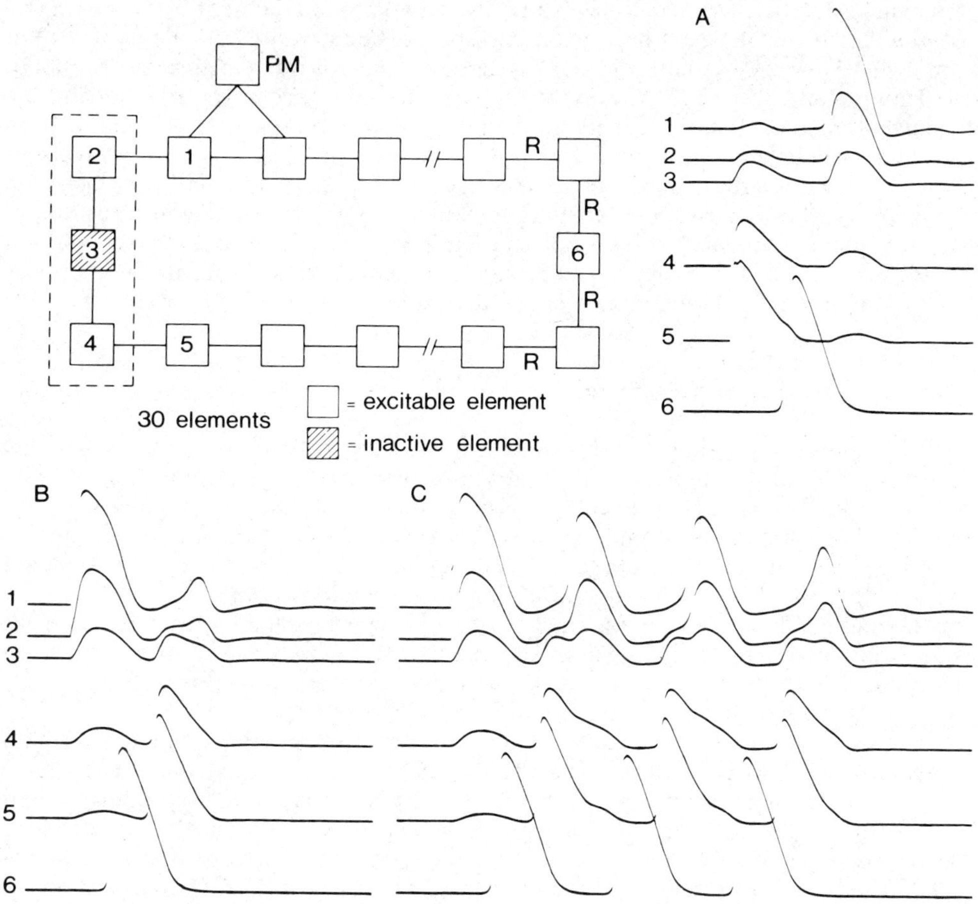

Figure 13. Enhancement of latent automaticity through an inexcitable gap. Elements 2–4 represent an inexcitable region with bidirectional conduction block. A long string of excitable elements connects both sides of the gap. Variation of the coupling resistances R in this loop results in variation of the conduction delay through the loop. A pacemaker element is added at one side of the gap in order to produce latent automaticity. Tracings correspond to elements numbered 1–6. Panel *A*: Element 5 is stimulated. Only a local response results in element 1. The activation is conducted through the loop, activating element 6 on its way, and reaches the other side of the gap where it is blocked. A subthreshold after-potential is visible in element 1. Panel *B*: Stimulation of element 1. Conduction through the gap fails but element 5 is reached through the loop. The afterdepolarization of element 1 is enhanced by the local response through the gap. Panel *C*: After a slight decrease of the conduction velocity in the loop the afterdepolarization in element 1 reaches threshold, resulting in a short run of extrasystoles.

the gap. When either side of the gap was stimulated, the activation front could reach the opposite side through this loop. At one side of the gap, a pacemaker element was added. This element could not fire spontaneously because of its tight coupling with two relatively large nonpacemaker cells, but it did show subthreshold oscillatory activity following activations. In panel A, a stimulus was applied to element 5. There was no conduction over the gap, only a local response being visible in element 1, but somewhat later the activity reached the opposite side of the gap through the loop, activating element 6 on its way. Note the subthreshold depolarization following the action potential in element 1. In panel B, element 1 was stimulated. Again conduction across the gap failed, and again the opposite side was activated later on by a wavefront that traveled through the loop. On reaching element 5, this wavefront was blocked in the gap, but the local response ensuing in elements 1 and 2 was now in a position to magnify the subthreshold after-depolarization in this region. In panel B, this did not result in activation of element 1, but when the conduction velocity in the loop was slightly depressed (panel C) a run of premature beats ensued.

What Can We Learn from Simulation Studies?

Computer simulations clearly cannot prove anything about mechanisms that play a role in a physiologic substrate. That part must be reserved for careful experimental evaluations. But what they can do is useful enough to grant them a place in our methodologic apparatus. First, simulations are useful to test our understanding of physiologic mechanisms. Failure to simulate a phenomenon we think we understand often helps us to detect a flaw in our arguments. Second, their heuristic value can be considerable. The "latent automaticity" concept, which emerges from the present simulation study, provides a good example. It may or may not turn out to be of importance in the intact heart, but experimental evidence settling this question either way would help us to understand what is really happening.

In any case, some of the manifestations of latent automaticity are suggestive at the present stage for its possible role in acute regional ischemia. Latent automaticity may become overt when injury is present (Fig. 12) or when triggering by properly timed local responses occurs (Fig. 13); both phenomena can be easily imagined to occur in acutely ischemic circumstances. Furthermore, it bears a close relation to the firmly established concept of "triggered activity" (Wit and Cranefield, 1976). In fact, it points to the possibility that triggered automaticity may occur not only as a local membrane phenomenon, but also as a result of coupling between cells of different propensity.

Our experimental results suggest that pacemaker activity is located in the Purkinje fibers at the healthy side of the ischemic border. Their automaticity may be promoted by catecholamine release and by stretch, caused by systolic bulging of the ischemic area (Kaufmann and Theophile, 1967). On the other hand, the extracellular potassium concentration at the healthy side of the border is 4.5 mM in our experiments, a value expected to counteract the induction of automaticity.

It is not yet clear which mechanisms are responsible for the early ectopic activity in acute regional ischemia. The present simulation study suggests latent automaticity as a good candidate, but further work will be needed too replace speculation by sound theoretical insight.

SUMMARY

Simultaneous DC recordings of 60 extracellular electrograms from isolated hearts of pigs and dogs permitted us to map the activation sequence during spontaneous ventricular arrhythmias in the early phase of myocardial ischemia following occlusion of the left anterior descending coronary artery. We found that the earliest activity during spontaneous ventricular premature beats occurred in nonischemic tissue close to the border zone. The ectopic beats occurred frequently just after a deep negative T wave in the ischemic area. No evidence was found for activity bridging the gap between late activity in the ischemic zone and early ectopic activity in the normal zone. Whenever Purkinje activity was found, it preceded myocardial activity in single premature beats, as well as in the initial beats of spontaneous ventricular tachycardias. From these findings we concluded that a focal mechanism in the normal Purkinje fibers close to the border was responsible for these arrhythmias, and that that mechanism was probably induced by injury currents. This conclusion was further strengthened by computer simulation studies, which provided clues about the role of cell coupling in the appearance of overt automaticity.

At a later stage of spontaneous ventricular tachycardias, reentry plays an important role. We observed circus movements with a diameter of 1 to 2 cm. Upon degeneration of the tachycardia into ventricular fibrillation, the wavefronts fragmentated in multiple reentrant circuits with a diameter of about 5 mm, although the individual circuits were seldom completed. Lidocaine prevented the occurrence of fibrillation in most cases. It accelerated the complete loss of excitability in the ischemic cells and thereby reduced the time during which conditions were favorable for multiple reentry.

REFERENCES

Allessie MA, Bonke FIM, Schopman FJG (1977) Circus movement in rabbit atrial muscle as a mechanism of tachycardia. III "The leading circle" concept: A new model of circus movement in cardiac tissue without the involvement of an anatomical obstacle. Circ Res **41**:9–18

Bickley WG (1948) Finite difference formulae for the square lattice. Quart J Mech **1**:35–42

Cardinal R, Janse MJ, van Eeden I, Werner G, Naumann d'Alnoncourt C, Durrer D (1981) The effects of lidocaine on intracellular and extracellular potentials, activation and ventricular arrhythmias during acute regional ischemia in the isolated porcine heart. Circ Res **49**: 792–806

Cranefield PF (1975) The Conduction of the Cardiac Impulse. Mt Kisco, NY, Futura Publishing Co

Garrey W (1914) The nature of fibrillary contraction of the heart—its relation to tissue mass and form. Am J Physiol **33**:397–414

Gul'ko FB, Petrov AA (1972) Mechanism of the formation of closed pathways of conduction in excitable media. Biofizika **17**:271–282

Hamlin RL, Burton RR, Leverett SD, Burns JW (1975) Ventricular activation process in minipigs. J Electrocardiol **8**:113–116

Holland RP, Brooks H (1976) The QRS complex during myocardial ischemia: an experimental analysis in the porcine heart. J Clin Invest **57**:541–550

Janse MJ, Cinca J, Morena H, Fiolet JWT, Kléber AG, de Vries JP, Becker AE, Durrer D (1979) The "border zone" in myocardial ischemia: an electrophysiological, metabolic and histochemical correlative study in the pig. Circ Res **44**:576–588

Janse MJ, van Capelle FJL, Morsink H, Kléber AG, Wilms-Schopman F, Cardinal R, Naumann d'Alnoncourt C, Durrer D (1980) Flow of "injury" current and patterns of excitation during early ventricular arrhythmias in acute regional myocardial ischemia in isolated porcine and canine hearts. Circ Res **47**:151–165

Kaplinsky E, Ogawa S, Balke CU, Dreifus LS (1979) Two periods of early ventricular arrhythmias in the canine acute myocardial infarction model. Circulation **60**:397–403

Kaufmann R, Theophile U (1967) Automatie-fördernde Dehnungseffekte an Purkinje-Fäden, Pappilarmuskeln und Vorhoftrabekeln von Rhesus-Affen. Pflüg Arch **297**:174–189

Lie KL, Wellens HJJ, van Capelle FJL, Durrer D (1974) Lidocaine in the prevention of primary ventricular fibrillation. N Engl J Med **291**:1324–1326
Moe GK, Rheinboldt WC, Abildskov JA (1964) A computer model of atrial fibrillation. Am Heart J **67**:200–220
van Capelle FJL, Durrer D (1980) Computer simulation of arrhythmias in a network of coupled excitable elements. Circ Res **47**:454–466
Wit AL, Cranefield PF (1976) Triggered activity in cardiac muscle fibers of the simian mitral valve. Circ Res **38**:85–98

Discussion

DE MELLO: What is the coupling situation between the ischemic and the normal region of the heart? How does coupling persist when it has been shown that in hypoxia you do get an appreciable increase in the longitudinal resistance?

VAN CAPELLE: Well, note that we are working at very early stages of ischemia and that in this situation there has not been time for any partial or complete sealing of communications, so that longitudinal intercellular resistance should still be quite low.

PAES DE CARVALHO: Do you propose that a slow-response mechanism operates within the infarcted area? Some of the action potentials shown in this area were very slow and showed humps.

VAN CAPELLE: The responses observed in the ischemic area are certainly slow. We do not know whether they are "true" slow responses or just depressed fast responses.

PAES DE CARVALHO: With respect to your mathematical and computer model, do you characterize that as a fast or a slow conducting model?

VAN CAPELLE: The computer model can be characterized as a very slowly conducting model. The reason for that is a technical one. We could not mimic in so many units a very fast upstroke and very slow plateau and repolarization phases, because of technical limitations of the time setting of our model. So, we had to do it with a time scale such that the upstroke was also slow even though not as slow as the repolarization phase.

MÉNDEZ: I am glad to find out that the mathematical model put forward by Moe et al. (Am Heart J 67:200, 1964) has finally received demonstration in your records. Both the model and your experimental data show that fibrillation is caused by a number of wavelets roaming through the cardiac syncytium.

RAMÓN: I am wondering why in your experiments the extrasystole is started not at the ischemic region but elsewhere beyond its boundaries.

VAN CAPELLE: Our experiments indicate that the extrasystole comes from the healthy side of the border, possibly from Purkinje fibers. We believe that currents of injury across the border have something to do with it. We do not know whether these currents act directly as a stimulating current or whether they act indirectly by provoking or enhancing automaticity in the healthy region. We are inclined to believe the latter.

Chapter 27

Reentrant Excitation in the Infarcted Canine Ventricle

Andrew L. Wit, Maurits A. Allessie, Felix I.M. Bonke, John J. Fenoglio, Jr., Wim Lammers and Joep Smeets

That an impulse could circulate in the heart and reexcite the same tissue over and over again (a process called *circus movement* or *reentrant excitation*) thereby causing cardiac arrhythmias was suggested to McWilliam in 1887 by his observations on the nature of ventricular fibrillation (McWilliam, 1887). Until that time, it was generally believed that all abnormalities in the rhythm of the heart were due to enhanced impulse initiation de novo from hyperexcitable heart muscle. The suggestion that an impulse could circulate was soon forgotten and not revived until nearly 20 years later, when Alfred Mayer began studies on the causes of rhythmic pulsations in the bell of the Medusa (Mayer, 1906; 1908). It was his studies along with those of Mines and Garrey, between 1912 and 1914, that elucidated most of the mechanisms we know today, by which an excitatory wave can continue to propagate and reexcite (reenter) tissue it has previously excited (Mayer, 1906; 1908; Mines, 1913; 1914; Garrey, 1914; 1924).

The success of Mayer, Mines, and Garrey in demonstrating reentrant excitation was derived from the simplicity of their experimental models, which were simple and large rings of excitable tissue (Wit and Cranefield, 1978). They could follow the movement of the slow contractile wave visually, and because the wave was conducting through a circumscribed pathway it was not difficult to follow it around the pathway (Fig. 1). As the final proof of reentry, they showed that the impulse died out when the ring was cut through at one point.

The major difficulties in experimental design and analysis fell on subsequent investigators, whose aim it was to demonstrate that reentrant excitation was a cause of abnormal rhythms in the intact heart. The experimental models became more complex, and it became more difficult to adhere to the criteria for proving the presence of circus movement as established by Mines (1913; 1914). Mines's criteria are as follows: *(1)* An area of unidirectional block must be demonstrated so that the impulse

---

Dr. Fenoglio is a recipient of a Research Career Development Award, Grant No. 5-KO4-HL 00185, from the National Heart, Lung and Blood Institute, National Institutes of Health.

Supported in part by Grant HL 12738 from the National Institute of Health (USA) and by Grant 13-22-24 from the Stichting Voor Fundamenteel Geneeskundig Onderzoek (FUNGO), The Netherlands.

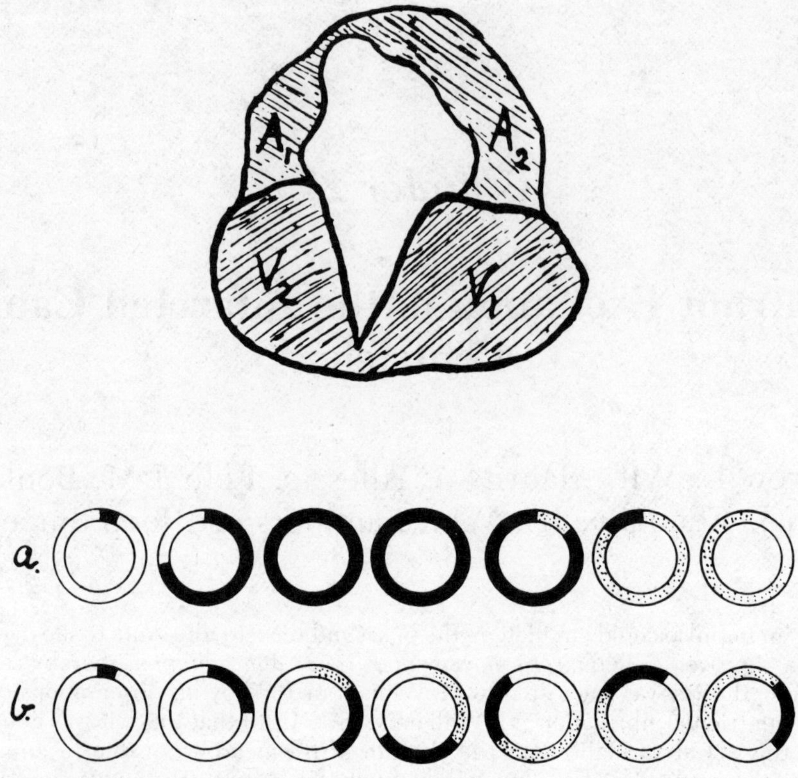

Figure 1. Top: Mines diagram of his ring preparation comprised of the auricle (A) and ventricle (V) of the tortoise heart, in which he observed circulating excitation. During this circulating rhythm contraction proceeded in the order V_1, V_2, A_1, A_2. Bottom *A* and *B*: Mines explanation of the mechanism for circulating excitation. *A* shows the events that occur if the impulse travels too rapidly in one direction around the loop, unidirectional block being present in the other direction. The conducting impulse represented by the darkly shaded area, is initiated by a stimulus and travels rapidly around the loop only to return to its point of origin prior to recovery of excitability of this region (3rd and 4th diagrams from the left). As a result the impulse dies out as shown in the 5th and 6th diagrams, and the tissue remains refractory (stippled area). In the 7th diagram the tissue begins to regain excitability as shown by disappearance of the stippled area. *B* shows that reentry will occur if conduction is slowed and the duration of the refractory period is decreased. A stimulated impulse (darkly shaded area) conducts slowly in one direction, leaving in its wake refractory tissue (stippled area). Since conduction is slow and the refractory period is short, by the time the impulse has returned to its site of origin (5th and 6th diagrams from the left), this region has recovered excitability so the impulse can continue to circulate. (Reproduced from Mines GR: On dynamic equilibrium in the heart. J Physiol [Lond] **46**:350–383, 1913 with permission from the publisher.)

conducts in one direction. *(2)* The movement of the excitatory wave should be observed to progress through the pathway and to return to its point of origin (see Fig. 1). And *(3)*, according to Mines (1913; 1914) "The best test for circulating excitation is to cut through the ring at one point. If impulses continue to arise in the cut ring, circus movement as a cause can be ruled out."

In this report we present the initial results of our studies on reentrant excitation in the canine ventricles during ventricular tachycardia caused by myocardial infarction. We recorded electrical activity from up to 192 sites within a small region (3½ × 4½ cm) where arrhythmias were arising and were able to show unidirectional conduction block and to follow propagation of the impulse through reentrant pathways.

METHODS

The Canine Model of Ventricular Tachycardia

Ventricular tachycardias can be induced in the canine heart by stimulated premature ventricular impulses or by rapid stimulation of the ventricles 3 to 7 days after complete occlusion of the left anterior descending coronary artery near its origin (Kaplinsky et al., 1972; El Sherif, 1977; Karagueuzian et al., 1979). These induced tachycardias usually are short in duration. Previous studies have shown that the origin of many of the tachycardia impulses is in the epicardial muscle that survives on the surface of the anterior and lateral left ventricular walls over the infarcted region (El Sherif et al., 1977; Wit et al., 1981). In this study, we have determined the excitation pattern in this epicardial muscle during the tachycardias and their initiation.

We caused infarction of the anterior left ventricle by completely occluding the left anterior descending coronary artery of six dogs, in two stages, as described by Harris (1950). The animals were then permitted to recover from surgery. On the following day spontaneous ventricular arrhythmias were present but they disappeared after 48 hours (Harris, 1950). The experiments were carried out on the 3rd to 5th day following occlusion of the coronary artery. At this time, the dogs were anesthetized with pentobarbital (15 to 20 mg/kg, i.v.) and were ventilated with a mixture of nitrous oxide and oxygen. The chest was opened by a midsternotomy, the pericardium opened, and a pericardial cradle made to support the heart. A catheter was placed in the femoral artery to record blood pressure. A pentapolar plaque electrode was sutured to the base of the right ventricle near the origin of the left anterior descending coronary artery for bipolar stimulation. Figure 2 shows one of the techniques that we used to induce ventricular tachycardia. The ventricles were driven at a constant rate with rectangular pulses, 2 msec in duration and at twice the diastolic threshold. Premature stimuli (2 msec in duration and quadruple the diastolic threshold) were introduced through the same stimulating electrode after every 15 to 20 driven impulses; first late in the ventricular cycle, and then the coupling interval between the premature stimuli and the basic impulses was decreased in steps of 10 msec or less. The basic drive was inhibited for a period of 10 to 15 sec following premature stimulation to permit nondriven repetitive activity (tachycardia). Nonsustained, ventricular tachycardias lasting 1 to 15 sec were induced in all dogs by stimulated premature impulses near or on the descending limb of the T wave of the previous impulse (Fig. 2). Excitation patterns were mapped during induction of these tachycardias. Another way by which we induced tachycardia was to drive the ventricles at a rapid rate for 1 to 10 sec. Then, when the driving stimulus was suddenly turned off, rapid tachycardias often occurred (see Fig. 15).

Electrode Array and Recording System

Some of the nonsustained ventricular tachycardias induced by the stimulated premature impulses or by rapid ventricular stimulation arose in the narrow sheet of epicardial muscle that survives over the infarct on the anterior and lateral ventricular

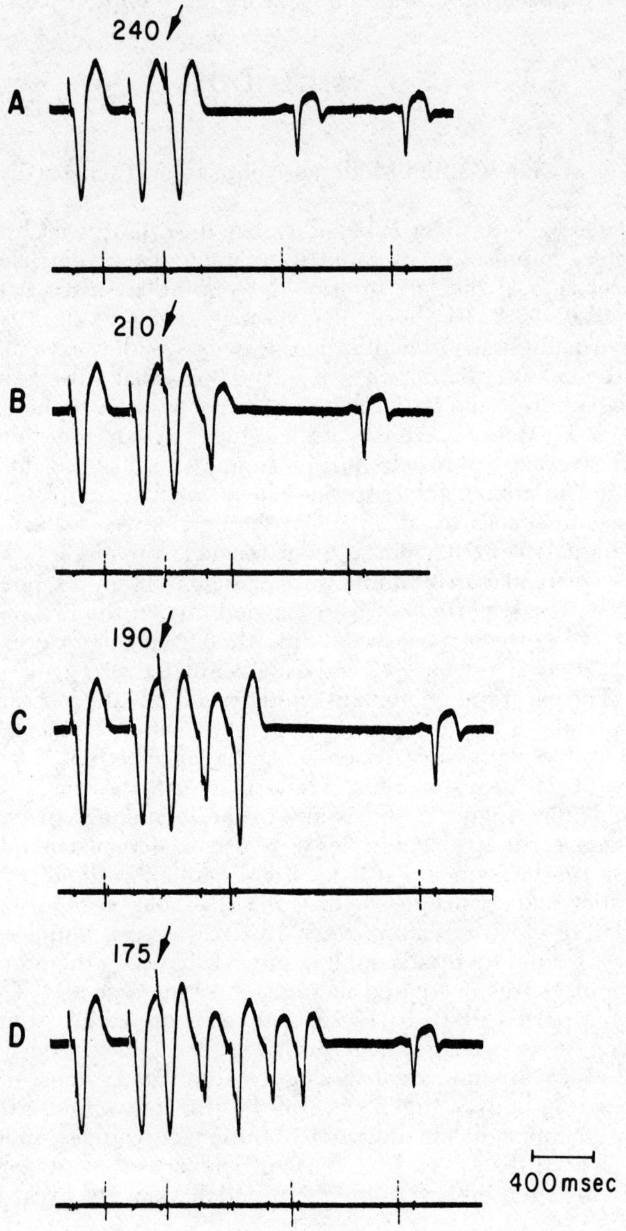
240
A
210
B
190
C
175
D
400msec

walls (El Sherif, 1977; Wit et al., 1980; 1981). To determine the pattern of excitation in this muscle, we used a plaque electrode array constructed from a 2-mm-thick sheet of plexiglass which was molded to fit the curvature of the anterolateral left ventricle (Fig. 3). The plaque was oval with diameters of 3.5 and 4.5 cm. Holes, 0.5 mm in diameter, were drilled every 2 mm in the plexiglass, and in each hole was glued the end of a Teflon-coated silver wire. These ends were polished flush to the surface of the plaque. The ends of the wires formed the electrode contact when the plaque was placed on the ventricles. The plaque contained 384 such electrodes, which were connected by flexible insulated wire to 8 48-pin Cannon plugs. The contacts were paired to make 192 bipolar electrodes; each pole of a bipolar pair was 2 mm apart, and there was a distance of 2 mm separating each bipolar pair. This plaque electrode array was placed on the anterolateral ventricle (Fig. 3) and held there lightly by hand during the induction of ventricular tachycardias.

We recorded bipolar electrograms simultaneously from the 192 sites on the ventricle with a multiplexing system that was developed in the Department of Physiology at The University of Limburg, The Netherlands. Figure 4 diagrams the essential components of this system. The leads from each of the 192 electrodes were led into individual autoranging amplifiers, enabling each signal to be amplified separately. Separate amplification of each signal was necessary because of their variable magnitude, particularly in the ischemic area. The optimal amplification factor of all amplifiers could be set simultaneously, just prior to induction of tachycardia, by a single switch and then locked in. Because the amplitude of the electrograms during rapid tachycardias often was different than it was during sinus rhythm or basic drive of the ventricles, the gain of all amplifiers could be simultaneously reset after tachycardia induction. The filters of the amplifiers were set at 2 and 400 Hz. After preamplification, the 192 signals were multiplexed and digitized. Three multiplexers were used, each of which multiplexed 64 signals. Each signal was sampled every 0.5 msec or five times the maximum frequency of 400 Hz, resulting in 2000 samples/sec/signal. The multiplexed signals were then digitized, by an 8-bit analog-to-digital converter. The multiplexed and digitized data were converted to analog pulses using Pulse Code Modulation with the Miller Code and recorded on three tracks of analog tape at 120 inches/sec with a wide-band Ampex PR 2300 recorder. A digital time code and the surface electrocardiogram were simultaneously recorded on additional tape tracks.

Figure 2. Effects of ventricular premature stimulation on ventricular rhythm of a dog 3 days after permanent coronary artery occlusion. In each panel the upper trace is the ECG recording obtained from subcutaneous electrodes across the chest wall. The lower trace is an atrial electrogram. The ventricles are being driven at a cycle length of 400 msec. In panel *A* a stimulated premature impulse (arrow) at a coupling interval of 240 msec is followed by a pause of 600 msec and then by sinus rhythm. In panel *B* the coupling interval of the stimulated premature impulse (arrow) is 210 msec; it is followed by a single nonstimulated ventricular depolarization and after a pause of 800 msec sinus rhythm ensues. In panel *C*, the coupling interval of the premature impulse is 190 msec (arrow); this is followed by two nonstimulated ventricular depolarizations, and after a pause of 1030 msec sinus rhythm occurs. In panel *D*, the coupling interval of the applied premature impulse is 175 msec (arrow); this is followed by a short period of tachycardia consisting of four nonstimulated depolarizations. After a pause of 540 msec sinus rhythm resumes. (Reproduced from Karagueuzian et al: Protracted ventricular tachycardia induced by premature stimulation of the canine heart after coronary artery occlusion and reperfusion. Circ Res **44**:333–846, 1979 with permission from the publisher.)

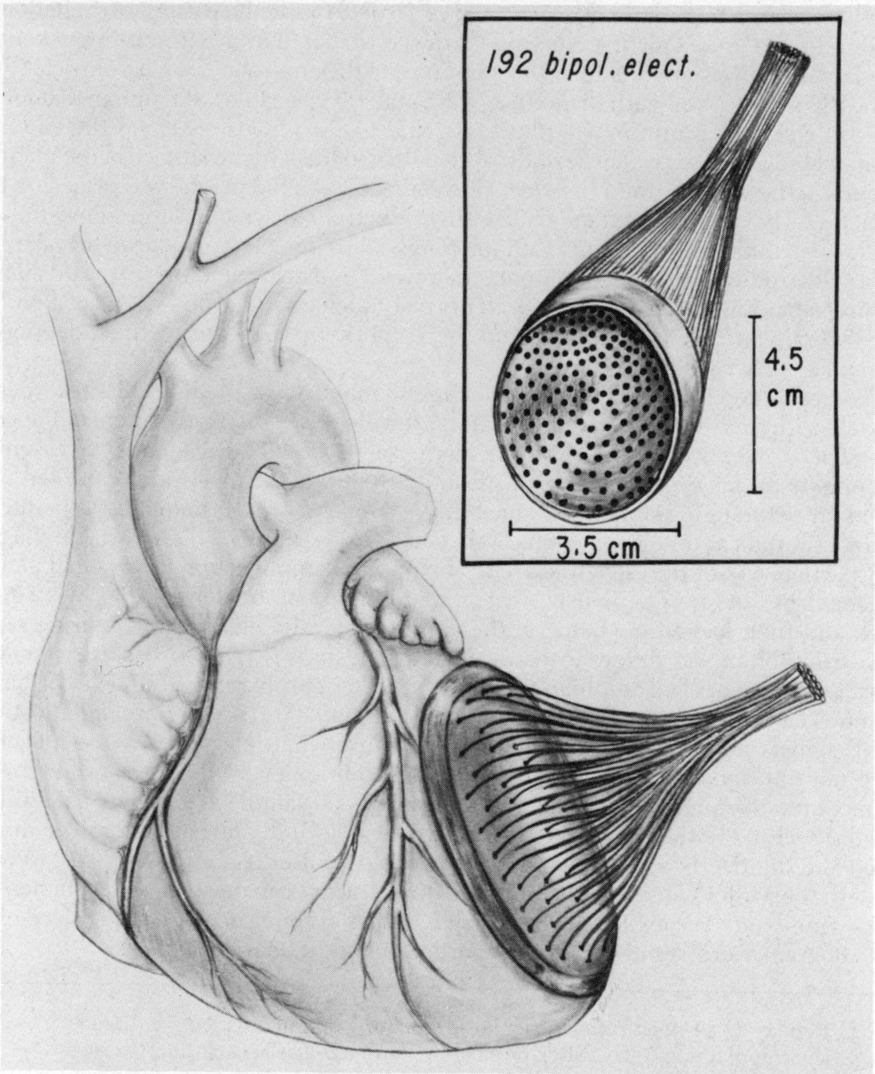

Figure 3. The plaque electrode array used to map activation of the epicardial muscle over the infarct. The inset at the upper right shows the curved under-surface of the electrode array containing 384 electrode contacts at equally spaced intervals. The leads from the electrodes to the amplifiers come out the top of the plaque and form a flexible cable. Below is an illustration of the plaque array on the anterior surface of the left ventricle, adjacent to the left anterior descending coronary artery which runs along the left margin of the electrode plaque. (Figs 3, 4, 6, 9–11, and 14 reproduced with permission from Wit et al., *Am. J. Cardiol.* 49:166–185, 1982.)

Actual data collection usually occurred for a total of 20 to 30 min during the course of a 4 to 5-hr experiment. Data analysis was not done during the experiment. To analyze the data, we initially played back the electrocardiogram and several selected electrograms with the time code on a Schwarzer pen recorder at a paper speed of 10 mm/sec. During playback of the tape, the pulse code-modulated signal was decoded

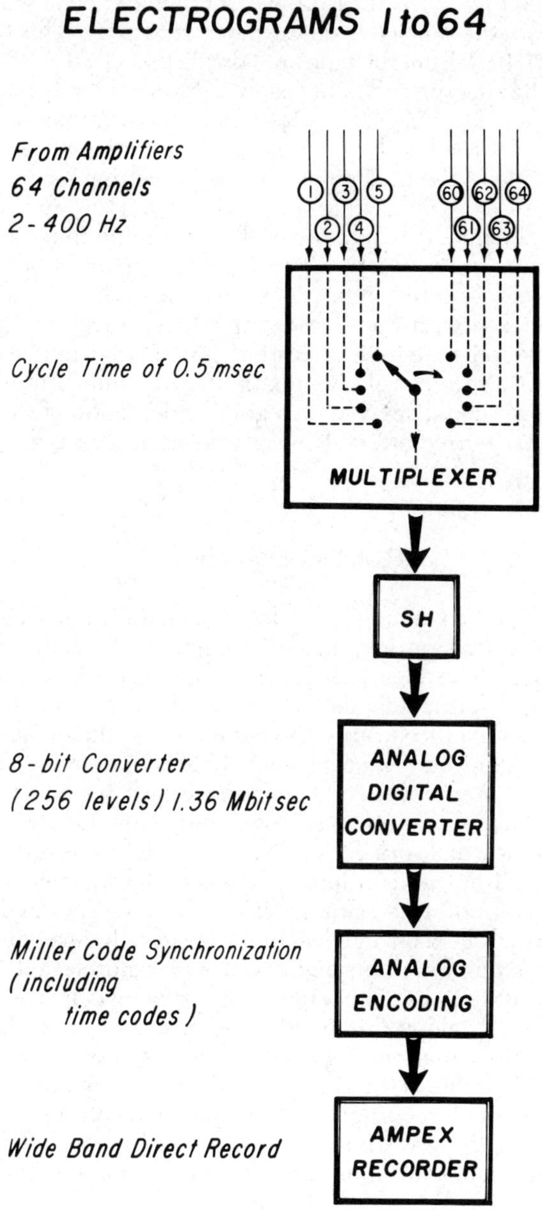

Figure 4. Block diagram of the recording system. Three multiplexers are used each of which multiplexes 64 channels. SH indicates a sample and hold circuit.

and converted to the original analog form by a digital-to-analog converter. The paper record provided a log of what had been done, what had happened, and when it had happened during the entire experiment. Selected time periods during the experiment were then chosen for detailed analysis. For example, to analyze the conduction pattern of the last of a series of basic drive impulses followed by a single premature impulse induced by a stimulus and the first several beats of the tachycardia induced by that premature impulse (see Figs. 7, 8, 12, 13), the exact time period at which these events occurred was noted from the time code on the paper recording. This time period of up to 3 sec then was played back from the tape onto the disk of a PDP 11/04 computer. The electrograms during the time period being analyzed were then displayed in groups of 10 to 15 on the CRT of a Tektronix graphics terminal, and the moment of activation was marked with a cursor. For the bipolar recordings, the moment of activation was taken as the greatest amplitude of the deflection. But, the electrograms recorded from the surviving epicardial muscle cells in the infarcted region were not always the sharp deflections that would enable us to unequivocally determine the exact time of activation. Some electrograms were up to 40 to 60 msec in duration, and they were sometimes comprised of multiple deflections (see Figs. 10, 11, 14). Nevertheless, when they were compared with the electrograms from surrounding sites, it almost always was possible to determine their activation time relative to that of the surrounding sites. These activation times relative to a reference time (stimulus artifact or Q wave on the ECG) were then displayed on a graphic depiction of the electrode array (Fig. 5). Isochrones at 10-msec intervals were drawn either by the computer or by hand.

Histological Study

The exact location of the plaque electrode array on the anterolateral left ventricle was marked by placing sutures around its entire circumference after the electrophysiologic study was finished. The dog was killed by removing the heart, which was placed in 10% neutral-buffered formaldehyde. After complete fixation, the region of the anterolateral wall marked by the sutures (the region where the plaque electrode array had been located) was removed. The oval-shaped block of tissue was cut transversely along its axis (from base towards apex) into five pieces, each of which was embedded by standard procedures for subsequent histologic study. Sections were cut 6-μ thick perpendicular to the epicardial surface, so that each section showed the full thickness of the ventricular wall from epicardium to endocardium. Selected sections were stained with hematoxylin-phloxine-safranin. From these sections we determined the thickness of the epicardial sheet of ventricular muscle usually surviving over infarcts in the canine heart and the number of surviving ventricular muscle cell "layers" comprising this sheet in different regions. The number of surviving cell layers was counted at 50 to 75 preselected points along the length of each section (from base to apex) and plotted on a graphic representation of the anterolateral ventricular epicardial surface (Fig. 6). This provided a profile of the anatomy of the surviving epicardial muscle from which electrograms had been recorded with the plaque electrode array, and enabled us to determine whether there were intact muscular connections between surviving epicardial muscle and deeper intramural muscle in the infarcted region.

RESULTS

Anatomy of the Infarcts

We report here the mapping data from two dogs that underwent coronary artery occlusion. The infarcted region where electrograms had been recorded was character-

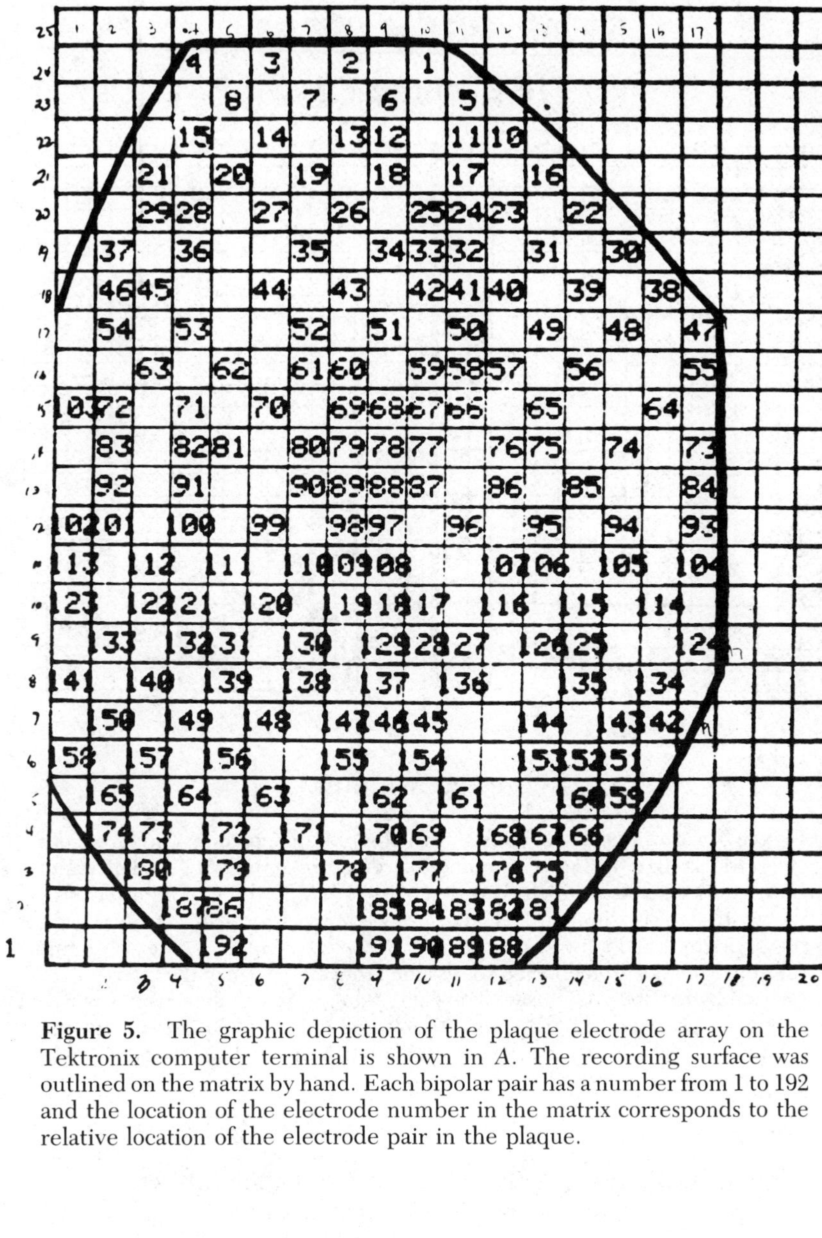

Figure 5. The graphic depiction of the plaque electrode array on the Tektronix computer terminal is shown in *A*. The recording surface was outlined on the matrix by hand. Each bipolar pair has a number from 1 to 192 and the location of the electrode number in the matrix corresponds to the relative location of the electrode pair in the plaque.

ized by a surviving sheet of epicardial muscle, which varied in thickness in most places from 0.01 to 0.1 mm (Fig. 6). The myocardium beneath the surviving epicardial sheet of muscle was entirely necrotic, with no apparent possibilities for impulse conduction, transmurally, from endocardial or intramural regions. Impulse conduction occurred mainly in a horizontal direction. In some of the experiments, not included here, up to one third of the outer ventricular wall survived the coronary artery occlusion, and thus the epicardial muscle over the infarct could be activated in a transmural as well as horizontal direction, making it more difficult to interpret excitation maps.

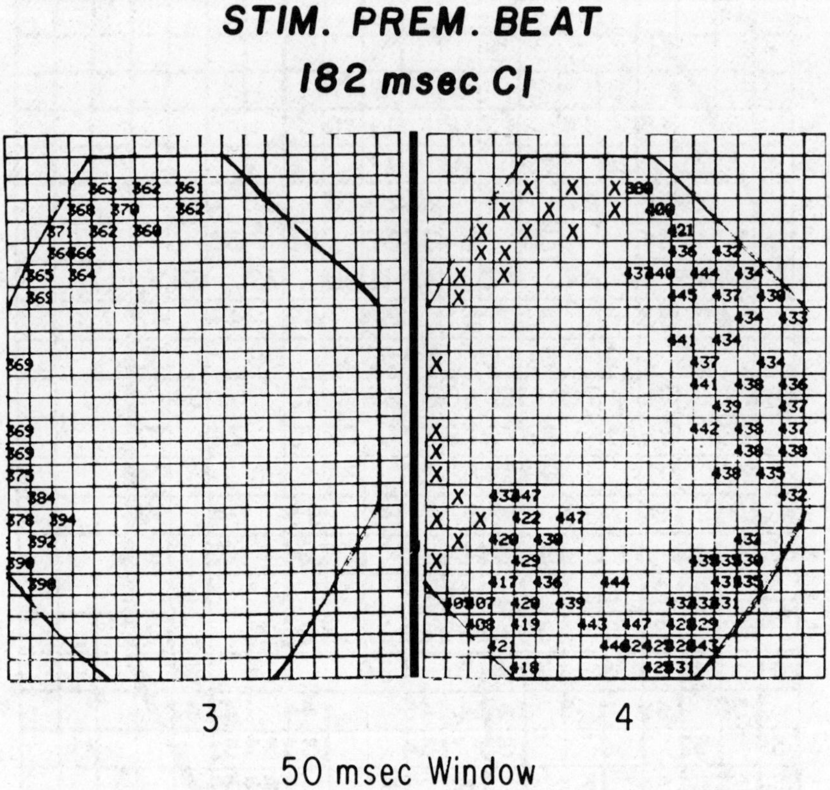

Figure 5 *(Continued).* In B is shown the plot of activation times, on the electrode matrix during a stimulated premature impulse. The left panel shows the electrodes which recorded activity within the first 50 msec after the ventricle was stimulated. The reference 0 was arbitrarily chosen during the basic rhythm 350 msec prior to this premature impulse. Relative to this reference point a group of electrodes along the left margin of the matrix were activated after 360−395 msec. The right panel shows the electrodes which recorded activity during the next 50 msec period (400−450 msec after the reference 0). The X's were drawn in by hand to indicate the electrodes which were activated in the left panel.

Excitation of Epicardial Muscle over the Infarct During Nonsustained Tachycardias

Circus Movement Caused by Premature Stimulation of the Ventricles

Detailed activation maps of the epicardial muscle over the infarcts were constructed from the time measurements made on electrogram recordings. Figures 7, 8, 12, and 13 show the excitation pattern of this region in one of the experiments during the basic drive of the ventricles, a stimulated premature impulse that induced a short period of tachycardia consisting of three impulses and the first two impulses of that tachycardia. The anatomy of the infarcted area in this experiment is shown in Figure 6.

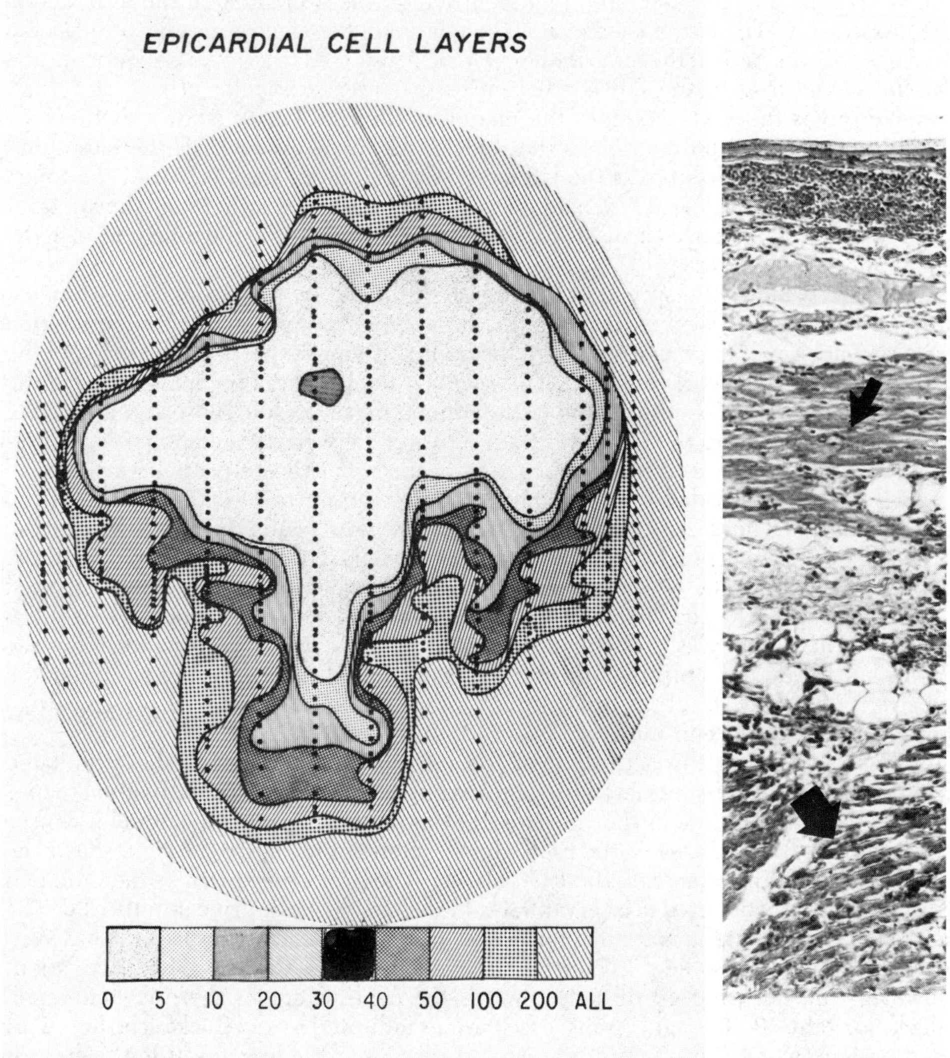

Figure 6. Graphic depiction of the thickness of the surviving epicardial sheet of muscle over an infarct in a region from which electrograms were recorded with the plaque electrode array (see Figs. 10, 11, 14). The oval represents the region where the electrode array was located. The top of the oval area is near the base of the left ventricle, the left margin is adjacent to the LAD, the bottom of the oval area is toward the apex and the right margin is toward the lateral left ventricle (see Fig. 3). Each pattern of shading indicates the number of surviving epicardial cell layers (thickness) according to the key at the bottom of the figure. Each dot represents a point where the number of cells was counted. Thus, there is an extensive center region where only 2–10 cell layers survived while, toward the margins, the surviving sheet is greater than 100 cell layers thick. The inset at the upper right is a photomicrograph of the intact epicardial cells in this infarcted region (small arrow).

The figures are arranged in the following way; the oval region in each panel represents the area of the anterior and lateral left ventricular free wall beneath the oval plaque electrode array. The top of each oval is the margin of the electrode array or infarcted area towards the base of the anterior left ventricle (referred to as the basal margin), the margin of the oval to the left is adjacent to the interventricular groove and LAD (referred to as the LAD margin), the margin of the oval below is towards the apex (apical margin), and the margin to the right in the figures is towards the lateral left ventricular wall (referred to as the left lateral margin) (also, see Fig. 3). At the top of each panel in Figures 7, 8, 12, and 13 is the same electrocardiogram showing the period of ventricular tachycardia; the shaded areas correspond to the time period in the excitation maps below.

Figure 7 shows the spread of the impulse initiated by the basic drive stimulus, through the epicardial muscle over the surface of the infarct. Earliest excitation occurred in a small region at the top of the figure, 10 to 20 msec after the onset of the QRS (see shaded area on the ECG). This region is the border of the infarct toward the base of the heart and is in the vicinity of the stimulating electrode. A broad region along the margin adjacent to the LAD was then activated between 20 and 30 msec. Subsequent excitation occurred in a sequence indicating that the activation wave spread laterally in the epicardial muscle from the LAD margin, toward the middle of the infarcted area. There are several regions of very slow conduction; one where the 30-msec isochrone is nearly adjacent to the region activated between 40 and 50 msec, and another where the 50-msec isochrone is nearly adjacent to the region activated between 80 and 90 msec. This may even be a zone of conduction block. The central region of the infarct was probably also excited by wave fronts propagating from the basal, left lateral and apical margins. Total excitation of the entire region under the electrode array required 80 to 90 msec. There is also no evidence for epicardial breakthrough from deep muscle.

Figure 8 shows the activation of the infarcted region during the stimulated premature impulse that initiated the nonsustained tachycardia. The activation map is divided into two continuous time periods; the map at the left shows the initial 120 msec of conduction (striped area on the ECG above) whereas the map to the right shows the next 40 msec (stippled area on the ECG above). The premature impulse that initiated the tachycardia conducted in a very different way than the basic drive impulse did. The left panel shows that the margin of the infarct along the LAD and towards the base was activated initially between 40 and 60 msec after the onset of the QRS. Activation, however, did not proceed directly towards the central region; there is conduction block along the 40-, 50-, and 60-msec isochrones indicated by the thick black line. Part of the block along the 40- and 50-msec isochrones extending towards the base is probably outside the field of the recording electrodes, as we have indicated in the schematic diagram shown in Figure 9. Activation then occurred toward the apex, along the margin of the infarct adjacent to the LAD, and reached the apical border at the 110-msec isochrone. Along the basal and left lateral margins, there appeared to be conduction block between the 50- and 120-msec isochrones. The activation wave entering the infarcted region at the left lateral margin at 120 msec appeared to have conducted outside the recording field of the electrode around this region of block, as shown schematically in Figure 9. The right panel shows that after conducting around the margins of the infarct, excitation occurred towards the center from the apical and left lateral borders, and then back towards the margin along the LAD, which was reached between 140 and 150 msec. The region shown by the arrows, which was initially excited by the premature impulse at 50 to 60 msec, was reexcited by the reentering impulse at 160 msec. The margin of the infarct above and below this region

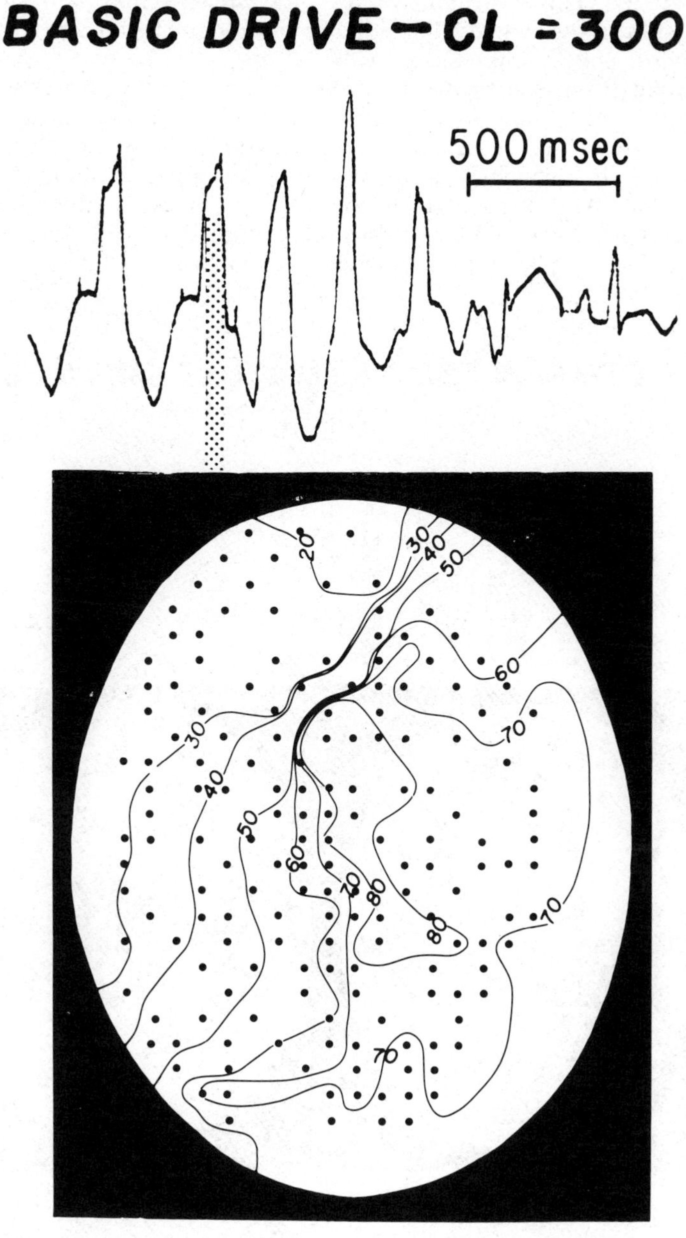

Figure 7. Activation map of the anterior surface of the left ventricle constructed from the timing of electrograms recorded with the plaque electrode during basic drive stimulation, in a dog with a 3 day old infarction. The oval area represents the region of the anterior left ventricle under the plaque electrode (see Fig. 3). The orientation is described in the text. Each dot on the map indicates the location of a recording site where an activation time was measured. At the top of the figure is the electrocardiogram. The shaded area is the time period shown in the activation map below.

was not reexcited. This returning impulse probably reexcited the ventricles to cause the first impulse of the tachycardia, although it could not be followed after it reexcited the LAD border of the infarcted area.

Recordings from ten of the electrodes in the reentrant pathway during this stimulated premature impulse are shown along with the electrocardiogram in Figure 10. The locations of these electrodes are indicated in the schematic diagram of Figure 9. Electrode 102 (which is shown both at the top and the bottom of the figure) was located near the LAD margin of the infarct (Fig. 9). This region was initially excited by the stimulated premature impulse at 60 msec. Figure 10 shows that electrograms were recorded at the other sites progressively later in time as the impulse propagated

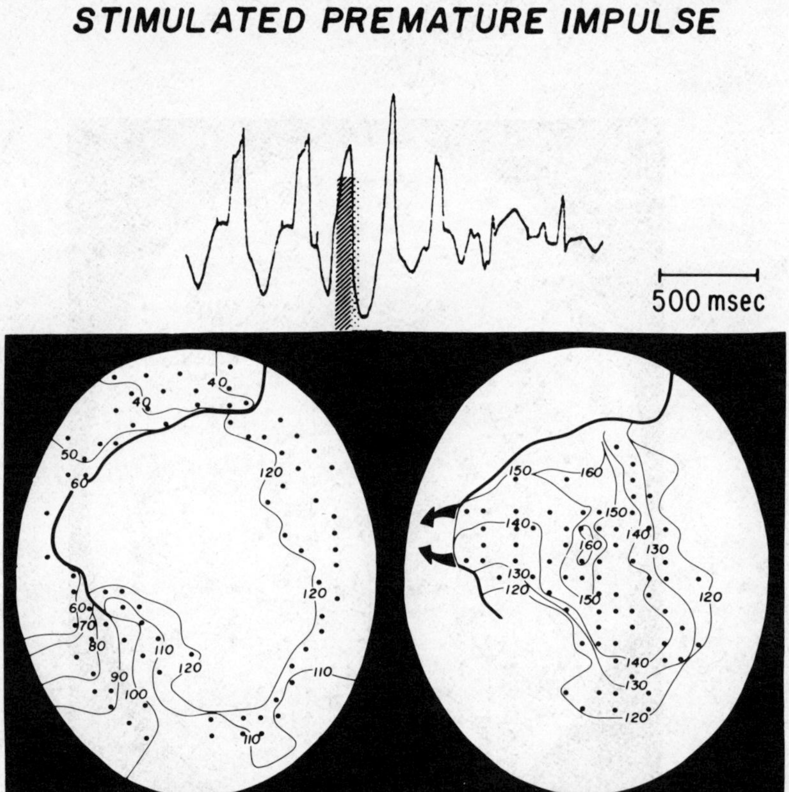

Figure 8. Activation maps of the anterior surface of the left ventricle constructed from the timing of electrograms recorded with the plaque electrode, during the stimulated premature impulse which initiated a short period of ventricular tachycardia. The general format is the same as Fig. 7. The map to the left includes the 1st 120 msec after the onset of the premature QRS complex, and corresponds to the time period indicated by the striped area on the ECG above. The map to the right includes the subsequent 50 msec, corresponding to the time period indicated by the stippled area on the ECG.

towards the apex and then back toward the LAD margin. The region under electrode 102 was then reexcited by the reentering impulse 100 msec after it was initially excited by the stimulated premature impulse.

Unidirectional conduction block is one of the requisites for the occurrence of reentry (Wit and Cranefield, 1978), and the reentry of the stimulated premature impulse in Figures 8 to 10 occurred because of the broad area of block along the 40 to 60 msec isochrones. This area of block prevented the central region from being activated directly by the premature impulse, and therefore provided an excitable pathway for subsequent retrograde activation, which led to reentry. The cause of the unidirectional block in this experiment is not known. Selected electrograms recorded across this zone of conduction block are shown in Figure 11. Compared with the other electrodes, electrode 103 was located more towards the LAD border, in the area activated at 60 msec (see Fig. 9 for the location of the electrodes). It is clear that the premature impulse excited muscle at this recording site, as indicated by the deflection in the electrogram trace labeled P. Electrodes 83 and 82 were located in the region where conduction block of the premature impulse occurred. The recording in 83 shows a slow wave, which occurred soon after the "P" deflection in 103. This slow wave may have resulted from *(1)* very slow conduction of the premature impulse just prior to block, *(2)* electrotonic interaction of the region under the electrode, which may be at the site of block, with the region proximal to the site of block (electrode 103), or *(3)* a combination of both slow conduction and electrotonic effects. Electrode 82 was distal to the site of block and showed only a very low-amplitude, slow deflection, reflecting perhaps some slight electrotonic interaction with the region proximal to the block. In addition, electrodes 82, 83 and 103 show excitation by the returning impulse. The region where electrode 103 was located was excited both by the stimulated premature impulse and by the reentering impulse 90 msec later.

After the stimulated premature impulse returned to reexcite the LAD border of the infarct at 160 msec (Fig. 8) and presumably the ventricles causing the first beat of the tachycardia, the epicardial muscle over the infarct was not activated again for another 90 msec. At this time (250 msec after the onset of the QRS of the stimulated premature impulse and 10 msec after the QRS wave of the first tachycardia impulse), activation again occurred along the LAD margin (Fig. 12). Because only a limited area of the ventricle was covered by the plaque electrode array, we were not able to follow the propagation of the impulse that left the infarcted region at 160 msec, through some other part of the reentrant pathway prior to its return to the area under the electrode at 250 msec.

This returning activation wave also blocked along the LAD margin of the infarcted area, along the 260-msec isochrone (Fig. 12). The site of block is very similar to that for the stimulated premature impulse. Excitation then progressed along the LAD margin of the infarct toward the apex, reaching it at 300 msec. At the same time that the LAD margin of the infarct was being activated, the left lateral margin of the infarct was also activated by another wave front entering this region at 270 msec. This activation wave may have resulted from an impulse spreading along the basal margin of the infarct and outside the recording field of the plaque electrode as diagrammed in Fig. 9B. Activation then progressed from the apex and left lateral margin toward the center of the infarcted region. Figure 12 only shows the spread of activation to the 350-msec isochrone. The left panel in Figure 13 shows continuation of activation from this 350-msec isochrone to the LAD margin of the infarct, which was reached at 410 msec, just prior to the occurrence of the second impulse of the tachycardia (darkly shaded area on the ECG above). After returning to the LAD border at 410 msec, activation waves conducted around the margins of the infarcted region both towards the base and

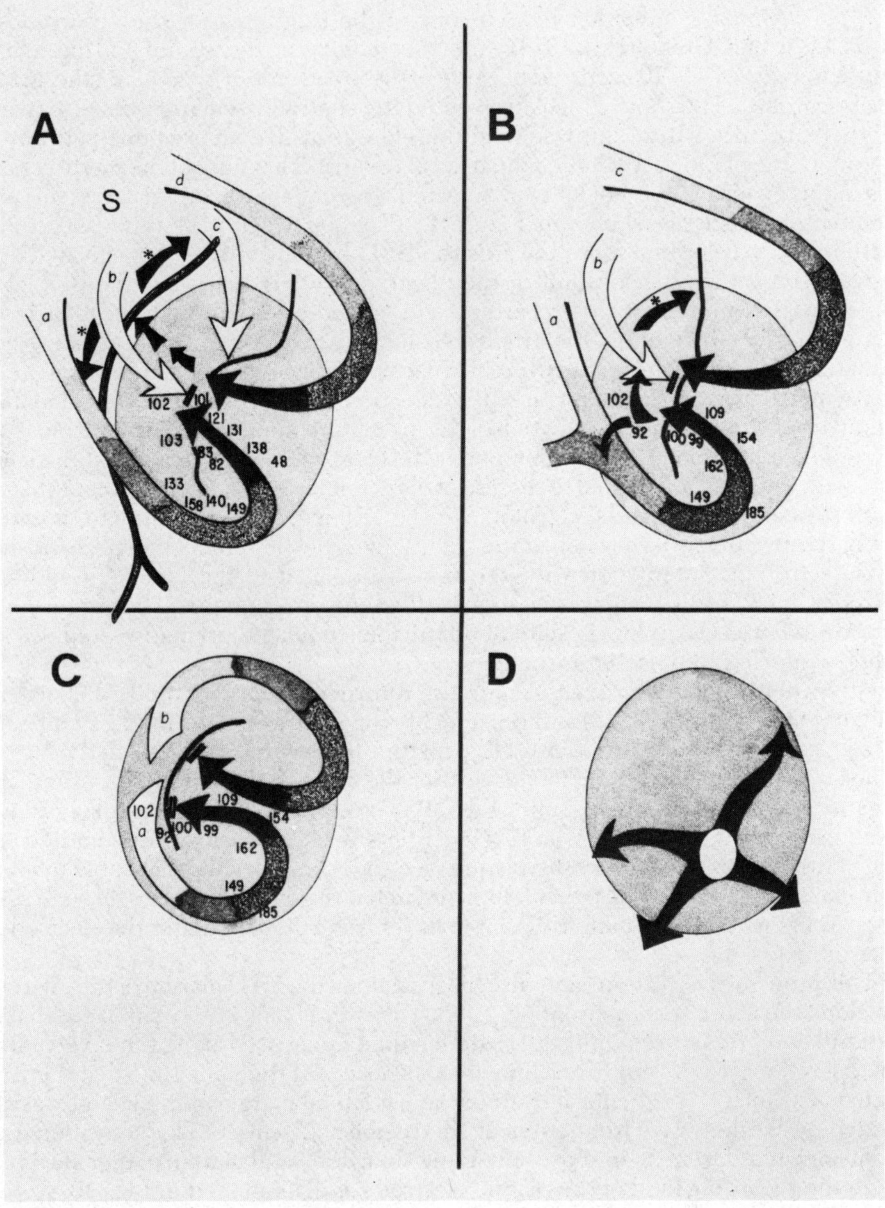
A
S
a
b
c
d
*
*
102
101
121
131
103
183
82
138
48
133
158
140
149
B
a
b
c
*
102
92
100
99
109
154
162
149
185
C
b
a
102
92
100
99
109
154
162
149
185
D

the apex and collided at the left lateral margin at 520 msec. The map to the right in Figure 13, which shows the next 40 msec, indicates that conduction then occurred back towards the center and LAD margin of the infarct. But, the entire wave front blocked along the 540- to 560-msec isochrones, and the impulse did not reach the LAD margin or reenter the ventricles. This conduction block occurred during the second tachycardia impulse and ended circus movement in this region of the ventricle.

Figure 14 shows selected electrograms recorded from the reentrant pathways during the first and second impulses of the tachycardia. The locations of these electrodes are also shown in Figure 9, B and C. Electrode 102, which is shown both at the top and the bottom of the figure, was in the region at the LAD margin activated at 260 msec in Figure 12; as conduction occurred through the reentrant pathway during the first tachycardia impulse (T1) electrograms were recorded from electrodes 102 to 92 in the sequence shown in the figure, and then electrode 102 was reexcited at 410 msec. The circulating impulse again activated the infarcted region in a similar manner during the second tachycardia (T2, electrograms in traces 102 through 109 show this), and the conduction block that terminated circus movement at 560 msec can be seen to occur between electrodes 109 and 92, where the amplitudes of the electrograms progressively diminished until there was no activation. The last tachycardia impulse (T3) had a QRS morphology very different from the previous two impulses. This last impulse did not result from circus movement in the epicardial muscle over the infarct (see Fig. 9D).

Circus Movement Caused by Rapid Stimulation of the Ventricles

Rapid stimulation of the ventricles also can cause ventricular tachycardias in hearts with 3- to 5-day old infarcts (Kaplinsky et al., 1972, El Sherif et al., 1977), as

---

Figure 9. Diagrammatic depiction of the reentrant circuits leading to the nonsustained tachycardia in Figs. 7, 8, 12, 13. The oval area represents the region where the plaque electrode was located. The numbers within this area in panels *A*, *B* and *C* indicate the approximate location where electrograms shown in Figs. 10, 11 and 14 were recorded. *S* in panel *A* is the relative location of the stimulating electrode. The arrows in each panel indicate the direction and pattern of impulse propagation in the surviving epicardial muscle. In *A*, conduction of the stimulated premature impulse is shown (corresponding to the maps in Fig. 8). Wave fronts *(a)* and *(d)* conducted around the margins of the infarct while *(b)* and *(c)* blocked after they entered the infarcted region from the border with the LAD (area of block is indicated by thick black line); *(a)* and *(d)* then reentered into this region of initial block toward the LAD margin (black arrows, asterisks) causing the first tachycardia impulse. In *B*, conduction during the first tachycardia impulse is shown (corresponding to the maps in Figs. 12 and 13). The wave front, represented by arrows *(a)*, *(b)* and *(c)* again blocked toward the LAD margin at the thick black line (arrow *b*), and conducted around the margins of the infarct (arrows *a* and *c*, and then back towards the LAD, resulting in reentry (black arrows). In *C*, conduction during the second impulse of tachycardia is shown (corresponding to the maps in Fig. 13). Wave fronts *(a)* and *(b)* resulted from the reentering impulse shown in Panel *B*; the impulses conducted again around the margins of the infarct and then blocked at the dark line without reentry. In *D*, conduction during the last impulse of tachycardia is shown. The impulse originated in the small oval area towards the apex and conducted away from this region; there is no evidence of circus movement.

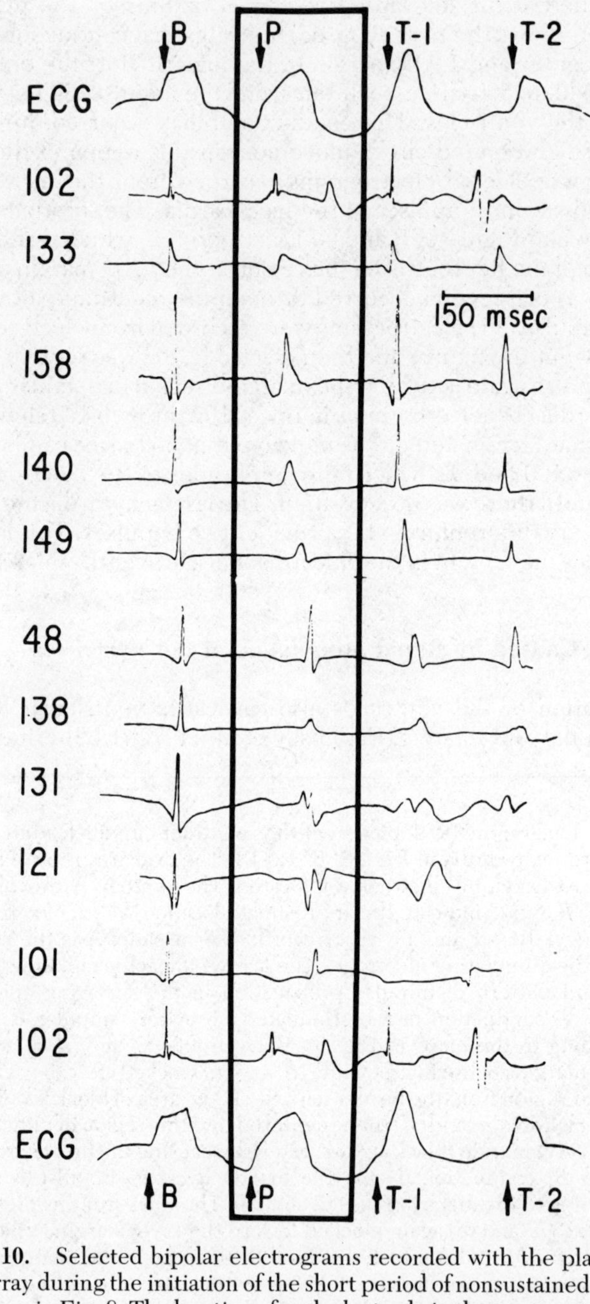

Figure 10. Selected bipolar electrograms recorded with the plaque electrode array during the initiation of the short period of nonsustained tachycardias shown in Fig. 8. The location of each electrode in the reentrant pathways is shown in the diagram of Fig. 9. The same electrocardiogram is shown at both the top and the bottom of the figure; *B* indicates the last of a series of basic drive impulses, *P* is the stimulated premature impulse and T1 and T2 are the first two impulses of tachycardia. The recordings from electrode 102 are shown at both the top and bottom of the figure. The electrograms enclosed within the area outlined by the rectangle were recorded during the stimulated premature impulse.

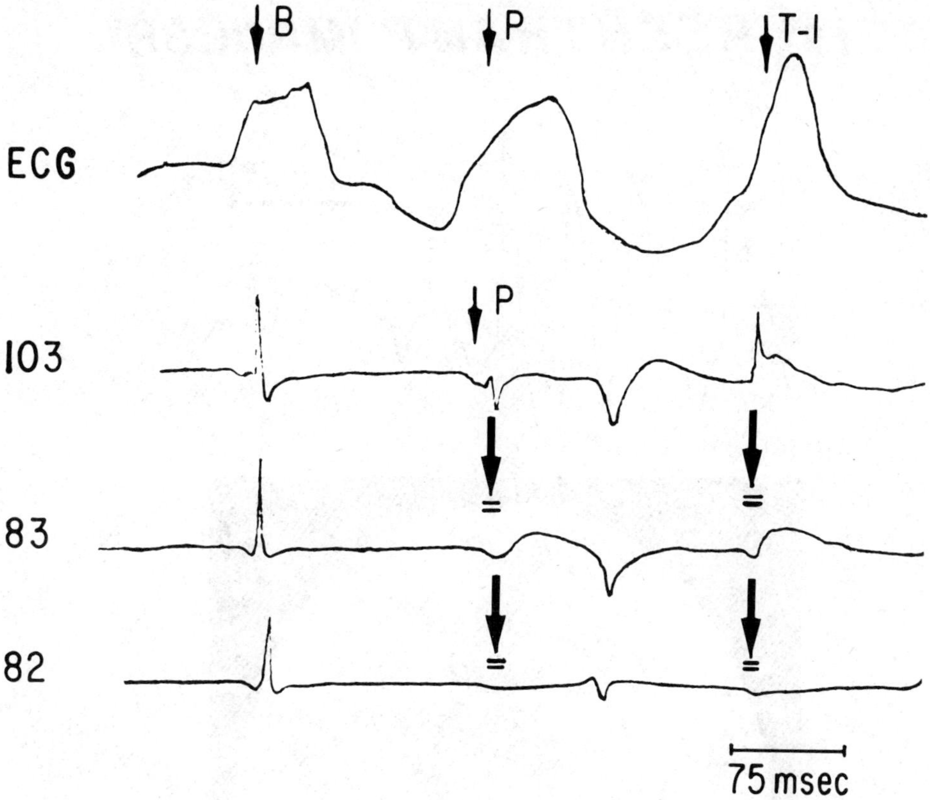

Figure 11. Selected bipolar electrograms recorded with the plaque electrode array in the region where conduction of the premature impulse, that initiated the tachycardia (in Fig. 8), blocked. The location of the electrodes is shown in the diagram of Fig. 9. At the top is the electrocardiogram which shows the last basic drive impulse (B), the stimulated premature impulse (P), and the first tachycardia impulse (T1). Electrode 103 was located proximal to the block, electrodes 83 and 82 were located at or distal to the zone of block.

shown in Figure 15. After a period of sinus rhythm (cycle length, 630 msec) the ventricles were driven for 2 sec, in this experiment, at a cycle length of 200 msec. This period of rapid drive was followed by a ventricular tachycardia consisting of 15 impulses. The excitation pattern of the epicardial muscle over the infarct during the second and third impulses of the tachycardia is shown in Figure 16. Earliest excitation in the left panel occurred along the lateral left ventricular margin, 170 to 180 msec after the reference time, which is the beginning of the QRS of the first tachycardia impulse. Excitation then progressed from this margin towards the center of the infarcted region, but there was an area of conduction block along the 200-, 220-, and 210-msec isochrones (indicated by the dark black line), which extended from the margin at the base, approximately halfway towards the apex. Below this region of block, there was conduction from the left lateral and apical margins towards the center until another region of

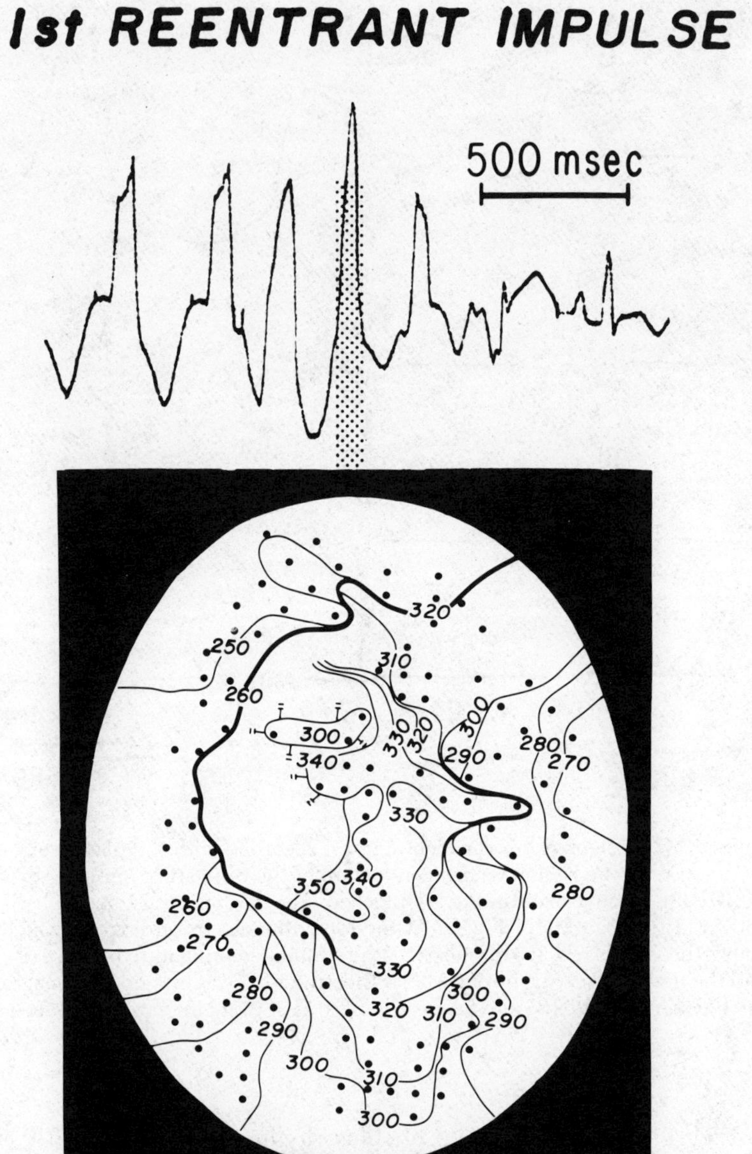

Figure 12. Activation map of the anterior surface of the left ventricle constructed from the timing of electrograms recorded with the plaque electrode, during the 1st nondriven impulse of the tachycardia. The map corresponds to the time period indicated by the shaded area in the ECG above. The format is the same as for Fig. 7. Activation is shown only until the 350 msec isochrone. Fig. 13 shows the continuation of activation.

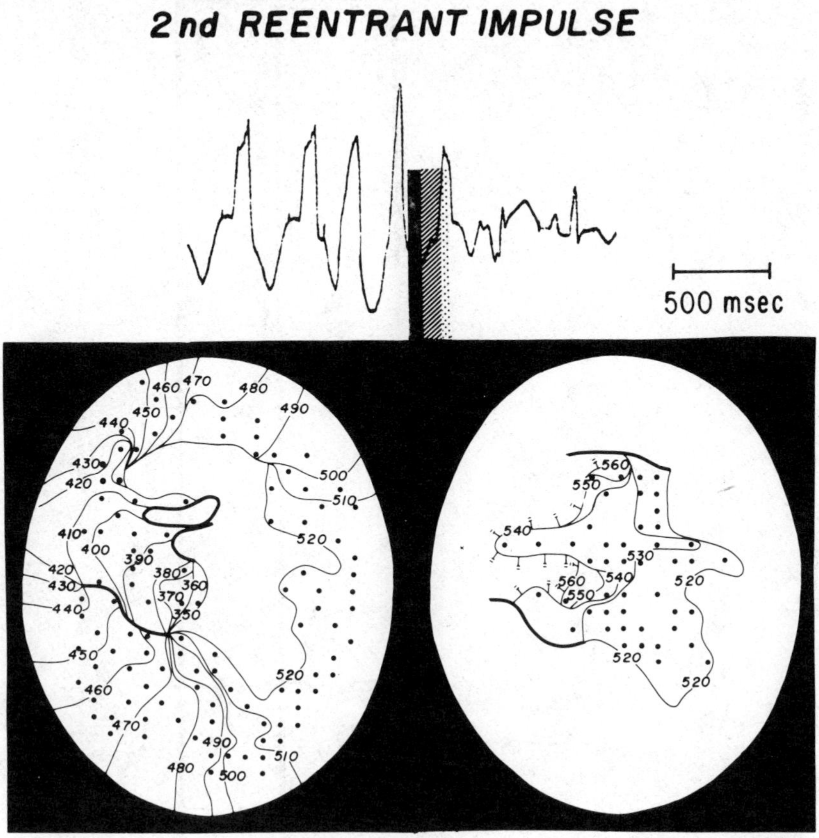

Figure 13. Activation maps of the anterior surface of the left ventricle constructed from the timing of electrograms recorded with the plaque electrode during the 2nd impulse of the tachycardia. The activation times are contiguous to those shown in Fig. 12. The map at the left corresponds to the time period indicated by the heavily shaded and striped areas on the ECG, isochrones 350 to 410 correspond to the time period indicated by the darkly shaded area, isochrones 410–520 correspond to the time period indicated by the striped area. The map at the right shows activation during the next 50 msec, corresponding to the time period indicated by the stippled area on the ECG. The format is the same as for Fig. 7.

block was encountered at the 260- to 270-msec isochrones (indicated in the figure by the shaded area). Excitation skirted this region of block around the edge towards the apex and near the LAD margin and then proceeded towards the base of the heart (isochrones 270 to 310); the region adjacent to the first area of block described above (at the 200-msec isochrone) was activated at 310 msec. The time elapsing during propagation of the impulse through the infarcted region was sufficient to enable conduction to continue into the area where this initial block occurred, as shown in the right panel of Figure 16. This excitation map shows a time period that partially overlaps that of the left panel and that continues from the time when the excitation map in the left panel ended. It also shows excitation progressing from 270 to 310 msec, but then it shows that

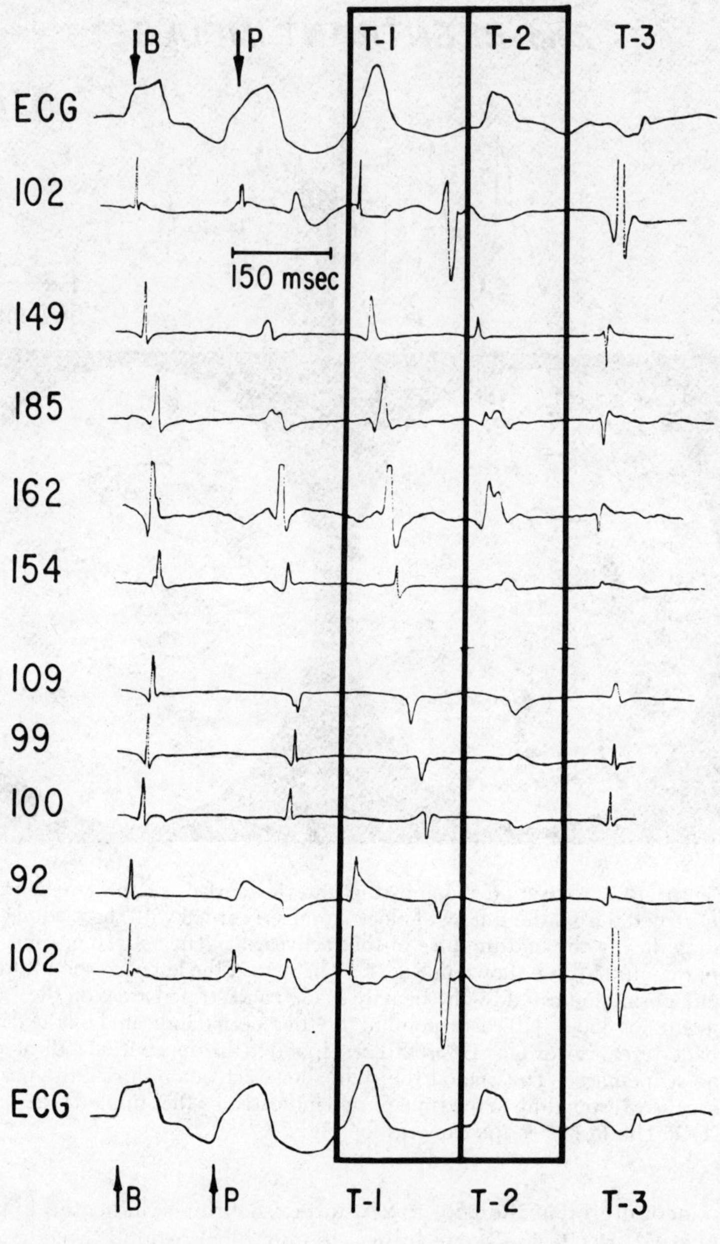

Figure 14. Selected bipolar electrograms recorded with the plaque electrode array during the short period of nonsustained tachycardia shown in Figs. 12 and 13. The location of each electrode in the reentrant pathway is shown in the diagrams of Fig. 9. The same electrocardiogram is shown at the top and bottom of the figure. B indicates the last of a series of basic drive impulses, P is the stimulated premature impulse, and T1, T2, and T3 are the tachycardia impulses. The electrograms recorded from electrode 102 are shown at the top and bottom of the figure. The electrograms recorded during the initial 2 tachycardia beats are enclosed within the areas outlined by the rectangles.

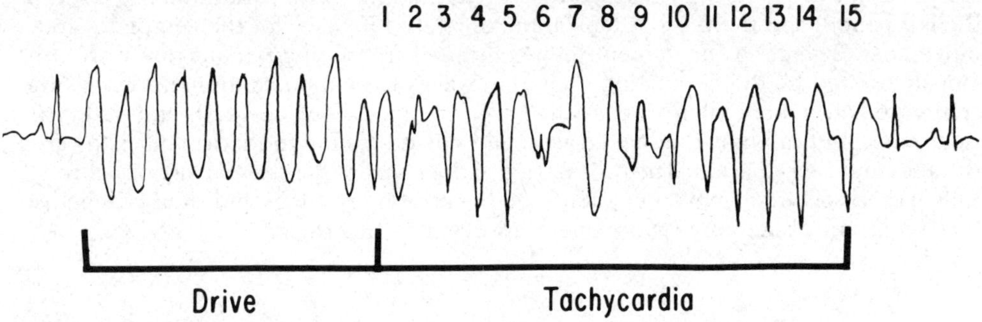

Figure 15. Tachycardia induced by a short period of rapid ventricular drive at a cycle, length of 200 msec. The tachycardia lasted 15 impulses (which are numbered) and its spontaneous termination was followed by sinus rhythm.

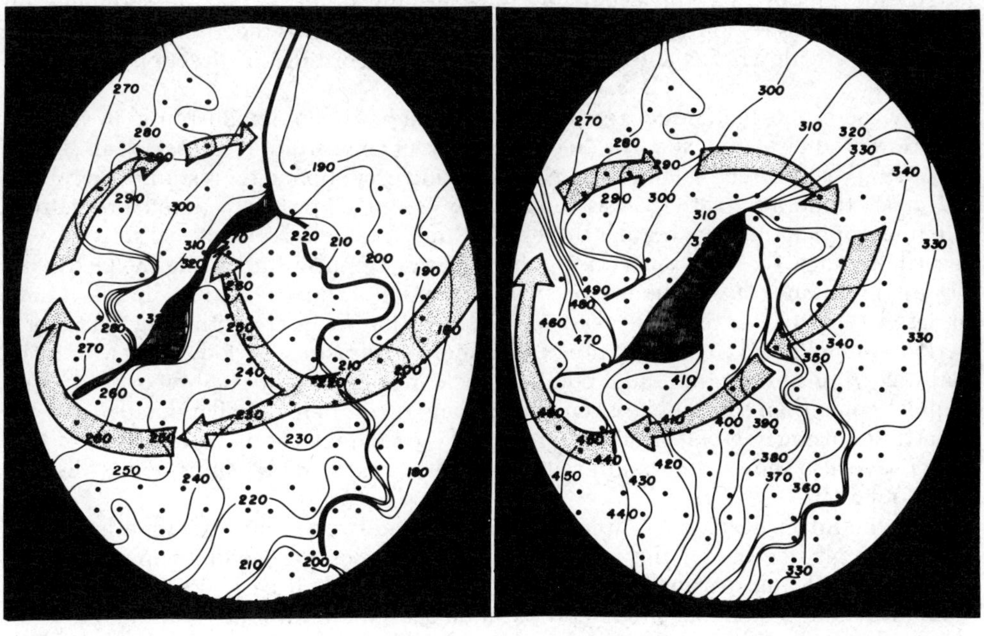

Figure 16. Activation maps of the anterior surface of the left ventricle constructed from the timing of electrograms recorded with the plaque electrode during the 2nd and 3rd impulses of the tachycardia shown in Fig. 15. The map at the left shows activation beginning 180 msec after the onset of the QRS of the 1st tachycardia impulse, and lasting until 320 msec. The map at the right overlaps this time period, i.e., it begins at the 270 msec isochrone and shows activation until 480 msec. The format is the same as for Figure 7.

excitation continued around the basal margin to reexcite areas towards the lateral margin at 330 to 340 msec. These were the areas initially excited at around 200 msec (in the left panel), and therefore it took approximately 130 msec for the complete circus movement. The circus movement then continued, reexciting regions that were previously excited by the circulating excitation wave. Excitation continued towards the center region, where there was a small area of block along the 410- and 420-msec isochrones, indicated by the shaded area, and skirted around the area of block towards the apex and LAD margin. The time period of the map ends at the 490 msec isochrone. This pattern of circus movement continued several more times and then changed so that reentrant excitation was no longer apparent in this region.

DISCUSSION

One way to demonstrate reentry is to show that the excitatory wave conducts through a pathway that leads it back to its starting point, so that the impulse reexcites regions it has previously excited (Mines, 1913; 1914). This can be done by recording electrical activity at a large number of sites within the region where circular conduction (circus movement) may be occurring and carefully determining the sequence of excitation. In this region, the number of sites where activity is recorded must be large enough to provide a reasonable degree of certainty concerning the direction of impulse propagation.

By use of this technique, reentrant excitation has been demonstrated in several experiments on isolated, superfused preparations of myocardium. Allessie et al. (1973; 1976; 1977) have directly demonstrated circulating excitation in their studies on rabbit left atria. Repetitive activity was induced by a single, properly timed premature stimulus applied during a regular driven rhythm. Extracellular electrical activity was recorded from at least 300 sites during the initiating impulse and during the tachycardia to determine the sequence of atrial activation. The premature impulse that initiated repetitive activity blocked in one direction in fibers with long refractory periods and followed a course in fibers with shorter refractory periods along a circular pathway, returning to the initial point of block after excitability had recovered. The impulse could then continue to circulate for many revolutions. Similar detailed activation studies using microelectrode recordings of intracellular action potentials from 130 fibers have also shown reentrant excitation in the isolated rabbit sinus node (Allessie and Bonke, 1979).

In the intact heart, such direct demonstration of reentrant excitation has been more difficult because of the increased number of possible conduction pathways, compared with that of small isolated preparations. Several early studies by Lewis (1920; 1925) suggested that circular propagation of excitation around the venae cavae of the dog heart caused experimental flutter and fibrillation, but Lewis used few recording sites, and his recordings were not obtained from a large segment of the proposed reentrant circuit, that is, the left atrium. Similarly, in some subsequent studies on reentrant excitation in the atria, the number of recordings has been insufficient to positively define the exact pathway of impulse propagation (Kimura et al., 1954; Hayden et al., 1967). Recently, Boineau et al. (1980) have constructed epicardial atrial activation maps from 72 to 96 bipolar recordings and demonstrated activation patterns suggestive of circus movement during atrial flutter in the canine heart.

In the ventricles, the thick walls provide a third dimension for impulse conduction (transverse conduction from epicardium to endocardium), in addition to horizontal conduction. Therefore determination of excitation patterns resulting in reentry is even more difficult than in the atria. Nevertheless, de Baaker et al (1979), using a grid of 48 electrodes on the epicardial surface of the canine right ventricle to study propagation of impulses during the induction of tachycardia and fibrillation after local hypothermia, showed some activation patterns in the vicinity of the stimulating electrode that were interpreted to be circus movement. Janse et al (1980) have also shown circulating excitation on the epicardial surface of the pig heart shortly after coronary artery occlusion (also see Chapter 26, this volume).

In our experiments, the unusual anatomy of the 3- to 5-day old infarcts eliminated, for the most part, the third dimension for impulse conduction that often makes interpretations of excitation maps in the ventricles a difficult problem. In the infarcts included in this study, there was homogenous necrosis of the free left anterior and lateral ventricular walls except for a surviving rim of epicardial ventricular muscle cells (see Fig. 6) and a surviving rim of endocardial Purkinje fibers (Friedman et al., 1975). Earliest epicardial excitation of the ventricles during nonsustained ventricular tachycardias induced by premature stimulation or stimulation at a rapid rate is often in this epicardial muscle or at the border of the infarcted and noninfarcted ventricle (El Sherif et al., 1977; Klein et al., 1979; Wit et al., 1980; 1981). The narrow rim of surviving epicardial muscle dictates that there be mostly lateral or horizontal spread of excitation waves in this region; there can be no excitation waves propagating in a transmural direction to excite this epicardial muscle from below.

Our results showed circus movement and reentry in the surviving epicardial rim of muscle during ventricular tachycardias initiated by stimulation of the ventricles. Numerous time-measurements enabled the isochrones in our activation maps to be constructed with a high degree of accuracy, at 10-msec intervals. Reentry occurred because *(1)* block of stimulated impulses provided an excitable pathway for the return of the reentering impulse, and *(2)* conduction of the impulse in the reentrant pathway was slow enough to permit recovery of regions excited previously. The conduction block of the stimulated premature impulse, shown in Figures 8 and 11, near the LAD margin, is the unidirectional block that is necessary for reentry to occur (Wit and Cranefield, 1978). Similar block occurred during the rapid stimulation of the ventricles, which caused the tachycardia shown in Figure 15. It is a unidirectional block in the sense that conduction did not occur in the direction from the LAD margin towards the center of the infarct zone, but conduction of the reentering impulse from the center to the LAD margin did occur. The same pattern of unidirectional block can be seen also in Figures 12 and 13 during the tachycardia; in Figure 12 there was block along the 260-msec isochrone in one direction, but in Figure 13 (left panel) the impulse conducted successfully through this same region in the opposite direction (isochrones 380 to 410). The unidirectional block of these impulses, therefore, provided the excitable pathway for the return of the reentering impulse. Because conduction from the LAD margin towards the center of the infarct zone occurred through part of this region during the basic drive (Fig. 7) whereas block occurred after the premature impulse (Fig. 8), the unidirectional block was functional rather than fixed. The slowed conduction of the stimulated premature impulses and the tachycardia impulses enable reentry to occur in such a circumscribed region where the length of the reentrant pathway was less than 9 cm; conduction velocity was between 0.05 and 0.2 m/sec in different regions.

The precise causes for conduction block and slow conduction in the epicardial muscle during circus movement remains to be determined, but there are some data showing that the muscle cells have reduced resting potentials, have relatively slow rates of phase-0 depolarization, and show rate-dependent variations in refractoriness (Lazzara and Scherlag, 1980). The orientation of the surviving epicardial muscle fibers according to the direction of impulse propagation may also be an important determinant of conduction properties (Spach et al., 1981; also see Chapter 9, this volume). The unidirectional conduction block may be caused by conduction of action potentials with low amplitudes and slow-upstroke velocities through low-resistant pathways, when the long axis of the muscle bundles are parallel to the direction of impulse propagation, whereas regions of slow conduction may be dictated by propagation of the impulse perpendicular to the direction of the muscle bundles (Spach et al., 1981). The possible influences of fiber geometry on reentry in infarcts have not yet been investigated.

Mines third criteria for proof of reentry was not satisfied in our study or in the other experimental studies previously cited; that is, cutting through the pathway in which the supposed reentrant impulse is conducting should abolish impulse initiation if it is really caused by reentry. As stated by Mines (1913; 1914), unless this is done, the possibility always remains that there is "a series of automatic beats originating in one point in the ring and traveling around it in one direction only owing to a complete block close to the point of origin of the rhythm on one side of this point."

REFERENCES

Allessie MA, Bonke FIM (1979) Direct demonstration of sinus node reentry in the rabbit heart. Circ Res **44**:557–568

Allessie MA, Bonke FIM, Schopman FJG (1973) Circus movement in rabbit atrial muscle as a mechanism of tachycardia. Circ Res **33**:54–62

Allessie MA, Bonke FIM, Schopman FJG (1976) Circus movement in rabbit atrial muscle as a mechanism of tachycardia. II. Role of nonuniform recovery of excitability in the occurrence of unidirectional block, as studied with multiple microelectrodes. Circ Res **39**:168–178

Allessie MA, Bonke FIM, Schopman FJG (1977) Circus movement in rabbit atrial muscle as a mechanism of tachycardia. III. The "leading circle" concept: a new model of circus movement in cardiac tissue without the involvement of an anatomical obstacle. Circ Res **41**:9–18

Boineau JP, Schuessler RB, Mooney CR, Muller CB, Wylds AC, Hudson RD, Borremans JM, Brocku CW (1980) Naturally and evoked atrial flutter due to circus movement in dogs. Role of abnormal atrial pathways, slow conduction, nonuniform refractory period distribution and premature beats. Am J Cardiol **45**:1167–1181

de Baaker JMT, Henning B, Merx W (1979) Circus movement in canine right ventricle. Circ Res **45**:374–377

El-Sherif N, Hope RR, Scherlag BJ, Lazzara R (1977) Reentrant ventricular arrhythmias in the late myocardial infarction period. I. Conduction characteristics in the infarction zone. Circulation **55**:686–702

Friedman PF, Fenoglio JJ, Jr, Wit AL (1975) Time course for reversal of electrophysiological and ultrastructural abnormalities in subendocardial Purkinje fibers surviving extensive myocardial infarction in dogs. Circ Res **36**:127–144

Garry WE (1914) The nature of fibrillary contraction of the heart. Its relation to tissue mass and form. Am J Physiol **33**:397–408

Garrey WE (1924) Auricular fibrillation. Physiol Rev **4**:215–250

Harris AS (1950) Delayed development of ventricular ectopic rhythms following experimental coronary occlusion. Circulation **1**:1318–1329

Hayden WG, Hurley EJ, Rytand DA (1967) The mechanism of canine atrial flutter. Circ Res **20**:496–505

Janse MJJ, van Capelle FJL, Morsink H, Kleber AG, Wilms Schopman F, Cardinal R, Naumann d'Almoncourt C, Durrer D (1980) Flow of "injury" current and patterns of excitation during early ventricular arrhythmias in acute regional myocardial ischemia in isolated porcine and canine hearts: Evidence for two different arrhythmogenic mechanisms. Circ Res **47**:151–165

Kaplinsky E, Yahini JH, Neufeld HN (1972) On the mechanism of sustained ventricular arrhythmias associated with acute myocardial infarction. Cardiovasc Res **6**:135–142

Karagueuzian HS, Fenoglio JJ, Jr, Weiss MB, Wit AL (1979) Protracted ventricular tachycardia induced by premature stimulation of the canine heart after coronary artery occlusion and reperfusion. Circ Res **44**:833–846

Kimura E, Kato K, Maurao S, Ajioakia H, Koyama S, Omiya A (1954) Experimental studies on the mechanism of the circular flutter. Tohoku J Exptl Med **60**:197–207

Klein GJ, Ideker RE, Smith WM, Harrison LA, Kasell J, Wallace AG, Gallagher JJ (1979) Epicardial mapping of the onset of ventricular tachycardia initiated by programmed stimulation in the canine heart with chronic infarction. Circulation **60**:1375–1384

Lazzara R, Scherlag BJ (1980) Role of the slow current in the generation of arrhythmias in ischemic myocardium. In The Slow Inward Current and Cardiac Arrhythmias, edited by DP Zipes, JC Bailey and V Eharrar. The Hague, Martinus Nijhoff, pp 399–416

Lewis T, Feil HS, Stroud WD (1920) Observations upon flutter and fibrillation. Part II. The nature of auricular flutter. Heart **7**:191–233

Lewis T (1925) The mechanism and graphic registration of the heart beat. London, Shaw

Mayer AG (1906) Rhythmical pulsation in Scyphomedusae. Carnegie Inst. Wash. Publ No 47, 1906

Mayer AG (1908) Rhythmical pulsation in Scyphomedusae: II. Carnegie Inst. Wash. Papers, Tortugar Lab. **1**:113–131. Carnegie Inst. Wash. Publ. No. 102 part VII, 1908

McWilliam JA (1897) Fibrillar contraction of the heart. J Physiol (Lond) **8**:296–310

Mines GR (1913) On dynamic equilibrium in the heart. J Physiol (Lond) **46**:350,383

Mines GR (1914) On circulating excitations in heart muscle and their possible relation to tachycardia and fibrillation. Trans Roy Soc Can Ser 3, Sect IV, **8**:43–52

Spach MS, Miller WT, III, Geselowitz DB, Barr RC, Kootsey JM, Johnson EA (1981) The discontinuous nature of propagation in normal canine cardiac muscle: Evidence for recurrent discontinuities of intracellular resistance that affect the membrane currents. Circ Res **48**: 39–54

Wit AL, Cranefield PF (1978) Reentrant excitation as a cause of cardiac arrhythmias. Am J Physiol (Heart Circ Physiol) **4**:H1–H17

Wit AL, Allessie MA, Bonke FIM, Lammers W, Smeets J (1980) Excitation of the infarcted canine heart during initiation of ventricular tachycardia by premature impulses. Circulation **62** Suppl II, 195

Wit AL, Allessie MA, Bonke FIM, Lammers W, Smeets J, Fenoglio JJ, Jr (1982) Electrophysiological mapping to determine the mechanism of experimental ventricular tachycardia initiated by premature impulses: Experimental approaches and initial results demonstrating reentrant excitation. Am J Cardiol **49**:166–185

Discussion

PAES DE CARVALHO: Do partially depolarized cell groups in the infarcted regions show slowly moving activity of the slow-response type? Even though hypoxia and metabolic inhibition have been shown to depress the slow response, its occurrence in the infarcted region might still be observed, because, at least in the early stages of ischemia, you must have viable adrenergic innervation, with the possibility of catecholamine release and potentiation of slow responses. Now, if there are slow responses roaming around, you can have several degrees of local block or very prolonged local delays of the type that Masuda and Cukierman have shown in their chapters. We might therefore find places where the subthreshold response may smolder for up to 500 msec before a slow response appears.

WIT: This is a problem we are very much interested in. We do not actually know what the cellular electrophysiology of this surviving epicardial layer is. We can record reasonably fast surface electrograms from it during sinus rhythm, so I am not sure how depressed the cells are; this is a question that we would certainly have to answer. In the situation where circus movement was produced at high driving rates, we did try some calculations of conduction velocity within the infarcted region, and it came out to be something like 0.1 m/sec, which is not extraordinarily slow. But, in different regions within the ischemic area there may be different conduction velocities, and this has to be taken into consideration. The 0.1-m/sec value is an overall value for the trip around the reentry circuit, but as you have seen, the isochrones are not evenly spaced. In some circus movements we find very unusual surface electrograms that may be indicative of what you are suggesting; in these situations, we can sometimes record very slow prolonged surface complexes in places where during the basic drive or during a single premature response fairly sharp complexes would be observed. What we have to do is to put microelectrodes in the regions where this is occurring so as to get some hint whether a mechanism such as you suggest can occur.

Index